PRE-COURSE/POST-COURSE ASSESSMENT

 **W9-BSB-065**

Name: _____ Date: _____

As you complete the key fitness/wellness lab assessments in this course, record your results in the "Pre-Course Assessment" column. At the end of the course, re-do the labs, record your results in the "Post-Course Assessment" column, and see the progress you have made!

Lab	Pre-Course Assessment	Post-Course Assessment
Lab 3.2: Assessing Your Cardiorespiratory Fitness Level	**3-minute step test** 1 minute recovery HR:_____ (bpm) Fitness rating: _____ **1-mile walk test** VO₂ max: _____ Fitness rating: _____ **1.5-mile run test** VO₂ max: _____ Fitness rating: _____	**3-minute step test** 1 minute recovery HR:_____ (bpm) Fitness rating: _____ **1-mile walk test** VO₂ max: _____ Fitness rating: _____ **1.5-mile run test** VO₂ max: _____ Fitness rating: _____
Lab 4.1: Assessing Your Muscular Strength	**Chest press** S/BW ratio: _____ Rating: _____ **Leg press** S/BW ratio: _____ Rating: _____	**Chest press** S/BW ratio: _____ Rating: _____ **Leg press** S/BW ratio: _____ Rating: _____
Lab 4.2: Assessing Your Muscular Endurance	**20RM assessment** Chest press 20RM weight lifted: _____ Leg press 20RM weight lifted: _____ **Push-up assessment** Repetitions: _____ Rating: _____ **Curl-up assessment** Repetitions: _____ Rating: _____	**20RM assessment** Chest press 20RM weight lifted: _____ Leg press 20RM weight lifted: _____ **Push-up assessment** Repetitions: _____ Rating: _____ **Curl-up assessment** Repetitions: _____ Rating: _____
Lab 5.1: Assessing Your Flexibility	**Sit-and-reach test** Reach distance (in or cm): _____ Rating: _____	**Sit-and-reach test** Reach distance (in or cm): _____ Rating: _____
Lab 6.1: How to Calculate Your BMI	BMI: _____ kg/m² Weight classification: _____	BMI: _____ kg/m² Weight classification: _____
Lab 6.2: Measure and Evaluate Your Body Circumferences	Waist: _____ Hip: _____ WHR Ratio: _____ Upper arm: _____ (right) _____ (left) Forearm: _____ (right) _____ (left) Thigh: _____ (right) _____ (left) Calf: _____ (right) _____ (left) Neck: _____ Disease risk rating for WHR: _____ Disease risk rating for WC: _____	Waist: _____ Hip: _____ WHR Ratio: _____ Upper arm: _____ (right) _____ (left) Forearm: _____ (right) _____ (left) Thigh: _____ (right) _____ (left) Calf: _____ (right) _____ (left) Neck: _____ Disease risk rating for WHR: _____ Disease risk rating for WC: _____
Lab 6.3: Estimate Your Percent Body Fat (Skinfold Test)	Sum of 3 skinfolds: _____ % body fat estimate: _____ Rating: _____	Sum of 3 skinfolds: _____ % body fat estimate: _____ Rating: _____
Lab 7.3: Improving Your Nutrition	Dairy intake: _____ cups Protein-rich foods intake: _____ oz. Vegetables intake: _____ cups Fruits intake: _____ cups Grains intake: _____ oz.	Dairy intake: _____ cups Protein-rich foods intake: _____ oz. Vegetables intake: _____ cups Fruits intake: _____ cups Grains intake: _____ oz.
Lab 8.1: Calculating Energy Balance and Setting Energy Balance Goals	Estimated calorie intake: _____ Estimated calorie expenditure: _____ Calorie balance (intake minus expenditure): _____	Estimated calorie intake: _____ Estimated calorie expenditure: _____ Calorie balance (intake minus expenditure): _____
Lab 8.3: Your Weight Management Plan	% body fat: _____ Weight: _____ lb. BMI: _____ kg/m²	% body fat: _____ Weight: _____ lb. BMI: _____ kg/m²
Lab 9.1: How Stressed Are You?	Score: _____ Stress level: _____	Score: _____ Stress level: _____
Lab 10.1: Understanding Your CVD Risk	Family risk for CVD, total points: _____ Lifestyle risk for CVD, total points: _____ Additional risks for CVD, total points: _____	Family risk for CVD, total points: _____ Lifestyle risk for CVD, total points: _____ Additional risks for CVD, total points: _____

BEHAVIOR CHANGE ¦ CONTRACT

Choose a health behavior that you would like to change, starting this quarter or semester. Sign the contract at the bottom to affirm your commitment to making a healthy change and ask a friend to witness it.

My behavior change will be:

_____

My long-term goal for this behavior change is:

_____

Barriers I must overcome to make this behavior change are (things I am currently doing or situations that contribute to this behavior or make it harder to change):

1. _____

2. _____

3. _____

The strategies I will use to overcome these barriers are:

1. _____

2. _____

3. _____

Resources I will use to help me change this behavior include:

A friend/partner/relative _____

A school-based resource _____

A community-based resource _____

A book or reputable website _____

In order to make my goal more attainable, I have devised these short-term goals:

Short-Term Goal _____ **Target Date**_____ **Reward** _____

Short-Term Goal _____ **Target Date**_____ **Reward** _____

Short-Term Goal _____ **Target Date**_____ **Reward** _____

When I make the long-term behavior change described above, my reward will be:

Reward _____ **Target Date**_____

I intend to make the behavior change described above, I will use the strategies and rewards to achieve the goals that will contribute to a healthy behavior change.

Signed _____ **Date**_____

Witness _____ **Date**_____

Helping students
find the path to lifelong fitness

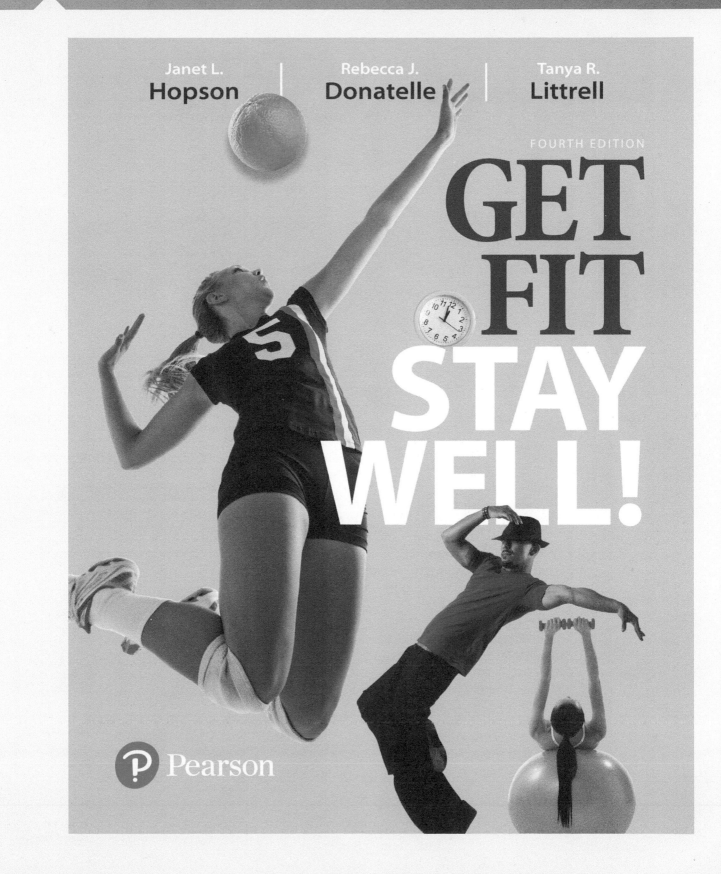

Janet L.
Hopson

Rebecca J.
Donatelle

Tanya R.
Littrell

FOURTH EDITION

GET
FIT
STAY
WELL!

Ⓟ **Pearson**

Tools to help students adopt healthy habits today . . .

Putting It All Together

YOUR TOTAL FITNESS PROGRAM

Activate, Motivate, & Advance YOUR FITNESS

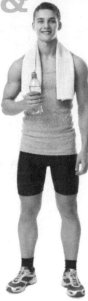

Pull all your fitness programs together to create a comprehensive personal program—one that meets your own long-term goals. First, identify which exercises work for you and which ones you'd like to modify (refer to Figure 4.10 on pages 137–150, Figure 5.7 on pages 185–190, and Figure 5.8 on pages 191–192). Then, look at the following sample programs. Start at your current level and modify for your own preferences and rate of improvement.

ACTIVATE!
Warm-Up & Cool-Down

Warming-up prior to exercise is crucial! Start with gentle cardiorespiratory exercises for 5 to 10 minutes. After breaking a light sweat, add dynamic movements that increase your range of motion.

After your exercise session, cool down by moving at a slower pace until your heart rate and temperature fall to comfortable levels. Finish your cool-down with a few stretches.

Total Fitness Programs

Adjust intensity, volume, and training days to suit your personal fitness level and schedule.

P-1

NEW! Putting It All Together: Fitness Program Building on what students learn in Chapters 1–5 , the Putting It All Together: Fitness Program helps students to create an overall comprehensive fitness program that both incorporates the elements of fitness concepts discussed throughout the book and allows students to implement change today.

NEW! Integrated Labs and Programs Where relevant, when students assess themselves in an end of chapter lab or a chapter exercise, the authors guide them to their appropriate starting level in the **Activate, Motivate, and Advance Programs,** on yoga, running, flexibility, and meditation, giving students the ability to do the lab activity in class and then enhance their own lifelong wellness by implementing the program on a daily basis at the appropriate starting level.

Section V: Cardiorespiratory Training Program Design

Plan a four-week cardiorespiratory training program, using resources available to you (facility, instructor, text). Complete the following training calendar (A = activity, I = intensity, T = time).

To get started: Review Programs 3.1 to 3.3 on pages 103–110 for running, cycling, and swimming. Choose a Beginning program if your Lab 3.2 fitness ratings are Fair or lower or the activity is new for you. Aim for an Intermediate program if your Lab 3.2 fitness ratings are Good, and try an Advanced program if your ratings are Excellent or above and you are used to this activity.

Four-Week Cardiorespiratory Training Program						
Sun	Mon	Tues	Wed	Thurs	Fri	Sat
Date: _____	Date: _____	Date: _____	Date: _____	Date: _____	Date: _____	Date: _____
A:	A:	A:	A:	A:	A:	A:
I:	I:	I:	I:	I:	I:	I:
T:	T:	T:	T:	T:	T:	T:
Date: _____	Date: _____	Date: _____	Date: _____	Date: _____	Date: _____	Date: _____
A:	A:	A:	A:	A:	A:	A:
I:	I:	I:	I:	I:	I:	I:
T:	T:	T:	T:	T:	T:	T:
Date: _____	Date: _____	Date: _____	Date: _____	Date: _____	Date: _____	Date: _____
A:	A:	A:	A:	A:	A:	A:
I:	I:	I:	I:	I:	I:	I:
T:	T:	T:	T:	T:	T:	T:
Date: _____	Date: _____	Date: _____	Date: _____	Date: _____	Date: _____	Date: _____
A:	A:	A:	A:	A:	A:	A:
I:	I:	I:	I:	I:	I:	I:
T:	T:	T:	T:	T:	T:	T:

Section VI: Tracking Your Program and Following Through

1. **Goal and Program Tracking:** Use the following chart or a web/app activity log to monitor your progress. Change the activity, intensity, or time of your workout plan to reflect your progress as needed.

2. **Goal and Program Follow-Up:** At the end of the course or at your short-term goal target date, reevaluate your cardiorespiratory fitness and ask yourself the following questions:

   a. Did you meet your short-term goal or your goal for the course? If so, what positive behavioral changes contributed to your success? If not, which obstacles blocked your success?

   _____

   b. Was your short-term goal realistic? What would you change about your goals or training plan?

   _____

And tomorrow.

NEW! Chapter 15, Maintaining Lifelong Fitness and Wellness

This chapter is now available in the printed text as well as the eText. The addition of the chapter within the printed text emphasizes the theme that the choices that students make today will impact the rest of their lives.

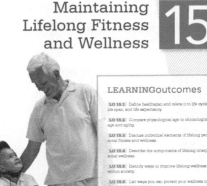

Hallmark! GetFitGraphics

GetFitGraphic infographics highlight compelling topics in visually stunning presentations. For the 4th edition, these figures have been streamlined and updated with the latest information and data. **New!** Two new GetFitGraphics are included in this edition: Fit Body, Fit Brain? (Chapter 1) and What is Sitting Syndrome? (Chapter 2).

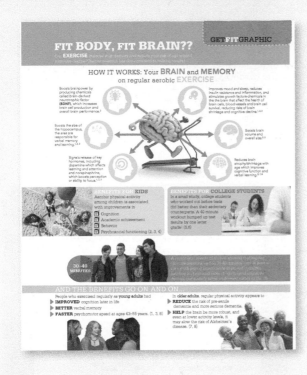

NEW! Study Plan tied to Learning Outcomes

Numbered learning outcomes now introduce every chapter and are tied directly to chapter sections, giving students a roadmap for their reading. Each chapter concludes with a Study Plan, which includes new summary points of the chapter and provides review questions to check understanding, all tied to the chapter's learning outcomes and assignable in MasteringHealth.

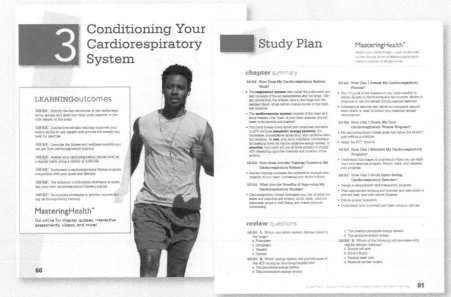

Continuous Learning
Before, During, and After Class

BEFORE CLASS

Mobile Media and Reading Assignments Ensure Students Come to Class Prepared

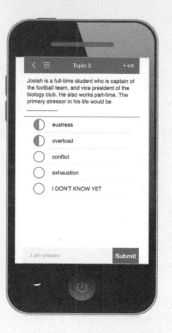

NEW! Dynamic Study Modules help students study effectively by continuously assessing student performance and providing practice in areas where students struggle the most. Each Dynamic Study Module, accessed by computer, smartphone, or tablet, promotes fast learning and long-term retention.

NEW! Interactive eText 2.0 mobile app gives students access to the text whenever they can. eText features include:

- Now available on smartphones and tablets.
- Seamlessly integrated videos and other rich media.
- Accessible (screen-reader ready).
- Configurable reading settings, including resizable type and night reading mode.
- Instructor and student note-taking, highlighting, bookmarking, and search.

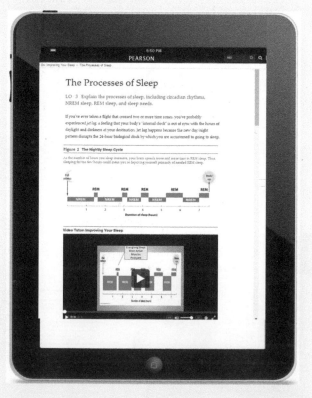

NEW! Pre-Lecture Reading Quizzes are easy to customize and assign

Reading Questions ensure that students complete the assigned reading before class and stay on track with reading assignments. Reading Questions are 100% mobile ready and can be completed by students on mobile devices.

with MasteringHealth™

DURING CLASS

Engage Students with Learning Catalytics

Learning Catalytics, a "bring your own device" student engagement, assessment, and classroom intelligence system, allows students to use their smartphone, tablet, or laptop to respond to questions in class.

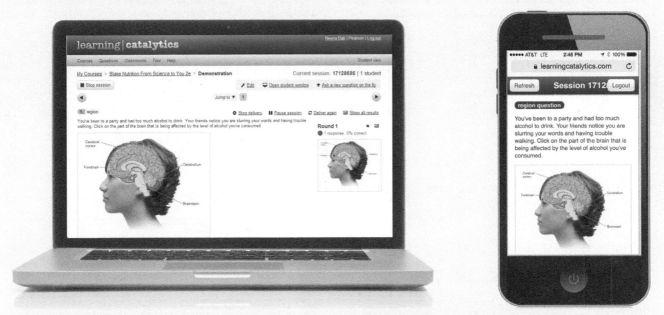

AFTER CLASS

MasteringHealth Delivers Automatically Graded Health and Fitness Activities

NEW! Interactive Behavior Change Activities—Which Path Would You Take Have students explore various health choices through an engaging, interactive, low-stakes, and anonymous experience. These activities show students the possible consequences of various choices they make today on their future health.

These activities are assignable in Mastering with follow-up questions.

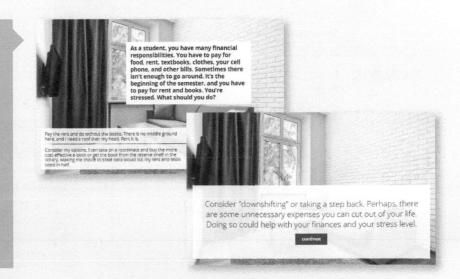

Continuous Learning
Before, During, and After Class

AFTER CLASS

Other Automatically Graded Health and Fitness Activities Include . . .

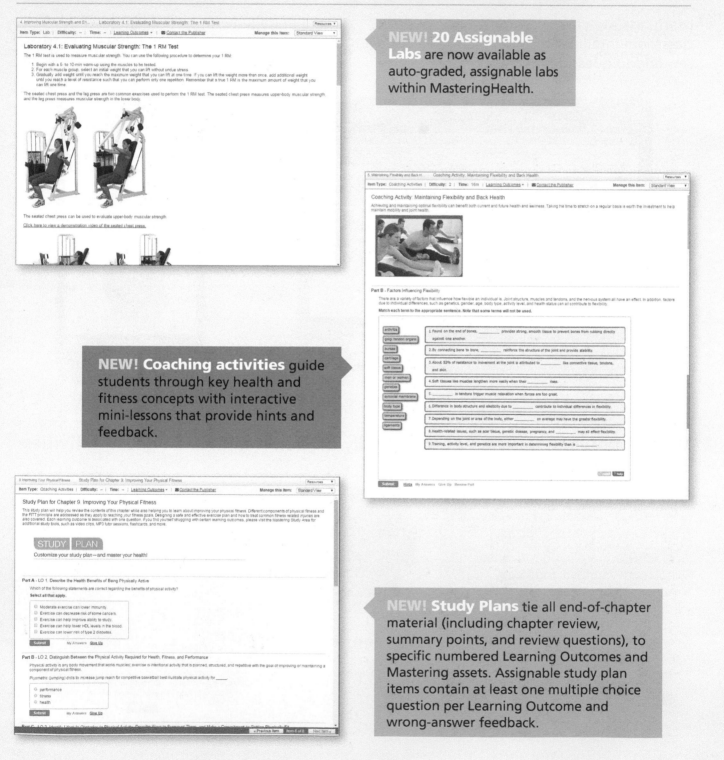

NEW! 20 Assignable Labs are now available as auto-graded, assignable labs within MasteringHealth.

NEW! Coaching activities guide students through key health and fitness concepts with interactive mini-lessons that provide hints and feedback.

NEW! Study Plans tie all end-of-chapter material (including chapter review, summary points, and review questions), to specific numbered Learning Outcomes and Mastering assets. Assignable study plan items contain at least one multiple choice question per Learning Outcome and wrong-answer feedback.

with MasteringHealth™

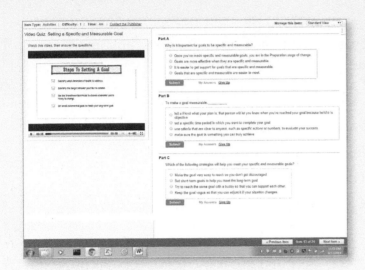

Behavior Change Videos are concise whiteboard-style videos that help students with the steps of behavior change, covering topics such as setting SMART goals, identifying and overcoming barriers to change, planning realistic timelines, and more. Additional videos review key fitness concepts such as determining target heart rate range for exercise. All videos include assessment activities and are assignable in MasteringHealth.

NEW! ABC News Videos bring health to life and spark discussion with up-to-date hot topics from 2012–2015. Activities tied to the videos include multiple choice questions that provide wrong-answer feedback to redirect students to the correct answer.

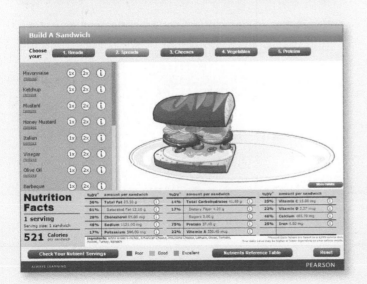

Updated! NutriTools Coaching Activities in the nutrition chapter allow students to combine and experiment with different food options and learn firsthand how to build healthier meals.

Resources for YOU, the Instructor

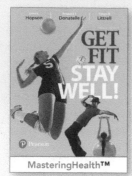

MasteringHealth™ provides you with everything you need to prep for your course and deliver a dynamic lecture, in one convenient place. Resources include:

Media Assets for Each Chapter

- *ABC News* Lecture Launcher videos
- Behavior Change videos
- PowerPoint Lecture Outlines
- PowerPoint clicker questions and Jeopardy-style quiz show questions
- Files for all illustrations and tables and selected photos from the text

Test Bank

- Test Bank in Microsoft Word, PDF, and RTF formats
- Computerized Test Bank, which includes all the questions from the printed test bank in a format that allows you to easily and intuitively build exams and quizzes.

Teaching Resources

- Instructor Resource and Support Manual in Microsoft Word and PDF formats
- Teaching with Student Learning Outcomes
- Teaching with Web 2.0
- Learning Catalytics: Getting Started
- Getting Started with MasteringHealth

Student Supplements

- Take Charge of Your Health Worksheets
- Behavior Change Log Book and Wellness Journal
- Eat Right!
- Live Right!
- Food Composition Table

Measuring Student Learning Outcomes?
All of the MasteringHealth assignable content is tagged to book content and to Bloom's Taxonomy. You also have the ability to add your own learning outcomes, helping you track student performance against your learning outcomes. You can view class performance against the specified learning outcomes and share those results quickly and easily by exporting to a spreadsheet.

GET
FIT
STAY
WELL!

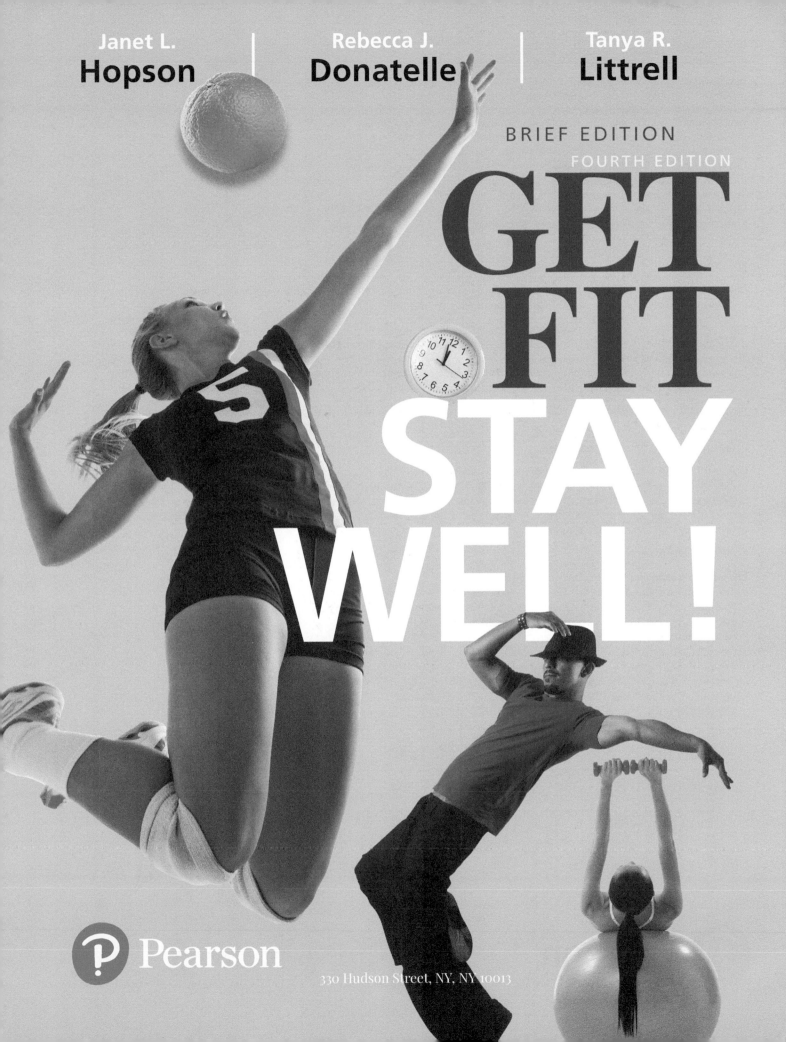

Janet L. **Hopson**

Rebecca J. **Donatelle**

Tanya R. **Littrell**

BRIEF EDITION

FOURTH EDITION

GET FIT STAY WELL!

 Pearson

330 Hudson Street, NY, NY 10013

Senior Portfolio Manager: Michelle Yglecias
Content Producer: Susan Malloy
Managing Producer, Science: Nancy Tabor
Courseware Sr. Analyst: Alice Fugate
Courseware Analyst: Jay McElroy
Courseware Editorial Assistant: Nicole Constantine
Production Management and Compositor: iEnergizer Aptara®, Ltd.
Project Manager: Sherrill Redd, iEnergizer Aptara®, Ltd.
Cover and Interior Designer: Gary Hespenheide, Hespenheide Design
Rights & Permissions Project Manager: Laura Murray
Rights & Permissions Management: Ben Ferrini
Photo Researcher: Danny Meldung, Photo Affairs, Inc.
Manufacturing Buyer, Higher Ed.: Stacey Weinberger
Executive Product Marketing Manager: Neena Bali
Senior Marketing Manager: Mary Salzman
Mastering Content Producer, Health & Nutrition: Lorna Perkins

Cover Photo Credit: victoriaKh/Shutterstock, Mike Kemp/Getty Images, View Stock/Getty Images, Elnur Amikishiyev/Alamy Stock Photo, Blend Images - Erik Isakson/Getty Images, Coprid/Shutterstock.

Library of Congress Cataloging-in-Publication Data
Names: Hopson, Janet L., author. | Donatelle, Rebecca J., 1950- author. | Littrell, Tanya R., author.
 Title: Get fit stay well! / Janet L. Hopson, M.A., San Francisco State University,
Rebecca J. Donatelle, PH.D., Oregon State University, Tanya R. Littrell, PH.D.,
Portland Community College.
 Description: Fourth edition. | Boston : Pearson, [2018] | Includes bibliographical references and index.
 Identifiers: LCCN 2016041755| ISBN 9780134392066 | ISBN 013439206X
 Subjects: LCSH: Physical fitness—Textbooks. | Health—Textbooks.
 Classification: LCC RA781.H65 H67 2017 | DDC 613.7—dc23
 LC record available at https://lccn.loc.gov/2016041755

6 2019

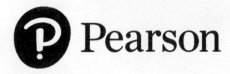

ISBN 10: 0-134-45228-3; ISBN 13: 978-0-134-45228-9 (Brief edition)

To the memory of Ruth and David Hopson, who taught me, by example and encouragement, to love fitness activity.—JLH

To the strong, intelligent, loving, and hard-working women who have motivated me and taught me to care about the important things—especially my mom, Agnes E. Donatelle.—RJD

To the memory of my loving grandmother Doretta Littrell Lawrence, a dance, fitness, and physical education professional who influenced many lives and inspired us all.—TRL

About the Authors

Janet L. Hopson, M.A.

Author and university lecturer, Janet L. Hopson has written or co-authored many books, including two popular non-fiction books on human pheromones and human brain development, and eight textbooks on general biology and wellness for college and high school students. Ms. Hopson teaches science writing at San Francisco State University. She holds B.A. and M.A. degrees from Southern Illinois University and the University of Missouri. She has won awards for magazine writing, and her articles have appeared in *Smithsonian, Psychology Today, Science Digest, Science News, Outside, Scientific American Mind*, and others. She is married and enjoys reading, traveling, gardening, golfing, swimming, tennis, and equestrian sports.

Rebecca J. Donatelle, Ph.D.

Dr. Rebecca J. Donatelle is a professor emeritus in public health at Oregon State University, having served as the department chair, Coordinator of the Public Health Promotion and Education Programs, and faculty member and researcher in the College of Health and Human Sciences. She has a Ph.D. in community health/health behavior, an M.S. in health education, and a B.S. with majors in both health/physical education and English. Her main research and teaching focus has been on the factors that increase risk for chronic diseases and the use of incentives and social supports in developing effective interventions for high-risk women and families. Her research has been published in numerous journals, and she has been a consultant, guest speaker, and presenter at professional conferences throughout the country. Dr. Donatelle is also the author of the highly successful introductory health textbooks *Access to Health, Health: The Basics*, and *My Health: An Outcomes Approach*. When she isn't writing textbooks, she spends her time playing acoustic guitar, gardening, keeping up with her Westies, and camping with friends in Oregon's quiet wooded areas.

Tanya R. Littrell, Ph.D.

Dr. Tanya R. Littrell is the Faculty Department Chair of the Fitness Technology Program at Portland Community College in Portland, Oregon. She has her Ph.D. in exercise physiology, M.S. in human performance, and a minor in nutrition from Oregon State University. She started her educational path with a B.S. in physical education and minor in biology from the University of Oregon. Dr. Littrell teaches exercise physiology, fitness assessment, fitness and aging, and general fitness in the Fitness Technology and Physical Education departments at PCC. She has been teaching lifetime fitness classes for undergraduates since 1998 and before that worked as a fitness director, instructor, and personal trainer. When Dr. Littrell isn't in the classroom, preparing to teach, coordinating the program, or writing, you can find her on the trails running or mountain biking, hiking, traveling, or spending quality time with family and friends.

Brief Contents

Contents

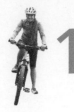

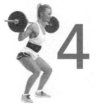

3 Conditioning Your Cardiorespiratory System 66

How Does My Cardiorespiratory System Work? 67

An Overview of the Cardiorespiratory System 67
Three Metabolic Systems Deliver Essential Energy 70
The Cardiorespiratory System at Rest and during Exercise 71

How Does Aerobic Training Condition My Cardiorespiratory System? 72

Aerobic Training Increases Oxygen Delivery to Your Muscles 72
Aerobic Training Improves the Transfer and Use of Oxygen 72
Aerobic Training Improves Your Body's Ability to Use Energy Efficiently 73

What Are the Benefits of Improving My Cardiorespiratory Fitness? 73

Cardiorespiratory Fitness Decreases Your Risk of Disease 73
Cardiorespiratory Fitness Helps You Control Body Weight and Body Composition 74
Cardiorespiratory Fitness Improves Self-Esteem, Mood, and Sense of Well-Being 74
Cardiorespiratory Fitness Improves Immune Function 74
Cardiorespiratory Fitness Improves Long-Term Quality of Life 75

How Can I Assess My Cardiorespiratory Fitness? 75

Understand Your Maximal Oxygen Consumption 75
Test Your Submaximal Heart Rate Responses 76
Test Your Cardiorespiratory Fitness in the Field/Classroom 76

How Can I Create My Own Cardiorespiratory Fitness Program? 77

Set Appropriate Cardiorespiratory Fitness Goals 77
Learn about Cardiorespiratory Training Options 77
Apply the FITT Formula to Cardiorespiratory Fitness 78
Include a Warm-Up and Cool-Down in Your Workout Session 82

How Can I Maintain My Cardiorespiratory Program? 83

Understand the Stages of Progression 83
Record and Track Your Progress 84
Troubleshoot Problems Right Away 84
Periodically Reassess Your Cardiorespiratory Fitness Level 84
Reassess Your Goals and Program as Needed 84

How Can I Avoid Injury during Cardiorespiratory Exercise? 84

Design a Personalized, Balanced Cardiorespiratory Program 84
Wear Appropriate Clothing and Footwear 84
Pay Attention to Your Exercise Environment 85
Ensure Proper Hydration 86
Understand How to Prevent and Treat Common Injuries 87

Study Plan 91

LAB 3.1 Learn a Skill: Monitoring Intensity During a Workout 93
LAB 3.2 Assess Yourself: Assessing Your Cardiorespiratory Fitness Level 95
LAB 3.3 Plan for Change: Plan Your Cardiorespiratory Fitness Goals and Program 99
PROGRAM 3.1 A Running Program 103
PROGRAM 3.2 A Cycling Program 107
PROGRAM 3.3 A Swimming Program 110

4 Building Muscular Strength and Endurance 113

What Is Muscular Fitness? 114

How Do My Muscles Work? 114

An Overview of Skeletal Muscle 114

5 Maintaining Flexibility and Back Health 168

6 Understanding Body Composition 210

7 Improving Your Nutrition 232

8 Managing Your Weight 278

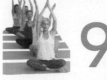

9 Managing Stress 311

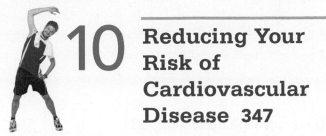

10 Reducing Your Risk of Cardiovascular Disease 347

Feature Boxes

Labs and Programs

Preface

You may have noticed that health, fitness, and wellness are always trending topics! Visit online news sites or turn on the TV and you will undoubtedly find information about the benefits of exercise, the health risks associated with sitting too much, or the results of a recent nutritional study. At the same time, if you are a college student taking a fitness and wellness course, you may feel a sense of disconnect between those stories and your own life. You might wonder: What has any of this got to do with me?

Our primary goal in writing this textbook was simple: To help students realize that the lifestyle choices you make now—regardless of your current age—have real and lasting effects on your lifelong wellness. We also wanted to address the many challenges related to exercise, stress, nutrition, and other issues facing today's students and to create a flexible, personalized fitness and wellness program that works with your own goals and life demands. Finally, we wanted to help students bridge a common fact of life: There is a gap between knowing what we *ought* to do (e.g., exercise more, eat healthier foods, quit smoking, etc.) and actually *doing it*. Throughout this textbook, we emphasize that effective behavior change is both an individual and gradual process, based on realistic expectations and achievable short-term and long-term goals. With these aims in mind, the following are some of the unique features you'll find in *Get Fit, Stay Well!*

New to This Edition

- *Putting It All Together: Your Total Fitness Program.* This program, following the main text content, builds on the fitness principles covered in Chapters 1–5 and guides you in putting it all together to meet your fitness goals. This special section provides customizable four-week programs for beginning, intermediate, and advanced exercisers that show cardiorespiratory fitness, muscle fitness, flexibility, and back health exercises laid out into one easy-to-follow plan.

- *GetFitGraphics.* These infographics highlight compelling topics in visually stunning presentations. For the fourth edition, we have streamlined and updated selected infographics with the latest information and data. We include all new GetFitGraphics in Chapters 1 and 2.

- *Study Plan Tied to Learning Outcomes.* Numbered learning outcomes now introduce every chapter and are tied directly to chapter sections, giving students a roadmap for their reading. Each chapter concludes with a Study Plan, which includes new summary points of the chapter and provides review questions and critical thinking questions to check understanding, both tied to the chapter's learning outcomes and assignable in MasteringHealth™. Also new in the Study Plan is Check Out These eResources, a section pointing students to the most up-to-date online resources relevant to the chapter content.

- *New APPLY IT!/TRY IT! questions.* Found at the end of case studies and various feature boxes, these questions encourage critical thinking and help students apply the material to their own lives. These often supply step-by-step coaching suggestions and help readers to create and refine goals for behavior change.

- *Integrated Labs and Programs.* Where relevant, when students assess themselves in an end-of-chapter lab or a chapter exercise, the authors guide them to their appropriate starting level in the Activate, Motivate, & Advance Programs on yoga, running, flexibility, and meditation. This gives students the ability to do the lab activity in class and then enhance their own lifelong wellness by implementing the program on a daily basis at the appropriate starting level.

- *Vibrant design and engaging visual presentation of content.* Fine-tuning of the text design includes making headings more visible, integrating learning outcomes into the material, and pulling out references—all to enhance navigation and visual appeal.

- *Ongoing content improvements.* This edition makes literally thousands of improvements and revisions to text, art, pedagogical materials, and references based on advances within the fitness and wellness fields and on feedback from educators and readers.

Chapter-by-Chapter Changes

The authors have updated the fourth edition line by line to provide students with the most current information plus references for further exploration. This includes all data and statistics throughout the text. We have reorganized portions of chapters to improve the flow of topics, and added, updated, and improved upon figures, tables, photos, and feature boxes. The following is a chapter-by-chapter listing of noteworthy changes, updates, and additions.

Chapter 1: Changing Personal Behaviors for Optimal Wellness

- New Diversity box comparing young adults to others in leading causes of death and preventable risks
- New GetFitGraphic focused on whether exercise improves mental functioning
- New Q&A box analyzing how improved wellness benefits society
- New Tools for Change box focused on what influences your behaviors and your efforts to change
- Revised Q&A box on how to find reliable health information
- Updated coverage on provisions of the Affordable Care Act that are relevant to students
- New information on the importance of journaling and electronic activity monitoring systems (EAMS) in improving exercise behaviors

Chapter 2: Understanding Fitness Principles

- New GetFitGraphic on "Sitting Syndrome"
- Updated Tools for Change box with a checklist of tips for getting up and moving
- New section on pregnancy and exercise (moved from Chapter 15)
- New Q&A box to help you decide whether technology will help you get more fit
- Updated Diversity box on physical activity for everyone

- Updated American College of Sports Medicine (ACSM) recommendations
- New figure to determine your physical activity stage of change
- Updated pre-exercise screening questionnaire in Lab 2.1
- New Lab 2.3 to check your daily activity levels (steps and mileage)

Chapter 3: Conditioning Your Cardiorespiratory System

- Updated and expanded case study
- Updated information regarding lactic acid/lactate
- New Q&A box about hot trends in fitness
- New Tools for Change box with step-by-step guidance in selecting the right athletic shoe

Chapter 4: Building Muscular Strength and Endurance

- Expanded section on resistance training benefits in aging
- New Tools for Change box on alternate muscle fitness training equipment
- New Q&A box on using eccentric training to help you get stronger

Chapter 5: Maintaining Flexibility and Back Health

- Updated box on alternate ways to increase your range of motion without "stretching"
- Updated sections on posture, "text neck," and risky activities and occupations for back pain

Chapter 6: Understanding Body Composition

- Updated BMI figures showing obesity classes
- Expanded discussion and photos of bioelectrical impedance analysis (BIA) assessment

Chapter 7: Improving Your Nutrition

- Numerous changes based on the new Dietary Guidelines for Americans 2015–2020

- Reorganized and expanded sections on special dietary needs, nutrition throughout the life cycle, and food safety
- Updated Tools for Change box on tips for outings to restaurants and Q&A box on whether to take supplements
- Streamlined and improved Tables 7.2 and 7.3 on vitamins and minerals
- New Table 7.6 on eating fruits and vegetables for healthful antioxidants
- New Figure 7.7 on food labeling requirements and changes
- Updated Lab 7.2 using current ChooseMyPlate.gov tracking tools

Chapter 8: Managing Your Weight

- New case study
- New Table 8.1 comparing name-brand diets
- New GetFitGraphic on weight loss myths
- New Figure 8.1 on trends in adult overweight and obesity; Figure 8.3: new obesity map of the US, and Updated Q&A box on diet drugs and surgery
- New coverage of the psychology of food craving and the role of gut microbes in weight gain

Chapter 9: Managing Stress

- New GetFitGraphic on stress caused by college debt
- New Q&A box on stress and emotional wellness
- New Tools for Change Box on solutions for Internet stress
- New Figure 9.3 on allostatic load
- New content on connections between stress and topics including inflammation, sugar consumption, and social networking
- New content on the role of gut microbes in stress response
- New coverage of stress in international students

Chapter 10: Reducing Your Risk of Cardiovascular Disease

- Significantly revised boxes: Q&A on salt, sugar, and CVD risk; Diversity box on college students and hypertension; Diversity box on men, women, and

CVD; Tools for Change box on eating for heart health; and Q&A box on diet drugs and surgery
- Updated information on connections between CVD risk and plaque, e-cigarettes, sugar, and genetics

Other Key Features

- *Unique Case Studies presented in each chapter* introduce a "character" who reflects the concerns, questions, and thought processes that students are likely to have themselves. Try It! and Apply It! questions at the end of the case studies encourage critical thinking and help students consider how the material applies to their own lives.
- *Labs employ a unique three-pronged approach:* (1) skill-acquisition labs, (2) self-assessment labs, and (3) action-plan labs. The labs not only measure a student's current level of fitness/wellness, but also teach practical lifelong skills and encourage real behavior change. All labs are also available online in interactive PDF and/or auto-graded format and are assignable through MasteringHealth. Additional self-assessment labs are offered online in the Study Area in MasteringHealth.
- *Reflection questions* appear at the end of the labs, asking students to reflect on the choices they made or their results from the assessments.
- *The most modern strength-training presentation available* includes photos of more than 100 strength-training and flexibility exercises featuring actual college students, modern gym equipment, and options for students with limited access to equipment. Videos of the exercises in the book, as well as many alternate exercises, are available online in MasteringHealth.
- *A strong emphasis on behavior change appears throughout the text.* Try It!/Apply It! features suggest immediate action, while Tools for Change boxes provide tools for longer-term change. The Plan for Change labs ask students to write out an action plan for behavior change.
- *Q&A boxes* investigate common questions and concerns students may have in relation to chapter topics.

- *Diversity boxes* address topics relevant to diverse student populations, acknowledging that age, race, gender, disability, and individual life circumstances can result in specific fitness and wellness needs.

- *A running glossary* helps students easily review and master key terms.

- *Research citations* demonstrate the accuracy, currency, and scientific grounding for information presented in the text.

- *A pre- and post-course progress worksheet* included at the beginning of the book and available online allows students to assess their progress on key fitness/wellness assessments.

MasteringHealth for Instructors and Students

MasteringHealth is an online homework, tutorial, and assessment program designed to work with this text to engage students and improve results. Interactive, self-paced tutorials provide individualized coaching to help students stay on track. With a wide range of activities available, students can actively learn, understand, and retain even the most difficult concepts.

- *Pre-Lecture Reading Quizzes* ensure that students complete the assigned reading before class and stay on track with reading assignments. Reading Questions are 100 percent mobile ready and can be completed by students on mobile devices. They're also easy-to-customize and assign, saving instructors valuable time.

- *Dynamic Study Modules* help students study effectively on their own by continuously assessing their activity and performance in real time. Here's how it works: Students complete a set of questions with a unique answer format that also asks them to indicate their confidence level. Questions repeat until the student can answer them all correctly and confidently. Once completed, Dynamic Study Modules explain the concept using materials from the text. These are available as graded assignments prior to class, and accessible on smartphones, tablets, and computers. NEW! Instructors can now remove questions from Dynamic Study Modules to better fit their course.

- *eText 2.0* is now optimized for mobile:
  o Available on smartphones and tablets.
  o Can be downloaded for most iOS and Android phones/tablets from the Apple App Store or Google Play.

  o Seamlessly integrated videos and other rich media.
  o Accessible (screen-reader ready).
  o Configurable reading settings, including resizable type and night reading mode.
  o Instructor and student note-taking, highlighting, bookmarking, and search.
  o eText 2.0 mobile app offers offline access on your iOS or Android phones/tablets.

- *Learning Catalytics*™ helps you generate class discussion, customize your lecture, and promote peer-to-peer learning with real-time analytics. As a student response tool, Learning Catalytics uses students' smartphones, tablets, or laptops to engage them in more interactive tasks and thinking.
  o NEW! Upload a full PowerPoint® deck for easy creation of slide questions
  o NEW! Team names are no longer case sensitive
  o Help your students develop critical thinking skills
  o Monitor responses to find out where your students are struggling
  o Rely on real-time data to adjust your teaching strategy
  o Automatically group students for discussion, teamwork, and peer-to-peer learning

- *Interactive Behavior Change Activities—Which Path Would You Take?* direct students to explore various health choices through an engaging, interactive, low-stakes, and anonymous experience. These assignable activities show students the possible consequences of various choices they make today on their future health.

- *25 Auto-gradable Labs* are now available as auto-graded, assignable labs within MasteringHealth, saving instructors' time.

- *Tough Topics Coaching Activities* guide students through key health and fitness concepts with interactive mini-lessons that provide hints and feedback, ensuring that learners comprehend the material.

- *Behavior Change Videos* are concise whiteboard-style videos that help students with the steps of behavior change, covering topics such as setting SMART goals, identifying and overcoming barriers to change, planning realistic timelines, and more. Additional videos review key fitness concepts such as determining target heart rate range for exercise. All videos include assessment activities and are assignable in MasteringHealth.

- **ABC News** *Videos* bring health to life and spark discussion with up-to-date hot topics from 2012 to 2015. Activities tied to the videos include multiple-choice questions that provide wrong-answer feedback to redirect students to the correct answer.

- *NutriTools Coaching Activities* in the nutrition chapter have been updated and allow students to combine and experiment with different food options and learn firsthand how to build healthier meals.

- *The Test Bank* in MasteringHealth includes multiple choice, true/false, and short-answer questions, allowing you to easily and intuitively build exams and quizzes. Questions are tagged to Bloom's taxonomy and global and book-specific student learning outcomes.

- *Additional instructor resources*—including PowerPoint® lecture outlines; PowerPoint clicker and Jeopardy-style quiz show questions; and .jpeg files for illustrations, tables, and selected photos from the text—further bolster the in-class experience.

- *Measuring Student Learning Outcomes?* All of the MasteringHealth assignable content is tagged to book content and to Bloom's taxonomy. Instructors also have the ability to add their own learning outcomes, helping to track student performance against their learning outcomes. Share results quickly and easily by exporting them to a spreadsheet.

- *The Study Area of MasteringHealth* is organized by learning areas: *See It* includes *ABC News* videos on important health topics and more than 100 exercise videos. *Hear It* contains MP3 chapter review files and audio case studies. *Do It* contains critical-thinking questions and web links. *Review It* contains study quizzes for each chapter. *Live It* will help jump-start students' behavior-change projects with assessments and resources to plan change.

Teaching Toolkit (Download Only)

The Teaching Toolkit resources replace the former printed Teaching Toolbox by providing everything you need to prep for your course and deliver a dynamic lecture in one convenient place. Download all of these resources from the Instructor Resources tab in MasteringHealth:

For Lecture Prep

- *ABC News* Lecture Launcher videos
- PowerPoint® lecture outlines
- PowerPoint® clicker questions and Jeopardy-style quiz show questions
- Files for all illustrations and tables and selected photos from the text
- Test Bank:
  - Test Bank in Word® and RTF formats
  - Computerized Test Bank, which includes all the questions from the test bank in a format that allows you to easily and intuitively build exams and quizzes
- Instructor's Resource Support Manual
  - Organized by chapter, this useful guide includes objectives, lecture outlines, critical thinking and in-class discussion questions, references to figures, and *ABC News* Lecture Launcher video discussion questions, as well as teaching tips.
- Introduction to MasteringHealth
- Introductory video for Learning Catalytics
- Great Ideas: Active Ways to Teach Health & Wellness: This manual provides new ideas for classroom activities related to specific health and wellness topics, as well as suggestions for activities that can be adapted to various topics and class sizes.
- Teaching with Student Learning Outcomes
- Teaching with Web 2.0: How can you integrate blogs, Twitter, RSS feeds, and other relevant social media into your health and wellness class? Get ideas here for classroom and project activities that can be adapted to various topics and class sizes.

For Use with Students

- Take Charge of Your Health Worksheets: A total of 50 additional self-assessment exercises
- Behavior Change Log Book and Wellness Journal: This assessment tool helps students track daily exercise and nutritional intake and create a long-term nutritional and fitness prescription plan. It also includes a Behavior Change Contract and topics for journal-based activities.
- Eat Right! Healthy Eating in College and Beyond: This handy, full-color booklet provides students with

practical guidelines, tips, shopper's guides, and recipes that turn healthy eating principles into blueprints for action. Topics include healthy eating in the cafeteria, dorm room, and fast food restaurants; planning meals on a budget; weight management; vegetarian alternatives; and how alcohol impacts health.

- Live Right! Beating Stress in College and Beyond: Live Right! gives students useful tips for coping with stressful life challenges both during college and for the rest of their lives. Topics include sleep, managing finances, time management, coping with academic pressure, and relationships. This book also presents an objective overview of some

of the health-oriented products now being advertised.

- Food Composition Table

Contributors to Instructor Resources

We thank the authors of the instructor supplements: Allison Nye (Cape Fear Community College) and Adam Thompson (Indiana Wesleyan University), who updated and revised the Test Bank, and Denise Wright (Southern Editorial), whose team updated and revised the Instructor's Resource Support Manual and PowerPoint Lecture Outlines, Quiz Shows, and Clicker Questions. Your work ensures that instructors have the resources that they need to teach effectively.

Acknowledgments

From Janet Hopson

Preparing a new edition of a college program such as *Get Fit, Stay Well!*—plus all of its accompanying study and instructional materials—is an exciting and gratifying adventure but also an enormous undertaking. The authors' efforts are just part of a complex, well-integrated, and coordinated effort. We would like to thank the following members of the Pearson team: Courseware Senior Analyst Alice Fugate, who handled with skill and grace the daily demands of upgrading, updating, and shepherding our author team through this new edition and all its innovations; Content Producer Susan Malloy and Project Manager Sherrill Redd, who so ably guided and coordinated our ongoing efforts; Senior Portfolio Manager Michelle Cadden Yglecias, who skillfully and diplomatically steered our team through major plan decisions; Barbara Yien, Frank Ruggirello, Sandra Lindelof, and Deirdre Espinoza, who all championed and greatly improved this book in its early stages; Claire Alexander, who so nimbly functioned as development editor in earlier editions; our superb marketing manager Neena Bali; the talented composition and production team at Aptara; Gary Hespenheide and Hespenheide Design, who are responsible for this book's dynamic design and cover; former student Geoffrey Kober, who tirelessly aided our research of the scientific literature; and Heidi Arndt and Nicole Constantine, who cheerfully and creatively smoothed our pathway as portfolio management assistants. Finally, and in many ways primarily, I would like to thank Rebecca Donatelle and Tanya Littrell for their superb knowledge, experience, authorship, and steadfast support.

From Rebecca Donatelle

After working on several college textbooks over the years, one thing has become very clear to me: The publishing house you choose to work with is the single most important factor in producing a quality textbook that is going to be successful in the marketplace. Pearson has assembled a truly remarkable group of top-notch acquisition, editorial, production, marketing, sales, and ancillary staff to help nurture a text through its development and growth. I am fortunate to have had the opportunity to work with individuals who worry the details and possess an incredible degree of creativity and professionalism. You are truly THE BEST . . . thank you so much to each and every one of you. I would especially like to thank Michelle Yglecias, Senior Portfolio Manager, for her steady hand, attention to overall project management, and personalized approach in bringing GFSW to fruition. Managing all of the layers of writing, development, and changes that occur in an organization is a tough job and Michelle did an outstanding job. I would also like to thank Susan Malloy for her terrific oversight of day-to-day project details and challenges. Susan's years of experience and understanding of the process and the players is unique in the field. She has worked on several of my books over the years and I always smile when she is involved in one of my projects. I know that she will worry the details and ensure a quality project! She is a rare gem of wisdom and dedication to excellence in the fast-changing publishing world today. Also, I would like to thank Cathy Murphy, who was the original developmental manager on this project. Her organizational skills, hard work, and dedication to early project guidance and initiation were exemplary. As per usual, Alice Fugate did an outstanding job in her capacity as developmental editor. Her

Acknowledgments (continued)

thoughtful and thorough reviews and editorial commentary helped bring this project to fruition and kept the wheels turning in ensuring a market-leading product. Thanks, Alice! Finally, I would like to thank Sherrill Redd, project manager for this edition of GFSW. Sherrill's organizational skills, communication skills, and thoughtful suggestions provided the guidance that made our work easier in the final stages of the project. Additionally, I would like to thank my amazing co-authors, Jan and Tanya. From conceptualization to creative thought processes, hard work, painstaking attention to the science and art of writing a high-quality, well-written college text—these two are the best!

From Tanya Littrell

I would like to first and foremost thank my family and friends for all of their support through the long hours of creating and revising this textbook. Next, I would like to thank my co-authors, Janet Hopson and Becky Donatelle. These two individuals are committed to producing the highest quality and most usable textbook in this genre and working with them is an honor. We have had some incredible individuals at Pearson on this project over the years. In addition to Jan's complete list, I would like to thank Sandra Lindelof, Barbara Yien, Kari Hopperstead, and Erin Schnair for their guidance on the previous editions of this book. For this fourth edition, I had the privilege of working with Alice Fugate, Susan Malloy, Sherrill Redd, and Michelle Cadden Yglecias most directly. Collectively, I feel that their support and superior editorial and managerial skills are evident in this edition. I would also like to thank fellow faculty members at Portland Community College, who have been supportive throughout this project, in particular, Janeen Hull. Ms. Hull was the knowledgeable and creative mind behind the initial development of the Activate, Motivate, & Advance programs. For this fourth edition, she helped shape the fitness chapter revisions with extensive research of the current fitness trends and supporting scientific literature. My time at Oregon State University set the stage for my work on this project. I would like to thank Anthony Wilcox, Associate Professor, College of Public Health and Human Sciences at OSU, for giving me the teaching and supervisory experience that led to this opportunity.

Reviewers for the Fourth Edition

Many thanks to the hundreds of instructors and students who reviewed and class-tested the previous editions of this text, and to the following reviewers who contributed feedback for this revision:

Donna Dey (Austin Peay State University), Randolph Dietz (Our Lady of the Lake University), Jamie Dolieslager (Bethel University), Michael A. Dupper (University of Mississippi), Sharrie Horbold (Lane Community College), Justin Kraft (Missouri Western State University), Michelle LeCompte (University of Colorado at Colorado Springs), Laura Lewis (Meridian Community College), Melissa Madeson (Hardin-Simmons University), Constance McClain (Ventura College), Allison Nye (Cape Fear Community College), Linda J. Romaine (Raritan Valley Community College), Jason V. Slack (Utah Valley University), Adam Thompson (Indiana Wesleyan University), Virginia Trummer (University of Texas San Antonio), Kendra Zenisek (Ball State University)

Changing Personal Behaviors for Optimal Wellness

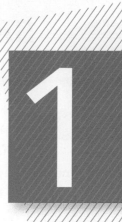

1

LEARNINGoutcomes

LO 1.1 Define wellness and identify where you are on the wellness continuum.

LO 1.2 Describe the dimensions of wellness and how they are interconnected.

LO 1.3 Explain the benefits of wellness for individuals and for society as a whole.

LO 1.4 Determine your stage in the behavior change process for one or more behaviors.

LO 1.5 Demonstrate skill at using the SMART goal-setting guidelines by creating a goal for changing one wellness behavior.

LO 1.6 Develop a behavior change contract with strategies you will use to plan, implement, and maintain your behavior changes, including the resources and supports that will ensure your success.

MasteringHealth™

Go online for chapter quizzes, interactive assessments, videos, and more!

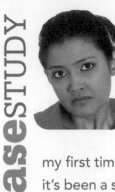

SERENA

"Hi, I'm Serena. I come from a small town in Arizona and just started my freshman year at a big university 1,500 miles from home. It's my first time living away from home, and it's been a struggle. My boyfriend and my friends are still in Arizona. My family has sacrificed a lot for me to be here. I probably shouldn't have taken so many classes for my first term. I'm hitting the books, but I can't seem to catch up. I'm sleeping only four hours per night and I'm tired all the time, feel like crying much of the time, and don't know how to get out of this slump. I don't have any friends yet because I don't take time to socialize. Several women on my floor have dropped out—too much partying during their first term! I feel like my life is out of control. What can I do?

Hear It!
To listen to this case study online, visit the Study Area in MasteringHealth™.

Can you relate to Serena's problems? You are not alone. In a large survey, college students reported stress, anxiety, sleep difficulties, frequent colds, depression, and work issues as key factors negatively affecting their academic performance (see **Figure 1.1**).[1] Add too much time on extracurricular activities, social media, pressure to get good grades, and issues with money, roommates, friends, and family and today's college students face considerable challenges! It's not surprising that when asked to rate their overall health or wellness, just over 52.8 percent of them (59.9 percent of men and 49.7 percent of women) described it as *very good or excellent*, leaving just over 32 percent to rate their health as merely *good* and the rest rating their health as only *fair or poor*.[2] Since young adulthood is the time when most people are in their prime health years, we should be seeing higher percentages of very good and excellent health. Finding ways to improve on these percentages and achieve higher levels of health and wellness is a key focus of this text.

wellness Achieving the highest level of health possible in each of several dimensions

physical fitness The ability to perform moderate to vigorous levels of physical activity without undue fatigue

LO 1.1 What Is Wellness and How Well Am I?

Wellness is an active process in which people take steps to become more aware of, and make choices toward, a healthy and fulfilling life.[3]

To understand wellness, let's first consider the concept of *health*. While historically the term *health* meant merely the absence of disease, experts today view it as an inclusive term that encompasses everything from environmental health to the health of individuals, populations, and communities. *Wellness* often conveys a more personalized perspective on health defined as the achievement of the highest level of health possible in physical, social, intellectual, emotional, spiritual, and environmental dimensions.[4] It describes a vibrant state in which individuals take responsibility for improving and maintaining their health, and are capable of adapting and effectively moving forward through life's challenges. Wellness is a process in which people actively work to be the best that they can be, to contribute to society, and to live up to their potential. In contrast, *health* is a broader term that includes the individual dimensions of wellness but has a major focus on community, health policy, health systems, and social and environmental factors affecting health.

In this book, we will sometimes use the terms *health* and *wellness* interchangeably. However, *wellness* typically refers to a more individualized, dynamic concept, requiring self-evaluation, thoughtful planning, and effort, but with the potential to bring great rewards. Central to wellness is **physical fitness**, or simply *fitness,* the ability to perform moderate to vigorous levels of physical activity without undue fatigue. Fitness is just one dimension of wellness, but we give it special attention in this book because it influences so many of the other dimensions and because the tools for improving fitness are readily available while you are a college student—a period in your life when you are able to make decisions and establish personal habits that will benefit you right now and for a lifetime.

Where Am I on the Wellness Continuum?

Improving your wellness—moving toward that vibrant multidimensional state—is an ambitious but

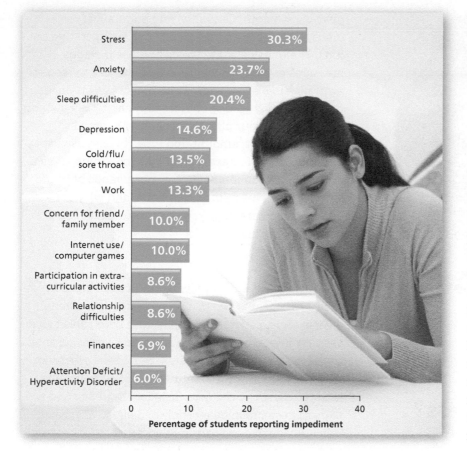

FIGURE **1.1** Major factors affecting student wellness and academic performance.

Data from American College Health Association, *American College Health Association—National College Health Assessment II: Reference Group Executive Summary, Fall 2015* (Hanover, MD: American College Health Association, 2016).

affect your wellness. Additionally, having access to high-quality medical care, nutritious food, good exercise facilities, and social support networks enhance positive behaviors. Unfortunately, some people are more at risk for health risks due to their macro social and physical environments.[5] Although early adulthood is a period in life when you are most likely to reach your physiological health peak with fewer risks of lifestyle-related chronic illness, far too many young adults are "works in progress" when it comes to optimal wellness. This may be the ideal time to insure that your efforts reap positive rewards.

The first step? Assess how close you are now to your long-term goals. We can picture wellness as a continuum of greater or lesser total soundness of body and mind (**Figure 1.2**). Understanding your current place on the **wellness continuum** is important for setting goals and changing wellness behaviors.

achievable goal. The wellness patterns you establish during this course can change your life, affecting your fitness, success in relationships and career, susceptibility to disease, and the quality and quantity of your years. However, no single college course can address every health concern or guarantee a lifetime of wellness. Your age, socioeconomic status, education, neighborhood, personal history, genetic susceptibility to disease/disability, and physical environment all

> **wellness continuum** A spectrum of wellness states from irreversible damage to optimum wellness

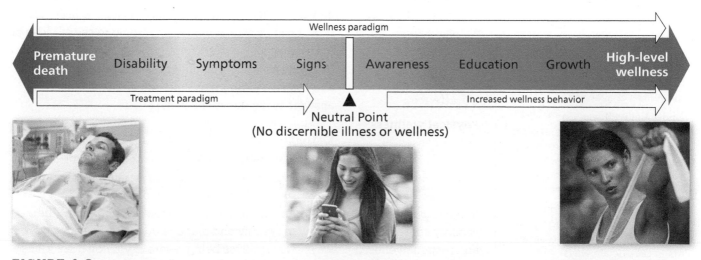

FIGURE **1.2** The illness-wellness continuum

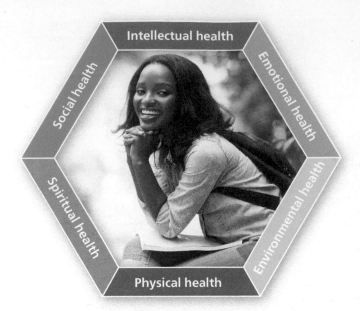

FIGURE **1.3** Wellness is an optimal level of health in six interconnected dimensions of human experience.

LO 1.2 What Are the Dimensions of Wellness?

We can think of wellness as consisting of six primary dimensions (physical, social, intellectual, emotional, spiritual, and environmental) (**Figure 1.3**). Because wellness is a process, you may experience faster growth in one dimension than in others. The dimensions are interconnected, meaning that positive effort in one area can help you make progress in others and move you toward greater overall health and well-being.

physical wellness A state of physical health and well-being that includes body size and shape, body functioning, measures of strength and endurance, and resistance to disease

social wellness A person's degree of social connectedness and skills, leading to satisfying interpersonal relationships

intellectual wellness The ability to think clearly, reason objectively, analyze, and use brain power to solve problems and meet life's challenges

emotional wellness The ability to control emotions and express them appropriately at the right times; includes self-esteem, self-confidence, and other emotional qualities

emotional intelligence The ability to identify and manage your own emotions and those of others in productive ways

Physical Wellness

Physical wellness encompasses all aspects of a sound body, including body size, shape, and composition; sensory sharpness and responsiveness; body functioning; physical strength, flexibility, and endurance; resistance to diseases and disorders; and recuperative abilities. The physical state we call *fitness* includes measures of physical wellness and allows a person to exert physical effort without undue stress, strain, or injury. Your day-to-day choices and habits can support or undermine your physical wellness. Examples include your diet; amount and types of exercise; sleep patterns; level of stress; use of tobacco, drugs, or alcohol; participation in unsafe sex; observance of traffic laws; wearing helmets or seat belts; and whether you access healthcare (e.g., regular checkups, vaccinations, and treatment).

Social Wellness

Social wellness is the ability to have satisfying interpersonal relationships and maintain connections through diverse social networks. This includes being able to successfully interact with others, adapt to a variety of social situations, and act appropriately, regardless of setting. Whether you are shy and introverted or outgoing and extroverted, social wellness includes the ability and willingness to communicate clearly and effectively; establish intimacy through trust and acceptance; ask for and give support; maintain friendships over time; and interact within groups, such as on the job or in the community.

Intellectual Wellness

Intellectual wellness is the ability to use your brain power effectively to solve problems and meet life's challenges. It allows you to think clearly, quickly, creatively, and critically; use good reasoning and make careful decisions; and learn from your successes and mistakes. However, it is more than pure intellect. It involves being open-minded and non-judgmental; exposing yourself to new ideas, beliefs' and people; being able to listen and think about others, opinions and trying to see all sides of an issue; having a thirst for knowledge and information; being culturally competent and multiculturally aware; and acknowledging that there are often no simple answers to big questions in life.[6]

Emotional Wellness

Emotional wellness refers to the ability to control your emotions and express them appropriately at the right times. An aspect of emotional wellness that gained increasing attention is **emotional intelligence**—the ability to identify and manage our emotions in positive ways. This involves being aware of your own emotions and triggers for them, being able to calm others (and yourself) when overly reactive, and being able to listen to others' frustration or grief.[7]

Unfortunately, emotional wellness and overall mental health are growing concerns on campus. Several reports that stress, anxiety, and depression are soaring on college campuses have surfaced, with campuses scrambling to help students cope with multiple demands.[8] It may surprise you to know that nearly 50 percent of mental illness begins by age 14, and 75 percent of lifetime mental health problems begin before age 24.[9] College students are particularly vulnerable as evidenced by the fact that 64 percent of those who drop out of college do so because of mental or emotional health issues.[10] Improving emotional wellness requires developing positive *self-esteem*; *self-efficacy* (confidence); coping with stress, anger, and negativity; and developing an appropriate balance of emotional dependence and independence. Importantly, it also requires that people who have problems recognize that they need help, know where to go for help, and can access those services.

Spiritual Wellness

For some people, **spiritual wellness** may involve a belief in a supreme being or a way of life prescribed by a particular religion. For others, spiritual wellness is a feeling of oneness with others and with nature, and a sense of meaning or value in life. Developing spiritual wellness may deepen one's understanding of life's purpose; allow a person to feel part of a greater spectrum of existence; and promote feelings of love, joy, peace, contentment, and wonder over life's experiences. It may also provide a means of coping with challenges that seem overwhelming.

Environmental Wellness

While we often think of the word *environment* in terms of nature, environmental wellness is much more all-encompassing. It includes the macro environment we live and work in, the schools we attend, and the communities and neighborhoods where we spend much of our time. **Environmental wellness** entails understanding how the environment can positively or negatively affect you and your role in preserving, protecting, and improving the world around you.

Related Dimensions of Wellness

Occupational and *financial wellness* overlap with other wellness areas, and are sometimes considered their own dimensions. For our purposes, we include them as a related category under the larger environmental wellness dimension. Your wellness in these areas can dramatically

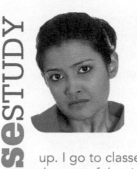

SERENA

"I am the first one in my family to go to college. My mom and dad are divorced and my mom took on another part-time job to help pay for tuition. I really want her to be proud of me, but I'm finding it hard to keep up. I go to classes, eat on the run, and study the rest of the time. Yesterday, I got the first "C" in my life! My anxiety is growing and I'm feeling overwhelmed. Maybe I'm not "college material." Yesterday, I dozed through two of my classes and didn't hear much of the lecture. I also have a cold I can't shake. I know I should exercise and eat better, but there is never enough time. My diet is lousy and I drink way too much coffee! I can't tell my mom because she would only worry, and my high school friends seem to be drifting away."

APPLY IT! Do you recognize any of Serena's issues in yourself or other students? Which dimensions of wellness are problems for Serena? Where would you place her on the wellness continuum? Where would you place yourself? What steps could she take to improve her situation?

TRY IT! **Today,** identify your strongest wellness dimensions, your weakest ones, and the first one you would like to improve. **This week,** create a wellness balance chart and plan the balance you would like to achieve (see **Lab 1.2**). **In two weeks,** chart any improvements and readjust your plan, if necessary.

Do It!
Access these labs at the end of the chapter or online at MasteringHealth™.

Hear It!
To listen to this case study online, visit the Study Area in MasteringHealth™.

affect your overall wellness. If you ask family members and friends about their current problems, many will identify their jobs or finances as top stressors in their lives. In fact, according to a recent survey of job satisfaction, 55 percent of American workers reported being dissatisfied with their jobs—with the youngest workers (those under age 25) reporting the highest level of dissatisfaction ever recorded![11]

spiritual wellness A feeling of unity or oneness with people and nature and a sense of life's purpose, meaning, or value; for some, a belief in a supreme being or religion

environmental wellness An appreciation of how the external environment can affect oneself, and an understanding of the role one plays in preserving, protecting, and improving it

Occupational wellness is the level of happiness and fulfillment you experience in your work as well as possible hazards or health risks you face on the job. An important component of occupational wellness is whether an individual feels valued and that their opinions matter. Contrary to what people often think, job satisfaction and motivation are not closely tied to high wages. When your goals align with those of your employer and you feel you are contributing, occupational wellness is more likely.[12]

Financial wellness is the ability to successfully balance your financial needs and wants with your income, debts, savings, and investments. If you cannot pay your bills, it can be hard to think of much else and this dimension can overshadow and unbalance the others. Students who successfully navigate financial challenges will experience less stress and have a greater chance of improved wellness. (See Chapter 9 for more information about the relationship between stress and finances, and strategies for coping with money-related problems.)

Balancing Your Wellness Dimensions

You may have healthy relationships, but no fondness for exercise. Perhaps your spiritual life is rich, but you have trouble juggling academic demands. Virtually everyone is stronger in some dimensions of wellness than others and these may fluctuate wildly during various times in life. Trying to improve all six wellness dimensions is a lifelong goal. One approach is to go slow and set achievable goals, focusing on those dimensions with the most pressing need, while working on the others in a steady, but relaxed and motivated way. Your brain and body, your thoughts and emotions, your actions and reactions, your relationship to yourself and others—all are interconnected and integrated. Likewise, the dimensions of wellness are interrelated. For example, increasing your exercise and activity and improving your eating habits may help you improve in other areas, such as sleep quality, stress and mood, body composition, and decreased risks for type 2 diabetes.[13]

occupational wellness A level of happiness and fulfilment in work, including harmony with personal goals, appreciation from bosses and co-workers, and a safe workplace

financial wellness The ability to balance and manage financial needs and wants with income, debts, savings, and investments

***healthy* life expectancy** The years a person can expect to live without disability or major illness

LO 1.3 Why Does Wellness Matter?

Wellness has many benefits for both individuals and society.

Good Wellness Habits Can Help You Live a Longer, Healthier Life

In spite of significant increases in recent years, the average life expectancy at birth for males is 76.4 years and for females 81.2 years in the United States, well below at least 40 other countries in the world. Although we spend the most for health care, we lag in life expectancy and infant mortality—two key indicators of overall health status.[14] Importantly, our average ***healthy* life expectancy**—the years a person can expect to live without disability or major illness—is about 68 for males and 71 for females (**Figure 1.4**).[15]

See It!
Watch "101 Year Old's Secret to Longevity" at MasteringHealth™.

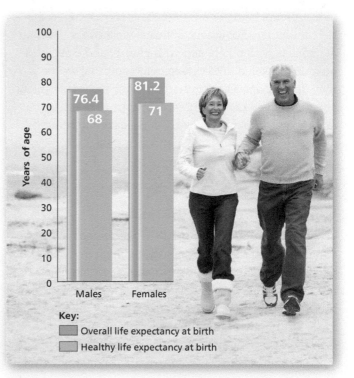

FIGURE **1.4** Healthy life expectancy is the number of years a person lives in good health. Healthy years are an important wellness goal.

Data from J. A. Salomon et al., "Healthy Life Expectancy for 187 Countries, 1990–2010: A Systematic Analysis for the Global Burden Disease Study, 2010," *Lancet* 380, no. 9859 (2012): 2144–62, doi: 10.1016/S0140-6736(12)61690-0; C. Murray et al., "Global, Regional, and National Disability-Adjusted Life Years (DALYs) for 306 Diseases and Injuries and Healthy Life Expectancy (HALE) for 188 Countries, 1990–2013: Quantifying the Epidemiological Transition," *Lancet* (2015), doi: http://dx.doi.org/10.1016/S0140-6736(15)61340-X; World Health Organization, "Global Health Observatory Data Repository: Life Expectancy Data by Country," 2013, http://apps.who.int/gho/data/view.main.680?lang=en

Young Adults Have Preventable Risks

Look closely at the causes of death for people ages 15 to 24, and you'll find that more died from accidents than from most other causes combined (**Table 1.1**).[16] By making better wellness choices—such as wearing seat belts and bike helmets, and avoiding risky behaviors such as driving under the influence of drugs or alcohol—you can reduce your risk of premature death in an accident.

For all age groups, significant proportions of the five leading causes of death are related to risk factors that are *modifiable*—meaning that you can often control them. These risks include high blood pressure, tobacco use, alcohol use, high cholesterol, obesity, low fruit and vegetable intake, and physical inactivity.

In fact, compelling new research highlights the continued importance of physical activity in youth and early adulthood as a potent risk reduction strategy for many of our chronic diseases. Improving fitness in these early years may be particularly important in reducing risks of heart disease and diabetes later in life.[17]

Living a **sedentary** life also increases the danger of **hypokinetic diseases**—conditions that can be triggered or worsened by too little movement or activity, such as obesity, back pain, arthritis, and high blood pressure. In fact, watching television or sitting at a desk for six hours per day could shorten your life by five years, while engaging in sufficient leisure-time

> **sedentary** Physically inactive; exerting physical effort only for required daily tasks and not for leisure-time exercise
>
> **hypokinetic diseases** Conditions that can be triggered or worsened by too little movement or activity, such as obesity, back pain, arthritis, and high blood pressure

TABLE 1-1 Leading Causes of Death in the United States, 2014

Rank	Ages			All Ages
	15-24	25-34	35-44	
1	Unintentional Injury 11,836	Unintentional Injury 17,357	Unintentional Injury 16,048	Heart Disease 614,348
2	Suicide 5,079	Suicide 6,569	Malignant Neoplasms 11,267	Malignant Neoplasms 591,699
3	Homicide 4,144	Homicide 4,159	Heart Disease 10,368	Chronic Low Respiratory Disease 147,101
4	Malignant Neoplasms 1,569	Malignant Neoplasms 3,624	Suicide 6,706	Unintentional Injury 136,053
5	Heart Disease 953	Heart Disease 3,341	Homicide 2,588	Cerebrovascular 133,103
6	Congenital Anomalies 377	Liver Disease 725	Liver Disease 2,582	Alzheimer's Disease 93,541
7	Influenza & Pneumonia 199	Diabetes Mellitus 709	Diabetes Mellitus 1,999	Diabetes Mellitus 76,488
8	Diabetes Mellitus 181	HIV 583	Cerebrovascular 1,745	Influenza & Pneumonia 55,227
9	Chronic Low Respiratory Disease 178	Cerebrovascular 579	HIV 1,174	Nephritis 48,146
10	Cerebrovascular 177	Influenza & Pneumonia 549	Influenza & Pneumonia 1,125	Suicide 42,773

Source: Data from Centers for Disease Control and Prevention, National Vital Statistics System–National Center for Health Statistics, WISQARS, "Ten Leading Causes of Death by Age, United States, 2014," March 2015, www.cdc.gov/injury/wisqars/pdf/leading_causes_of_death_by_age_group_2014-a.pdf

FIT BODY, FIT BRAIN??

Can **EXERCISE** improve your memory and reduce your risk of age-related cognitive decline? Recent research has demonstrated promising results!

HOW IT WORKS: Your **BRAIN** and **MEMORY** on regular aerobic **EXERCISE**

Boosts brainpower by producing chemicals called *brain-derived neurotrophic factor* (**BDNF**), which increases brain cell production and overall brain performance.[2]

Improves mood and sleep, reduces insulin resistance and inflammation, and stimulates growth factors-chemicals in the brain that affect the health of brain cells, blood vessels and brain cell survival, reducing risks of brain shrinkage and cognitive decline.[1, 2, 3]

Boosts the size of the hippocampus, the area is responsible for verbal memory and learning.[1, 2, 3]

Boosts brain volume and overall size.[2, 3]

Signals release of key hormones, including *dopamine* which affects learning and attention and *norepinephrine*, which boosts perception or ability to focus.[1, 2, 3]

Reduces brain atrophy/shrinkage with age which improves cognitive function and verbal learning.[2, 7, 8]

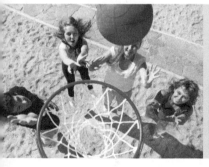

BENEFITS FOR **KIDS**
Aerobic physical activity among children is associated with improvements in

- ☑ Cognition
- ☑ Academic achievement
- ☑ Behavior
- ☑ Psychosocial functioning (2, 3, 4)

BENEFITS FOR **COLLEGE STUDENTS**
In a small study, college students who worked out before tests did better than their sedentary counterparts. A 40-minute workout bumped up test results by one letter grade! (5,6)

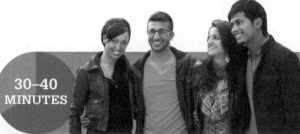

30–40 MINUTES

A systematic review of studies showed that regular exercise sessions lasting 30-40 minutes over at least a six-month period significantly improved cognitive function and reduced rates of age-related cognitive decline, particularly when performed earlier in life. (3)

AND THE BENEFITS GO ON AND ON...

People who exercised regularly as **young adults** had
- ▶ **IMPROVED** cognition later in life
- ▶ **BETTER** verbal memory
- ▶ **FASTER** psychomotor speed at ages 43–55 years. (1, 3, 8)

In **older adults**, regular physical activity appears to
- ▶ **REDUCE** the risk of pre-senile dementia and more serious dementia.
- ▶ **HELP** the brain be more robust, and even at lower activity levels, it may slow the risk of Alzheimer's disease. (7, 8)

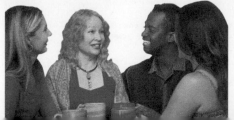

activity could lengthen it by nearly that much.[18] **Figure 1.5** illustrates health benefits of regular physical activity.

The American College of Sports Medicine recommends that all healthy adults between the ages of 18 and 65 strive for at least 150 minutes of moderate exercise per week (or 75 minutes of vigorous exercise or a combination of the two).[19]

However, in 2014, 25.4 percent of adults and 15.2 percent of youth reported no physical activity in the last month.[20] Only 20.6 percent of adults met the recommended guidelines for aerobic and muscle strengthening activity.[21] The high percentages of overweight and

See It!
Watch "New Study Shows Exercise May Build Brain Power" at MasteringHealth™.

obese adults provide more evidence that most Americans are too inactive.[22] Indeed, we are one of the most sedentary and overweight nations on earth.[23]

Good Wellness Habits Benefit Society as a Whole

If Americans could raise their levels of wellness, they would have fewer health issues, be more productive, and spend less money on health care. In fact, the country as a whole would benefit. While the focus of this text is primarily about you, it is important to remember that your actions ultimately affect others (see Q&A: How Does Improved Wellness Benefit Society? on page 11).

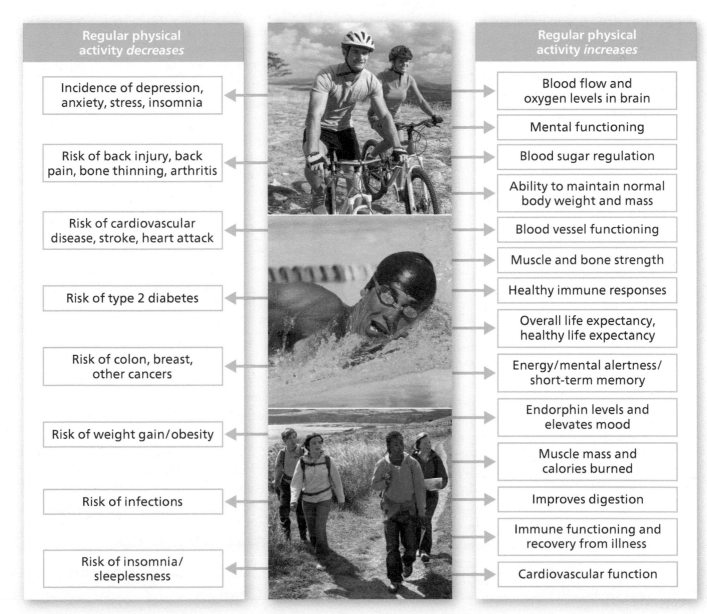

Regular physical activity *decreases*	Regular physical activity *increases*
Incidence of depression, anxiety, stress, insomnia	Blood flow and oxygen levels in brain
Risk of back injury, back pain, bone thinning, arthritis	Mental functioning
Risk of cardiovascular disease, stroke, heart attack	Blood sugar regulation
Risk of type 2 diabetes	Ability to maintain normal body weight and mass
Risk of colon, breast, other cancers	Blood vessel functioning
Risk of weight gain/obesity	Muscle and bone strength
Risk of infections	Healthy immune responses
Risk of insomnia/sleeplessness	Overall life expectancy, healthy life expectancy
	Energy/mental alertness/short-term memory
	Endorphin levels and elevates mood
	Muscle mass and calories burned
	Improves digestion
	Immune functioning and recovery from illness
	Cardiovascular function

FIGURE **1.5** Regular physical activity results in both short- and long-term health benefits.

The Surgeon General of the United States has summarized its health priorities in *Healthy People 2020*, a report that outlines four broad goals: (1) attain high-quality, longer lives free of preventable disease, disability, injury, and premature death; (2) achieve health equity, eliminate disparities, and improve the health of all groups; (3) create social and physical environments that promote good health for all; and (4) promote quality of life, healthy development, and healthy behaviors across all life stages.[24] Accordingly, the Surgeon General advises Americans to eat better diets, be more physically active, not smoke, limit alcohol, and avoid drugs—all of which are wellness behaviors. Imagine if society would make a concerted effort to embrace principles of wellness—a world where people respected others and the environment; valued diversity and cultural differences; worked toward physical health; tried to improve/maintain mental and emotional health; and prioritized the well-being of others. If each person focused on improving their wellness and we enacted policies and programs to protect the vulnerable and all living things, the net result might far surpass any goals outlined in government documents. Motivating each of you to be the change agents that will help achieve wellness goals is an important focus of this text.

Several areas need our attention. The high cost of health care and health insurance is a major concern for Americans. In 2014, Americans spent $3 trillion on health care, which averages to more than $9,523 for every man, woman, and child.[25] Further, although Americans spend more on health care than other countries of the world, their health is worse than in most other industrialized nations.[26]

In 2010, Congress passed the *Patient Protection and Affordable Care Act (PPACA)*, also known as *Obamacare*, to provide a means for all Americans to obtain affordable health care and to encourage more to seek preventive care and adopt wellness behaviors.[27] Young adults age 19 to 34 benefited most from ACA, with uninsured rates declining from 28 percent to 18 percent in this group. One of the key ACA provisions allows parents to keep young adults on their existing insurance policies through age 26. Because of this, more than 3 million additional 19- to 25-year-olds now have health insurance.[28] In addition, because one in six young adults has a chronic illness like cancer, diabetes, or asthma, these individuals can no longer be denied coverage for a pre-existing condition.[29]

Healthy People 2020 A report by the US Surgeon General that outlines four broad national goals for improving the health and well-being of Americans by the year 2020, based upon current statistics

behavior change An organized, deliberate effort to alter or replace an existing habit or pattern of activity

stages of behavior change From the transtheoretical model, a set of states most people pass through in their awareness of, determination to alter, and efforts to replace existing habits or actions

---

LO 1.4 How Can I Change My Behavior to Improve My Wellness?

If you are like most people, you made a New Year's resolution on January 1, worked hard to adopt some new behavior until about January 10, started slipping back to your old habits by the 15th, and forgot about the whole thing by the 31st! Sound familiar? You had good intentions; however, like most people, "things" got in the way. In contrast, some people seem to have "iron wills" and do exactly what they set out to do. Why? Who wins at successful behavior change and who can't seem to stay on track?

See It!
Watch "Life-Changing Resolutions" at MasteringHealth™.

In truth, there are no simple answers to this question. **Behavior change** is a complex process in which many factors converge to influence your success or failure. It isn't as simple as being weak willed and unable to follow through. The key to successful behavior change is to identify risks, anticipate potential barriers to change, and plan carefully to ensure success!

Stages of Behavior Change: It Doesn't Happen Overnight

To prepare for behavior change, we must go through a series of mental and emotional stages over a period of months. Take a careful look at your current habits, be specific about exactly what and why you want to change, and accept that you are going to have to work for what you want.

The rest of this chapter takes you through a series of practical steps designed to help you succeed at your new wellness goals. The steps are inspired by the *transtheoretical model of behavior change*, a blueprint for altering your own behavior developed by psychologists James Prochaska and Carlo DiClemente.[30]

Step One: Understand the Stages of Behavior Change

The transtheoretical model of behavior change delineates six **stages of behavior change**: precontemplation,

Q&A How Does Improved Wellness Benefit Society?

Individual health risks don't just affect us as individuals; they ultimately affect society as a whole. In addition to pain, suffering, and loss of life, soaring rates of obesity, poor dietary habits, and sedentary lifestyles result in huge increases in health care costs, insurance premiums, and losses in productivity. These are then passed on as increased costs to businesses and consumers. This jeopardizes the economic stability of our nation and puts us at a competitive disadvantage with other countries of the world, among other issues. Consider the following:

DRAIN ON SOCIETY

- Five major chronic diseases, most of which have key lifestyle contributors, add significantly to our US economic burden. Estimated costs include:

Cancer	$504 billion
Diabetes	$228 billion
Heart disease	$210.1 billion
Hypertension	$497.1 billion
Stroke	$63.1 billion

- The above five diseases contributed more than $1.5 trillion of the health care costs in 2014. Put in perspective, that amount could wipe out the US trade deficit for 2014 or pay a big chunk of our national debt.

- People who are ill or caring for ill friends and family cost businesses significantly in terms of *presenteeism* (coming to work despite feeling ill, distracted, or unable to perform). These losses are several times more than the losses from actual sick leave.

Combined costs of lower productivity, sick leave, and health care add significantly to prices for every product and service. By improving our health and reducing these costs, our economy would become healthier, too. As the health of a population improves, workers become more productive, opportunities improve, educational level rises, and crime rates and other social issues improve. As the economy grows stronger, there are more jobs available. People live more productive years.

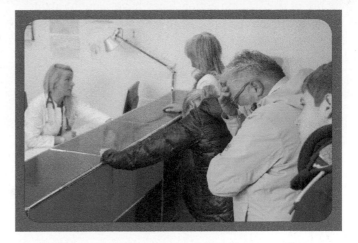

BENEFITS OF BEHAVIOR CHANGE: EXAMPLES OF ACTIONS YOU CAN TAKE

- A person with diagnosed diabetes has an average medical expenditure of nearly $14,000 per year, approximately 2.3 times higher than someone without diabetes. A person with prediabetes can reduce the risk for health problems via diet and exercise. For every one-point reduction in HbA1C (a three-month average of blood sugar levels), there are 40 percent reductions in microvascular problems (nerves in hands and feet, blindness or vision problems, kidney disease, etc.) and up to $1,400 savings per year. Lowering body mass index by 5 percent or more can have a significant impact on blood glucose levels overall, possibly preventing prediabetes and diabetes.

- The major risk factors for the above five chronic diseases are smoking, unhealthy diet, and sedentary lifestyle. If these factors were eliminated, at least 80 percent of heart disease, stroke, and type 2 diabetes and 40 percent of cancers could be prevented.

Sources: A. Chatterjee et al., "Checkup Time: Chronic Disease and Wellness in America," Milken Institute (2015); W. Yang et al., "Economic Costs of Diabetes in the US in 2012," *Diabetes Care* 36, no. 4 (2013): 1033–46; National Association of Chronic Disease Directors, "Why Public Health Is Necessary to Improve Healthcare," accessed September 2015, www.chronicdisease.org/?page-WhyWeNeedPH2impHC.

---

contemplation, preparation, action, maintenance, and termination. According to this model, behavior change usually involves a gradual process of *awareness, preparation*, and then *action*. Understanding this process can help you proceed more deliberately to identify and successfully change a problem behavior. Remember that the steps of this model are general and people often slip backwards before they get to the action, maintenance, and termination stages.

Precontemplation People in the precontemplation stage have no current intention of changing. They may have tried to change an old habit and given up, or they may be in denial and unaware of the problem.

Contemplation In this stage, people recognize that they have a problem and begin to contemplate the need to change within six months or so. People can languish in this stage for months or years, however, realizing that they have a negative wellness pattern, yet lacking the time, energy, or commitment to make the change.

Preparation Most people at this stage are within a month or so of taking action. They have thought about what they might do and may even have come up with a plan. Rather than thinking about why they can't begin, they have started to focus on what they can do.

Action In this stage, people begin to execute their action plans. Unfortunately, many people try to take shortcuts; they start behavior change here rather than going through the earlier stages. However, without making a plan, publicly stating the desire to change, enlisting other people's help, and setting specific, realistic goals, they are likely to fail.

Maintenance In the maintenance stage, people work to prevent a relapse into old habits through a conscious application of wellness tools and techniques. Maintenance requires vigilance, attention to detail, and long-term commitment. You are in the maintenance stage after you have incorporated the new action and have continued it for six months or longer without relapse into old habits.

Relapse While not an original stage of behavior change, relapse is something that happens periodically for most people trying to change behaviors. Common causes of relapse include overconfidence, daily temptations, stress or emotional distractions, and putting yourself down.

Termination At the termination stage, the new behavior is ingrained; you are maintaining it and are no longer at risk for relapse. The new behavior has become a part of the way you live and thus the temptation to return to former behaviors is greatly reduced.

Step Two: Increase Your Awareness

Become aware of what is required to achieve wellness. Before getting started, it's important to think about how well Americans are in general and how you compare.

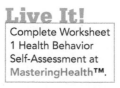
Live It!
Complete Worksheet 1 Health Behavior Self-Assessment at MasteringHealth™.

Staying Physically Fit Nowhere does the phrase "use it or lose it" apply more fully than to your physical fitness. Only 49.2 percent of adults 18 and over met the 2008 Physical Activity Guidelines for Americans and a mere 20.8 percent met the 2008 guidelines for both aerobic and strength training last year even as we face an epidemic of overweight and obesity.[31]

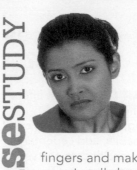

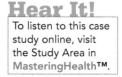
Eating Healthy Foods In spite of massive efforts toward change, the American diet continues to be suboptimal. Our diet is high in excess calories, many of which are nutrient poor.[32] Important factors are the availability of unhealthy foods (including on college campuses); aggressive marketing campaigns that promote unhealthy foods; and the short-term pleasure we get from eating rich, salty, soft, and sweet foods.[33] However, good nutrition habits have many wellness benefits, including increased energy, greater stamina, better weight management, stronger disease resistance, and reduced risk of chronic illness.

Managing Your Weight Sixty-nine percent of American adults have a body weight and mass (fat-to-lean

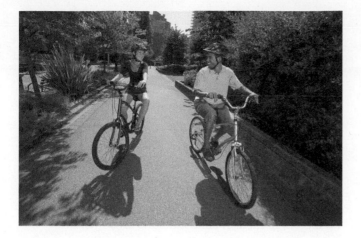

ratio) above recommended ranges. Although college students are less likely to be overweight or obese than all adults nationally, more than 52 percent of undergraduates are trying to lose weight at any given time and many are not meeting national recommendations for exercise.[34] Since excess weight can contribute to numerous physical, emotional, and social wellness issues, modifying your activity levels and improving diet can significantly improve overall wellness.

Managing Your Stress Most students find college stressful. The lifestyle changes and competing demands of academics, work, and social commitments can take an emotional and physical toll. Chronic, unresolved stress has been linked to a wide range of negative outcomes, including disruptions in thinking and memory, disturbed sleep, depression, impaired immunity to infections, weight gain, emotional volatility, poor coping skills, and academic and social problems. (See Chapter 9 on stress and wellness.)

Building Social Capital and Social Support for Life's Challenges Taking time for others and working to build social support and social capital are important to overall wellness. **Social support** includes four major support areas: *emotional* (close friends/family/loved ones who demonstrate caring, trust, security, support), *instrumental* (tangible aid/service, e.g., someone who will help you study for a test; babysit or pet sit for you while you go to the gym; loan you money to help pay for books), *informational* (advice, suggestions, perspective on a situation, services), and *appraisal* (provides feedback, reality check/honesty).

    Social capital is a broader term that includes elements of society/community such as support networks, social trust, and feeling of belonging in a group where there is a history or common bond you can rely on.

Knowing which individual and community/campus resources and supportive systems you can access is a key to planning for challenges.

Avoiding Drugs, Smoking, and Alcohol Abuse

Using drugs, smoking, and abusing alcohol are all ways of manipulating the brain chemically. Unfortunately, the use and abuse of these substances carries high risks for illness and injury, suicide, and mental health problems, and can undermine multiple dimensions of wellness.

Practicing Accident, Injury, and Disease Prevention

Prevention has several practical meanings for wellness behavior. It can mean preventing injuries and the accidents that account for most deaths among young adults. It can mean self-care such as daily dental hygiene and regular body checks for skin and tissue changes (i.e., tracking moles and performing breast self-exams). And it can mean preventing disease through medical checkups and vaccinations and key lifestyle changes.

    How do you compare to others when it comes to the above wellness indicators?

Step Three: Contemplate Change

As we have discussed, research has confirmed that people are more successful when they prepare for change emotionally and mentally rather than starting right in on the change itself. For example, people who believe they can change their physical activity levels and make specific plans to do so are significantly more successful at launching new exercise patterns.[35]

Examine Your Habits and Patterns What current behavior would you like to change? **Lab 1.1** will help you identify habits that lower your wellness. When considering a habit, ask yourself the following:

- How long has it been going on?
- How often does it happen?
- How serious are the consequences of the habit or problem?
- What are some of my reasons for continuing this problematic behavior?
- What kinds of situations trigger the behavior?
- Are other people involved in this habit? If so, in what way?

Do It!
Access these labs at the end of the chapter or online at MasteringHealth™.

social support Includes emotional, instrumental, informational, and appraisal forms of support from others

social capital Support systems and networks, trust, and sense of belonging/fitting in

Habits involve deliberate choice but are also influenced by automatic, subconscious processes as well as many other factors. Age, sex, race, income, family background, education, personal beliefs, and access to health care all increase or decrease the likelihood of developing certain health habits. For example, people are more likely to eat snacks after being exposed to numerous junk food advertisements in the media. While smokers are addicted to the tobacco and nicotine in cigarettes, they may also become hooked by the smoking ritual such as holding the cigarette or playing with their lighter.[36]

Identify factors that encourage negative behaviors or block positive ones. Analyzing the factors that reinforce your current habit patterns can also help you understand why you developed and maintained unwanted habits and where you need to make changes in order to succeed.

Assess Your Beliefs and Attitudes
Your attitudes about health and wellness affect your daily choices. When reaching for another cigarette, smokers, for example, sometimes tell themselves, "I'll stop tomorrow" or "only old people die from smoking." These beliefs allow them to continue smoking. One well-known model explaining why some people act to change behavior and others do not is explained by the original **Health Belief Model** and its newer, expanded version. According to this model:[37]

- You must *believe* that your current behavior makes you *susceptible* to a health threat. The more you think the threat could harm you (*perceived severity*) and the more you think your changed behavior can *benefit you*, the more likely you will be to act to change behaviors. However, if you perceive that there are too many *barriers* keeping you from action and certain *modifying factors* in your environment (culture, education, history, access) make change seem difficult, and you don't have the appropriate *cues to action* (from media, events, illness, friends), you might be less likely to take action.

- You must believe that you are susceptible to developing the health problem. For example, losing a parent to lung cancer could make a person work harder to stop smoking. However, thinking that only "old people" die of cancer could make young smokers think they are not susceptible and they don't need to act now. Being addicted to tobacco can make change more difficult, especially if your friends all smoke.

Reading the evidence that points to increased risks for increased rates of cancer among those who've smoked since youth, and lower rates among quitters may lead you to seek help on campus. If smoking cessation counseling is available and friends are supportive, you may be more likely to quit. What beliefs underlie your current pattern of wellness habits, both positive and negative?

Assess Your Motivation
What is your **motivation**, or inducement, to change a wellness behavior? For some, a rewarding result, such as looking better, can motivate change. For others, a sense of accomplishment or just feeling better every day may do it. (See Tools for Change: What Influences Your Behaviors?)

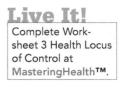

Live It!
Complete Worksheet 3 Health Locus of Control at MasteringHealth™.

Motivations can be external (come from someone or something outside yourself) or internal (come from inside yourself), but in either case they are part of your sense of self. The degree to which you are confident in your own abilities is your **self-efficacy**.

Your conviction that you can control events and factors in your life is your **locus of control**. An *internal* locus of control gives you a strong belief in your ability to effect change. An *external* locus of control leads you to see other people and things as controlling what you do.

A person with a strong sense of self-efficacy and internal locus of control has a better chance of following through with a decision to change wellness behavior. For example, suppose you wish to bring your weight down to a healthy range. If your parents are both overweight, you may think "my weight is controlled by my genes" and be resigned to being overweight. However, by gathering information about weight management, by identifying behaviors that are within your power to change (such as food choices, eating habits, and exercise), by acknowledging their importance, and seeing others be successful at a given weight loss strategy, you may be able to identify with their successes and feel that you can do it too. You can boost your own

---

Health Belief Model Focuses on motivation to change behavior based on perceived susceptibility and severity of risk, and perceived benefits of making a change as key components

motivation One's inducement to do something, such as change a current behavior

self-efficacy The degree to which one believes in his or her ability to achieve something

locus of control Belief that control over life events and changes come primarily from outside of oneself (external locus of control) or from within (internal locus of control)

CHANGE

What Influences Your Behaviors?

While behaviors are influenced by a complex web of interactive variables, some of the most important factors are listed below. As you look at each one of these, try to think about what positive and potentially negative elements might serve to influence your ability to be successful. For example, if you live in an unsafe neighborhood and can't walk outside by yourself, that might be a negative environmental factor; however, if your campus has a great fitness facility that is free to students, that might be a positive asset in helping you make changes.

Your Environment: Parental/family values, culture, socioeconomic status, neighborhood, schools, access to health care, learned behaviors/habits, and finances can all influence your success. Think about your assets: those positive skills, talents, and behaviors that you already have and the people and organizations you can tap into for help along the way.

Social Support: Think about those friends/family/loved ones who demonstrate caring through each of the various forms of social support. If you were stranded on a dark road at 1 AM, who could you call to help you? Who would help you if you couldn't afford a safe place to live? Cultivating social support, nurturing friendships and being there for others makes it more likely others will be there for you. Also, when others aren't there, knowing how to access community supports in times of crisis is a key to wellness.

Social Capital: Are you currently part of a campus group, social group, church or community group? How can you start to build social capital? Is there a group you identify with and feel a part of?

Habits: Been a couch potato for many years with a full DVR and a family of TV characters you identify with? Those habits are going to be harder to break. Recognizing both your good and bad habits when it comes to your health is a good place to start thinking about a planned change. Make a list of areas you think may be difficult for you and which things you are already doing right.

Prioritize key ones for change and key ones that you want to build upon.

Health Status: Overweight? Obese? Already have problems with your knees and/or back? Experiencing symptoms of a chronic disease? All of these factors can influence your behavior change plan. Thinking about how to maximize your physical health resources to start slow and at a pace that is realistic for you is going to be key.

Self-Efficacy: What is your track record in terms of commitment to change? Have you been successful at things you've set out to do differently? What factors helped you be successful? How confident are you that you will be successful in meeting your own goals?

Knowledge: How much do you know about changing this behavior? Have you done your homework? If you don't have the information, talk to those who have been successful and seem to be on the right track. Ask others for help and seek out your best resources.

Genetics: Do you know your own family background and risks when it comes to health? Diabetes, CVD, cancer in the grandparents, parents, or siblings? When did they develop their health problems? Any thoughts on risks that you might have that are similar to their risks?

Beliefs: How worried are you that if you don't take action to change this behavior, you will end up with a significant health threat? How sure are you that if you DO change your behavior, that the behavior will result in a positive outcome?

Motivation: How motivated are you right now to really do this? Are you motivated *intrinsically*, meaning that you are doing it because it matters to you, that you really enjoy something and think it's important; or *extrinsically*, because you are doing what someone else wants you to do or to impress others? A bit of self-reflection may help you figure out why you really want to change and what unique things would help you stay motivated. Keep the enjoyment in the action. Have you built motivational factors into your plan for change?

self-efficacy by experiencing small initial successes that increase your confidence and your feelings of internalized control.

Choose a Target Behavior Select one habit, or **target behavior**, as your initial focus for change. It is a much better strategy to start small and build on success than to try for too much and end up failing. To choose potential target behaviors, ask yourself these questions:

- *What do I want?* What is your ultimate goal? To lose weight? Exercise more? Reduce stress? Sleep better? Have a lasting relationship? Whatever it is, you need a clear picture of your target outcome and how you will measure success!

- *Which change is my greatest priority at this time?* People often decide to change several things at once. Suppose you are gaining unwanted weight. Rather than saying, "I need to eat less and start exercising," identify one specific behavior that contributes significantly to this problem and tackle that first. "I will only eat healthy, low-calorie snacks this week." Or, "I will walk for 15 minutes" every day this week."

- *Why is this important to me?* Think through why you want to change. Are you doing it because of your health? To improve your academic performance? To look better? To win someone else's approval? It's best to target a behavior because it's right for you rather than because you think it will help you win others' approval.

- *Fill in the details.* Rather than using a generality ("I need to eat better"), consider specific behaviors that relate to the general problem. What are your unhealthy eating habits? Do you eat too few fruits and vegetables? Do you have fast food for lunch every day? Is a high-calorie coffee drink part of your daily regimen? Identify a specific behavior you would like to change.

Step Four: Prepare for Change

Once you have assessed your current status and chosen a target behavior, you are ready to make specific preparations. For instance, watching others successfully change their behavior can give you ideas and encouragement for your own changes. This process of modeling, or learning from role models, can be very helpful. Suppose you have trouble talking to strangers or new acquaintances and want to improve your communication skills. Try observing friends whose social skills you admire and note how they make conversation. What techniques help make them successful communicators?

target behavior One well-defined habit chosen as a primary focus for change

barriers to change Stumbling blocks faced in the efforts to alter a current behavior

LO 1.5 Set "SMART" Goals

Your wellness goals should be both achievable and in line with what you truly want. Achievable, truly desired goals increase motivation, and this, in turn, promotes success.

To set successful goals, try using the SMART system. SMART goals are *specific*, *measurable*, *action-oriented*, realistic, and *time-oriented*.[38] A vague goal is "Get into better shape by exercising more." A SMART goal is:

- *Specific*—"Increase my overall strength level by purchasing a gym membership or hiring a personal trainer"

- *Measurable*—"Increase the amount of weight I can safely lift by a specified amount each week, starting with a weight I can lift at least 10 times without fatigue"

- *Action-oriented*—"Go to the gym three times per week for at least 30 minutes each time over the next month"

- *Realistic*—"Increase the weight I can lift and number of reps I can lift by 10 percent in 6 months (not 100 percent)"

- *Time-oriented*—"Try my new weight program for one month, then reassess; do the same after two months"

Anticipate and Overcome Barriers to Change Anticipate **barriers to change**, or possible stumbling blocks, to help you prepare for behavior change. Like other groups, college students struggle with weight. Diet-control failure is based on several barriers to change, including ready availability of high-calorie fast foods. Anticipating these temptations and packing nutritious snacks for hunger pangs can help you stay on track with your dietary goals. Barriers to behavior change include:

- *Overambitious goals.* Most people cannot lose weight, stop smoking, and begin running three miles a day all at the same time. Don't try for dramatic change within an unrealistically short time frame—such as losing 20 pounds in one month. Habits are best changed one at a time, taking small, progressive steps; rewarding successes; and being patient with yourself.

- *Self-defeating beliefs and attitudes.* Believing that you are too young to worry about fitness and wellness can bar you from making a solid commitment to change. Likewise, thinking you are helpless to change your

Q&A How Can I Find Reliable Wellness Information?

Fitness and wellness are important American preoccupations—and major industries as well. It can be hard to distinguish legitimate information from thinly disguised advertising. Here are some tips.

Look for unbiased, legitimate reviews.

Don't be duped by phony reviews provided by companies hired by e-tech companies to make their products look good. Stick with reviews by reputable sources such as Consumers Union/Consumer Reports or research groups reporting results of rigorous trials and published in reputable journals.

Look for organizations without a direct interest in your wallet.

Examples are health-related agencies of the state and federal governments (e.g., Centers for Disease Control and Prevention or Food and Drug Administration); major colleges and universities; big-name hospitals and medical centers (e.g., Mayo Clinic or Cooper Institute); and well-known non-profit organizations (e.g., American College of Sports Medicine or American Medical Association). Cross-check any information you gather from other sources against these known and reliable sources to see whether facts and figures are consistent.

If the media quote a research report, look up the research itself.

Consider details of the study, noting whether the researcher works for a large, recognizable university, government agency, or research institute; whether the study had human subjects or inferred conclusions from lab animals; and whether the conclusions were based on hundreds of research subjects or just a few.

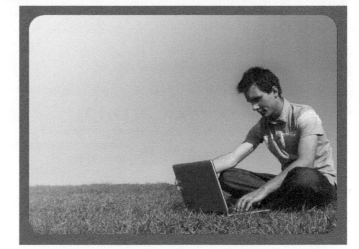

Take fitness advice only from experts who represent reliable sources.

Well-meaning friends often have misinformation, and promoters of products and services are usually biased.

Read consumer health newsletters published by distinguished universities, research institutes, and non-profit organizations.

Examples include the *Harvard Health Letter*, *Mayo Clinic Health Letter*, and *Nutrition Action Health Letter*.

Finally, use established, widely respected websites to learn more about fitness and wellness topics. See the eResources section on page 20 for examples of reliable websites.

Note: *Web links are always subject to change. Visit the Study Area in* MasteringHealth *to view updated Web links for each chapter.*

---

weight, smoking, or fitness habits could undermine your efforts. Greater self-efficacy and more positive expectations may help.

- *Failing to accurately assess your current state of wellness.* You might assume that you are strong and flexible, for example, when you are actually below average for your age. Failing to gather enough data on wellness risks and benefits can also be a barrier that weakens your commitment.

- *Lack of support and guidance.* Supportive friends are a good start. You should also seek guidance from your fitness and wellness instructor; from counselors and other campus resources; from up-to-date, trusted health sources on the Internet; and from health

professionals. (See Q&A How Can I Find Reliable Wellness Information?)

LO 1.6 Make the Commitment and Be Accountable

The final stage in behavior change is to make a commitment and take action and keep it up! A formal written document called the **behavior change contract** functions as:

- a promise to yourself

> **behavior change contract** A formal document that clarifies the goals and steps needed to change a current habit or habit pattern

- a public declaration of intent
- an organized plan that lays out start and end dates and daily actions
- a list of barriers or obstacles you may encounter
- a place to brainstorm strategies for overcoming those impediments
- a collected set of sources of support
- a reminder of the rewards you plan to give yourself for sticking with the program

In **Lab 1.3** you will create a behavior change contract as part of your fitness and wellness plan.

Do It!
Access these labs at the end of the chapter or online at MasteringHealth™.

Visualize New Behavior Athletes often use a mental practice called *imagined rehearsal* or *visualization* to reach their performance goals. Picturing themselves accomplishing an action in their minds ahead of time helps prepare them for real competition. Visualization can help you imagine the way a current negative behavior unfolds, and then allows you to practice in advance what you will say and do to counter it.

Control Your Environment If you are trying to quit drinking, going to a bar could lead you to resume an undesired behavior. Going to dinner and a movie with a sympathetic friend, on the other hand, could help reinforce your abstinence. If you are trying to lose weight but need to eat out, choose a restaurant that has healthy options you enjoy. Think about which people and settings tend to trigger your unwanted behavior, and then stay away from them as much as possible and set up supportive situations instead.

Change Your Self-Talk Your *self-talk*—that is, the way you think and talk to yourself—matters. Think about what you say to yourself when something goes badly or when something succeeds. Stay positive. Be firm, but remember to cut yourself some slack. Be as nice to yourself in your self-talk as you would be to a good friend who was having similar difficulties.

countering Substituting a desired behavior for an undesirable one

journaling Keeping a written record of personal experiences, interpretations, and results

electronic activity monitoring systems (EAMS) Wearable devices or trackers that measure activity, sleep, and other diet and exercise details

Learn to "Counter" **Countering** is another term for substituting a desired behavior for an undesirable one. You may want to stop eating junk food, for example, but quitting "cold turkey" just isn't realistic. Instead, compile a list of substitute foods and places to get them. Then, have your healthy options ready before your mouth starts watering at the smell of pizza.

Practice "Shaping" *Shaping* is a stepwise process of making a series of small changes, starting slowly and mastering one step before moving on to the next. Suppose you want to start jogging three miles every other day, but right now you get tired and winded after a trip around the block! Shaping would dictate a process of slow, progressive steps such as walking 30 minutes at a comfortable pace every day for a week; then gradually increasing your time and speed on a progressive schedule until you eventually are able to reach your goal in the third week.

Reward Yourself Set up a system of rewards to help you stay on track. A reward can be consumable (a cookie or gourmet meal), active (going to a concert or playing Frisbee), a new possession (new clothes or downloading a movie), an incentive (a friend treats you to a special event), or social (receiving praise or a hug). It can also be intrinsic, meaning the new behavior feels so enjoyable it becomes its own reward. Whatever your motivational rewards may be, build a few into your plan.

Use Journaling and EAMS Tracking as Wellness Tools Throughout the labs in this textbook, you will examine your current wellness habits and analyze them through writing. **Journaling**, or writing personal experiences, interpretations, and results in a journal or notebook, is an important skill for behavior change. Journaling can help you monitor your daily efforts, measure how much you have learned, record how you feel about your progress, and note ideas for improving your program.

Live It!
Complete Worksheet 2 Weekly Behavior Change Evaluation at MasteringHealth™.

Interactive computerized tracking and mobile journaling programs are increasingly popular. **Electronic activity monitoring systems (EAMS)**—wearable devices or trackers that measure activity, sleep, and other diet and exercise details—are part of a new generation of monitoring and motivational strategies that can be very helpful. (See the eResources feature at the end of each chapter in this book).

Study Plan

chapter summary

LO 1.1 What Is Wellness and How Well Am I?

- Wellness means people actively engage in efforts to be the best that they can be, contribute to society, and work to live up to their potential.

LO 1.2 What Are the Dimensions of Wellness?

- Wellness includes six major interconnected dimensions: *physical*, *social*, *intellectual*, *emotional*, *spiritual*, and *environmental health*.

- Balance among and between wellness dimensions is a lifelong process and should also be a lifelong goal.

LO 1.3 Why Does Wellness Matter?

- Positive wellness habits, particularly during youth and early adulthood, can help increase your *life expectancy*, determine your *healthy life expectancy*, and reduce risks for chronic diseases.

LO 1.4 How Can I Change My Behavior to Improve My Wellness?

- Influences such as *environment, social support, social capital, habits, health status, self-efficacy, knowledge,* *genetics, beliefs,* and *motivations* can help you come up with a plan.

- The stages of change/transtheoretical model includes the *pre-contemplation, contemplation, preparation, action, maintenance, relapse,* and *termination* stages. The Health Belief Model includes perceived susceptibility and severity of risk as well as your belief in benefits of possible action, and other variables.

LO 1.5 "SMART" Goals

- Use strategies such as *visualizing the new behavior, controlling your environment, changing your self-talk, practicing shaping, rewarding yourself,* and *journaling or using EAMS tracking* and other actions to help you achieve your goal.

- Make sure your SMART goals are *specific, measureable, action-oriented, realistic,* and *time-oriented.*

LO 1.6 Making the Commitment and Being Accountable

- Develop a behavior change contract with your goal and specific strategies.

review questions

LO 1.1 1. How does *wellness* differ from *health*?
   a. Wellness is the absence of disease.
   b. Wellness is the achievement of the highest level of health possible in physical, social, intellectual, emotional, environmental, and spiritual dimensions.
   c. Wellness and health are equivalent.
   d. Health is a more individualized, dynamic concept than wellness.

LO 1.1 2. Which of the following is the leading cause of death among Americans aged 20 to 24?
   a. Accidents
   b. Heart disease
   c. Stroke
   d. Cancer

LO 1.1 3. What is meant by the term *healthy life expectancy*?
   a. How many years a person can expect to live at birth
   b. How many years a person can expect to live without disability or major illness
   c. A realistic attitude toward how long a person can expect to live
   d. A positive attitude about how many years a person believes he or she has to live

LO 1.2 4. Which of the following statements is CORRECT?
   a. *Instrumental support* refers to the advice, suggestions, and perspective on situations type of social support.
   b. *Social capital* refers to the social networks, trust and feelings of belonging, and security/bonds that you can rely on.
   c. *Extrinsic motivation* refers to being motivated by your own thoughts, beliefs, and because something matters to you personally.
   d. *Self-efficacy* is a rigid behavioral construct and it cannot be changed by history or experience.

LO 1.3 **5.** Which of the following are potential benefits of wellness?

a. Young adults should be in their prime health years and may benefit now from positive changes in lifestyle.

b. Health care costs are soaring and individual efforts to reduce health risks can have positive impacts on costs and reduce the economic burden of disease.

c. Dimensions of wellness are interconnected and when one area is a problem, such as the environment, everyone is affected either directly or indirectly.

d. All of the above are potential benefits.

LO 1.3 **6.** Which of the following is CORRECT about the Patient Protection and Affordable Care Act?

a. Uninsured rates among older adults have improved the most out of any age group.

b. The 19- to 26-year-old group has seen the greatest improvements in number of uninsured of any group.

c. Under this act fewer people are able to access key preventive care services and increased numbers are being denied coverage for pre-existing conditions.

d. Young adults are cut off from family insurance plans by age 18 and must find insurance on their own or face fines.

LO 1.4 **7.** Which of the following is a stage of the transtheoretical model of behavior change?

a. Increased wellness

b. Preparation

c. Emotional intelligence

d. Motivation

LO 1.5 **8.** Which of the following is NOT part of developing SMART goals for planned behavior change?

a. Staged

b. Measureable

c. Action-Oriented

d. Realistic

e. Time-Oriented

LO 1.6 **9.** What is "shaping"?

a. A stepwise process of change, designed to change one small piece of a target behavior at a time

b. A model of behavior change that uses mental imaging to reshape the brain's signals

c. A journaling strategy

d. A way of learning behaviors by watching others perform them

critical thinking questions

LO 1.1 **1.** What does it mean to be well? What are the benefits of wellness?

LO 1.3 **2.** What are the benefits of wellness for you at this stage of your life and for society as a whole? Why should wellness matter?

LO 1.3 **3.** Which habits (wellness-related or not) have you tried to change in the past? Why do you think your efforts succeeded or failed? Using the skills for behavior change described in this chapter, outline your plan for successful change.

LO 1.4 **4.** Using the stages of change (transtheoretical) model, discuss what you might do (in stages) to help a friend stop smoking. Why is it important that a person be ready to change before trying to change?

LO 1.5 **5.** Describe the SMART goal-setting guidelines and how you would use them to set goals for one behavior that you would like to change.

LO 1.6 **6.** Which risk-lowering choices do you incorporate into your lifestyle? Choose two or three of them and discuss the factors that are currently influencing you to have issues with that behavior. How can you reduce effects of influences as you make changes?

check out these eResources

- **Centers for Disease Control and Prevention** Federal government agency that publishes a wide range of information on health conditions and prevention. **www.cdc.gov**
- **Consumer Reports** Subscription website (and print magazine) that reports on impartial tests of products and services. **www.consumerreports.org**
- **Food and Drug Administration** Federal agency that monitors the safety of foods, medicines, and other products. **www.fda.gov**

- **National Center for Health Statistics** Division of the Centers for Disease Control and Prevention that maintains statistics on health issues. **www.cdc.gov/nchs**
- **World Health Organization** International organization devoted to studying and reporting health issues around the globe. **www.who.int**

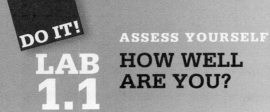

DO IT!
LAB 1.1

ASSESS YOURSELF
HOW WELL
ARE YOU?

MasteringHealth™

Name: _____   **Date:** _____

Instructor: _____   **Section:** _____

Purpose: This lab will help you assess your current level of wellness in each of the six dimensions and identify which wellness areas to target for behavior change.

Directions: Complete sections I–VI. For each item, indicate how often you think the statements describe you by checking the box under the relevant score. After each section, total your scores for that section and write your score in the space provided. After completing all sections, you will summarize, analyze, and reflect on your results in section VII.

Section I: Physical Wellness

	Never 1	Rarely 2	Sometimes 3	Often 4	Always 5
1. I listen to my body and make adjustments or seek professional help when something is wrong.					✓
2. I keep my weight within the normal BMI range and make adjustments to not let my weight get out of control.					✓
3. I engage in moderate physical activity for at least 30 minutes, five times or more per week.					
4. I do exercises for muscular strength and endurance at least two to three times per week.				✓	
5. I do stretching and limbering exercises at least five times per week.				✓	
6. I do yoga, Pilates, tai chi, or other exercises for balance and core strength two or three times per week.				✓	
7. I feel good about the condition of my body. I have lots of energy and can get through the day without being overly tired.			✓		
8. I get adequate rest at night and wake on most mornings feeling ready for the day ahead.		✓			
9. My immune system is strong, and my body heals quickly when I get sick or injured.				✓	
10. I eat nutritious foods daily and avoid junk food.				✓	
Total for Section I: Physical Wellness = _____44_____					

Section II: Social Wellness

	Never 1	Rarely 2	Sometimes 3	Often 4	Always 5
1. I am open, honest, and get along well with others.		✓			
2. I participate in a variety of social activities and enjoy all kinds of people.			✓		
3. I try to be a better person and work on behaviors that have caused friction in the past.			✓		
4. I am open and accessible to a loving and responsible relationship.					✓
5. I have someone I can talk to about private feelings.					✓
6. When I meet people, I feel good about the impression they have of me.				✓	
7. I get along well with members of my family.		'	✓	✓	
8. I consider the feelings of others and do not act in hurtful or selfish ways.			✓		
9. I try to see the good in my friends and help them feel good about themselves.				✓	
10. I am good at listening to friends and family who need to talk.				✓	
Total for Section II: Social Wellness = _____					

Section III: Intellectual Wellness

	Never 1	Rarely 2	Sometimes 3	Often 4	Always 5
1. I carefully consider options and possible consequences as I make choices.			✓		
2. I am alert and ready to respond to life's challenges in ways that reflect thought and sound judgment.				✓	
3. I learn from my mistakes and try to act differently the next time.					
4. I am open minded, try to listen to others' opinions, and try to be non-judgmental.			✓		
5. I manage my time well rather than letting time manage me.				✓	
6. I follow directions or recommended guidelines and act in ways likely to keep myself and others safe.					✓
7. I consider myself to be a wise health consumer and check for reliable sources of information before making decisions.				✓	
8. I have at least one personal-growth hobby that I make time for every week.					
9. My credit card balances are low, and my finances are in good order.					
10. I examine my own perceptions and then check evidence to see whether I was correct or acted in a biased, irrational manner.					
Total for Section III: Intellectual Wellness = _____					

Section IV: Emotional Wellness

	Never 1	Rarely 2	Sometimes 3	Often 4	Always 5
1. I find it easy to laugh, cry, and show emotions such as love, fear, and anger, and I try to express them in positive ways.					
2. I avoid using alcohol or drugs as a means to forget my problems or relieve stress.					
3. My friends regard me as a stable, well-adjusted person whom they trust and rely on for support.					
4. When I am angry, I try to resolve issues in non-hurtful ways rather than stewing about them.					
5. I try not to worry unnecessarily, and I try to talk about my feelings, fears, and concerns rather than letting them build up.					
6. I recognize when I'm stressed and take steps to relax through exercise, quiet time, or calming activities.					
7. I view challenging situations and problems as opportunities for growth.					
8. I feel good about myself and believe others like me for who I am.					
9. I try not to be too critical or judgmental of others.					
10. I am flexible and adapt to change in a positive way.					
Total for Section IV: Emotional Wellness = _____					

Section V: Spiritual Wellness

	Never 1	Rarely 2	Sometimes 3	Often 4	Always 5
1. I take time alone to think about life's meaning and where I fit in to the greater whole.					
2. I believe life is a gift we should cherish.					
3. I look forward to each day as an opportunity for further growth.					
4. I experience life to the fullest.					
5. I take time to enjoy nature and the beauty around me.					
6. I have faith in a greater power, nature, or the connectedness of all living things.					
7. I engage in acts of care and goodwill without expecting something in return.					
8. I look forward to each day as an opportunity to grow and be challenged in life.					
9. I work for peace in my interpersonal relationships, my community, and the world at large.					
10. I have a great love and respect for all living things and regard animals as important links in a vital living chain.					
Total for Section V: Spiritual Wellness = _____					

Section VI: Environmental Wellness

	Never 1	Rarely 2	Sometimes 3	Often 4	Always 5
1. I am concerned about environmental pollution and actively try to preserve and protect natural resources.					
2. I buy recycled paper and purchase biodegradable products whenever possible.					
3. I recycle my garbage, reuse containers, and try to minimize the amount of paper and plastics that I use.					
4. I consider whether my clothes are truly dirty before washing them to save on water and reduce detergent in our water sources.					
5. I try to reduce my use of gasoline and oil by limiting my driving.					
6. I write my elected leaders about environmental concerns.					
7. I turn down the heat and wear warmer clothes at home in cold weather and use air conditioning sparingly in heat.					
8. I use green products for cleaning house and washing clothes whenever possible.					
9. I go paperless and use a laptop/notebook and/or use both sides of the paper when taking notes and doing assignments.					
10. I consciously try to reduce my water usage for showers, shaving, or brushing my teeth.					
Total for Section VI: Environmental Wellness = _____					

Section VII: Reflection—Your Personal Wellness Continuum

1. Enter your totals for sections I–VI below:

Physical Wellness _____   Emotional Wellness _____

Social Wellness _____   Spiritual Wellness _____

Intellectual Wellness _____   Environmental Wellness _____

2. **Understanding your scores:**

Scores of 35–50: Outstanding! Your answers show that you are aware of the importance of these behaviors in your overall wellness, and that you are putting your knowledge to work by practicing good habits that should reduce your overall risks.

Scores of 30–34: Your wellness practices in these areas are very good, but there is room for improvement. What changes could you make to improve your score?

Scores of 20–29: Your wellness risks are showing. Find information about the risks you face and why it is important to change these behaviors.

Scores below 20: You may be taking unnecessary risks to your wellness. Identify each dimension and, whenever possible, seek additional resources for changing your behavior, either on your campus or through your local community health resources.

3. Which dimension did you score highest on? Which dimension did you score lowest on? Were you surprised by these results?

_____

_____

4. Discuss the potential health implications of your scores on the individual dimensions and your overall score.

_____

_____

LAB 1.2 CHART YOUR PERSONAL WELLNESS BALANCE

MasteringHealth™

Name: _____ Date: _____

Instructor: _____ Section: _____

Purpose: To learn how to chart your current personal wellness balance and identify the wellness areas in which you would like to improve.

Materials: Results from Lab 1.1

Directions: Follow the instructions below.

Section I: Your Personal Wellness Balance

1. Create a personal wellness balance chart with your scores from sections I–VI of Lab 1.1. Allocate a larger "piece of the pie" for dimensions of wellness where your scores are higher and a smaller slice for dimensions with lower scores. Another option—allocate a larger slice for areas where you spend most of your time during a week.

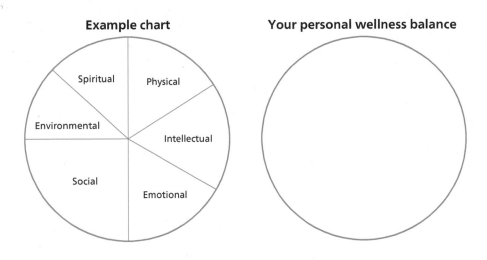

Example chart

Your personal wellness balance

2. Now create your goal wellness balance chart. Change your current balance chart to reflect your desired scores in each wellness dimension, or to reflect the optimal percentage of time you would like to allocate to each dimension.

Goal wellness balance chart

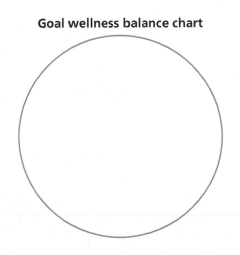

Section II: Reflection

Reflect on your wellness balance charts, your answers, and your wellness continuum (from the Try It! on page 5). What are your major areas of concern regarding your wellness? What two or three behaviors could you change easily to improve your wellness? Which one needs attention first?

_____

_____

_____

_____

_____

_____

_____

_____

_____

_____

_____

_____

_____

_____

_____

_____

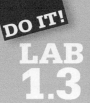
CREATE A BEHAVIOR CHANGE CONTRACT

MasteringHealth™

Name: _____ **Date:** _____

Instructor: _____ **Section:** _____

Purpose: To introduce students to the process of writing a behavior change contract and planning for new lifestyle behaviors. This introduction will serve as a model for other behavior change plans in subsequent chapters.

Directions: Complete the following sections.

Section I: Personal Wellness Review

1. Review your answers from Lab 1.1 and Lab 1.2.

2. Consider the stages of change (precontemplation, contemplation, preparation, action, maintenance) and evaluate your readiness to make a behavior change.

3. Choose a target behavior to change. For this behavior, you should be in the contemplation or preparation stages. Write the behavior below.

My behavior to change is _____

Section II: Short- and Long-Term Goals

1. **Long-Term Goal:** Long-term goals are those set for six months to a year or more. These goals should be achievable and may take many steps and an extended time to accomplish. Use SMART (specific, measurable, action-oriented, realistic, time-oriented) goal-setting guidelines. After writing out your long-term goal, choose an appropriate target date and a reward for completing your goal.

    a.   Long-Term Goal: _____

    b.   Target Date: _____

    c.   Reward: _____

2. **Short-Term Goals:** Short-term goals are those you want to achieve in fewer than six months. These goals will often help you reach your long-term goal. They may also be part of your long-term goal. Again, use SMART goal-setting guidelines. After writing your short-term goals, choose appropriate target dates and rewards.

    a.   Short-Term Goal #1: _____

    b.   Target Date: _____

    c.   Reward: _____

    a.   Short-Term Goal #2: _____

    b.   Target Date: _____

    c.   Reward: _____

Section III: Behavior Change Obstacles and Strategies

1. Below are three obstacles to changing this behavior (things I am currently doing or situations that contribute to this behavior or make it harder to change):

   a. _____

   b. _____

   c. _____

2. Here are three strategies I will use to overcome the three obstacles:

   a. _____

   b. _____

   c. _____

Section IV: Getting Support

1. Resources I will use to help me change this behavior:

   a. A friend/partner/relative: _____

   b. A school-based resource: _____

   c. A community-based resource: _____

   d. A book or reputable website: _____

2. How will you use these supportive resources to help you with your goals?

   _____

   _____

Section V: Contract, Tracking, and Follow-Up

1. **Contract:** I intend to make the behavior change described above. I will use the strategies and rewards to achieve the goals that will contribute to a healthy behavior change.

   Signed _____ Date _____

   Witness _____ Date _____

2. **Tracking:** Tracking progress toward your goals is very important to ensure successful behavior change. As you move through this course, you will be asked to monitor your progress on several of your health, wellness, and fitness goals. Accurate and regular record-keeping is important.

3. **Follow-Up:** When reaching your target date, it is important to follow up and reassess your program. During this course, you will be answering questions such as: Did you accomplish your goal? Do you need to set a new and more challenging goal? Do you need to alter your goals or program to make it more realistic? This section in your labs is important to modify your goals and your program and to set future goals.

Understanding Fitness Principles

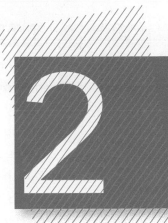
2

LEARNINGoutcomes

LO 2.1 Describe the three primary levels of physical activity and their benefits.

LO 2.2 Articulate the importance of each health-related component of fitness.

LO 2.3 Identify the role that the skill-related components of fitness play in overall physical fitness.

LO 2.4 Explain how following the fitness principles of overload, progression, specificity, reversibility, individuality, and recovery will increase your fitness program success.

LO 2.5 Describe how much and the types of physical activity you should do for optimal health and wellness.

LO 2.6 Incorporate general strategies for exercising safely.

LO 2.7 Identify individual attributes that should be taken into account before beginning a fitness program.

LO 2.8 Individualize and implement strategies that will help you get started on your fitness and exercise goals.

MasteringHealth™

Go online for chapter quizzes, interactive assessments, videos, and more!

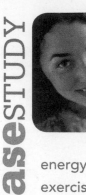

LILY

"Hi, I'm Lily. After a summer of lazing around, I am ready to get back into shape. I'm hoping to put some serious time and energy into it, but the last time I started exercising, I tried to do too much and ended up injured. How do I keep from doing the same thing this time? How much exercise do I really need? And what does it actually mean to be fit, anyway—does it just mean being able to walk or run a certain distance, or is there more to it than that?"

Hear It!

To listen to this case study online, visit the Study Area in MasteringHealth™.

F itness is a critical component of overall wellness. Being physically fit can improve your mood and sleep, give you more energy, help you maintain a healthy weight, lower stress levels, and reduce your risk of infectious and chronic diseases. All of these benefits can, in turn, help you live a longer, healthier life.

In this chapter, we cover the basic principles of fitness, address the question of how much exercise you need, introduce general guidelines for exercising safely, and discuss individual factors to consider when designing your personal fitness program. Most important, we'll introduce tools and strategies that will help you get moving right away!

LO 2.1 What Are the Three Primary Levels of Physical Activity?

Physical fitness is the ability to perform moderate to vigorous levels of physical activity or exercise without undue fatigue. **Physical activity** technically means any bodily movement produced by skeletal muscles that results in an expenditure of energy, whereas **exercise** specifically refers to planned or structured physical activity done to achieve and maintain fitness.

Physical activity is often measured in metabolic equivalents, or **MET** levels. A MET level of 1 equals the energy you use at rest or while sitting quietly. A MET

level of 2 equals two times the energy used at a MET level of 1, while a MET level of 3 equals three times the energy used at a MET level of 1, and so forth. Levels of physical activity can be grouped into three primary categories: (1) *light/lifestyle/physical activities* (<3 METS), (2) *moderate physical activities* (3 to 6 METS), and (3) *vigorous physical activities* (>6 METS). **Figure 2.1** illustrates examples of each of these MET levels and the benefits associated with them.

LO 2.2 What Are the Health-Related Components of Physical Fitness?

The five **health-related components of physical fitness** are *cardiorespiratory endurance, muscular strength, muscular endurance, flexibility,* and *body composition*. Minimal competence in each of these areas is necessary for you to carry out daily activities, lower your risk of developing chronic diseases, and optimize your health and well-being.

Cardiorespiratory Endurance

Cardiorespiratory endurance (also called *cardiovascular fitness/endurance, aerobic fitness,* and *cardiorespiratory fitness*) is the ability of the cardiovascular and respiratory systems to provide oxygen to working muscles during sustained exercise. Adequate cardiorespiratory endurance decreases your risk of dying from both cardiovascular and non-cardiovascular diseases.[1] Increased cardiorespiratory endurance is associated with positive changes in your brain[2] and improves your ability to enjoy recreational activities for an extended period of time.

Muscular Strength

Muscular strength is the ability of your muscles to exert force. Think of it as your ability to lift a

physical fitness A set of attributes that relate to one's ability to perform moderate to vigorous levels of physical activity without undue fatigue

physical activity Any bodily movement produced by skeletal muscles that results in an expenditure of energy

exercise Physical activity that is planned or structured, done to improve or maintain one or more of the components of fitness

MET The standard metabolic equivalent used to estimate the amount of energy (oxygen) used by the body during physical activity; 1 MET = resting or sitting quietly

health-related components of physical fitness Components of physical fitness that have a relationship with good health

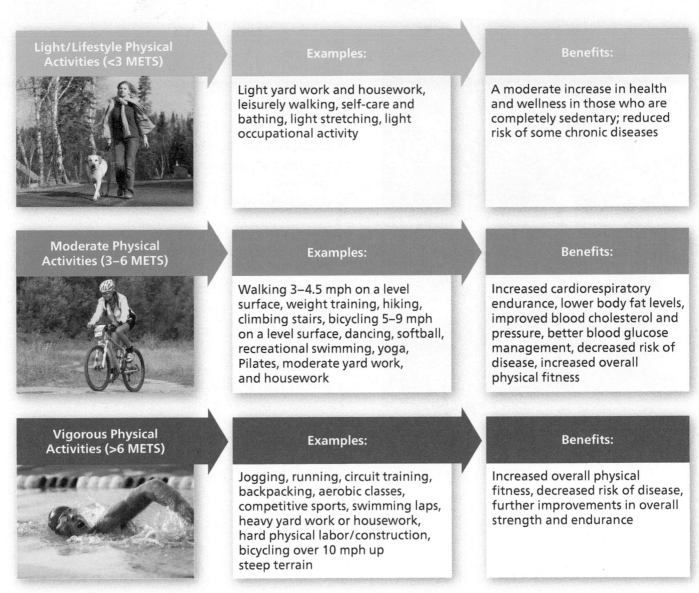

Light/Lifestyle Physical Activities (<3 METS)	Examples:	Benefits:
	Light yard work and housework, leisurely walking, self-care and bathing, light stretching, light occupational activity	A moderate increase in health and wellness in those who are completely sedentary; reduced risk of some chronic diseases
Moderate Physical Activities (3–6 METS)	Examples:	Benefits:
	Walking 3–4.5 mph on a level surface, weight training, hiking, climbing stairs, bicycling 5–9 mph on a level surface, dancing, softball, recreational swimming, yoga, Pilates, moderate yard work, and housework	Increased cardiorespiratory endurance, lower body fat levels, improved blood cholesterol and pressure, better blood glucose management, decreased risk of disease, increased overall physical fitness
Vigorous Physical Activities (>6 METS)	Examples:	Benefits:
	Jogging, running, circuit training, backpacking, aerobic classes, competitive sports, swimming laps, heavy yard work or housework, hard physical labor/construction, bicycling over 10 mph up steep terrain	Increased overall physical fitness, decreased risk of disease, further improvements in overall strength and endurance

FIGURE **2.1** Examples and benefits of light/lifestyle physical activity, moderate physical activity, and vigorous physical activity.

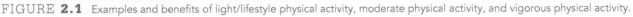

heavy weight. Improved muscular strength decreases your risk of low bone density and musculoskeletal injuries.[3] To improve muscular strength, you need to tax your muscles in a controlled setting. This typically involves a weight room, as well as supervision to avoid injury.

Muscular Endurance

Muscular endurance is the ability of your muscles to contract repeatedly over time. Along with cardiorespiratory endurance, muscular endurance allows you to participate in recreational sports without undue fatigue. For example, to play a continuous game of basketball, you need good cardiorespiratory endurance to move up and down the court for the entire 90 minutes—and you need good muscular endurance to keep guarding, blocking, and shooting the ball effectively.

Flexibility

Flexibility is the ability to move your joints in a full range of motion. Maintaining a minimal level of flexibility increases your ability to do the activities you enjoy. Although we don't know whether stretching reduces overall injury rates, it may reduce specific muscle and tendon injuries.[4] Having an adequate joint range of motion can be especially important to prevent neck and back pain when you are older and help prevent the decreased physical function associated with aging.[5]

Body Composition

Body composition refers to the relative amounts of fat and lean tissue in your body. Lean tissue consists of muscle, bone, organs, and fluids. A healthy body composition has adequate muscle tissue with moderate to low

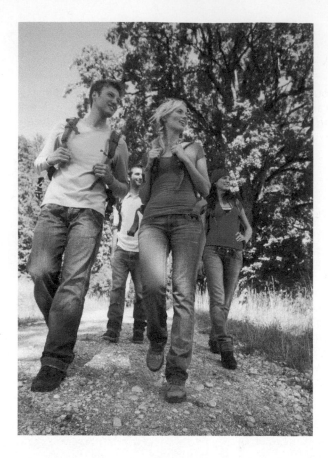

and allows you to maintain your independence as you get older. The six skill-related components of fitness are:

- **Agility:** The ability to rapidly change the position of your body with speed and accuracy
- **Balance:** The maintenance of equilibrium while you are stationary or moving
- **Coordination:** The ability to use both your senses and your body to perform motor skills smoothly and accurately
- **Power:** The ability to perform work or contract muscles with high force quickly
- **Speed:** The ability to perform a movement in a short period of time
- **Reaction time:** The time between a stimulus and the initiation of your physical reaction to that stimulus

Although heredity largely determines skill-related fitness, regular training can improve it significantly.[6] To improve skill-related components of fitness, athletes and exercisers need to target the skills important to their specific sport or exercise. For instance, a runner can benefit from increasing power for hill running, whereas a tennis player can benefit from improved agility and reaction time.

Improving your sport skills can be as easy as regularly participating in a sport or activity. Playing football will increase reaction time and power, while dancing will increase balance, agility, and coordination. Another way to increase these skills is to perform drills that mimic sport movements or target the skill-related components of fitness. Such drills may involve specialized equipment. For example, quickly navigating obstacles such as hurdles or cones can help you improve your speed, agility, and coordination.

amounts of fat tissue. The recommendations for fat percentages vary based upon your gender and age. Increased levels of fat put you at risk for diabetes, heart disease, and certain cancers.

LO 2.3 What Are the Skill-Related Components of Physical Fitness?

In addition to the five health-related components of fitness, physical fitness involves attributes called the **skill-related components of fitness**. Often termed *sport skills*, these are qualities that improve your ability to perform athletic, exercise, and daily functional tasks. Athletes target these to gain a competitive edge, but everyone benefits from increasing their sport skills. Maintaining a minimal level in each of these areas reduces your risk of falling

skill-related components of fitness Components of physical fitness that have a relationship with enhanced motor skills and performance in sports

principles of fitness General principles of exercise adaptation that guide fitness programming

overload Subjecting the body or body system to more physical activity than it is accustomed to

LO 2.4 What Are the Principles of Fitness?

To design an effective fitness program, consider the basic **principles of fitness** (also called *principles of exercise training*). These guiding principles explain how the body responds or adapts to exercise training.

Overload

The principle of **overload** states that in order to see improvements in your physical fitness, the amount or dose of training you undertake must be more than your body or specific body system is accustomed to. This applies to any component of physical fitness discussed earlier. For example, to increase your flexibility, stretch a little farther than you are used to.

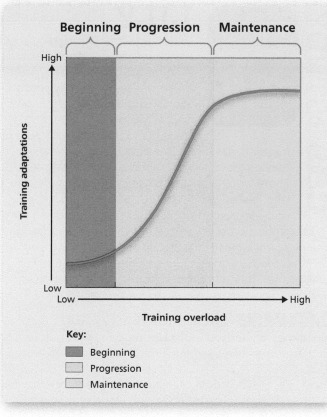

Beginning Progression Maintenance

Training adaptations

High

Low

Low ————————————————→ High

Training overload

Key:
- Beginning
- Progression
- Maintenance

FIGURE **2.2** After adjusting to new training overloads at the beginning of your exercise program, you will see larger adaptations and improvements during the progression phase. As you approach your goal or genetic limits, your increases in overload will not result in further adaptations. This is a sign that you have reached a plateau and should maintain (if satisfied) or adjust your program for further improvement.

Training Effects Consistent overloads or stresses on a body system will cause an *adaptation* to occur (**Figure 2.2**). An adaptation is a change in the body as a result of an overload. In exercise, this is called a *training effect*. For example, if you normally run two laps around a track, you may feel tired and out of breath the first time you run four laps. After a few weeks of running four laps, adaptations in your cardiorespiratory and muscular systems will allow you to cover that distance with greater ease.

Dose-Response The amount of adaptation you can expect is directly related to the amount of overload or training dose that you complete. This is called the *dose-response relationship.* An increase in your "dose," or amount of training, will result in increased responses or adaptations to that training. How much response or adaptation you can expect depends upon the body system trained, the health or fitness outcome measured, and your individual physical and genetic characteristics.

Diminished Returns According to the concept of *diminished returns* (also called the *initial values*

principle), the rate of fitness improvement diminishes over time as fitness levels approach genetic limits. Genetic limits are determined by your potential for improvement given your biological makeup. Initial fitness levels also determine the amount of improvement that you can achieve from exercise training. If you are sedentary and far from your genetic limits, you have a greater potential for fitness improvements than people who are active and closer to their genetic limits already.

Progression

The principle of **progression** states that in order to effectively and safely increase fitness, you need to apply an optimal level of overload to the body within a certain time period. Simply stated, you need to increase your workout levels enough to see results, but not so much that you increase your risk of injury. Your body will then progressively adapt to the overloads presented to it. To make sure that you are not progressing too quickly, follow the "**10 percent rule**": increase your exercise frequency, intensity, or duration by no more than 10 percent per week.

Specificity

The principle of **specificity** states that a body system will improve only if the physical activity stresses or progressively overloads that specific body system. To follow this principle, make sure that you are training targeted muscle groups specific to your sport and your program is structured to meet your goals. For instance, if you are planning to walk a marathon, you should primarily *walk* during your training. If, instead, you decide to swim laps for most of your training, you may increase your cardiorespiratory fitness, but you will not be specifically training your lower body muscles to walk 26 miles.

Reversibility

All fitness gains are reversible, according to the principle of **reversibility**. This is the "use it or lose it" principle. If you do not stay physically active, your fitness levels will slip. Most people take breaks in their exercise

progression A gradual increase in a training program's intensity, frequency, and/or time

10 percent rule Increasing one aspect of your training program (frequency, intensity, or duration) by no more than 10 percent per week to ensure progression and injury prevention

specificity The principle that only the body systems worked during training will show adaptations

reversibility The principle that training adaptations will revert toward initial levels when training is stopped

programs from time to time due to illness, travel, social commitments, work, or holidays, but know that when you do, it takes only one to two weeks to start losing your hard-earned fitness gains.[7] In fact, most of your fitness improvements could be gone in a few months.[8] In addition, a new or older exerciser will lose fitness faster than a trained athlete or younger person, and we lose cardiorespiratory fitness faster than muscle fitness.[9] The good news is that you can reduce the number of exercise sessions per week as long as you keep the intensity up (see the HIIT GetFitGraphic in Chapter 3).[10] This strategy will help you maintain your fitness during those busy times.

Individuality

The principle of **individuality** states that adaptations to a training overload may vary greatly from person to person due to genetics and other individual differences. Two people may participate in the same training program but have very different responses. While you cannot control your genetic makeup, understanding how you respond to exercise is important. A person who responds well to a training program is considered a *responder*. One who does not respond well is considered a *non-responder*. Of those individuals who show improvements, some may respond better to increases in total amount of physical activity, while others may show more improvement with increases in exercise intensity. Figuring out your individual responses to certain exercise programs is a trial-and-error process. Complete regular fitness assessments and training logs to track your progress. (See Q&A Can Technology Help Me Get More Fit?) Adjust your program accordingly to meet your goals.

Rest and Recovery

The principle of **rest and recovery** (also called the *principle of recuperation*) is critical to ensuring continued fitness improvement. Your body needs time to recover from the increased physiological and structural training stresses that you place on it during a progressive exercise program. In *resistance training* (also called *weight training*), most of the training adaptations actually take place during the rest periods between workouts. Constant training day after day with insufficient rest periods can lead to **overtraining**. If you are exercising consistently and start feeling more fatigue and muscle soreness than usual during and after exercise, you could be doing too much. Reduce your exercise duration or intensity and rest for a day or two. To prevent overtraining and gain optimal benefits, schedule one to three rest days per week for cardiorespiratory fitness training and every other day for strength training. Another important tip is to alternate hard workout days with easier workout days during your weekly plan.

individuality The variable nature of physical activity dose-response or adaptations in different persons

rest and recovery Taking a short time off from physical activities to allow the body to recuperate and improve

overtraining Excessive volume and intensity of physical training leading to diminished health, fitness, and performance

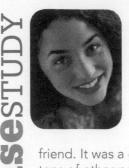

LO 2.5 How Much Exercise Is Enough?

How much exercise or physical activity do you really need? The answers will vary, depending on which sources you turn to and on your individual fitness goals. Most agree that the first step is to avoid

Q&A Can Technology Help Me Get More Fit?

Yes! Researchers have found that college students who use exercise video games, such as Wii Fit™, have more intention to continue over traditional exercise programs.[1] In addition to video games, there are a number of other technological advances that can motivate you to stay active and heathy. You can use a simple pedometer to track your steps per day or you can invest in a wearable activity tracker. You can use a free website to plan and log your fitness program on your computer or download an app to your smartphone with embedded workouts and tracking.

APPLY IT! Consider these things when choosing what will work best for you:

- **Purpose**—How will you use the technology? Do you want workout planning, exercises, *and* tracking all available? Some programs, apps, and trackers also have a social component where you can share workouts with friends and compete for top times. For activity trackers, decide what you want to monitor. Most track movement/steps and calories, but some can also record sedentary time, heart rate, oxygen levels, perspiration levels, and body heat. Some will even alert you if you've been inactive too long. In fact, some doctors use wearable activity monitors to track patient data before and after medical procedures.[2]

- **Money**—Wearable activity trackers generate more than $5 billion in the United States [3], which isn't surprising since most cost well over $100. If you don't want to invest that much, you can buy a simple pedometer for less than $20, and there are numerous free fitness websites and apps.

- **Activities**—Make sure the app or device is accurate for your type of activity. For example, wearables on the wrist are best for activities with arm movement and are not good for cycling or sensing the movement of your fidgety legs. If you are a swimmer, be sure to get one that's waterproof.

- **Ease of Use/Compatibility**—Try out the website, app, or tracker before investing much time or money. It should be easy to use and compatible with your computer and/or phone.

TRY IT! Do your research and find the best product for your needs and budget. Whether you decide to stay low-tech or jump into the high-tech fitness world, the important thing is that it motivates you to move!

Sources:
1. A. Garn, B. Baker, E. Beasley, and M. Solomon, "What Are the Benefits of a Commercial Exergaming Platform for College Students? Examining Physical Activity, Enjoyment, and Future Intentions," *Journal of Physical Activity and Health* 9, no. 2 (2012): 311–18.
2. E. Dwoskin and J. Walker, "Can Data from Your FitBit Transform Medicine?" *Wall Street Journal*, June 24, 2014, accessed August 11, 2015.
3. Ibid.

---

inactivity, particularly sitting too much. Sitting is associated with a greater risk of chronic health problems and diseases, like heart disease and diabetes, and the more you sit, the higher your risk.[11] See the GetFit-Graphic on page 36 for more information on the dangers of sitting too much. So, although *any* amount of physical activity is helpful, you should also aim to decrease your daily sitting time (think: standing computer/work stations or a treadmill desk!).

Start by making sure that you meet the minimal activity level recommendations given next. For additional health benefits and fitness improvements, follow the guidelines in the Physical Activity Pyramid and the FITT Principle.

> **Live It!**
> Complete Worksheet 26 How Much Do I Move? at MasteringHealth™.

Minimal Physical Activity Level Guidelines

Guidelines for physical activity and exercise are issued by organizations that rely on credible scientific research to develop their recommendations. These organizations are *government agencies* (e.g., the President's Council on Physical Fitness and Sports), *professional organizations* (e.g., the American College of Sports Medicine), or *private organizations* (e.g., the American Heart Association). In 2008, the US Department of Health and Human Services issued the first-ever national physical activity guidelines designed to "provide achievable steps for youth, adults, and seniors, as well as people with special conditions to live healthier and longer lives."[12] The recommendations are echoed by other leading organizations, such as the World Health Organization and American College of Sports Medicine.[13]

As a nation, Americans are gradually getting better at meeting these guidelines, but there is still room to improve. From 1997 to 2014, only 21 percent of adults met the minimal guidelines for both aerobic and muscle strengthening activities.[14] College-aged adults (18 to 24 years) did a little better, with 31 percent meeting the guidelines. However, the percentages drop as people age. Fewer than 15 percent of people 65 years and older reported enough aerobic and muscle strengthening activities in 2014 to meet the guidelines.

WHAT IS SITTING SYNDROME?

People around the globe are sitting more and more—and it is making us less healthy and literally killing us!

OVER 7 HOURS OF SITTING on average leads to:

61% greater risk of mortality—after accounting for age, diet, smoking and moderate physical activity levels![1]

More than double the risk of diabetes and heart events[2]

▶ *Is it more risky for WOMEN?*
Women who sit have a

10% greater risk of cancer[3]

and are 3 times more likely to be depressed than active women.[4]

I EXERCISE—ISN'T THAT **ENOUGH?**
The statistics above show that even after accounting for physical activities—*sitting is harmful!* Being physically active doesn't mean that you sit LESS than your sedentary counterparts.[5] However, being fit can REDUCE the negative effects of sitting on your health.[6]

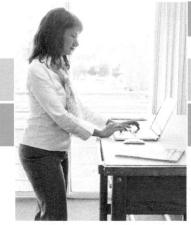

STAND UP!!
Standing up for 3 hours instead of sitting down can burn

750 more calories (kcals) per week

over 30,000 more kcals per year, or about *8 lbs of FAT!*[7]

That could be the equivalent of running 10 marathons per year! As an added benefit, standing after eating improves your blood glucose levels, potentially reducing your risk of diabetes as well.

STAND TO LIVE?
Higher levels of standing = lower mortality rates, especially in those who are sedentary.8

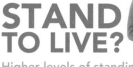

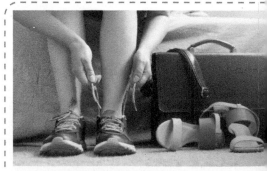

HOW MUCH WILL IT HELP TO GET ACTIVE?
If you are less active now, replace 1 hour of sitting with 1 hour of exercise per day =
42% decrease in mortality risk.

Replace with 1 hour of light, non-exercise activity per day =
30% reduction in mortality risk.[9]

If you are active already, you'll still see your risk of dying **decrease by**
9% if you replace sitting time with purposeful exercise.

Even a 2-minute walk in the middle of a work or study session can help—people who interrupt sedentary time with movement "breaks" have narrower waistlines and a low[er] risk of cardiovascular disease and diabetes.[10]

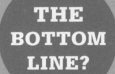 **THE BOTTOM LINE?** ▷ **GET UP** ▷ **GET MOVING** ▷ 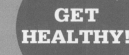 **GET HEALTHY!**

The good news is that Americans have already met the *Healthy People 2020* target for the number of adults getting both aerobic and muscle strengthening exercise. The bad news is that still leaves 79 percent not getting enough.[15] How close are you to meeting these recommendations? Look at the guidelines in **Table 2.1** to find out.

The Physical Activity Pyramid Guides Weekly Choices

The Physical Activity Pyramid (**Figure 2.3** on page 38) visually summarizes physical activity and exercise guidelines for optimal health and wellness.

- The pyramid's bottom layer represents light or lifestyle activities that you should strive to incorporate into your everyday life. Light physical activity every day, such as walking and gardening, is a great way to start and to ensure a strong "base" to your pyramid!

- The next layer of the pyramid represents moderate-to-vigorous aerobic and/or sports activities that you should do three to five times per week to build cardiorespiratory endurance and fitness. Overall, aim to accumulate at least 150 minutes of moderate physical activity each week, such as quick walking or flat bicycling, or 75 minutes of vigorous activity each week, such as swimming or jogging.

- The third layer of the pyramid represents strength training and flexibility—building exercises that you should do at least two days per week.

- The top layer of the pyramid represents sedentary activities, like computer or other screen time, that will ideally receive the least amount of time in favor of more active pursuits.

The Tips for Getting Up and Moving box on page 40 suggests ways to incorporate more physical activity into your daily life.

TABLE 2-1 Physical Activity Guidelines for Americans			
	Key Guidelines for Health*	For Additional Fitness or Weight Loss Benefits*	PLUS
Adults	150 min/week moderate-intensity OR 75 min/week of vigorous-intensity OR Equivalent combination of moderate- and vigorous-intensity (i.e., 100 min moderate-intensity +25 min vigorous-intensity)	300 min/week moderate-intensity OR 150 min/week of vigorous-intensity OR Equivalent combination of moderate- and vigorous-intensity (i.e., 200 min moderate-intensity +50 min vigorous-intensity) OR More than the previously described amounts	Muscle strengthening activities for all the major muscle groups at least 2 days/week
Older Adults	If unable to follow above guidelines, then as much physical activity as your condition allows	If unable to follow above guidelines, then as much physical activity as your condition allows	In addition to muscle strengthening activities, those with limited mobility should add exercises to improve balance and reduce risk of falling
Children and Adolescents	60 min or more of moderate- or vigorous-intensity physical activity daily	Add vigorous-intensity physical activities within the 60 daily minutes at least 3 days/week	Include muscle and bone strengthening activities with the 60 daily minutes at least 3 days/week. Activities should be age-appropriate, enjoyable, and varied

*Notes: Avoid inactivity, some activity is better than none; accumulate physical activity in sessions of 10 minutes or more at one time; and spread activity throughout the week.

Source: "2008 Physical Activity Guidelines for Americans: Be Active, Healthy, and Happy!" from the Office of Disease Prevention and Health Promotion, U.S. Department of Health and Human Services website, 2008, www.hhs.gov

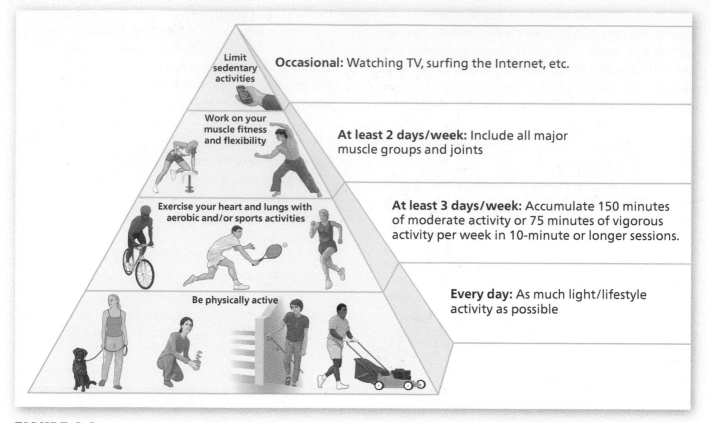

FIGURE **2.3** The Physical Activity Pyramid presents recommended levels of activity for optimal health and wellness.

The FITT Formula Can Help You Plan Your Program

The **FITT formula** acronym stands for frequency, intensity, time, and type. Consider these factors when planning your personal exercise program.

- **Frequency** is the number of times per week that you will perform an exercise.

- **Intensity** refers to how hard you will exercise. For aerobic activities, intensity is often measured in terms of how much the given activity increases your heart rate. For resistance activities, intensity is represented in the amount of resistance or weight lifted as a percentage of your maximal ability for that exercise (percentage of 1RM; repetition maximum).

- **Time** is the amount of time that you will devote to a given exercise. It can be the total amount of time you spend on an aerobic or a sport activity, the number of sets and repetitions for a resistance exercise, or the amount of time you spend holding a stretch for a flexibility exercise.

- **Type** refers to the kind of exercise you will do. Within each of the components of fitness, there are many types of exercises that will increase fitness levels. Your type, or **mode**, of exercise will be determined by your preferences, physical abilities, environment, equipment, and personal goals.

See **Figure 2.4** for a summary of the FITT guidelines for cardiorespiratory endurance, muscular fitness, and flexibility. If you are beginning a fitness program for the first time, you may want to start with the physical activity guidelines in Table 2.1. When you are ready, add appropriate levels of the Physical Activity Pyramid and then customize your program using the FITT formula to suit your personal goals.

To keep from getting injured, start small and progress gradually. In future chapters, we'll cover specific exercise progressions for cardiorespiratory, resistance, and stretching exercise programs. Next, let's look at additional considerations to stay injury-free.

LO 2.6 What Does It Take to Exercise Safely?

More than 7 million Americans receive medical attention for sports-related injuries each year, with the greatest numbers of injuries affecting 5- to 24-year-olds.[16] To reduce your risk of injury, follow the guidelines below.

FITT formula A formula for designing a safe and effective program that specifies frequency, intensity, time, and type of exercise

mode The specific type of exercise performed

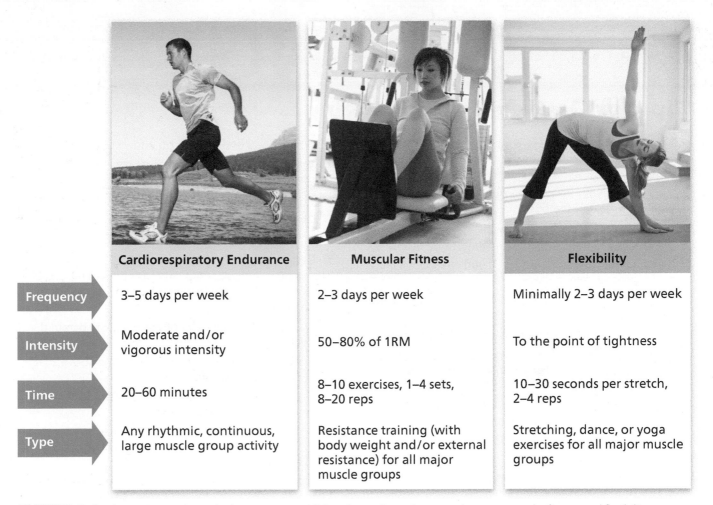

Cardiorespiratory Endurance	Muscular Fitness	Flexibility
Frequency 3–5 days per week	2–3 days per week	Minimally 2–3 days per week
Intensity Moderate and/or vigorous intensity	50–80% of 1RM	To the point of tightness
Time 20–60 minutes	8–10 exercises, 1–4 sets, 8–20 reps	10–30 seconds per stretch, 2–4 reps
Type Any rhythmic, continuous, large muscle group activity	Resistance training (with body weight and/or external resistance) for all major muscle groups	Stretching, dance, or yoga exercises for all major muscle groups

FIGURE **2.4** The FITT principle applied to summary guidelines for cardiorespiratory endurance, muscular fitness, and flexibility.

Data from American College of Sports Medicine, *ACSM's Guidelines for Exercise Testing and Prescription*, 9th ed. (Baltimore: Lippincott Williams & Wilkins, 2014).

Warm Up Properly Before Your Workout

A proper warm-up consists of two phases: a general warm-up and a specific warm-up. In a *general warm-up*, your goal is to warm up your body by doing 5 to 10 minutes of light physical activity similar to the activities you will be performing during exercise. During this period of time (called the *rest-to-exercise transition*), you are preparing your body to withstand the more vigorous exercise to come. Your core body temperature should rise a few degrees, and you should break a slight sweat. This movement and temperature rise will increase your overall blood flow, ready your joint fluid and structures, and improve muscle elasticity.

A *specific warm-up* should include three to five minutes of dynamic **range-of-motion** movements. Move muscles and joints in a manner similar to what you will be doing during the activity set. Move

range-of-motion The movement limits that limbs have around a specific joint

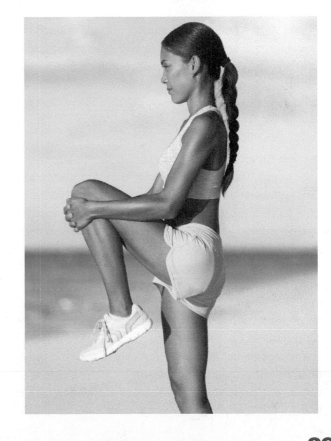

CHANGE

Tips for Getting Up and Moving

You can improve your fitness level simply by adding more physical activity to your daily life and reducing your sitting time. Below are a few simple ways to do that:

☐ Walk or ride your bike to campus instead of driving your car or taking the bus.

☐ Park your car farther from your destination or get off the bus at an earlier stop and walk.

☐ If you have a dog, walk it daily. If you already do that, add a second daily walk!

☐ Walk to the store with a backpack when you need just a few items.

☐ Carry a basket while grocery shopping instead of pushing a cart.

☐ If you have children, play actively with them—sweet laughter is a reward.

☐ If you have a desk job or study for long periods of time, get up and walk around often.

☐ Waiting for files to download? Do push-ups, curl-ups, or squats during that time.

☐ Create a standing work area for your computer or books to reduce your sitting time.

☐ Walk around while talking on the phone.

☐ On hold? Use that time to do a few stretches!

☐ Study while exercising! Complete class readings or study notes while on a stationary bike.

☐ Watch TV or movies from an exercise bike or treadmill.

☐ Stretch or do exercises while watching movies or during TV commercial breaks.

TRY IT!

1. Examine the Physical Activity Pyramid and think about how your weekly physical activity matches up to its recommendations.

2. Next, draw your personal physical activity pyramid reflecting your current level of activity.

3. Put a check mark next to the simple tips above that you can start doing **next week.**

4. Write out one or two new exercise activities that you can try in the next **two weeks.**

5. Now, draw a new goal personal physical activity pyramid incorporating your new active lifestyle choices (#3) and your new activities (#4).

6. Reflect upon your goal pyramid in **three weeks.** Were you able to incorporate your new behaviors and activities? Why or why not?

---

joints through a full range of motion but in a relaxed and controlled manner. If you want to add light stretching to your warm-up, do so at the end of your specific warm-up.

Cool Down Properly After Your Workout

After you finish your workout, cool down in a manner that is appropriate for the activity that you performed. This *exercise-to-rest transition* should last anywhere from 5 to 15 minutes. If your heart rate and temperature rose during your workout, perform a *general cool-down* to bring your heart rate, breathing rate, and temperature closer to resting levels. This cool-down is usually a less vigorous version of the activity you just performed. For example, if you jogged for 25 minutes, your general cool-down may consist of 10 minutes of walking.

If you have just finished a resistance-training program, perform a *specific cool-down* by stretching the muscles you have exercised. A specific cool-down can be performed after a general cool-down for aerobic activities and right after exercise for resistance training activities.

Take the Time to Properly Learn the Skills for Your Chosen Activity

There are hundreds of different activities that you can do to increase your health and fitness, each requiring a specific set of physical skills. You might choose activities, such as walking or jogging, that require little skill and have short learning curves, or you might prefer activities such as fencing or hockey that require more complex skills.

Whatever you choose, make sure you learn the physical skills required for that activity to enhance your enjoyment and avoid injury. If you are just beginning a sport for the first time—for example, skiing—do not immediately approach the sport the way a more experienced athlete would. Take lessons, start on the beginner slopes, and give yourself time to safely enjoy your chosen activity.

Consume Enough Energy and Water for Exercise

Deciding how much to eat and drink prior to exercise can be tricky. You need enough energy to work out, but you should not exercise on a full stomach. Eating a small meal 1½ to 2 hours before exercise is a good way to make sure that you have energy (but not an upset stomach) during the workout. A light snack 30 to 60 minutes before your workout is acceptable as well.

Dehydration is more likely than food intake to affect your exercise performance. During the hours before your workout, be sure to drink enough water so that you do not feel thirsty going into your exercise session. Guidelines for drinking before, during, and after exercising should be tailored to the individual and the exercise session.[17] General guidelines are 17 to 20 oz. of fluid two to three hours before exercise and 7 to 10 oz. of fluid 10 to 20 minutes prior to exercise.[18] During your workout, hydrate when you feel thirsty, and increase the amount of water you consume as you start to sweat more profusely. See Chapter 3 for more information about the effects of under- and over-hydration in cardiorespiratory exercise.

Select Appropriate Footwear and Clothing

Consider this: During one mile of running, your feet will typically strike the ground 1,000 times. Over weeks of training, that translates to a great deal of wear and tear on your feet and lower body. Needless to say, proper footwear is critical to a safe and successful training program—regardless of the activity you choose.

While some sports require specialized footwear, most beginning exercisers just need one pair of good, all-around athletic shoes. The most important considerations are proper fit, support, and cushioning. Always try on shoes before purchasing them, and, if possible, spend a few minutes mimicking the activity you will be doing in them. The best shoes are not always the most expensive, but purchase the highest-quality footwear you can afford. Ask for assistance from knowledgeable salespeople and see the Chapter 3 Tools for Change box Select the Right Shoe for You on page 85 for more on footwear selection.

Clothing for exercise can be very simple (shorts and a t-shirt) or very technical (clothing with special treatments for protection against harsh weather). The most important thing is to dress appropriately for your chosen activity. Your clothing should be comfortable and not restricting to your range of motion. Women may wish to wear supportive athletic bras, and men may want to

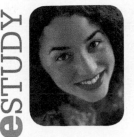

caseSTUDY

LILY

"I've started exercising again! Since my knees are still a little bit touchy, I've decided to start out with a walking program and build back up to jogging. I'm starting with a beginning walking program for four weeks. I want to focus on being consistent with my exercise and eventually get through the intermediate walking program, which is five days per week. I really like the way my body feels after my walks, so I'm not tempted to run a 5K again any time soon. If I can keep this new routine going, I should be ready to walk a 5K or maybe even a 10K in a few months!"

APPLY IT! What kinds of things would you advise Lily to do to reduce her chances of injury? Review the walking programs at the end of the chapter and decide if Lily is meeting the FITT formula for cardiorespiratory endurance.

TRY IT! **Today**, write down what you might do the same as or different from Lily in your exercise program. **This week**, figure out the system that you will use to record your activities (journal, log, smartphone, etc.) and start tracking what you do!

Hear It!
To listen to this case study online, visit the Study Area in MasteringHealth™.

wear supportive compression shorts or undergarments. If you exercise outdoors, consider the temperature and dress accordingly. The longer you plan to exercise, the more carefully you should think about what to wear for a successful workout.

LO 2.7 What Individual Factors Should I Consider When Designing a Fitness Program?

There is no such thing as a "one-size-fits-all" physical fitness program. Different individuals have different needs, and general recommendations need to be adapted to fit those individual needs. Factors to consider include your age, weight, current fitness level, and any disabilities and special health concerns.

Age

Healthy individuals of all ages can become more active. However, older

dehydration A process that leads to a lack of sufficient fluid in the body, affecting normal body functioning

adults may require additional precautions to prevent injury. Men over age 45 and women over age 55 should look closely at their health and cardiovascular risks before starting a vigorous exercise program.[19] Moderate aerobic activity, muscle-strengthening exercises, and flexibility work are all recommended activities for older adults. Include balance exercises to help prevent falls and injury.

Weight

Overweight people are at a higher risk of musculoskeletal injuries due to increased stress on their muscles and joints, and they should take precautions. If you are overweight, consider a cross-training routine with a mix of moderate weight-bearing (e.g., walking and stair-climbing) and non-weight-bearing (e.g., bicycling and water exercise) activities. Start your exercise program slowly to give your muscles and joints time to adjust to the new stresses placed upon them. Supportive but flexible footwear is very important for success in weight-bearing activities. If you feel pain in your lower-body joints during exercise, shift to more non-weight-bearing activities until your body adapts by getting stronger, and you've lost some body weight.

Some overweight individuals feel uncomfortable with typical exercise gyms. If this is you, seek out a low-key workout facility—you may even find one that caters to people who are overweight—or try appropriate exercise videos at home for a few months. You can also look for community centers with fitness facilities and classes, seek out a class specifically designed to target weight loss, and/or start a walking program around your neighborhood.

If you are underweight, perform enough strength-training and weight-bearing activities to keep your muscles and bones strong.

Current Fitness Level

Design a program that suits your current fitness level. If you already exercise regularly, consider increasing the frequency or intensity of your workouts for more fitness gains. If you are sedentary and just beginning to think about exercise, don't run a 5K race without training for it!

Disabilities or Temporary Physical Limitations

If you have mobility restrictions, poor balance, dizziness, injuries, short-term illness, or other physically limiting conditions, you can still incorporate activity into your daily life with alternative or adaptive exercises. Many colleges, community centers, parks and recreation facilities, and fitness centers offer adaptive courses, equipment, and adaptive-trained instructors. After obtaining medical clearance, ask your physician or physical therapist about facilities close to you. The Physical Activity and Sport for Everyone box on page 43 provides additional suggestions.

Special Health Concerns

Certain medical conditions may require you to exercise under medical supervision. Anyone with a diagnosed metabolic, cardiovascular, kidney, or lung disease needs to obtain medical clearance before beginning an exercise program.[20] If you have special health concerns, seek the advice of a qualified medical professional about exercising safely.

Individuals with significant bone or joint problems can benefit from lower-impact activities, such as swimming, water exercise, bicycling, walking, or low-impact aerobics. Resistance training that strengthens muscles and joints and helps maintain bone density is also important to incorporate.

If you are taking any prescription medications, ask your doctor whether there are side effects that you should consider before exercising. In addition, beware of over-the-counter medications and other products that may cause drowsiness (for instance, antihistamines, certain cough/cold medicines, and alcohol) because this will impair your reaction time, coordination, and balance.

Pregnancy

If you are pregnant, don't start an intense exercise or weight-loss program. Instead, aim to keep moving throughout your pregnancy. Most active women can continue pre-pregnancy activities if there are no other health concerns. By keeping active, you'll experience better cardiorespiratory function, less weight gain and discomfort, and a more stable mood. You will also reduce your risk of hypertension and gestational diabetes.

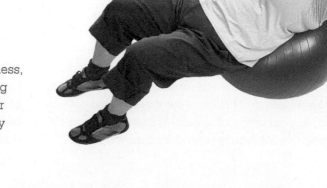

DIVERSITY
Physical Activity and Sport for Everyone

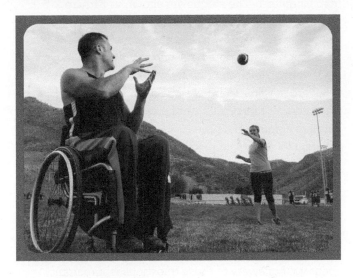

Over 53 million (more than 22 percent) of US adults reported having a disability in 2013. Physical mobility issues account for 13 percent—making it the most common type of disability—and altered cognitive function ranked second at 10 percent.[1] Women, minorities, people over 65 years, and those with a lower economic and/or education level were more likely to report a disability. Since being disabled is associated with higher levels of smoking and physical inactivity, it is important to reduce barriers to activity for everyone.

The US Department of Health and Human Services recommends that adults with disabilities follow the 2008 Physical Activity Guidelines for Americans, adjusting as necessary for varying abilities and physician recommendations.[2] Unfortunately, only about 10 percent of persons with disabilities meet these guidelines.[3]

The good news? There are many options available for modifying physical activities and helping all people achieve their health and fitness goals. For example, most strength-training machines are used from a seated position and can be operated by people in wheelchairs. Rubber exercise bands can serve as alternative strength-building aids. In addition, many companies offer modified sports equipment for people with disabilities. Handcycles allow someone to ride a bike using arm power, specialized flotation devices enable waterskiing and swimming activities, and several kinds of seated skis and snowboards make the mountain slopes accessible. People with physical limitations can play a long list of sports, including track and field, volleyball, tennis, golf, soccer, basketball, bowling, archery, tai chi, and karate, just to name a few.

In fact, every four years the Paralympic Games host over 4,000 athletes from more than 170 countries. They compete in 22 different sports, including the newly added canoeing and triathlon.[4] The athleticism displayed at the games demonstrates that physical limitations do not have to hinder the achievement of even the highest levels of physical fitness. With personal motivation, support from friends and family, and assistance from medical and fitness professionals, persons with disabilities can enjoy physically active lives.

Sources:
1. Centers for Disease Control and Prevention, "Prevalence of Disability and Disability Type among Adults—United States, 2013," *Morbidity and Mortality Weekly Report* 64, no. 29 (2015): 777-83.
2. Office of Disease Prevention and Health Promotion, US Department of Health and Human Services, *2008 Physical Activity Guidelines for Americans: Be Active, Healthy, and Happy!* ODPHP Publication no. U0036 (Washington, DC: US Department of Health and Human Services, 2008).
3. J. S. Schiller, J. W. Lucas, and J. A. Peregoy, "Summary Health Statistics for US Adults: National Health Interview Survey, 2011," *National Center for Health Statistics, Vital Health Stat*, no. 256 (2012).
4. Official website of the Paralympic Movement, August 2015, www.paralympic.org

---

Exercise benefits your child too. It improves stress tolerance and enhances brain development.[21] Research shows you can even decrease your child's risk of lifelong chronic diseases by staying active and eating a healthy diet while pregnant.[22] The American College of Obstetricians and Gynecologists presents these guidelines for safe exercise during pregnancy.[23]

- Get your doctor's approval for exercise.
- Seek out a pregnancy fitness exercise program with qualified instructors.
- Choose activities that are safe for you and your fetus. Avoid high-intensity sports, activities with fall risk,

and environments with extreme temperatures and barometric pressure changes (e.g., scuba diving).

- Aim for 150 minutes per week of moderate exercise.
- Monitor your exercise intensity during workouts and adjust to moderate levels as needed.
- In your third trimester, avoid exercises in which you lie on your back; these may restrict blood flow to the fetus.
- Do three to five sets of *kegel* or pelvic-floor exercises each day by tightening the pelvic-floor muscles 10 times in a row and holding each squeeze for 5 to 15 seconds. These can reduce postpartum incontinence and recovery time.

LO 2.8 How Can I Get Started Improving My Fitness Behaviors?

You know that exercise is good for you, but starting a fitness program and sticking with it over the long term can be a real challenge! If you are unsure how to start, you may have the impulse to just jump right in, do something your friends are doing, or try something you saw on TV or in a magazine. This haphazard approach often leads to disappointment and frustration—not to mention muscle soreness and even injury. A better approach is to:

- Think carefully about your exercise motivations, goals, and needs
- Select activities that will meet those needs (and that you enjoy!)
- Apply the FITT formula to each of those activities
- Make a conscious long-term commitment to your exercise program

To begin, fill out **Lab 2.1** to assess your readiness to become more physically active and to determine whether you should see a health care provider before you begin. Next, review the Stages of Behavior Change from Chapter 1. The stages are shown in **Figure 2.5**, where you can determine your Physical Activity Stage of Change and work toward the next stage. Lastly, as you plan your fitness program, ask yourself: What motivates me? What obstacles are in my way? What are reasonable fitness goals that I can set for myself? Am I prepared to commit to a fitness program?

Do It!
Access these labs at the end of the chapter or online at MasteringHealth™.

Understand Your Motivations

What are your main motivations for fitness and physical activity? Do you participate in sports? Are you active with friends? Why or why not? Which of your activities are the most fun, and what makes them so? Thinking about your answers to these questions is important because if you understand your motivations for exercise,

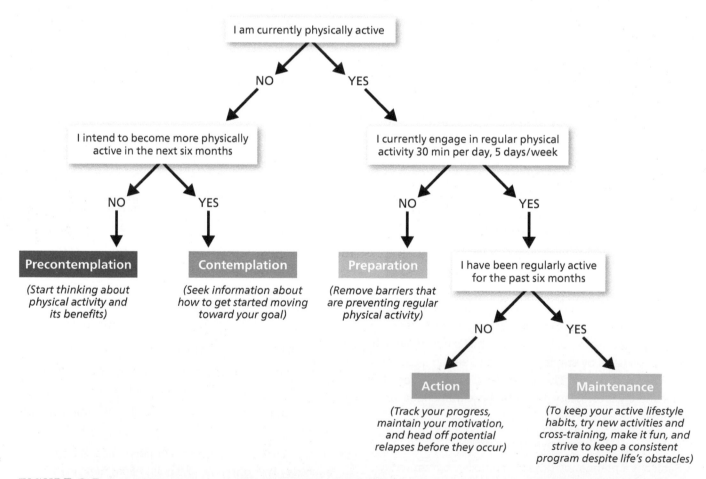

FIGURE **2.5** Answer the questions in the flowchart above to figure out your personal stage of change. Then, reflect on the suggestions under your stage for moving to the next stage (until you reach Maintenance).

Source: B. H. Marcus and B. A. Lewis, "Physical Activity and the Stages of Motivational Readiness for Change Model," *President's Council on Physical Fitness and Sports Research Digest* 4, no.1 (2003): 1–8.

you can plan activities in a way that makes you more likely to stick with them. Below are some of the most common reasons people decide to exercise, along with tips for maximizing your chances of long-term success.

- *I want to be healthier.* Sometimes a negative health event—like a loved one having a heart attack or stroke—will galvanize you into thinking about your own health. If this is your main motivation for starting your fitness program, try to design a program centered on physical activities that you find *easy to incorporate* in your day-to-day life. If you don't like gyms, don't sign up for one! Instead, select an activity that you genuinely enjoy and will do on most days, such as walking with a friend or family member.

- *I want to have fun.* What types of things make you happy? Can those be turned into active pursuits? Read or watch a movie while you ride an exercise bike or stretch. Recruit friends for a hike to catch up on your social time while being active, too. Join an intramural sports team on campus. If you seek out activities that you enjoy, you can have fun and the beneficial "side effect" of fitness. No matter what your choice of activity, consistent physical activity can lift your mood[24] and your ability to have more fun!

- *I want to meet new people or exercise with friends.* Participating in a fitness program can be a great way to socialize and being accountable to another person is a good way to keep a new exerciser coming back. Researchers confirm that the social aspect of sports and activities—a sense of belonging to a team, a gym, or simply a group of friends who like to play Frisbee in the park—helps people enjoy fitness activities and stick with them.[25] Look for classes, clubs, or teams that you can join with friends or where you can meet new people with similar interests.

- *I like the challenge of setting goals and doing well in competition.* If this sounds like you, regardless of what activity you choose, be sure to set realistic, attainable goals. You may find a clearly defined target—such as an upcoming 5K race—to be just what you need to get started, so sign up!

- *I want to lose some weight.* If weight loss is your main motivation, consider your nutrition and diet along with your fitness plan. Choose activities that burn plenty of calories and that you will enjoy doing often.

- *I would like to have a stronger, more toned body.* If this is your primary reason, select your favorite aerobic activity, begin strength training, or take a sport-specific class.

Anticipate and Overcome Obstacles

If you are not currently active, why not? Are you too busy? Do you simply dislike exercise? You can probably identify several things that keep you from being as active as you want to be.

Obstacles, or **barriers to physical activity**, can be categorized as either environmental or personal.

Environmental barriers include both physical and social factors that may make it harder for you to exercise. Do you feel safe exercising around your campus? Does the weather stop you from exercising? Are facilities closed during the hours that you need them? Do your friends prefer sedentary hobbies? These environmental factors can greatly affect your exercise habits.

Likewise, *personal barriers* can play a role in whether you are successful. Typical personal barriers include lack of self-motivation, injury, starting fitness levels, body weight issues, disability, relationship difficulties, financial limitations, or psychological problems such as depression or anxiety. Older-than-average students, students with children, and those who work long hours while attending school often face unique challenges as they work to improve their fitness. The Overcoming Common Obstacles to Exercise box provides strategies for overcoming specific obstacles. **Lab 2.2** at the end of this chapter helps you assess your motivations and identify your obstacles.

Do It! Access these labs at the end of the chapter or online at MasteringHealth™.

Make Time for Exercise

People often state that they don't exercise because they don't have enough time. That might be the case—or they

barriers to physical activity Personal or environmental issues that hinder your participation in regular physical activity

Overcoming Common Obstacles to Exercise

Below are strategies for overcoming common obstacles to exercise.

Obstacle: Lack of Time

- Monitor your daily activities for one week. Identify at least three 30-minute time slots you could use for physical activity.
- Add physical activity to your daily routine. For example, walk or ride your bike to work or shopping, walk your dog, exercise while you watch TV, and so on.
- Select activities requiring minimal time, such as walking, jogging, or stair-climbing.

Obstacle: Social Influence

- Explain your interest in physical activity to friends and family. Ask them to support your efforts.
- Invite friends and family members to exercise with you. Plan social activities involving exercise.
- Develop new friendships with physically active people. Join a group, such as the YMCA or a hiking club.

Obstacle: Lack of Energy

- Schedule physical activity for times in the day or week when you feel energetic.
- Convince yourself that if you give it a chance, physical activity will increase your energy level; then try it.

Obstacle: Lack of Willpower

- Plan ahead. Make physical activity a regular part of your schedule and write it on your calendar.
- Invite a friend to exercise with you on a regular basis and write it on your calendar.
- Join an exercise group or class.

Obstacle: Fear of Injury

- Learn how to warm up and cool down to prevent injury.
- Learn how to exercise appropriately considering your age, fitness level, skill level, and health status.
- Choose activities involving minimum risk.

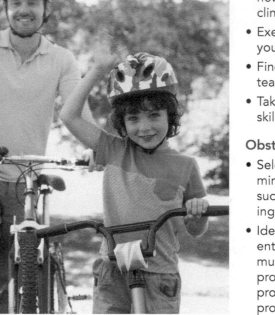

Obstacle: Lack of Skill

- Select activities requiring no new skills, such as walking, climbing stairs, or jogging.
- Exercise with friends who are at your skill level.
- Find a friend who is willing to teach you some new skills.
- Take a class to develop new skills.

Obstacle: Lack of Resources

- Select activities that require minimal facilities or equipment, such as walking, jogging, jumping rope, or calisthenics.
- Identify inexpensive, convenient resources in your community (community education programs, park and recreation programs, campus and worksite programs, etc.).

TRY IT! **Today**, write one activity that you could add for each of the following goals. What do you anticipate to be your primary obstacles for each activity?

	Activity	Obstacle
• more social contact	_____	_____
• more fun	_____	_____
• for five minutes a day	_____	_____

Write down how you will get around each of your obstacles, post reminders around your home, and try out each activity at least once **this week**.

After **two weeks,** evaluate your new activities. Do you look forward to them? Are they becoming part of your regular routine? Did your obstacles disappear or at least become easier?

Source: Adapted from Centers for Disease Control and Prevention, "Physical Activity for Everyone: Overcoming Barriers to Physical Activity," March 2013, www.cdc.gov; US Department of Health and Human Services, *Promoting Physical Activity: A Guide for Community Action*, 2nd ed. (1999).

may simply be assigning exercise a lesser priority in their life than other activities, such as watching TV or texting friends. While socializing and scheduling downtime in a busy life *are* important, consider how much time you spend on sedentary pursuits. Then consider the benefits to your health and sense of well-being if you replaced some of that sedentary time with physical activity.

To successfully stick with a fitness program, prioritize exercise the same way that you prioritize your classes, homework, job, and social life. Schedule your exercise sessions into your calendar. Prove to yourself that you are serious about getting fit by *making* time for exercise. Practice prioritizing active pursuits over sedentary ones by completing the Online Lab: Changing Your Sedentary Time into Active Time in the Mastering-Health Study Area.

Select Fun and Convenient Activities

Even if you have set aside time to exercise, you may not always *want* to. If you are accustomed to a sedentary lifestyle, it can be difficult to tear yourself away from the computer or get off the couch. One way to counter a lack of motivation is to choose fun activities. If your workout is a form of play, you will look forward to it time and time again.

Choosing the best type of exercise is also about convenience. Despite your good intentions and high level of motivation, if it's not convenient for your existing lifestyle and commitments, you will have a hard time sticking with it. Think about things you already do that can be expanded or changed to count as exercise and physical activity. Do you have a dog? Try walking your dog faster or work up to jogging. Do you walk from the bus stop to campus? Walk faster or take a route that is longer or incorporates a hill.

Activities can be classified into three general categories or types: lifestyle physical activities, exercise training options, and sports and recreational activities. **Figure 2.6** illustrates examples of moderate to vigorous activities from which you can choose.

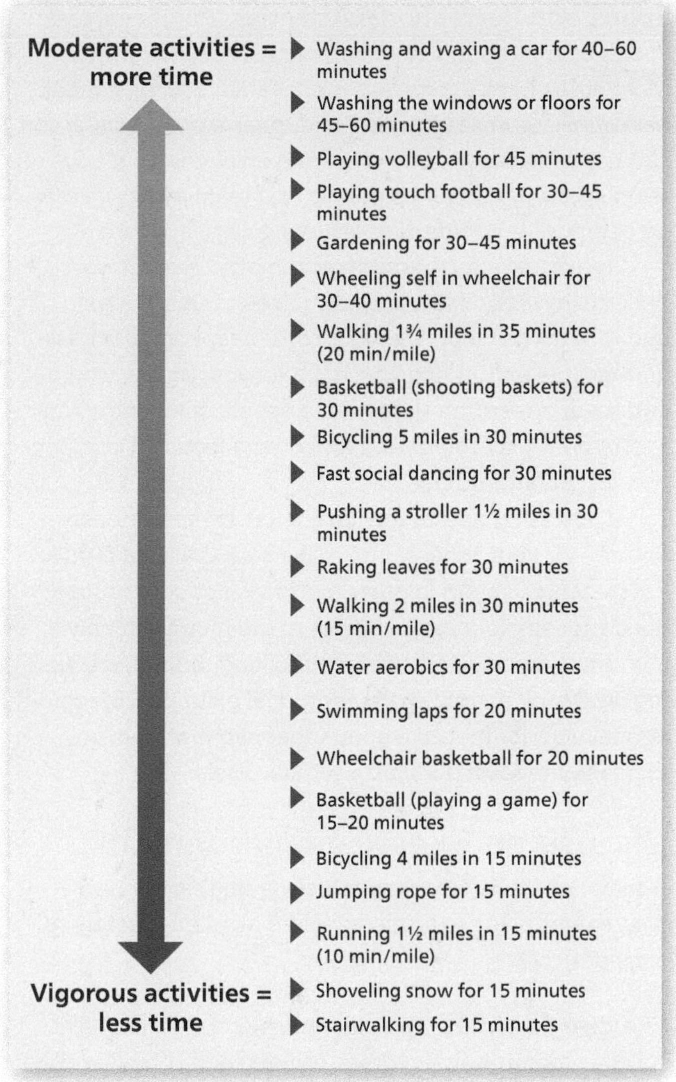

Lifestyle Physical Activities Lifestyle physical activities, sometimes called leisure-time physical activities, are those that you perform during daily life. These include things such as walking or biking to class. Lifestyle physical activities can be light, moderate, or vigorous, depending on the task and how long it takes. For instance, watering your garden for 15 minutes may be a light activity, but raking leaves for four hours can be vigorous.

A good way to increase your daily "dose" of lifestyle physical activity is to actively commute whenever you

Moderate activities = more time

- Washing and waxing a car for 40–60 minutes
- Washing the windows or floors for 45–60 minutes
- Playing volleyball for 45 minutes
- Playing touch football for 30–45 minutes
- Gardening for 30–45 minutes
- Wheeling self in wheelchair for 30–40 minutes
- Walking 1¾ miles in 35 minutes (20 min/mile)
- Basketball (shooting baskets) for 30 minutes
- Bicycling 5 miles in 30 minutes
- Fast social dancing for 30 minutes
- Pushing a stroller 1½ miles in 30 minutes
- Raking leaves for 30 minutes
- Walking 2 miles in 30 minutes (15 min/mile)
- Water aerobics for 30 minutes
- Swimming laps for 20 minutes
- Wheelchair basketball for 20 minutes
- Basketball (playing a game) for 15–20 minutes
- Bicycling 4 miles in 15 minutes
- Jumping rope for 15 minutes
- Running 1½ miles in 15 minutes (10 min/mile)
- Shoveling snow for 15 minutes
- Stairwalking for 15 minutes

Vigorous activities = less time

FIGURE **2.6** Examples of moderate to vigorous physical activities.

Source: Data from Centers for Disease Control and Prevention, "A Report of the Surgeon General: Physical Activity and Health At-A-Glance, 1996," accessed May 2013, www.cdc.gov

can. Think about how you can walk or ride your bike to class, work, social events, or run errands, and start doing it regularly! Complete Lab 2.3 to evaluate how many steps you take in a day. What you find might surprise you.

Do It!
Access these labs at the end of the chapter or online at MasteringHealth™.

Exercise Training Options When planning a fitness program, most people think of typical exercise options. These include cycling, running, weight training, indoor cardio workouts, fitness classes, yoga, tai chi, lap swimming, and water aerobics. These activities are great for specifically increasing your fitness. Consider including a few sports and recreational activities every now and then to keep yourself motivated and your body challenged.

Sports and Recreational Activities Traditional team sports offer a great deal of fun, motivation, and fitness. Most cities have sports leagues for adult soccer, softball, basketball, ultimate Frisbee, and other team sports. If you like the camaraderie of a team and enjoy the challenge of team sports, you may be able to find team sports classes on campus, at community centers, and in sports clubs.

Individual sports activities can offer great fitness benefits as well. Court sports such as tennis, squash, and racquetball increase your cardiorespiratory fitness and muscle endurance and improve your agility, coordination, and reaction time. Some people enjoy individual sports purely for recreation and others focus on competition for fun and fitness.

If you are going to rely on a sport or recreational activity for your fitness, just make sure that it is *regular*. For instance, skiing is great, but does not constitute a good fitness program if you get to the mountain only a few times a year. Golf, mountain biking, hiking, ice skating, and rock climbing are additional examples of recreational and competitive sports that can maintain or increase fitness if done on a regular basis.

Choose an Exercise Environment

A major obstacle for many people is finding a suitable, convenient place to work out. Here are some factors to consider:

Exercise Facilities You can find exercise facilities at colleges, community centers, athletic and fitness clubs, parks, YMCAs, corporate fitness centers, and schools. Choose a convenient location because the farther it is from your home, the less likely you are to use it. Other factors to consider are variety of classes, quality of cardio and weight equipment, hours that are compatible with your schedule, and ease of parking (if you drive) or bus access. Additionally, you may be looking for a swimming pool, basketball and racquetball courts, locker rooms, showers, or spa.

Cost can be a big factor. Large facilities will likely be more expensive than a basic fitness center. Community centers and parks often offer reasonable day or multiday fees. Almost all facilities offer day passes for a fee or even free passes to check out the facility. Try out the facility for several days before you invest. Determine whether you like the atmosphere, equipment, and instructors, and whether you feel safe and comfortable there.

If you have not taken advantage of your college facilities yet, you may be missing out on a good deal. As a student, you can typically get access to classes, courts, leagues, equipment, and even personal trainers. College

is the perfect time to try out new sports and fitness activities.

Neighborhood When people live in safe neighborhoods where it is easy to exercise, they are more likely to be active.[26] This is becoming a bigger issue as growing cities and suburbs lead to an increase in urban sprawl. Some experts even suggest that urban sprawl is partially to blame for the rise in obesity in the United States. For example, researchers in New Jersey found that residents of sprawling counties were less likely to walk during leisure time, more likely to have high blood pressure, and weighed more than residents living in compact urban areas.[27]

This relates to the type of "built environment" around you. Living near streets that encourage physical activity (with sidewalks, bike lanes, street lights, slower traffic) and parks with bike and walking paths increases your ability to stay active.[28]

Weather The impact of weather will, of course, depend on where you live and the time of year. If you are prepared, you can exercise in most weather conditions. Check weather reports before heading out. Pay attention to your body once you get outside. If you feel too hot when exercising outside, slow down, move into the shade, and consider suspending your workout for the day. Limit your exercise time in the rain if you become too wet and cold.

Safety Do you feel safe walking to the local gym to exercise? Do you feel comfortable jogging around your neighborhood? In order to maintain a regular exercise routine, you need to feel safe and comfortable in your surroundings. Consider the suggestions below for exercising safely:

- Any time you do activities outside, tell someone about your plans and always bring your ID, phone, and emergency contact information. Install a safety app on

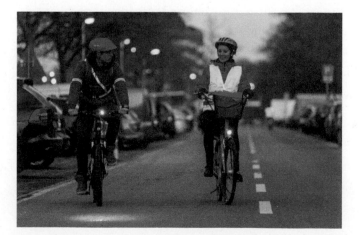

your phone to give you quick access to emergency responses (siren, 911 call, GPS coordinates to contacts) and/or alerts triggered by inactivity, which can be important if you are injured.

- Stay alert. Keep your eyes off your phone. When listening to music, wear only one ear bud so you can hear approaching people, dogs, and traffic.

- If your neighborhood is not safe, exercise with a friend or training group or drive to a different location. If you are traveling and unfamiliar with the area, ask around and stick to safe places.

- If you are exercising at night or around traffic, use lights, wear bright reflective clothing, and aim for streets that are less busy. Face traffic when walking or running, especially when no sidewalks exist.

- If you are heading into a wilderness area, go with a friend or at least let someone know specifically where you are going and when you will return. Know your route and carry a map, a cell phone, and a spare tube/pump/tools (if you're biking). Also bring basic safety supplies, including food and water for at least a day, a flashlight or headlamp, first-aid supplies, a pocketknife, and a space or emergency blanket.

- Exercise facilities are typically safe. If you have any concerns, talk to the manager and get an escort to your car.

Set Reasonable Goals, Plan Rewards, and Commit

Setting realistic goals can mean the difference between success and failure. People often start a fitness program and think they can start running a few miles right away—which may be unrealistic.

The best advice? Have a plan, start small, and build! Just five minutes every other day doing push-ups and abdominal curl can really help increase your muscle strength and endurance. Over time and with your increasing fitness, you will naturally want to increase your time. Before you know it, you have developed a habit of working on your upper body and core muscles for 20 minutes three to four times per week.

Setting reasonable goals includes considering everything that you have assessed about yourself: fitness level, motivations, and exercise barriers. If you are new to exercise, structure your goals around the sample exercise plans in Activate, Motivate, & Advance Your Fitness: A Walking Program in this chapter (page 63).

Plan Your Rewards Rewards are highly individual and the key is to come up with ones that reinforce your new,

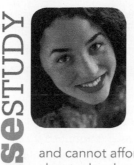
more active lifestyle. New exercisers often rely on **external exercise rewards** (also called extrinsic)—at least initially. External exercise rewards can be anything from a new workout wardrobe to a celebratory dinner to the admiration and praise of your peers or fitness instructor. **Internal exercise rewards** (also called intrinsic) commonly involve feeling better about yourself, having more energy, and increased life satisfaction from exercising. As you incorporate regular exercise into your life, you may find that internal rewards become more important to you.

Long-term exercisers often report that internal exercise rewards are their primary motivation. In fact, exercise releases endorphins in your body that can fill you with a sense of well-being,[29] so that physical activity itself is the reward. Exercisers who have internal motivations are more apt to stick with a regular fitness

external exercise rewards
Rewards for exercise that come from outside of a person (trophy, compliment, day at the spa)

internal exercise rewards
Rewards for exercise that are based upon how one is feeling physically and mentally (sense of accomplishment, relaxation, increased self-esteem)

program, whereas too much external motivation is associated with lower activity levels.[30] So, do it for yourself! Figure out your internal motivations and use them to get yourself moving.

Make a Personal Commitment to Regular Exercise

The first step to changing your exercise behaviors is deciding to do it. The harder step is to commit to that decision. Examine what a more active lifestyle would mean to you and write out your personal commitment statement: a list of reasons to commit to fitness. Review this list regularly until your new behaviors become routine.

Remember that changing behavior takes perseverance. If you feel your commitment waning, reread your personal commitment statement and remind yourself of the reasons you began your program in the first place. Don't be hard on yourself. Allow yourself a few setbacks along the way. Take them *in stride*, and don't let those setbacks stop you from reaching your ultimate goals.

See It!
Watch 3 Big Mistakes Sabotaging Your Workout at MasteringHealth™.

Study Plan

chapter summary

LO 2.1 Three Levels of Physical Activity

- (1) light/lifestyle/physical activities (<3 METS), (2) moderate physical activities (3 to 6 METS), and (3) vigorous physical activities (>6 METS)

LO 2.2 Health-Related Components of Physical Fitness

- **Cardiorespiratory endurance** is the ability of the cardiovascular and respiratory systems to provide oxygen to working muscles during sustained exercise.
- **Muscular strength** is the ability of your muscles to exert force.
- **Muscular endurance** is the ability of your muscles to contract repeatedly over time.
- **Flexibility** is the ability to move your joints in a full range of motion.
- **Body composition** refers to the relative amounts of fat and lean tissue in your body.

LO 2.3 Skill-Related Components of Physical Fitness

- Skill-related components include agility, balance, coordination, power, speed, and reaction time.

LO 2.4 Fitness Principles

- The **overload** principle: to see improvement, you must do more training than your body is used to.
- The **progression** principle: to increase fitness levels safely and effectively, you need to gradually increase body system overloads over time.

- The **specificity** principle: a body system will improve only if that specific body system is stressed or overloaded by the activity you are doing.
- The **reversibility** principle: your fitness levels will slip if you do not maintain a minimal level of physical activity and exercise.
- The **individuality** principle: adaptations to a training overload may vary greatly from person to person.
- The **rest and recovery** principle: your body needs time to recover and adapt to the increased training stresses to avoid **overtraining**.

LO 2.5 How Much Exercise Is Enough?

- Aim for the minimal recommendations of 150 minutes of moderate physical activity each week (or 75 minutes of vigorous), plus muscular fitness exercises twice a week.

LO 2.6 How to Exercise Safely

- Warm up by doing light activity and dynamic movements. Cool down after exercise.
- Learn the physical skills required, consume enough energy and water, and select appropriate footwear and clothing.

LO 2.7 Individual Factors for Fitness Programming

- Adapt general recommendations to fit individual needs.

LO 2.8 Getting Started Improving Fitness Behaviors

- Select activities and exercise environments, apply the FITT formula, plan rewards, and commit to your new fitness behaviors!

review questions

LO 2.1 **1.** Examples of moderate physical activity include
  a. yard work, housework, and leisurely walking.
  b. cycling, weight training, and brisk walking.
  c. hard physical labor, jogging, and aerobics classes.
  d. playing competitive sports, cycling up a steep hill, and running.

LO 2.2 **2.** Which health-related component of fitness involves moving your joints through a full range of motion?
  a. Cardiorespiratory fitness
  b. Muscular endurance
  c. Flexibility
  d. Body composition

LO 2.3 **3.** Which skill-related component of fitness is most involved in braking quickly when a car in front of you stops suddenly?
  a. Agility
  b. Power
  c. Coordination
  d. Reaction time

review questions CONTINUED

LO 2.4 **4.** Which fitness principle refers to subjecting the body or body system to more physical activity than it is accustomed to?
a. Overload
b. Adaptation
c. Dose-response
d. Specificity

LO 2.4 **5.** The principle of individuality with respect to fitness states that
a. adaptations to training overload may vary widely from person to person.
b. all individuals respond the same way to exercise.
c. genetic makeup has nothing to do with individual responses to exercise.
d. non-responders are individuals who do not benefit from exercise.

LO 2.5 **6.** The 2008 Physical Activity Guidelines for Americans emphasize
a. vigorous physical activity every day of the week.
b. moderate physical activity for 150 minutes per week or vigorous physical activity for 75 minutes per week.
c. resistance training for 300 minutes per week.
d. limiting the amount of time you spend walking.

LO 2.6 **7.** A proper warm-up consists of
a. a few quick side bends.
b. stretches that you hold for one minute or more.

c. quick stair climbing.
d. a gradual increase in body temperature and easy movements in the muscles and joints.

LO 2.7 **8.** Experiencing knee pain can be categorized as having a(n) _____ barrier to physical activity.
a. social
b. scheduling
c. environmental
d. personal

LO 2.8 **9.** Which of the following is an example of an internal exercise reward?
a. Buying new workout clothing
b. Having fun while exercising
c. Placing third in your age group in the local 5K race
d. Taking a celebratory trip after meeting an exercise goal

LO 2.8 **10.** Enlisting a friend, classmate, or co-worker to be your workout buddy and hold you accountable is a good strategy for which common exercise obstacle below?
a. Lack of time
b. Travel
c. Weather conditions
d. Lack of willpower

critical thinking questions

LO 2.4 **1.** Give an example of how training overload can lead to adaptations and training effects.

LO 2.4 **2.** Describe the similarities and differences between the principle of diminished returns and the principle of progression.

LO 2.5 **3.** Imagine you are about to begin a fitness program centered on bicycling. Apply the FITT formula to describe how you might set up your program.

LO 2.6 **4.** If you are reluctant to increase your activity level due to fear of injury, what are five strategies that will help you overcome those fears and avoid injury?

LO 2.8 **5.** Exercise options include lifestyle physical activities, exercise training options, and sports/recreational activities. Think of at least one activity in each category that you can incorporate into your weekly schedule.

check out these eResources

- **ACSM** Exercise guidelines, position statements, certification, and physical activity advocacy news and information. **www.acsm.org**
- **Centers for Disease Control and Prevention, Physical Activity** Physical activity guidelines, statistics, videos, and walking program information. **www.cdc.gov/physicalactivity**
- **ExRx.net** A website with exercise programs, fitness testing calculators, general questions, and links to

additional resources. Click on the "Beginner's Page" if you are just getting started. **http://exrx.net**
- **TED Talks** Search for "Exercise" or "Amy Balcetis" to learn why some people find exercise more difficult than other people do. **www.ted.com**
- **WebMD** Click on "Living Healthy," then "Fitness & Exercise" for articles, slideshows, and quizzes about a variety of exercise topics. **www.webmd.com**

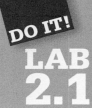
ASSESS YOURSELF

ASSESS YOUR PHYSICAL
ACTIVITY READINESS

MasteringHealth™

Name: _____ Date: _____

Instructor: _____ Section: _____

2016 PAR-Q+

The Physical Activity Readiness Questionnaire for Everyone

The health benefits of regular physical activity are clear; more people should engage in physical activity every day of the week. Participating in physical activity is very safe for MOST people. This questionnaire will tell you whether it is necessary for you to seek further advice from your doctor OR a qualified exercise professional before becoming more physically active.

GENERAL HEALTH QUESTIONS

Please read the 7 questions below carefully and answer each one honestly: check YES or NO.	YES	NO
1) Has your doctor ever said that you have a heart condition ☐ OR high blood pressure ☐?	☐	☐
2) Do you feel pain in your chest at rest, during your daily activities of living, **OR** when you do physical activity?	☐	☐
3) Do you lose balance because of dizziness **OR** have you lost consciousness in the last 12 months? Please answer **NO** if your dizziness was associated with over-breathing (including during vigorous exercise).	☐	☐
4) Have you ever been diagnosed with another chronic medical condition (other than heart disease or high blood pressure)? **PLEASE LIST CONDITION(S) HERE:** _____	☐	☐
5) Are you currently taking prescribed medications for a chronic medical condition? **PLEASE LIST CONDITION(S) AND MEDICATIONS HERE:** _____	☐	☐
6) Do you currently have (or have had within the past 12 months) a bone, joint, or soft tissue (muscle, ligament, or tendon) problem that could be made worse by becoming more physically active? Please answer **NO** if you had a problem in the past, but it *does not limit your current ability* to be physically active. **PLEASE LIST CONDITION(S) HERE:** _____	☐	☐
7) Has your doctor ever said that you should only do medically supervised physical activity?	☐	☐

☑ **If you answered NO to all of the questions above, you are cleared for physical activity.**
Go to Page 4 to sign the PARTICIPANT DECLARATION. You do not need to complete Pages 2 and 3.

▶ Start becoming much more physically active – start slowly and build up gradually.

▶ Follow International Physical Activity Guidelines for your age (www.who.int/dietphysicalactivity/en/).

▶ You may take part in a health and fitness appraisal.

▶ If you are over the age of 45 yr and **NOT** accustomed to regular vigorous to maximal effort exercise, consult a qualified exercise professional before engaging in this intensity of exercise.

▶ If you have any further questions, contact a qualified exercise professional.

⬤ **If you answered YES to one or more of the questions above, COMPLETE PAGES 2 AND 3.**

⚠ **Delay becoming more active if:**

✓ You have a temporary illness such as a cold or fever; it is best to wait until you feel better.

✓ You are pregnant - talk to your health care practitioner, your physician, a qualified exercise professional, and/or complete the ePARmed-X+ at **www.eparmedx.com** before becoming more physically active.

✓ Your health changes - answer the questions on Pages 2 and 3 of this document and/or talk to your doctor or a qualified exercise professional before continuing with any physical activity program.

 OSHF
Ontario Society for Health and Fitness

Copyright © 2016 PAR-Q+ Collaboration   1 / 4
01-01-2016

Source: www.csep.ca/cmfiles/publications/parq/parqplussept2011version_all.pdf

2016 PAR-Q+

FOLLOW-UP QUESTIONS ABOUT YOUR MEDICAL CONDITION(S)

1.   **Do you have Arthritis, Osteoporosis, or Back Problems?**

If the above condition(s) is/are present, answer questions 1a-1c   If **NO** ☐ go to question 2

1a.	Do you have difficulty controlling your condition with medications or other physician-prescribed therapies? (Answer **NO** if you are not currently taking medications or other treatments)	YES ☐ NO ☐
1b.	Do you have joint problems causing pain, a recent fracture or fracture caused by osteoporosis or cancer, displaced vertebra (e.g., spondylolisthesis), and/or spondylolysis/pars defect (a crack in the bony ring on the back of the spinal column)?	YES ☐ NO ☐
1c.	Have you had steroid injections or taken steroid tablets regularly for more than 3 months?	YES ☐ NO ☐

2.   **Do you currently have Cancer of any kind?**

If the above condition(s) is/are present, answer questions 2a-2b   If **NO** ☐ go to question 3

2a.	Does your cancer diagnosis include any of the following types: lung/bronchogenic, multiple myeloma (cancer of plasma cells), head, and/or neck?	YES ☐ NO ☐
2b.	Are you currently receiving cancer therapy (such as chemotheraphy or radiotherapy)?	YES ☐ NO ☐

3.   **Do you have a Heart or Cardiovascular Condition?** *This includes Coronary Artery Disease, Heart Failure, Diagnosed Abnormality of Heart Rhythm*

If the above condition(s) is/are present, answer questions 3a-3d   If **NO** ☐ go to question 4

3a.	Do you have difficulty controlling your condition with medications or other physician-prescribed therapies? (Answer **NO** if you are not currently taking medications or other treatments)	YES ☐ NO ☐
3b.	Do you have an irregular heart beat that requires medical management? (e.g., atrial fibrillation, premature ventricular contraction)	YES ☐ NO ☐
3c.	Do you have chronic heart failure?	YES ☐ NO ☐
3d.	Do you have diagnosed coronary artery (cardiovascular) disease and have not participated in regular physical activity in the last 2 months?	YES ☐ NO ☐

4.   **Do you have High Blood Pressure?**

If the above condition(s) is/are present, answer questions 4a-4b   If **NO** ☐ go to question 5

4a.	Do you have difficulty controlling your condition with medications or other physician-prescribed therapies? (Answer **NO** if you are not currently taking medications or other treatments)	YES ☐ NO ☐
4b.	Do you have a resting blood pressure equal to or greater than 160/90 mmHg with or without medication? (Answer **YES** if you do not know your resting blood pressure)	YES ☐ NO ☐

5.   **Do you have any Metabolic Conditions?** *This includes Type 1 Diabetes, Type 2 Diabetes, Pre-Diabetes*

If the above condition(s) is/are present, answer questions 5a-5e   If **NO** ☐ go to question 6

5a.	Do you often have difficulty controlling your blood sugar levels with foods, medications, or other physician-prescribed therapies?	YES ☐ NO ☐
5b.	Do you often suffer from signs and symptoms of low blood sugar (hypoglycemia) following exercise and/or during activities of daily living? Signs of hypoglycemia may include shakiness, nervousness, unusual irritability, abnormal sweating, dizziness or light-headedness, mental confusion, difficulty speaking, weakness, or sleepiness.	YES ☐ NO ☐
5c.	Do you have any signs or symptoms of diabetes complications such as heart or vascular disease and/or complications affecting your eyes, kidneys, **OR** the sensation in your toes and feet?	YES ☐ NO ☐
5d.	Do you have other metabolic conditions (such as current pregnancy-related diabetes, chronic kidney disease, or liver problems)?	YES ☐ NO ☐
5e.	Are you planning to engage in what for you is unusually high (or vigorous) intensity exercise in the near future?	YES ☐ NO ☐

   2 / 4

01-01-2016

2016 PAR-Q+

6.   **Do you have any Mental Health Problems or Learning Difficulties?** *This includes Alzheimer's, Dementia, Depression, Anxiety Disorder, Eating Disorder, Psychotic Disorder, Intellectual Disability, Down Syndrome*

         If the above condition(s) is/are present, answer questions 6a-6b   If **NO** ☐ go to question 7

6a.	Do you have difficulty controlling your condition with medications or other physician-prescribed therapies? (Answer **NO** if you are not currently taking medications or other treatments)	YES ☐ NO ☐
6b.	Do you have Down Syndrome **AND** back problems affecting nerves or muscles?	YES ☐ NO ☐

7.   **Do you have a Respiratory Disease?** *This includes Chronic Obstructive Pulmonary Disease, Asthma, Pulmonary High Blood Pressure*

         If the above condition(s) is/are present, answer questions 7a-7d   If **NO** ☐ go to question 8

7a.	Do you have difficulty controlling your condition with medications or other physician-prescribed therapies? (Answer **NO** if you are not currently taking medications or other treatments)	YES ☐ NO ☐
7b.	Has your doctor ever said your blood oxygen level is low at rest or during exercise and/or that you require supplemental oxygen therapy?	YES ☐ NO ☐
7c.	If asthmatic, do you currently have symptoms of chest tightness, wheezing, laboured breathing, consistent cough (more than 2 days/week), or have you used your rescue medication more than twice in the last week?	YES ☐ NO ☐
7d.	Has your doctor ever said you have high blood pressure in the blood vessels of your lungs?	YES ☐ NO ☐

8.   **Do you have a Spinal Cord Injury?** *This includes Tetraplegia and Paraplegia*

         If the above condition(s) is/are present, answer questions 8a-8c   If **NO** ☐ go to question 9

8a.	Do you have difficulty controlling your condition with medications or other physician-prescribed therapies? (Answer **NO** if you are not currently taking medications or other treatments)	YES ☐ NO ☐
8b.	Do you commonly exhibit low resting blood pressure significant enough to cause dizziness, light-headedness, and/or fainting?	YES ☐ NO ☐
8c.	Has your physician indicated that you exhibit sudden bouts of high blood pressure (known as Autonomic Dysreflexia)?	YES ☐ NO ☐

9.   **Have you had a Stroke?** *This includes Transient Ischemic Attack (TIA) or Cerebrovascular Event*

         If the above condition(s) is/are present, answer questions 9a-9c   If **NO** ☐ go to question 10

9a.	Do you have difficulty controlling your condition with medications or other physician-prescribed therapies? (Answer **NO** if you are not currently taking medications or other treatments)	YES ☐ NO ☐
9b.	Do you have any impairment in walking or mobility?	YES ☐ NO ☐
9c.	Have you experienced a stroke or impairment in nerves or muscles in the past 6 months?	YES ☐ NO ☐

10.   **Do you have any other medical condition not listed above or do you have two or more medical conditions?**

         If you have other medical conditions, answer questions 10a-10c   If **NO** ☐ read the Page 4 recommendations

10a.	Have you experienced a blackout, fainted, or lost consciousness as a result of a head injury within the last 12 months **OR** have you had a diagnosed concussion within the last 12 months?	YES ☐ NO ☐
10b.	Do you have a medical condition that is not listed (such as epilepsy, neurological conditions, kidney problems)?	YES ☐ NO ☐
10c.	Do you currently live with two or more medical conditions?	YES ☐ NO ☐

PLEASE LIST YOUR MEDICAL CONDITION(S) AND ANY RELATED MEDICATIONS HERE: _____

_____

GO to Page 4 for recommendations about your current medical condition(s) and sign the PARTICIPANT DECLARATION.

OSHF
Ontario Society for Health and Fitness

Copyright © 2016 PAR-Q+ Collaboration   3 / 4
01-01-2016

2016 PAR-Q+

☑ **If you answered NO to all of the follow-up questions about your medical condition, you are ready to become more physically active - sign the PARTICIPANT DECLARATION below:**

▶ It is advised that you consult a qualified exercise professional to help you develop a safe and effective physical activity plan to meet your health needs.

▶ You are encouraged to start slowly and build up gradually - 20 to 60 minutes of low to moderate intensity exercise, 3-5 days per week including aerobic and muscle strengthening exercises.

▶ As you progress, you should aim to accumulate 150 minutes or more of moderate intensity physical activity per week.

▶ If you are over the age of 45 yr and **NOT** accustomed to regular vigorous to maximal effort exercise, consult a qualified exercise professional before engaging in this intensity of exercise.

⬡ **If you answered YES to one or more of the follow-up questions about your medical condition:**

You should seek further information before becoming more physically active or engaging in a fitness appraisal. You should complete the specially designed online screening and exercise recommendations program - the **ePARmed-X+ at www.eparmedx.com** and/or visit a qualified exercise professional to work through the ePARmed-X+ and for further information.

⚠ **Delay becoming more active if:**

✓ You have a temporary illness such as a cold or fever; it is best to wait until you feel better.

✓ You are pregnant - talk to your health care practitioner, your physician, a qualified exercise professional, and/or complete the ePARmed-X+ **at www.eparmedx.com** before becoming more physically active.

✓ Your health changes - talk to your doctor or qualified exercise professional before continuing with any physical activity program.

● You are encouraged to photocopy the PAR-Q+. You must use the entire questionnaire and NO changes are permitted.
● The authors, the PAR-Q+ Collaboration, partner organizations, and their agents assume no liability for persons who undertake physical activity and/or make use of the PAR-Q+ or ePARmed-X+. If in doubt after completing the questionnaire, consult your doctor prior to physical activity.

PARTICIPANT DECLARATION

● All persons who have completed the PAR-Q+ please read and sign the declaration below.

● If you are less than the legal age required for consent or require the assent of a care provider, your parent, guardian or care provider must also sign this form.

I, the undersigned, have read, understood to my full satisfaction and completed this questionnaire. I acknowledge that this physical activity clearance is valid for a maximum of 12 months from the date it is completed and becomes invalid if my condition changes. I also acknowledge that a Trustee (such as my employer, community/fitness centre, health care provider, or other designate) may retain a copy of this form for their records. In these instances, the Trustee will be required to adhere to local, national, and international guidelines regarding the storage of personal health information ensuring that the Trustee maintains the privacy of the information and does not misuse or wrongfully disclose such information.

NAME _____   DATE _____

SIGNATURE _____   WITNESS _____

SIGNATURE OF PARENT/GUARDIAN/CARE PROVIDER _____

———— **For more information, please contact** ————
www.eparmedx.com
Email: eparmedx@gmail.com

Citation for PAR-Q+
Warburton DER, Jamnik VK, Bredin SSD, and Gledhill N on behalf of the PAR-Q+ Collaboration. The Physical Activity Readiness Questionnaire for Everyone (PAR-Q+) and Electronic Physical Activity Readiness Medical Examination (ePARmed-X+). Health & Fitness Journal of Canada 4(2):3-23, 2011.

Key References
1. Jamnik VK, Warburton DER, Makarski J, McKenzie DC, Shephard RJ, Stone J, and Gledhill N. Enhancing the effectiveness of clearance for physical activity participation; background and overall process. APNM 36(S1):S3-S13, 2011.
2. Warburton DER, Gledhill N, Jamnik VK, Bredin SSD, McKenzie DC, Stone J, Charlesworth S, and Shephard RJ. Evidence-based risk assessment and recommendations for physical activity clearance; Consensus Document. APNM 36(S1):S266-s298, 2011.
3. Chisholm DM, Collis ML, Kulak LL, Davenport W, and Gruber N. Physical activity readiness. British Columbia Medical Journal. 1975;17:375-378.
4. Thomas S, Reading J, and Shephard RJ. Revision of the Physical Activity Readiness Questionnaire (PAR-Q). Canadian Journal of Sport Science 1992;17:4 338-345.

The PAR-Q+ was created using the evidence-based AGREE process (1) by the PAR-Q+ Collaboration chaired by Dr. Darren E. R. Warburton with Dr. Norman Gledhill, Dr. Veronica Jamnik, and Dr. Donald C. McKenzie (2). Production of this document has been made possible through financial contributions from the Public Health Agency of Canada and the BC Ministry of Health Services. The views expressed herein do not necessarily represent the views of the Public Health Agency of Canada or the BC Ministry of Health Services.

OSHF
Ontario Society for Health and Fitness

Copyright © 2016 PAR-Q+ Collaboration 4 / 4
01-01-2016

Section IV: Reflection

1. After reviewing your answers to the questions in Sections I to III, do you feel ready to begin an exercise program? Why or why not?

_____

_____

_____

2. If you already exercise, what are you currently doing?

_____

_____

_____

3. If you exercised in the past but have stopped, what exercise did you do? Why did you stop?

_____

_____

_____

LAB 2.2 IDENTIFY YOUR PHYSICAL ACTIVITY MOTIVATIONS AND OBSTACLES

MasteringHealth™

Name: _____ Date: _____

Instructor: _____ Section: _____

Purpose: To identify your motivations for starting a physical activity, exercise, or sport (or maintaining your current fitness routine) and your obstacles to exercise, plus learn how to set up exercise-specific rewards to overcome those obstacles.

Section I: What Motivates You?

Assign a rating of 1 to 7 for each of the motivations listed below, using the following scale: 1 = not at all true for me, 7 = very true for me

I participate (or want to participate) in my physical activity or sport because:

_____ **1.** I want to be physically fit.

_____ **2.** It's fun.

_____ **3.** I like engaging in activities that physically challenge me.

_____ **4.** I want to obtain new skills.

_____ **5.** I want to maintain my weight and/or look better.

_____ **6.** I want to be with my friends.

_____ **7.** I like to do this activity.

_____ **8.** I want to improve existing skills.

_____ **9.** I like the challenge.

_____ **10.** I want to define my muscles so that I look better.

_____ **11.** It makes me happy.

_____ **12.** I want to keep up my current skill level.

_____ **13.** I want to have more energy.

_____ **14.** I like activities that are physically challenging.

_____ **15.** I like to be with others who are interested in this activity.

_____ **16.** I want to improve my cardiovascular fitness.

_____ **17.** I want to improve my appearance.

_____ **18.** I think it's interesting.

_____ **19.** I want to maintain my physical strength to live a healthy life.

_____ **20.** I want to be attractive to others.

_____ **21.** I want to meet new people.

_____ **22.** I enjoy this activity.

_____ **23.** I want to maintain my physical health and well-being.

_____ **24.** I want to improve my body shape.

_____ **25.** I want to get better at my activity.

_____ **26.** I find this activity stimulating.

_____ **27.** I will feel physically unattractive if I don't.

_____ **28.** My friends want me to.

_____ **29.** I like the excitement of participation.

_____ **30.** I enjoy spending time with others doing this activity.

Section II: Scoring Motivations

The following table lists the motivation categories for each question above. Fill in your scores for the questions above in the appropriate boxes (for example, in the box for "Q 2," enter the numerical value you answered for question #2). Then add the totals for each type of motivation. Your total scores reflect which category motivates you the most.

Interest/Enjoyment	Competence	Appearance	Fitness	Social
Q 2:	Q 3:	Q 5:	Q 1:	Q 6:
Q 7:	Q 4:	Q 10:	Q 13:	Q 15:
Q 11:	Q 8:	Q 17:	Q 16:	Q 21:
Q 18:	Q 9:	Q 20:	Q 19:	Q 28:
Q 22:	Q 12:	Q 24:	Q 23:	Q 30:
Q 26:	Q 14:	Q 27:		
Q 29:	Q 25:			
Total:	Total:	Total:	Total:	Total:

Source: Based on R. M. Ryan and C. M. Frederick, "Intrinsic Motivation and Exercise Adherence," *International Journal of Sport Psychology* 28 (1997); C. M. Frederick and R. M. Ryan, "Differences in Motivation for Sport and Exercise and Their Relationships with Participation and Mental Health," *Journal of Sport Behavior* 16 (1993).

Section III: Motivation Reflection

1. What were your highest and lowest motivators for physical activity or sport?

Highest: _____   Lowest: _____

2. Were you surprised by these results? Explain why or why not.

_____

3. How can you use your motivation preferences to increase your level of activity? (See the *Understand Your Motivations* section on page 44 in this chapter.)

_____

Section IV: What Keeps You from Being Active?

Listed below are common reasons that people give to describe why they do not get as much physical activity as they would like. Read each statement and indicate how likely you are to state the same reason.

How likely are you to say:	Very likely	Somewhat likely	Somewhat unlikely	Very unlikely
1. My day is so busy now, I just don't think I can make the time to include physical activity in my regular schedule.	3	2	1	0
2. None of my family members or friends like to do anything active, so I don't have a chance to exercise.	3	2	1	0
3. I'm just too tired after work to get any exercise.	3	2	1	0
4. I've been thinking about getting more exercise, but I just can't seem to get started.	3	2	1	0
5. I'm getting older, so exercise can be risky.	3	2	1	0
6. I don't get enough exercise because I have never learned the skills for any sport.	3	2	1	0
7. I don't have access to jogging trails, swimming pools, bike paths, etc.	3	2	1	0
8. Physical activity takes too much time away from other commitments—work, family, etc.	3	2	1	0
9. I'm embarrassed about how I will look when I exercise with others.	3	2	1	0
10. I don't get enough sleep as it is. I just couldn't get up early or stay up late to get some exercise.	3	2	1	0
11. It's easier for me to find excuses not to exercise than to go out to do something.	3	2	1	0
12. I know of too many people who have hurt themselves by overdoing it with exercise.	3	2	1	0
13. I really can't see learning a new sport at my age.	3	2	1	0
14. Exercise is just too expensive. You have to take a class or join a club or buy the right equipment.	3	2	1	0
15. My free periods during the day are too short to include exercise.	3	2	1	0
16. My usual social activities with family or friends do not include physical activity.	3	2	1	0
17. I'm too tired during the week, and I need the weekend to catch up on my rest.	3	2	1	0
18. I want to get more exercise, but I just can't seem to make myself stick to anything.	3	2	1	0
19. I'm afraid I might injure myself or have a heart attack.	3	2	1	0
20. I'm not good enough at any physical activity to make it fun.	3	2	1	0
21. If we had exercise facilities and showers at work, then I would be more likely to exercise.	3	2	1	0

Source: Centers for Disease Control and Prevention, "Barriers to Being Active Quiz," 2013, www.cdc.gov

Section V: Scoring Your Obstacles

Follow these instructions to score your answers in Section IV:

- Enter the circled number in the spaces provided, putting together the number for statement 1 on line 1, statement 2 on line 2, and so on.
- Add the three scores on each line. Your obstacles to physical activity fall into one or more of seven categories below. Circle any physical activity obstacles category with a score of 5 or above because this is an important obstacle for you to overcome.

_____ +	_____ +	_____ =	_____
1	8	15	**Lack of time**
_____ +	_____ +	_____ =	_____
2	9	16	**Social influence**
_____ +	_____ +	_____ =	_____
3	10	17	**Lack of energy**
_____ +	_____ +	_____ =	_____
4	11	18	**Lack of willpower**
_____ +	_____ +	_____ =	_____
5	12	19	**Fear of injury**
_____ +	_____ +	_____ =	_____
6	13	20	**Lack of skill**
_____ +	_____ +	_____ =	_____
7	14	21	**Lack of resources**

Section VI: Overcome Obstacles to Exercise

List two of your biggest personal obstacles to exercise. Next, come up with TWO strategies to overcome each one (see the Tools for Change box Overcoming Common Obstacles to Exercise on page 46 for ideas).

Obstacle #1: _____

Strategy for Obstacle #1: _____

_____

_____

Strategy for Obstacle #1: _____

_____

_____

Obstacle #2: _____

Strategy for Obstacle #2: _____

_____

_____

Strategy for Obstacle #2: _____

_____

_____

YOUR DAILY STEPS
AND MILEAGE (LO 2.8)

MasteringHealth™

Name: _____ Date: _____

Instructor: _____ Section: _____

Purpose: To practice using a pedometer or activity tracker to learn how many steps you take each day and translate that into miles.

Section I: Gathering Data/Calculations

1. Buy or borrow a pedometer or wearable activity tracker (see Q&A Can Technology Help Me Get More Fit? for more information on activity trackers). Wear it every day for a week, and fill out Worksheet A.

Worksheet A

	Monday	Tuesday	Wednesday	Thursday	Friday	Saturday	Sunday	Total Weekly Steps/Miles
Steps/Day								
Miles/Day*								

*If you have a wearable activity tracker, note the miles per day that your device records as well.
Average steps per day (total divided by 7) = _____
Average miles per day* (total divided by 7) = _____

2. Figure out your average **stride length**:

a. Walk 20 steps and measure the distance of your 20 steps = _____ (feet)

b. Divide your 20-step distance by 20 = _____ (Average stride length)

3. Figure out your number of **steps in a mile**:

a. Divide 5,280 (feet/mile) by your average stride length above = _____

4. Figure out your **mileage per day**:

a. Divide average steps per day by your steps in a mile = _____ (miles/day)

Section II: Reflection

1. If you have a wearable activity tracker, how close were your calculated miles per day (#4) and average miles recorded by the device (#1)? If they are different, why do you think this is?

_____

_____

2. You'll hear recommendations to walk 10,000 steps per day (about 5 miles), which may be unrealistic for new exercisers. How many miles would this be for you? (divide 10,000 steps by your steps in a mile)

_____

_____

3. Is 10,000 steps/day realistic for you? If not, suggest another number (either steps or miles) that you think you can attain in the next few weeks.

_____

_____

4. What are three ways that you can add more steps to your daily routine?

_____

_____

Are you ready to add more structured exercise to your week? See Program 2.1: A Walking Program at the end of this chapter for information, tips, and workout plans to help you get started!

Activate, Motivate, &Advance YOUR FITNESS

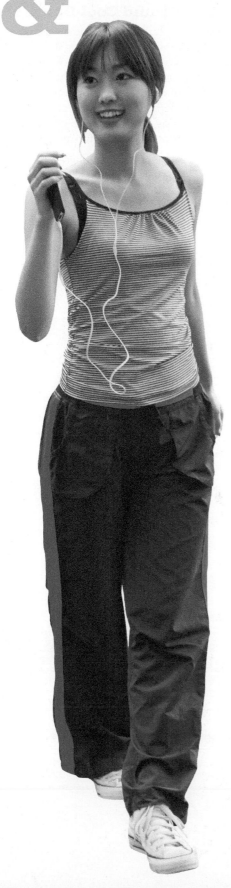

ACTIVATE!

Walking is the most popular fitness activity in the world! If you are not currently active, walking is one of the best ways to start.

What Do I Need for Walking?

SHOES: Obtain good-quality shoes by getting fitted at a local running and walking store. A good fit is one of the most important determinants of the right shoe for you.

CLOTHING: Wear comfortable, non-restrictive clothing and cushioned socks that prevent blisters (avoid all-cotton socks). If you are walking outside, wear light clothing in the heat, waterproof clothing in the rain and snow, or warm clothing in the winter. During the daytime, wear sunscreen, sunglasses, and a hat; if you are walking outside at sunrise, dusk, or dark, wear reflective clothing and/or vest and lights.

How Do I Start a Walking Program?

HEALTH WALKING TECHNIQUE AND SKILLS: Walking for *health* involves a basic walking stride with a focus on posture. Keep your head up and look straight ahead. Make sure that your shoulders are over your hips and you are not leaning too far forward or backward. Swing your arms easily at your sides, keeping your shoulders down and relaxed. Take natural strides and avoid stepping out too far. Focus on being "light" on your feet; particularly avoid slapping your toes down. Instead, control your feet and roll your foot forward.

FITNESS WALKING TECHNIQUE AND SKILLS: Increasing your walking pace for *fitness* involves a few adjustments to your walking stride. Follow the basic posture and foot recommendations above, but add the following changes. Bend your elbows at 90 degrees and swing your arms in time with your stride. Avoid letting your elbows "chicken-wing" out to the side; instead, keep your elbows close to you. Your hands (in a loose fist) should swing from your lower chest back to your hips. Remember that the faster you swing your arms, the faster your legs will go to keep up! Shorten your stride and take faster steps instead of longer steps. Keep your heel strike light, but exaggerate the roll through your foot even more. Forcefully press off your toes with each stride to propel you forward.

Walking Tips

STREET AND TRAIL WALKING: Plan safe and interesting walking routes considering traffic and available walking paths. You can use a mapping program or app to figure out your distance or to create a new route and calculate the distance. Pay attention to your own personal safety. See the safety tips within the chapter for guidance. Follow traffic laws and do not assume that a car or bike operator has seen you.

TRACK WALKING: Walking on a track provides a flat, stable surface with a measured distance. Most tracks are 400 meters around, with four laps being equal to a mile (on the innermost lane). Follow track etiquette by utilizing outside lanes for most of your training and leaving the inside lane (lane 1) for runners and sprinters or for timing yourself on a distance. If you are using the inside lane and a faster individual approaches behind you, move out to lane 2 or 3 to allow the person to pass on the inside.

TREADMILL WALKING: Familiarize yourself with the controls before starting. Learn to use the shut-off button (usually a large red button) and attach the emergency shut-off clip to your clothing. Keep your body upright and avoid using the handrails or leaning forward too much. Keep your body in the center of the treadmill near the console. Most treadmills have preprogrammed workouts, but you can also adjust the speed and incline manually. Start and stop by gradually increasing and decreasing the speed. When you finish, be careful exiting the treadmill; your legs may feel strange on the "non-moving" ground.

Walking Warm-Up and Cool-Down

A walking warm-up and cool-down include walking at a slower pace for 3 to 10 minutes. After breaking a slight sweat in the warm-up, you can add range-of-motion exercises and 10- to 15-second light stretches. When you finish your walk, you can hold stretches longer for improved flexibility. In particular, focus on stretching your upper and lower legs, hips, low back, and chest (see Chapter 5 for specific stretches to perform).

Adjust time, intensity, and days of the walks to suit your personal fitness level and schedule.

BEGINNER WALKING PROGRAM

If you have been sedentary for a long time and need to start slowly or if your cardiorespiratory fitness level in Lab 3.2 was Fair or Poor, start here.

GOAL: To walk 15 to 20 minutes continuously, three to four days a week

	Mon.		Tue.		Wed.		Thurs.		Fri.		Sat.		Sun.	
	T	I	T	I	T	I	T	I	T	I	T	I	T	I
Week 1	5	L			8	L			8	M				
Week 2	8	L			10	M			10	M	10	M		
Week 3	12	M			12	M			15	M	12	M		
Week 4	15	M			15	M			20	M	20	M		

T = Time. Total time is listed in minutes. Time does not include warm-up or cool-down time.
I = Intensity. Intensity is listed as Light/Lifestyle (L), Moderate (M), or Vigorous (V) (see Figure 2.1).

INTERMEDIATE WALKING PROGRAM

If you are able to walk 10 to 15 minutes continuously on three days a week or if your cardiorespiratory fitness level in Lab 3.2 was Good or Fair, start here.

GOAL: To walk 25 to 30 minutes continuously, four to five days a week

	Mon.		Tue.		Wed.		Thurs.		Fri.		Sat.		Sun.	
	T	I	T	I	T	I	T	I	T	I	T	I	T	I
Week 1	10	M			15	M			18	M				
Week 2	18	M			20	V			22	M	20	M		
Week 3	22	M	20	M	22	V			25	M	20	V		
Week 4	25	M	22	V	28	M			30	M	25	V		

T = Time. Total time is listed in minutes. Time does not include warm-up or cool-down time.
I = Intensity. Intensity is listed as Light/Lifestyle (L), Moderate (M), or Vigorous (V) (see Figure 2.1).

MOTIVATE!

Creating a plan and monitoring your progress are key motivators for any fitness behavior change. Use an exercise log or smart-phone app to track your walking program—make note of dates, times, distances, and intensity. With the right technology, you can also track heart rate, steps taken, and/or calories burned.

Sticking to a fitness plan can be tough, but there are plenty of things you can do to motivate yourself and overcome obstacles. Here are a few; see the Tools for Change box Overcoming Common Obstacles to Exercise on page 46 for more ideas.

- **Lack of time?** Look at your schedule and identify 15-minute time slots that you could use for walking—write in your "walking appointments." Add more walking in your daily activities (between classes, errands, etc.).
- **Motivated by numbers?** Keep track of the number of steps you take or daily calories you burn. Challenge yourself with mini-goals to increase your step count and/or calories expended.
- **Need a willpower boost?** Enlist a friend to walk with you—committing to another person can be a great motivator. Sign up for an upcoming charity walk and join a group that is training for it.
- **Dislike exercise?** Create an upbeat playlist of music to listen to while you walk—music can energize you and help you keep pace. Or download podcasts or audiobooks to listen to while you walk. Watch a favorite TV program or movie while treadmill walking. Switch up your route by walking in the woods or a shopping mall.

ADVANCE!

Ready for the next step? Once you have established your walking program, you may want to challenge yourself to take your activities to the next level. Below is a more advanced four-week program you can follow.

ADVANCED WALKING PROGRAM

If you are able to walk 20 to 25 minutes continuously on three days a week or if your cardiorespiratory fitness level in Lab 3.2 was Excellent or Good, start here.

GOAL: To walk 40 to 45 minutes continuously, five days a week

	Mon.		Tue.		Wed.		Thurs.		Fri.		Sat.		Sun.	
	T	I	T	I	T	I	T	I	T	I	T	I	T	I
Week 1	20	M			25	M			25	M				
Week 2	28	M			30	V			30	M	28	M		
Week 3	30	V	32	M	35	M			38	M	35	V		
Week 4	40	M	35	V	45	M			45	V	40	M		

T = Time. Total time is listed in minutes. Time does not include warm-up or cool-down time.
I = Intensity. Intensity is listed as Light/Lifestyle (L), Moderate (M), or Vigorous (V) (see Figure 2.1).

Note: These programs are designed for beginners and assume that all participants have been medically cleared for exercise via the procedures outlined in this chapter. Please also be sure that you have read and understood the basic fitness principles and procedures for starting a fitness program outlined in this chapter. This program is focused on the cardiorespiratory component of fitness, but remember that a well-rounded program will also include muscle strength, muscle endurance, flexibility, and back health components.

3 Conditioning Your Cardiorespiratory System

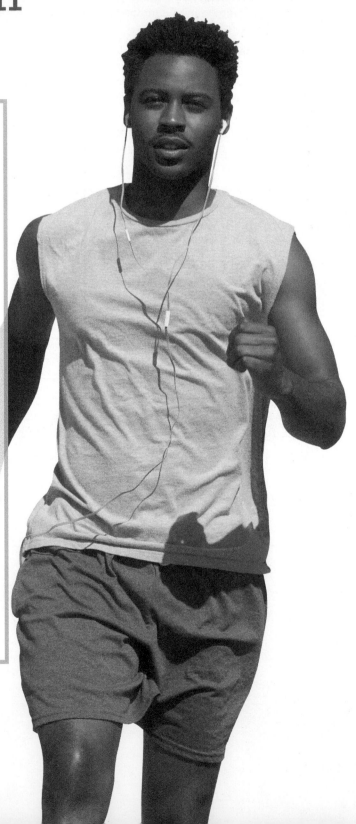

LEARNINGoutcomes

LO 3.1 Identify the key structures of the cardiorespiratory system and state how they work together to provide oxygen to the body.

LO 3.2 Outline how aerobic training improves your body's ability to use oxygen and provide the energy you need for exercise.

LO 3.3 Describe the fitness and wellness benefits you can get from cardiorespiratory training.

LO 3.4 Assess your cardiorespiratory fitness level on a regular basis using a variety of methods.

LO 3.5 Implement a cardiorespiratory fitness program compatible with your goals and lifestyle.

LO 3.6 Use behavior modification strategies to maintain your new cardiorespiratory fitness program.

LO 3.7 Incorporate strategies to prevent injuries during cardiorespiratory training.

MasteringHealth™

Go online for chapter quizzes, interactive assessments, videos, and more!

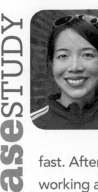

caseSTUDY

NAOMI

"Hi, I'm Naomi. In high school, I was on the cross-country team; I joined because a friend was doing it. I had fun, but I wasn't very fast. After high school, I spent a few years working and saving up money for college, so I'm a little older than most of my classmates. Unfortunately, I got out of shape during that time too. Even though people say I still look like a runner, I get winded going up stairs! I want to get back in shape again, but I'm not sure what to do. I'm close with my family, but none of them exercise. Some of my housemates are thinking about running in the mornings, but I work an early shift before classes. Should I just start running again on my own?"

Hear It!
To listen to this case study online, visit the Study Area in MasteringHealth™.

---

ardiorespiratory fitness is the ability of your cardiovascular and respiratory systems to supply oxygen and nutrients to large muscle groups to sustain continuous activity. It is a key component of your overall fitness and wellness. A healthy cardiorespiratory system can be the difference between having enough energy to sustain daily, recreational, and sports activities and becoming exhausted by performing even simple physical tasks.

When people decide to "get in shape," they often choose cardiorespiratory activities such as walking, jogging, or running. It is convenient to just put on a pair of athletic shoes and head out the door, but remember you need to consider many things to ensure that your cardiorespiratory fitness activities are safe and effective. In this chapter we provide a brief overview of how the cardiorespiratory system works. We also discuss the benefits of regular cardiorespiratory training. We then cover how to set goals for cardiorespiratory fitness and how to design and personalize a cardiorespiratory exercise program for your needs.

LO 3.1 How Does My Cardiorespiratory System Work?

The cardiorespiratory system is made up of the cardiovascular system and the respiratory system. Together,

these systems deliver essential oxygen and nutrients to your body's cells and tissues and remove carbon dioxide and wastes.

An Overview of the Cardiorespiratory System

The **respiratory system** (also called the *pulmonary system*) consists of the air passageways and the lungs; the **cardiovascular system** consists of the heart and blood vessels (arteries and veins) (see **Figure 3.1**).

cardiorespiratory fitness The ability of your cardiovascular and respiratory systems to supply oxygen and nutrients to large muscle groups in order to sustain dynamic activity

respiratory system The body system responsible for the exchange of gases between the body and the air

cardiovascular system The body system responsible for the delivery of oxygen and nutrients to body tissues and the delivery of carbon dioxide and other wastes back to the heart and lungs

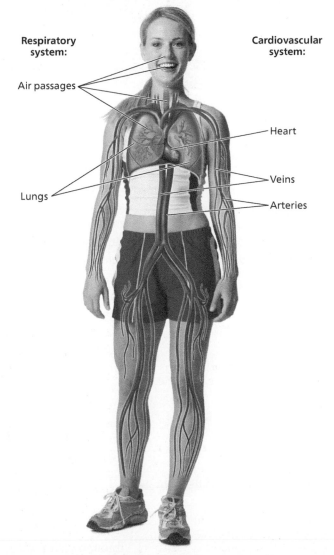

Respiratory system:
- Air passages
- Lungs

Cardiovascular system:
- Heart
- Veins
- Arteries

FIGURE **3.1** The cardiorespiratory system consists of the cardiovascular and respiratory systems.

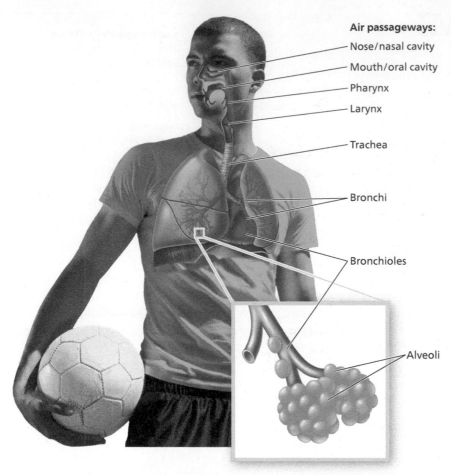

Air passageways:
- Nose/nasal cavity
- Mouth/oral cavity
- Pharynx
- Larynx
- Trachea
- Bronchi
- Bronchioles
- Alveoli

FIGURE **3.2** The respiratory system consists of the air passageways and the lungs.

swallow them. The inspired air travels down through the lower respiratory tract—the lower trachea, *bronchi,* and *bronchioles*—eventually reaching air sacs (*alveoli*) in the lungs, where gas exchange (i.e., the delivery of oxygen and the removal of carbon dioxide) occurs.

Lungs The air passageways in the lungs have extensive branching, similar to the branches on a tree. At the very ends of the smallest branches (the bronchioles) are alveoli, which are surrounded by small blood vessels, called *capillaries.* Because the walls of the alveoli and capillaries are very thin, oxygen moves easily from the alveolar sacs into the capillary blood. Blood vessels then transport oxygen to the heart and the rest of the body. Meanwhile, carbon dioxide moves from the capillaries into the alveoli and exits the body when you exhale. This exchange of oxygen and carbon dioxide is called **respiration**.

Heart The heart is a fist-sized pump consisting of four chambers: *right atrium, right ventricle, left atrium,* and *left ventricle* (**Figure 3.3** on page 69). Small *valves* regulate the rhythmic flow of blood between chambers and prevent the blood from flowing backward. The two **atria** are collecting chambers that receive blood from the body. The two **ventricles** pump blood out again. With each beat of the heart, the atria and ventricles fill and contract. The heart pumps blood through two different circulatory systems: in **pulmonary circulation**, blood circulates from the heart to the lungs and back; in **systemic circulation**, blood circulates from the heart to the rest of the body and back.

1. Blood returning to the heart from the body enters the heart through the right atrium (see Figure 3.3).
2. The right atrium pumps blood into the right ventricle. The right ventricle pumps blood through the **pulmonary artery** into the lungs.
3. Blood returning from the lungs enters the heart through the left atrium.
4. The left atrium pumps blood into the left ventricle. The left ventricle fills and contracts, pumping the blood out of the heart via the **aorta** and transporting it to the cells of the heart, brain, and body.

respiration The exchange of gases in the lungs or in the tissues

atria Upper chambers of the heart that collect blood from the body

ventricles Lower chambers of the heart that pump blood to the body

pulmonary circulation Blood circulation from the heart to the lungs and back

systemic circulation Blood circulation from the heart to the rest of the body and back

pulmonary artery The artery that carries blood from the right ventricle to the lungs

aorta The artery that carries blood from the left ventricle to the rest of the body

Air Passageways

Air enters your body via your nose and mouth. It then continues through your throat (*pharynx*), voice box (*larynx*), and windpipe (*trachea*) (see **Figure 3.2**). These upper respiratory passageways warm, humidify, and filter the air, promoting optimal gas exchange. Mucus and small, hairlike projections called *cilia* filter out unwanted particles in the air; you expel these particles through your nose or mouth, or you

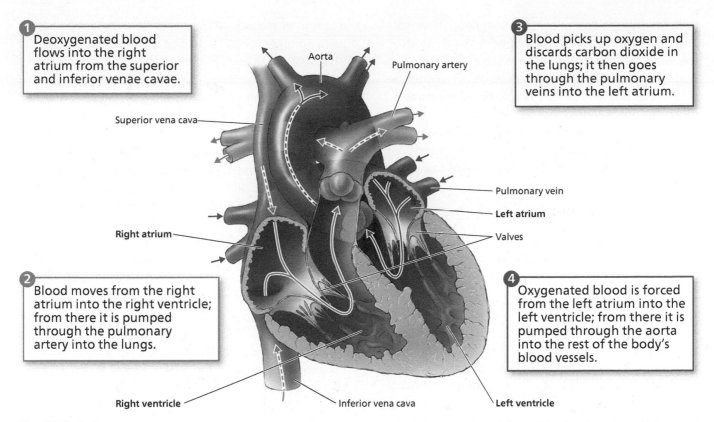

1 Deoxygenated blood flows into the right atrium from the superior and inferior venae cavae.

3 Blood picks up oxygen and discards carbon dioxide in the lungs; it then goes through the pulmonary veins into the left atrium.

Aorta

Pulmonary artery

Superior vena cava

Pulmonary vein

Left atrium

Right atrium

Valves

2 Blood moves from the right atrium into the right ventricle; from there it is pumped through the pulmonary artery into the lungs.

4 Oxygenated blood is forced from the left atrium into the left ventricle; from there it is pumped through the aorta into the rest of the body's blood vessels.

Right ventricle

Inferior vena cava

Left ventricle

FIGURE **3.3** The heart is a four-chambered pump. The right atrium and left atrium collect blood from the body. The right and left ventricles pump blood back out. In pulmonary circulation, blood circulates from the heart to the lungs and back. In systemic circulation, blood circulates from the heart to the rest of the body and back.

Contraction of the ventricles must be forceful enough to send blood out of the heart. To accomplish this task, the ventricles are more muscular than the atria. The left ventricle is the most muscular chamber because it must contract with enough force to send blood to the entire body.

The heart cycle consists of two phases: systole and diastole. During **systole**, the ventricles contract and blood is pumped out of the heart. During **diastole**, the ventricles relax and fill back up with blood from the right and left atria. Specialized heart tissue involuntarily and automatically starts the heart cycle. This tissue, located in the right atrium, is called the *pacemaker;* it determines how fast your heart beats. One "beat" of your heart consists of a full heart cycle. Through a stethoscope, you can hear your heartbeat as a "lub dub." The "lub" signals the end of the diastole phase (ventricular relaxation), and the "dub" signals the end of the systole phase (ventricular contraction). The number of times your heart beats in one minute is your **heart rate**.

Blood Vessels Blood vessels transport blood throughout your body. There are two types of blood vessels: **arteries** carry blood away from the heart, and **veins** carry blood back toward the heart. As arteries branch off from the heart, they divide into smaller blood vessels called *arterioles,* and then into even smaller blood vessels known as capillaries. As mentioned earlier, capillaries have thin walls that permit exchanges between cells and the blood. Oxygen and nutrients move from the blood to body cells, while carbon dioxide and waste products move from body cells to the blood for transport to the lungs and kidneys through veins and *venules* (small veins).

The pressure that blood exerts on the walls of blood vessels is called **blood pressure**. The blood pressure in arteries must be

systole The contraction phase of the heart cycle

diastole The relaxation phase of the heart cycle

heart rate The number of beats of the heart in one minute

arteries High-pressure blood vessels that carry blood away from the heart to the lungs or cells

veins Low-pressure blood vessels that carry blood from the cells or lungs back to the heart

blood pressure The pressure that blood in the arteries exerts on the arterial walls

high to drive the flow of blood to your cells. (In veins, blood pressure is close to zero.) Due to the strength of the heart contraction, pressure in the arteries is higher during systole. The pressure measured in the arteries during this phase is called **systolic blood pressure**. When the heart is relaxed, pressure in the arteries drops; this pressure is called **diastolic blood pressure**.

In addition to oxygen, working muscles need energy. Next, we discuss the three primary energy systems.

Three Metabolic Systems Deliver Essential Energy

All of the cells in your body need energy to function. The cellular form of energy is called *adenosine triphosphate,* or **ATP**. ATP must be constantly regenerated from energy stored in your body and from food. The energy stores in your body consist of fat in adipose tissues and muscles, glucose in the muscles and liver, and protein and **creatine phosphate** in muscles. The energy in food comes from fat, carbohydrates, and protein.

Your body breaks down stored and consumed nutrients to ATP via three metabolic energy systems: the *immediate, nonoxidative* (anaerobic), and *oxidative* (aerobic) systems. To varying extents, your body draws upon all three systems while you are active, depending on the intensity and duration of the activity. Let's examine each of these systems in detail.

---

systolic blood pressure Blood pressure during the systole phase of the heart cycle

diastolic blood pressure Blood pressure during the diastole phase of the heart cycle

ATP Adenosine triphosphate; the cellular form of energy

creatine phosphate A molecule that is stored in muscle cells and used in the immediate energy system to donate a phosphate to make ATP

anaerobic Without oxygen (nonoxidative)

lactic acid An end-product of the nonoxidative breakdown of glucose

lactate A negatively charged salt that is created when lactic acid dissociates a hydrogen ion (H^+)

The Immediate Energy System

For quick, immediate energy, your body first draws upon the ATP and creatine phosphate stored in your muscles. "Explosive" activities, such as a basketball jump shot, a 50-meter sprint, or a dive off a diving board, are all examples of actions fueled by this immediate energy system. However, your body depletes energy in your muscles within a matter of seconds: ATP in muscle cells is typically used up in less than 10 seconds, and creatine phosphate (which is used to make more ATP) is typically gone within 30 seconds. As a result, your body must rely on other energy systems in order to sustain longer activities.

The Nonoxidative (Anaerobic) Energy System

As soon as you start moving, the nonoxidative energy system begins breaking down glucose for energy. This system breaks down glucose quickly and *anaerobically* (without oxygen) to produce ATP. Although this system starts immediately, it does not supply the majority of your needed ATP until about 30 seconds into an activity. Examples of nonoxidative, **anaerobic** activities include a sprint down a soccer field, running up a steep hill, and swimming a 100-meter sprint in the pool.

You will likely experience muscular fatigue (a burning sensation in the muscles), with intense activities that use the nonoxidative energy system. This fatigue is primarily due to your body's limited glucose supply and the accumulation of acids in your muscles and blood. If you use up your accessible glucose during short intense activities, your muscles will no longer have the fuel they need to continue. Additionally, as you quickly break down glucose and ATP in exercise, your muscle cells produce acids. When these acids are produced more quickly than your body can clear them out, they accumulate in your muscles (and then spill over into your blood). Acids impair the ability of your muscles to contract quickly and forcefully over time, i.e. muscular fatigue.

Lactic acid is produced when glucose is broken down quickly under nonoxidative conditions—after which it is almost instantly changed to a free hydrogen ion (H^+) and **lactate**. That means it is lactate, not lactic acid, building up during intense exercise. Unfortunately lactic acid has gotten a "bad rap" over the years. Contrary to popular belief, the increase in lactic acid (lactate) is temporary. Your body clears it out within minutes or hours of exercise; longer and more intense exercise requires more time to clear. So, lactic acid (lactate) does *not* cause the muscle soreness you may feel a day or two after intense exercise and it isn't solely responsible for the increase in acids during intense exercise. In fact, lactic acid (lactate) is useful as a back-up energy source—certain body cells can reuse it for energy once it is cleared from the muscles and blood.

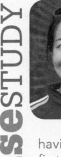

NAOMI

"I thought I would kick-start my plan to get back into shape by doing one of the workouts my high school coach had us do. I ran about a mile to a hill near campus. I tried to run up the hill a few times, but ended up having to walk. I decided that tackling hills my first time out was a mistake so I walked back home. My high school races were about three miles, so I was surprised at how much that one mile tired me out. I used to run a mile with no problem at all! I'm feeling a little frustrated because I let myself slip further out of shape than I thought."

APPLY IT! Which energy system do you think Naomi relied on most when running to the hill? What about when she tried to run up the hill? Do you think a better warm-up would have helped her?

TRY IT! **Today**, write out activities you would do for a 10-minute cardiorespiratory warm-up. **This week**, try your 10-minute warm-up and think about how the three energy systems are providing fuel to keep your muscles moving. **In two weeks**, log an entire workout session and outline the energy systems you are using.

Hear It!
To listen to this case study online, visit the Study Area in MasteringHealth™.

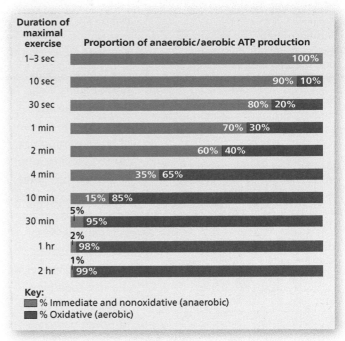

FIGURE **3.4** In the first two minutes of exercise, the body primarily uses ATP generated by the immediate and nonoxidative (anaerobic) energy systems. About three minutes into the exercise, the body begins to primarily use ATP generated by the oxidative (aerobic) energy system.

Figure 3.4 illustrates how the proportion of each energy system's contribution of ATP changes, depending on the duration of a given activity.

The Cardiorespiratory System at Rest and during Exercise

Your cardiorespiratory system must adapt in order to meet your body's needs during exercise.

Resting Conditions At rest, your body works to maintain **homeostasis**, a stable internal environment. During homeostasis, your oxygen and nutrient delivery matches the needs of your cells. Your body breaks down fat via the oxidative energy system in order to supply ATP to the body. Although you "burn" fat for energy, your total energy expenditure is low.

The nonoxidative energy system supplies your body with most of its ATP until about three minutes into an activity. At that point, the oxidative energy system becomes the primary provider of ATP.

The Oxidative (Aerobic) Energy System During the first three minutes of activity (even as the immediate and nonoxidative systems are supplying most of your ATP), your body is gradually increasing its *oxidative* production of ATP using oxygen in the **mitochondria** of your cells. The oxidative energy system is also called the **aerobic** energy system (*aerobic* means "with oxygen"). Mitochondria are often referred to as the "powerhouses of the cell" because most energy production occurs in these structures. The complete breakdown of fat, glucose, and protein occurs only in the mitochondria and the oxidative energy system yields more ATP from each energy source than any other system.

Aerobic activities are low- to moderate-intensity activities that are usually sustained for 20 minutes or longer. Examples of aerobic activities include cycling, walking, jogging, and water aerobics.

Response to Exercise Physical activity disrupts your body's homeostasis. During exercise, your body must increase blood flow to working muscles to maintain

mitochondria Cellular structures where oxidative energy production takes place

aerobic Dependent on oxygen (oxidative)

homeostasis A stable, constant internal environment

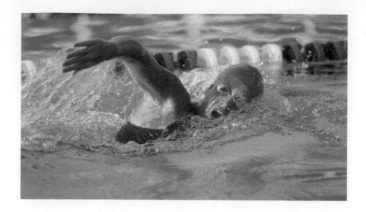

cardiac output The volume of blood ejected from the heart in one minute; expressed in liters or milliliters per minute

hemoglobin A four-part globular, iron-containing protein that carries oxygen in red blood cells

plasma The yellow-colored fluid portion of blood that contains water, proteins, hormones, ions, energy sources, and blood gases

stroke volume The volume of blood ejected from the heart in one heartbeat; expressed in liters or milliliters per beat

adequate oxygen and nutrient delivery. Your heart rate rises, and stronger heart contractions increase **cardiac output**—the amount of blood exiting your heart in one minute. Your breathing rate increases to transfer adequate oxygen into your blood for working muscles.

During exercise, the increased volume of blood moving from your heart into your blood vessels raises systolic blood pressure. The body directs this increased blood to contracting muscles and the vessels *dilate* (open wider) to accommodate the increased blood flow. This arterial dilation allows diastolic blood pressure to stay the same or even decrease during aerobic exercise. In addition, capillaries that were closed at rest open up to allow for oxygen and nutrient exchange with muscles.

When you begin to exercise, it takes a few minutes for your body to increase blood flow and fully engage the oxidative energy system. This is why your body relies on the faster immediate and nonoxidative energy systems in the first few minutes of exercise. The slower ATP production of the oxidative system also means that during your exercise session, you may have to draw upon the nonoxidative energy system more than once. For example, if you are jogging and suddenly sprint to the end of the street, your oxidative energy system may not be able to supply ATP quickly enough. Your body will then draw upon the nonoxidative system (which breaks down glucose quickly) to supply the additional ATP you need.

LO 3.2 How Does Aerobic Training Condition My Cardiorespiratory System?

Recall that aerobic activities are low- to moderate-intensity activities performed for an extended period of time (i.e., 20 minutes or longer). Regular aerobic training conditions your cardiorespiratory system by improving your body's ability to (1) deliver large amounts of oxygen

to working muscles, (2) transfer and use oxygen efficiently in the muscles, and (3) use energy sources for sustained muscular contractions. **Figure 3.5** summarizes these and other adaptations that occur over time with aerobic training.

Aerobic Training Increases Oxygen Delivery to Your Muscles

With regular aerobic training, your body gets better at delivering oxygen to working muscles. Your respiratory muscles become more efficient and you experience less fatigue. You can carry more oxygen in your blood, due to an increase in **hemoglobin**, the oxygen-carrying protein. Since the fluid portion of your blood, the **plasma**, also increases with aerobic training, you will see an increase in your total blood volume. Your heart will adapt to this greater volume by increasing the blood-holding capacity of your left ventricle. The ventricle will not only hold more blood, but (with training) it will also have stronger contractions. All of this will allow you to pump more blood out of your heart with every heartbeat, thus increasing your heart's **stroke volume**.

Aerobic Training Improves the Transfer and Use of Oxygen

Delivering oxygen to working muscles is only part of the picture. Your body also needs to transfer oxygen into the muscles and use it efficiently. Consistent aerobic training increases the number of capillaries in your muscles. This enhances blood flow to these muscles and improves oxygen transfer from the blood into the muscles. Once inside the muscle cells, oxygen is transported to mitochondria for use in the oxidative energy system. Mitochondria numbers increase within each muscle cell, improving oxygen use by muscles and subsequently improving oxidative production of ATP as well.

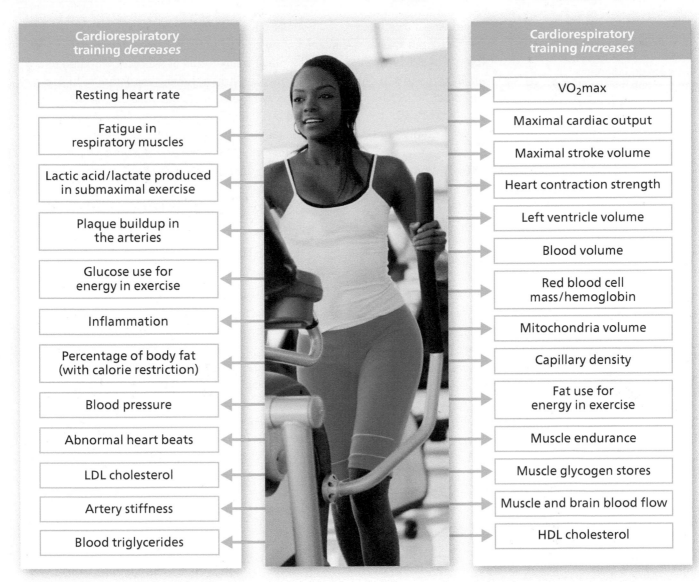

Cardiorespiratory training *decreases*	Cardiorespiratory training *increases*
Resting heart rate	VO₂max
Fatigue in respiratory muscles	Maximal cardiac output
Lactic acid/lactate produced in submaximal exercise	Maximal stroke volume
Plaque buildup in the arteries	Heart contraction strength
Glucose use for energy in exercise	Left ventricle volume
Inflammation	Blood volume
Percentage of body fat (with calorie restriction)	Red blood cell mass/hemoglobin
Blood pressure	Mitochondria volume
Abnormal heart beats	Capillary density
LDL cholesterol	Fat use for energy in exercise
Artery stiffness	Muscle endurance
Blood triglycerides	Muscle glycogen stores
	Muscle and brain blood flow
	HDL cholesterol

FIGURE **3.5** Regular cardiorespiratory training results in numerous adaptations to the cardiovascular, respiratory, and muscle systems and an increase in overall health and wellness.

Aerobic Training Improves Your Body's Ability to Use Energy Efficiently

Regular aerobic training increases your ability to store glycogen within muscles. When needed, glycogen can be broken down into glucose and used for energy during exercise. In fact, a minimal amount of glucose is needed during exercise to keep the oxidative energy system running efficiently.

Since fat is broken down for energy within the mitochondria, an increase in the number of mitochondria will improve your body's ability to use fat for energy, sparing glucose and glycogen stores. Improving your body's ability to burn fat may allow you to have some glucose "left over" for that last-minute sprint to the finish! Reduced nonoxidative glucose breakdown

also means less acid accumulates during exercise—which delays fatigue.

LO 3.3 What Are the Benefits of Improving My Cardiorespiratory Fitness?

There are many health-related reasons to improve your cardiorespiratory fitness.

Cardiorespiratory Fitness Decreases Your Risk of Disease

A low fitness level increases your risk for disease and early death. The good news is that you don't need to become extremely fit to see risk-reducing health

metabolic syndrome A clustering of three or more heart disease and diabetes risk factors in one person (high blood pressure, impaired glucose tolerance, insulin resistance, decreased HDL cholesterol, elevated triglycerides, overweight with fat mostly around the waist)

An increase in cardiorespiratory fitness can lower your resting heart rate and your blood levels of "bad" (LDL) cholesterol, and help prevent blood clots—all of which lower your risk of heart attack and stroke.

And it is never too early to start: in a study of preadolescent girls, higher cardiorespiratory fitness levels were associated with healthier arteries.[2] If children and adolescents sustain an active lifestyle and avoid obesity, they can avoid the stiffer, less healthy arteries that accompany a sedentary lifestyle in adulthood.[3]

Staying active and having higher cardiorespiratory fitness reduce your chances of developing **metabolic syndrome** (a group of obesity-related risk factors associated with cardiovascular disease and type 2 diabetes).[4] It can also lessen your risk of developing pre-diabetes and diabetes, since the regular muscular contractions that occur in aerobic exercise improve your body's ability to use insulin and glucose.[5]

benefits. An intermediate fitness level (being able to walk about three to four miles per hour) can significantly reduce early mortality from cardiovascular diseases, and it can lower heart disease risk factors as well.[1]

Regular physical activity stimulates hormones, anti-inflammatory agents, and immune responses that help protect against many forms of cancer. Compared to low cardiorespiratory fitness, having moderate or high cardiorespiratory fitness can lower your overall cancer mortality rate by 20 to 45 percent, regardless of your body fat level.[6] In fact, maintaining that fitness level over time may be more important for reducing your cancer risk than changing your body weight.[7]

Cardiorespiratory Fitness Helps You Control Body Weight and Body Composition

Cardiorespiratory training burns calories. By increasing your calorie expenditure through exercise, you can more effectively manage your body weight and keep your level of body fat low. You can even maintain your daily energy expenditure as you lose weight by performing regular aerobic exercise.[8] A high-intensity aerobic exercise session elevates your fat use for energy[9] and your metabolic rate, burning calories during the exercise session and long afterward.[10] You'll also burn many calories with moderate aerobic exercise by performing the activity for an extended period of time.

Cardiorespiratory Fitness Improves Self-Esteem, Mood, and Sense of Well-Being

Exercise makes you feel good! A single aerobic exercise session can improve mood and reduce tension and anxiety as a result of chemical changes in the brain and nervous system.[11] Since these benefits are primarily seen in regular exercisers,[12] don't be discouraged if you don't feel instantly "happy" after your first exercise session—stick with it! Long-term changes are even more dramatic. One study has shown that over the course of a 12-week aerobic fitness program, men and women reported improved self-concept, anxiety, mood, and depression scores, compared to a control group, and maintained their improved psychological health for a year.[13] Not surprisingly, exercise can also help reduce symptoms of depression.[14]

Cardiorespiratory Fitness Improves Immune Function

Light to moderate exercise can boost your immune system.[15] Regular, moderate aerobic exercise can reduce stress and improve your sleep (stress and sleep are both tied to immune system health). Although intense exercise can weaken the immune system temporarily, maintaining a high volume of aerobic exercise as you get older is associated with enhanced immune system functioning.[16]

Cardiorespiratory Fitness Improves Long-Term Quality of Life

Cardiorespiratory fitness has a protective effect against age-related cognitive declines.[17] Research even suggests that aerobic exercise training can increase brain volume and thus *improve* cognitive function and memory as you age.[18]

Increased cardiorespiratory fitness can also improve the quality of life for individuals with chronic diseases or other medical conditions. People living with HIV/AIDS can experience life-enhancing improvements in cardiorespiratory and overall physical functioning if they increase their levels of physical activity and/or exercise.[19] Cardiorespiratory fitness has also been linked to better quality of life for survivors of cancer,[20] heart attacks,[21] and strokes.[22] Of course, the best time to incorporate a cardiorespiratory program into your life is *before y*ou show signs of disease.

LO 3.4 How Can I Assess My Cardiorespiratory Fitness?

How fit is your cardiorespiratory system? Chances are you already have a general idea. If you are winded after walking up a short flight of stairs or have trouble walking quickly for more than 10 minutes, you likely have a low cardiorespiratory fitness level.

Monitoring your **resting heart rate** will help you track general changes in your fitness level. Recall that your heart rate is the number of times your heart beats in one minute. Your resting heart rate decreases as your cardiorespiratory system becomes more conditioned. With an increase in stroke volume, your heart does not have to beat as many times per minute to deliver the same amount of blood and oxygen to your body cells at rest.

When the heart contracts and pushes blood out, that wave of blood can be felt moving through the arteries. This is your **pulse**. To determine your heart rate, feel your pulse at specific arteries around the body. The most common locations used to check your pulse are the *carotid* and the *radial* arteries (see **Figure 3.6**). Gently press your index and middle fingers against your skin

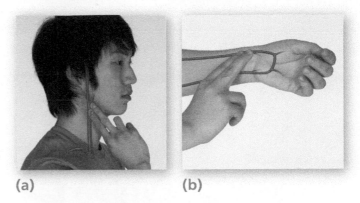

(a) **(b)**

FIGURE **3.6** To determine your heart rate, feel your pulse at either (a) the carotid artery or (b) the radial artery.

and count the beats that you feel. Avoid using your thumb when taking your pulse because the pulse in your thumb can alter your count. Use caution when feeling for your carotid pulse. Avoid pressing too hard or applying pressure to both sides of the neck at the same time. **Lab 3.1** walks you through how to use your pulse to record an accurate heart rate at rest and during exercise.

Do It!
Access these labs at the end of the chapter or online at MasteringHealth™.

Understand Your Maximal Oxygen Consumption

Your body's maximal ability to use oxygen during exercise is called **maximal oxygen consumption (VO_2max)**. Your VO_2max is the measure of your body's ability to deliver oxygen to the muscles and the muscles' ability to consume or use the oxygen. VO_2max numbers range from 20 to 94 ml/kg·min, with male athletes typically ranging from 50 to 70 ml/kg·min and female athletes ranging from 40 to 60 ml/kg·min. Your maximal oxygen consumption is largely determined by genetics and decreases as you get older. That said, you can improve your VO_2max 15 to 20 percent with training.

The most accurate VO_2max measurements are performed in a laboratory setting (see **Figure 3.7**). The test is usually completed on a treadmill or stationary bike and requires

resting heart rate The number of times your heart beats in a minute while the body is at rest; typically 50 to 90 beats per minute

pulse The pressure wave felt in the arteries due to blood ejection with each heartbeat

maximal oxygen consumption (VO_2max) The highest rate of oxygen consumption your body is capable of during maximal exercise; expressed in either liters per minute (L/min) or milliliters per minute per kilogram of body weight (ml/kg·min)

Submaximal tests in the laboratory predict your maximal effort level by assessing your heart rate response to exercising on a stationary bike or tread-mill. By testing your heart rate response to different exercise intensities, a technician can use your pre-dicted **maximal heart rate (HRmax)** to estimate your maximal exercise intensity and oxygen consumption. Your maximal heart rate is the fastest your heart will beat in exhaustive exercise (a number that decreases as you get older). One way to predict your HRmax is to subtract your age from the number 220. For example, if you are 18 years old, your predicted HRmax would be 220 − 18 = 202 beats per minute. This formula is not as accurate as maximal laboratory tests, but it is used in submaximal tests and target heart rate equations.

Test Your Cardiorespiratory Fitness in the Field/Classroom

Most college classes in health and fitness enroll too many students to perform laboratory testing. More appropriate for these classes are classroom or field tests of cardiorespiratory fitness. Like laboratory tests, these tests either predict your maximal oxygen consumption from submaximal test results or allow you to compare your results with norm tables. In **Lab 3.2** you will per-form three different assessments of cardiorespiratory fitness: the Queen's College step test, the 1-mile walking test, and the 1.5-mile running test.

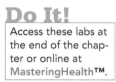
Do It! Access these labs at the end of the chapter or online at MasteringHealth™.

Queen's College Step Test In this test, you will step up and down on a 16.25-inch-high step bench. At the end of three minutes, take your recovery heart rate for 15 seconds. Use your results to calculate an estimated VO$_2$max and determine your fitness level for your age and sex. The faster your heart recovers from exercise, the better conditioned you are.

One-Mile Walking Test In this test, you will walk as fast as you can for one flat, measured mile. Record your finish time and your heart rate at the end of the one mile. Use your results to calculate an estimated VO$_2$max and determine your fitness level for your age and sex. A faster time and lower heart rate indicate a higher level of fitness.

1.5-Mile Running Test In this test, you will run 1.5 miles as fast as you can. If you cannot run the entire course, take walking breaks. Use your finish time to

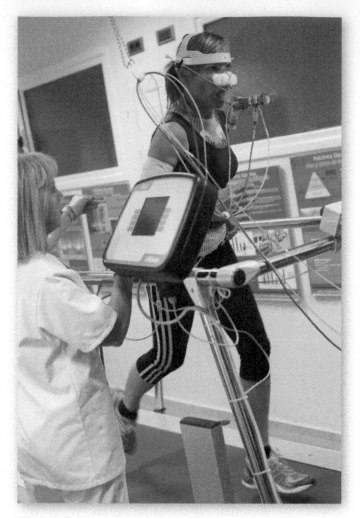
FIGURE **3.7** VO$_2$max can be most accurately measured in a laboratory setting, where direct gas analysis can determine the vol-ume of oxygen a person's body is using while exercising at maxi-mum capacity.

specialized equipment and technicians to ensure safety. The technicians measure the precise amount of oxygen that enters and exits the body during a maximal exer-cise session.

Test Your Submaximal Heart Rate Responses

An alternative to testing your true maximal oxygen con-sumption is to perform a *submaximal* test. Submaximal tests measure less than maximal responses to exercise that can be compared against norm charts or used to predict maximal values. Submaximal tests are safer, require less equip-ment and expertise, and are performed either in a laboratory or in a field/classroom setting.

maximal heart rate (HRmax) The highest heart rate you can achieve during maximal exercise

calculate your estimated VO_2max and determine your fitness level for your age and sex. A faster time indicates a higher level of fitness.

LO 3.5 How Can I Create My Own Cardiorespiratory Fitness Program?

Careful planning will help you reach your cardiorespiratory goals, prevent injuries, and ensure that you have fun while exercising!

Set Appropriate Cardiorespiratory Fitness Goals

Goal-setting for cardiorespiratory fitness should follow the SMART goal-setting guidelines (introduced in Chapter 1); effective goals are *specific, measurable, action-oriented, realistic,* and *time-oriented.* A vague goal, such as "Build a stronger cardiorespiratory system," is not as helpful as a specific goal. Try this instead: "Improve my cardiorespiratory fitness from a 'fair' to a 'good' rating on my three-minute step test, by exercising on the elliptical machine for 30 minutes three days a week over the next two months."

Use Lab 3.3 to set your own short- and long-term goals for cardiorespiratory fitness. Be realistic: If your goal is to run a marathon but you hate running, you will likely be setting yourself up for failure (unless your attitude toward running changes!). Choose goals that you can achieve, doing activities that you enjoy.

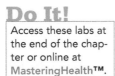

Do It!
Access these labs at the end of the chapter or online at MasteringHealth™.

Learn about Cardiorespiratory Training Options

A wide variety of cardiorespiratory training options are available.

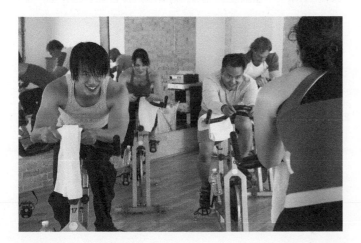

Classes If you enjoy the company of other people and like the motivating aspect of an instructor leading a workout, enroll in a group exercise class. Classes that incorporate either continuous movement or moderate-to high-intensity intervals will help you maintain or improve your cardiorespiratory fitness. You can find such classes in colleges, recreational centers, and fitness centers in almost every community. Class formats and instructors vary widely, so sample a few different classes and instructors before deciding on a regular class. Choose classes where the instructors are not only motivating, but also experienced, certified, and knowledgeable.

Indoor Workouts If you are not sure about working out in a group or with an instructor, you can design your own cardiorespiratory workout using indoor cardio equipment. You can find cardio equipment at most fitness centers or purchase it for home use. Indoor cardio workout equipment includes stationary bicycles, treadmills, elliptical trainers, stair-climbing machines, arm cycle ergometers, rowing machines, and jump ropes. If you are using a machine in a fitness facility, have an employee introduce you to the features, use, and safety. You might also consider running on an indoor track, swimming in a pool, deep-water jogging, or participating in a racquet sport.

Outdoor Workouts Many people pursue a combination of indoor and outdoor exercise routines, depending on the weather and the facilities available. Exercising outdoors can be very rewarding if you live in an area with interesting sights, safe routes, and beautiful trails. The options for outdoor cardio workouts are endless. Here are just a few ideas: walking, jogging, running, cycling, track workouts, trail running, hiking, tennis, cross-country skiing, open-water swimming, and inline skating.

Differing Workout Formats (Continuous, Interval, Circuit) Aerobic training is traditionally defined as *continuous* training—that is, you perform a rhythmic activity for a period of time (ideally 20 minutes or more). While this type of training may be the cornerstone of your cardiorespiratory training program, other workout formats can add variety, intensity, and additional benefits.

An **interval workout** alternates periods of higher-intensity exercise with periods of lower-intensity exercise or rest. An

interval workout A workout that alternates periods of higher-intensity exercise with periods of lower-intensity exercise or rest interval workout method allows you to increase the intensity of your workout to a level that you might not otherwise be able to sustain for a long period of time. If done correctly, this type of workout can further develop your body's aerobic training adaptations. High-intensity anaerobic intervals improve anaerobic conditioning but also have a greater injury potential. The GetFitGraphic Are Short Workouts Worth My Time? on page 79 reviews the benefits and basic principles of high-intensity interval training (HIIT).

A **circuit-training workout** involves moving from location to location in a circuit-training room and exercising for a certain amount of time (or number of repetitions) at each "station." You can enroll in a circuit-training class or circuit-train on your own. The circuit can contain alternating aerobic and weight-training activities, just weight stations, or just aerobic stations. The best circuit for cardiorespiratory conditioning is one with all aerobic exercise stations.

See Q&A Will These Fitness Trends Help Me? on page 80 for answers to questions you may have about popular workout programs such as fitness challenges, obstacle course runs, Tabata training, CrossFit, and cardio machine classes.

Apply the FITT Formula to Cardiorespiratory Fitness

After setting goals and selecting the types of cardiorespiratory exercise that you want to do, you must decide how much, how hard, and how long to exercise. Recall the FITT formula (introduced in Chapter 2): *f*requency, *i*ntensity, *t*ime, and *t*ype. Let's look at how each component of FITT applies to a cardiorespiratory fitness program.

Frequency According to the American College of Sports Medicine (ACSM), you should spend three to five days per week on cardiorespiratory conditioning. If you are exercising at higher-intensity levels, you can improve or maintain your VO$_2$max by working out only three days per week. If you are exercising at lower-intensity levels, you may need more than three days per week (five is recommended) to improve cardiorespiratory fitness.

If your goals include weight loss or disease prevention, you will benefit from exercising more often but at a lower intensity to prevent injuries and overtraining.

Intensity Your workouts should be intense enough to tax your cardiorespiratory system, but not so difficult as to discourage or injure you. You can measure the intensity of your exercise by various methods, including determining your heart rate, assessing your **perceived exertion**, and self-administering a **talk test**.

Determine Your Heart Rate Your heart rate provides an indication of how hard your cardiorespiratory system is working, since it is related to the amount of oxygen that your body is consuming. You can measure your heart rate by using a heart rate monitor or (as discussed earlier) by counting your pulse.

Heart rate monitors on cardio equipment require you to place your hands on the receiving pads for a few seconds. Personal heart rate monitors, with a chest strap transmitter and/or a wrist watch, are also widely available. Check out Q&A Can Technology Help Me Get More Fit? in Chapter 2 for more tips on using technology in your workouts.

Counting your pulse while you are exercising is an easy and low-cost way to measure your heart rate. Your heart rate decreases rapidly after stopping exercise; therefore, count your pulse for only 10 seconds, and try to keep moving as you count. Then multiply your 10-second count by six to convert to beats per minute (bpm).

What **target heart rate** should you aim for in a workout? The answer depends on your goals and fitness level. As you can see in **Table 3.1**, ACSM's recommendation for exercise intensity ranges from target heart

circuit-training workout A workout where exercisers move from one exercise station to another after a certain number of repetitions or amount of time

perceived exertion A subjective assessment of exercise intensity

talk test A method of measuring exercise intensity based on assessing your ability to speak during exercise

target heart rate The heart rate you are aiming for during an exercise session; often a range with high and low heart rates called your *training zone*

TABLE **3.1 ACSM's Training Guidelines for Cardiorespiratory Fitness**

Recommendations for the General Adult Population	
Frequency (days/week)	Moderate: 5
	Vigorous: 3
Intensity (how hard)	Moderate: 64–75% of HRmax
	Vigorous: 76–95% of HRmax
Time (how long)	Moderate: 30–60 min (150 min/week)
	Vigorous: 20–60 min (75 min/week)
Type (exercises)	Rhythmic, aerobic, large muscle group activity

Data from American College of Sports Medicine, *ACSM's Guidelines for Exercise Testing and Prescription*, 9th ed. (Baltimore: Lippincott Williams & Wilkins, 2014).

ARE SHORT WORKOUTS WORTH MY TIME?

IN SHORT, YES! Experts once believed that long aerobic workouts were more effective than short workouts for your health. Recent research shows that: (1) you don't have to exercise a long time to get benefits, and (2) short but a *high intensity* training can have a major impact on your health.

What are the BENEFITS of MULTIPLE SHORT WORKOUTS during the day?

Short workouts are better than one continuous workout at

- Lowering fats in the bloodstream.[1]
- Burning calories and balancing blood glucose/insulin levels (because metabolism increases after 10 minutes of exercise and persists for 60 minutes).[2]

What is HIGH-INTENSITY INTERVAL TRAINING (HIIT)?

HIIT is a workout strategy that alternates high intensity quick bursts of exercise activity with recovery periods of lower intensity exercise.

- 4 minutes of HIIT can lead to similar improvements in VO_2max and greater improvements in muscular endurance than 30 minutes of traditional endurance training.[3]

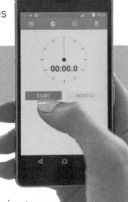

HOW DO YOU HIIT?

1 GET READY

Because of the **HIGHER INTENSITY** of some **HIIT PROTOCOLS, GO SLOW** if you aren't fit.

CHOOSE AN INTERVAL that you can perform for 15 seconds to 4 minutes at 80–95% of your maximum heart rate or a rating of 8–10 on the perceived exertion scale. Here are some common interval recommendations:

2 GET SET

JUST STARTING
1:3 ratio
30 sec high-intensity : 90 sec recovery

MODERATELY FIT
1:2 ratio
40 sec high-intensity : 80 sec recovery

ALREADY FIT
1:1 ratio
60 sec high-intensity : 60 sec recovery

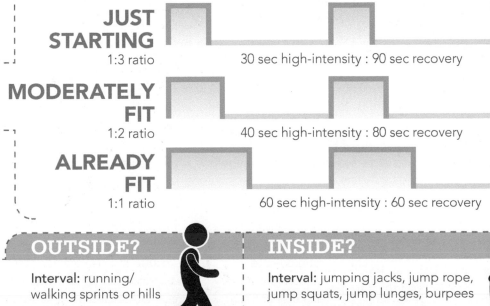

3 GO

OUTSIDE?

Interval: running/ walking sprints or hills

Recovery: jog/walk

INSIDE?

Interval: jumping jacks, jump rope, jump squats, jump lunges, burpees

Recovery: walk/jog in place

EXPAND YOUR OPTIONS by checking out the many **HIIT apps** available for your smartphone or device with preloaded interval workouts, timers, music, and tracking options.

Q&A Will These Fitness Trends Help Me?

Will "challenges" help me become more fit? Every now and then, we all need a challenge to kick up our motivation! 100 push-up challenges, 30-day ab challenges, 10,000 steps/day—there are many options to get you moving. Search out challenge motivators to help you start or bump up your cardio program, or any aspect of your fitness, for that matter. For even more accountability, challenge a friend or family member to take the "challenge" with you. Do an online search for fitness challenge ideas—or simply create your own.

Obstacle course races—should I try one? Warrior Dash, Tough Mudder, Spartan Race—just to name a few of the popular and fun new races you can do. All of these events have intense-sounding names for a reason—they are tough! If you are new to exercise, first establish a basic level of cardiorespiratory fitness and muscle endurance. Then, start training specifically for the race you are aiming to do. If you are trained and pay attention to safety procedures, you should have fun on race day. Bring your friends and a big plastic bag for your dirty race clothes!

What is Tabata training? What started out as a high-intensity training method for Japanese speed-skaters has turned into one of the most popular forms of high-intensity interval training (HIIT). Tabata training incorporates 20 seconds of all-out work, followed by 10 seconds of rest, repeated eight times (four minutes total). The original study showed that athletes using this regimen for six weeks improved both their VO_2max and their anaerobic capacity.[1] To incorporate Tabata today, download a Tabata-specific app for your smartphone that will guide your intervals.

Is CrossFit as intense as it looks? CrossFit is defined as "constantly varied functional movements performed at a fairly high intensity." Workouts are posted on the CrossFit website and performed in CrossFit gyms around the country. Competitive athletes test their skills and fitness in the CrossFit Games competition. CrossFit workouts are highly variable but focus on functional exercises that

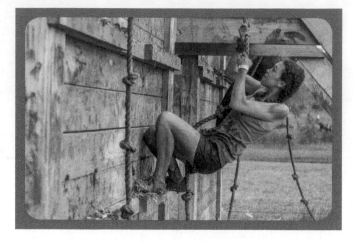

improve everyday activities. Some facilities emphasize more cardiorespiratory fitness-based training, along with basic CrossFit movements. CrossFit is intense, but as with any program, start where you are, modify as needed, and have fun along the way! Look online for CrossFit workouts and gyms close to you.

What are cardio machine classes all about? Prefer to work out indoors on cardio machines but like the motivation and support of a group class? Cycling classes have been popular for a long time, but treadmill and rowing classes are gaining popularity. In treadmill classes you'll get a mix of steady running, hill running, and intervals. Follow that up with muscle fitness exercises and stretching and you have a total body workout. Rowing classes are popular because the activity is low impact, similar to cycling, but offers upper and lower body muscle training at the same time. Using proper rowing technique is essential, so seek out that group class for some rowing skills and drills instruction! Check your local fitness clubs to find group treadmill and/or rowing classes.

1. I. Tabata et al., "Effects of Moderate-Intensity Endurance and High-Intensity Intermittent Training on Anaerobic Capacity and VO_2max," *Medicine & Science in Sports & Exercise* 28, no. 10 (1996): 1327–30.

---

rates of 64 percent to 95 percent of HRmax. Use the following guidelines to determine where within this range you should aim:

heart rate reserve (HRR) The number of beats per minute available or in reserve for exercise heart rate increases; maximal heart rate minus resting heart rate

• If your fitness level is low, follow the guidelines for moderate cardiorespiratory exercise or 64 to 75 percent of your

HRmax. Start below or at the low end of this range if you are very deconditioned or brand new to exercise.

• If your fitness level is moderate, aim for the vigorous exercise guidelines or 76 to 95 percent of your HRmax or choose to do a mix of moderate and vigorous exercise.

Table 3.2 also provides target heart rate guidelines for exercise, using the HRmax method based on your age. Another method of determining your target heart rate is to measure your **heart rate reserve (HRR)**, the

TABLE 3.2 Target Heart Rate Guidelines*

Age	Target HR Range (bpm)	10-Sec Count
18–24	139–179	23–30
25–29	135–174	22–29
30–34	132–169	22–28
35–39	129–165	21–28
40–44	125–160	21–27
45–49	122–156	20–26
50–54	118–151	20–25
55–59	114–147	19–25
60–64	110–142	18–24
65+	108–140	18–23

*Based upon the HRmax method, where 220 − age = HRmax and the training zone is 70 to 90 percent of HRmax (moderate to vigorous). Individuals with low fitness levels should start below or at the low end of these ranges.

difference between your resting and maximum heart rates. Lab 3.1 walks you through how to determine your HRR.

Do It! Access these labs at the end of the chapter or online at MasteringHealth™.

Perceived Exertion Another way to assess the intensity of your workout is by determining your perceived exertion: your perception of how hard you are working during exercise. In 1970, Gunnar Borg developed one of the best-known perceived exertion scales. His Rating of Perceived Exertion (RPE) scale is a subjective 15-point scale, from 6 through 20, that is related to heart rate responses to exercise.[23]

The Borg RPE scale can be a valuable tool when it is not easy or appropriate to use heart rate monitoring.

For example, if you participate in a water sport such as swimming, heart rate monitoring can be misleading; heart rates tend to slow down while you exercise in water due to increased hydrostatic pressure and decreased temperature. For this reason, you may prefer to use RPE to determine your exercise intensity.

Another perceived exertion scale is the OMNI Scale of Perceived Exertion. Although originally developed for children, adult versions now exist that provide a simple way to assess workout intensity on a 1 to 10 scale (see **Figure 3.8**). The OMNI scale is correlated with the Borg RPE scale and heart rate responses.[24] As you become more experienced with a particular cardiorespiratory activity and more attuned to how your body feels during exercise, your ability to use the perceived exertion scales accurately will improve.

The Talk Test The talk test method assesses how easily you can talk during exercise. While exercising at a *light* intensity, you should be able to talk easily and continuously. At a *moderate* intensity, you should be able to talk easily, but not continuously, during the activity. If you are too out of breath to carry on a conversation easily, you are working at a high or *vigorous* intensity. If you cannot talk at all, you are probably doing an anaerobic interval or sprinting.

To increase cardiorespiratory fitness, aim for a moderate intensity level for most of your workout or the highest level you can comfortably sustain for 20 to 30 minutes. You can incorporate short periods of light and vigorous activity for workout variety or interval training. **Table 3.3** summarizes the most common intensity scales for cardiorespiratory endurance exercise. Use the one that works best for you and the type of exercise you have chosen.

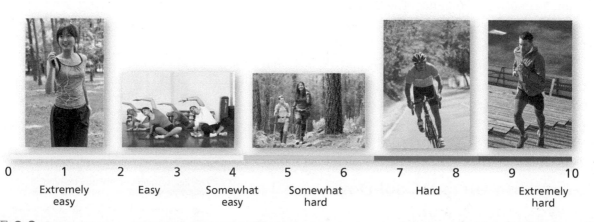

0	1	2	3	4	5	6	7	8	9	10
	Extremely easy		Easy		Somewhat easy	Somewhat hard		Hard		Extremely hard

FIGURE **3.8** Determine your exercise intensity on a 1 to 10 scale by assessing how you feel when exercising. Aim for ratings of 5, 6, 7, or 8 for most cardiorespiratory activities.

Source: Based on A. C. Utter et al., "Validation of the Adult OMNI Scale of Perceived Exertion for Walking/Running Exercise," *Medicine & Science in Sports & Exercise* 36, no. 10 (2004): 1776–80.

TABLE 3.3 Cardiorespiratory Intensity Scales*

General	Talk Test	OMNI	Borg RPE	% HRR	% HRmax
Light	Easy conversation	0	6	30	57
		1	7		
		2	8	35	60
			9		
		3	10		
		4	11	39	63
Moderate	Brief sentences and words	5	12	40	64
			13		
		6	14	59	75
Vigorous	A few words	7	15	60	76
			16		
		8	17	89	95
Anaerobic	Barely or not able to talk	9	18	90	96
			19		
		10	20	100	100

*The various methods to quantify exercise intensity in this table may not be equivalent to one another.

Data from American College of Sports Medicine, *ACSM's Guidelines for Exercise Testing and Prescription*, 9th ed. (Baltimore, MD: Lippincott Williams & Wilkins, 2014); Office of Disease Prevention and Health Promotion, US Department of Health and Human Services, "2008 Physical Activity Guidelines for Americans: Be Active, Healthy, and Happy!" ODPHP Publication no. U0036 (Washington, DC: US Department of Health and Human Services, 2008), www.health.gov; R. J. Robertson et al., "Validation of the Adult OMNI Scale of Perceived Exertion for Cycle Ergometer Exercise," *Medicine & Science in Sports & Exercise* 36, no. 1 (2004): 102–8; A. C. Utter et al., "Validation of the Adult OMNI Scale of Perceived Exertion for Walking/Running Exercise," *Medicine & Science in Sports & Exercise* 36, no. 10 (2004): 1776–80; G. Borg, *Borg's Perceived Exertion and Pain Scales* (Champaign, IL: Human Kinetics, 1998), 27–38.

cross-training The practice of using different exercise modes or types in your cardiorespiratory training program

warm-up The initial 5- to 10-minute preparation phase of a workout

cool-down The ending phase of a workout where the body is brought gradually back to rest

Time For optimal cardiorespiratory conditioning, your exercise sessions should be 20 to 30 minutes long. If you are just starting out, exercise continuously for as long as you can, and then work your way up to the minimum guideline of 20 minutes. The GetFit-Graphic Are Short Workouts Worth My Time? on page 79 examines how even workouts as short as 10 to 15 minutes can be beneficial.

Type For optimal motivation, training adaptation, and injury prevention, choose activities that you enjoy. Alternate these activities by the day or week for a **cross-training** effect. Cross-training helps you maintain muscle balance by working different muscle groups.

Include a Warm-Up and Cool-Down in Your Workout Session

A cardiorespiratory workout session should consist of three components: the **warm-up**, the cardiorespiratory conditioning set, and the **cool-down**. **Figure 3.9**

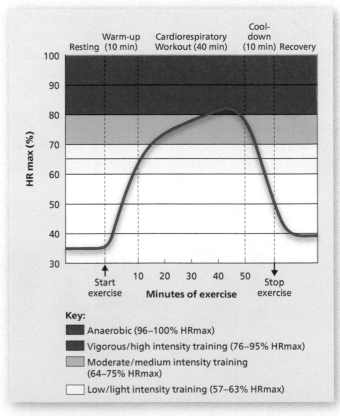

FIGURE **3.9** This graph charts a sample 60-minute cardiorespiratory workout, including a warm-up, cardiorespiratory fitness workout, and a cool-down.

illustrates a sample 60-minute workout showing each of these components. Remember that your warm-up should consist of light physical activity that mimics the movements of your conditioning set. For example, if you are planning to jog, an ideal warm-up would be to walk briskly. Likewise, your cool-down is ideally a less-vigorous version of your main exercise set. (Review Chapter 2 for more warm-up and cool-down guidelines.) When you are just starting an exercise program, perform longer warm-up (10 to 15 minutes) and cool-down (10 minutes or more) segments.

LO 3.6 How Can I Maintain My Cardiorespiratory Program?

How many times have you started a fitness program but quit after a few weeks? Sticking with your cardiorespiratory fitness program may be your biggest challenge! Next we'll discuss the stages of progression and the importance of tracking your progress and reassessing your needs.

Understand the Stages of Progression

When you are starting a new exercise program, it is easy to do too much too soon. A fitness program needs to be *progressive* for you to achieve results and avoid injury.

Start-Up In the *start-up* phase of a cardiorespiratory program, your progress may initially be slow, while your body adjusts to the new activity. During this stage, pay attention to how you feel during exercise so that you can make adjustments if necessary. Do you prefer exercising in the morning or in the evening? Is that aerobics class really right for you? In this first stage, your main concern should be fine-tuning your program until you settle on an activity and routine that are comfortable for you. Depending on your fitness level and experience, this stage can last anywhere from two to four weeks.

Improvement Once you have the "kinks" worked out of your program, you are ready to move into the *improvement* phase. In this stage, your body starts adapting to the cardiorespiratory exercise and your consistent participation will result in noticeable improvements. Some of these changes will be evident to you; some will not (refer to Figure 3.5). You should start feeling better during exercise, have more energy when not exercising, and feel that you can exercise for longer periods of time without fatigue. As in the initial stage, listen to your body so that you can make changes as needed.

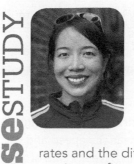

To prevent injuries, increase your workout by no more than 10 percent per week (the *10 percent rule*). That means that your weekly increases in frequency, intensity, or time should be no more than 10 percent total. For example, if you are jogging for 30 minutes per exercise session, next week you could safely increase each session to 33 minutes (a 10 percent increase in time). The improvement stage can last anywhere from three to eight months, depending on your program and goals.

Maintenance After months of hard work, you are at the fitness level you desire and you feel great! You have reached the *maintenance* stage. The key to this stage is to keep your program consistent. If you stop exercising, you can lose your newly achieved fitness level in only half the time it took you to acquire it. In fact, athletes can start losing cardiorespiratory fitness after just two weeks of inactivity. If you need to cut back but don't want to lose your hard-earned improvements, cut back on exercise time but not intensity level. It is easier to maintain cardiorespiratory fitness with shorter but more intense workouts. The maintenance stage lasts for as long as you continue your program.

Record and Track Your Progress

Do you remember how you felt during that spinning workout three weeks ago? What was the speed and incline of your treadmill workout last week? One of the best ways to stay focused in your fitness program is to record your activity and track your progress over time. In a workout journal or log, write down things such as the FITT components of your workout, how you felt during the workout, the time of day, and any other information that may be relevant. Record successes and setbacks—this will remind you of the progress you have made and help determine if your goals or workouts should be adjusted over time.

To get started, see the four-week cardiorespiratory training log in Lab 3.3. You can also use technology to record your workouts, motivate yourself for the next session, and track your progress over time. Check out the Q&A Can Technology Help Me Get More Fit? in Chapter 2 for more tips on using technology for fitness program tracking. You can also refer back to Lab 2.3 to practice using a pedometer or activity tracker to record your steps and/or miles during a workout.

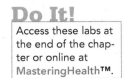

Do It!
Access these labs at the end of the chapter or online at MasteringHealth™.

Troubleshoot Problems Right Away

Everyone experiences obstacles or problems when starting an exercise program. You may not have enough time in your day, it may be difficult for you to physically get to your fitness facility, you may be feeling pain in your knee, and so on. While these issues may set you back temporarily, they should not keep you from reaching your goals. Address the obstacles right away and brainstorm solutions; the sooner you acknowledge a problem and address it, the sooner you can get back on track.

Periodically Reassess Your Cardiorespiratory Fitness Level

Although you will feel your progress by how your body responds to exercise, it is always nice to have quantitative measures of your progress. Complete the assessments in Lab 3.2 after three months of your new program and again at six months. Keep in mind that you will see the most improvements in assessments that are similar to your chosen workout activity (e.g., if you are

walking for fitness, you will see more improvement in the walk test than in the 1.5-mile run test). If you have not improved, evaluate your fitness program design and alter it if necessary.

Reassess Your Goals and Program as Needed

Once a target date arrives, review your goals for that date. Did you achieve what you set out to do? If not, list the reasons why. You may need to set more realistic goals and target dates, or select a different activity. If you need more motivation, consider finding a workout partner or working with a personal trainer. If you did reach your goal, set a new goal for maintenance or a more challenging goal to improve your fitness level even more. The sample running, cycling, and swimming programs at the end of this chapter (pages 103–112) can help you set new goals and develop new fitness plans.

LO 3.7 How Can I Avoid Injury during Cardiorespiratory Exercise?

The fastest way to disrupt a training program is to get injured. Reduce your risk by following common exercise injury prevention methods.

Design a Personalized, Balanced Cardiorespiratory Program

The most common injuries from cardiorespiratory fitness programs are from overuse, such as strains and tendonitis, particularly in the lower body. If you do too much too soon, you put yourself at risk for such injuries. Make sure your exercise program considers your current level of fitness and make your FITT targets realistic and achievable. You may also want to consider incorporating cross-training into your program. Doing one activity exclusively can result in uneven muscle development, making you more vulnerable to injury.

Wear Appropriate Clothing and Footwear

Use common sense when you are dressing for your chosen cardiorespiratory activity. If you are cycling outdoors, a helmet and bright clothing are essential. If you are running, walking, taking a group fitness class, or participating in a racquet sport, pay close attention to your footwear. You need shoes that will protect your feet and provide the right amount of support and cushioning. See

Select the Right Shoe for You

If you answer yes to any of the following, it's time to shop for new shoes!

☐ YES—I've had my athletic shoes for more than six months and use them every day (for walking around and/or exercise)

☐ YES—My feet, ankles, shins, hips, or lower back have been hurting after starting my cardio program.

☐ YES—I've barely used my athletic shoes, but I've had them more than a year (shoe cushioning can break down over time, even without use).

Use these tips to help guide you through the challenging shoe selection process:

1. Shop for shoes at a sporting goods or sport-specific store for the best selection and assistance.

2. Have a knowledgeable sales associate watch you walk or run to help you choose the best shoe for you.

3. Shop for shoes after a workout or at the end of the day when your feet are biggest.

4. Wear socks that you will wear when exercising.

5. Try on both the right and left shoes to ensure they both fit.

6. Shoes should feel comfortable as soon as you try them on.

7. Be sure you can freely wiggle all your toes.

8. Make sure that your heel doesn't slide up or down as you walk.

9. Lace shoes up correctly and walk/run around the store.

10. Choose a sport-specific shoe if you participate in a sport three or more times a week or will be doing high-intensity movements.

11. Select a shoe design based upon your foot type; complete the TRY IT! activity next to determine your foot type.

12. Stay away from fads (i.e., barefoot/minimalist or ultra-high cushion shoes, etc.) until you've assessed what works for your feet and chosen activity.

TRY IT!

THE WET TEST: Determine your **foot type** based upon the height of your arches:

1. Pour water into a shallow pan or dish and wet the bottom of your foot.

2. Step onto a brown grocery bag and look at your wet foot print.

3. Compare your foot print with the following photos to **circle your foot type**.

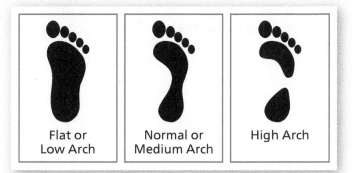

| Flat or Low Arch | Normal or Medium Arch | High Arch |

4. Use this guide when choosing new shoes:
   a. If you have a **flat** or **low arch**, purchase a motion-control shoe to correct pronation, the inward rolling of your foot.
   b. If you have a **normal** or **medium arch**, look for a stability or light pronation-control shoe.
   c. If you have a **high arch** and normal stride, a neutral shoe is probably best for you.

Sources:
1. American Academy of Orthopaedic Surgeons, "Ortho Info: Athletic Shoes," reviewed September 2015, www.orthoinfo.org/topic.cfm?topic=A00318
2. Runner's World, "Take the Wet Test: Learn Your Foot Type," reviewed September 2015, www.runnersworld.com/running-shoes/take-this-simple-test-to-learn-if-you-have-high-or-low-arches

the Tools for Change box Select the Right Shoe for You above for practical guidance on choosing footwear.

Pay Attention to Your Exercise Environment

Prevent Heat-Related Illness When exercising indoors, be sure the exercise room is well ventilated and cool enough to prevent you from overheating. When exercising outdoors in hot weather, take precautions to avoid heat-related illnesses such as **heat cramps**,

> **heat cramps** Severe cramping in the large muscle groups and abdomen caused by high fluid and electrolyte loss in sustained exertion in the heat

heat exhaustion, or **heat stroke**. Your risk of heat-related illness increases if you (1) exercise too hard for your fitness level, (2) exercise in high heat, humidity, and sunshine, (3) have a low fitness level overall, (4) lack adequate sleep, (5) are not accustomed to the environment, (6) have an underlying infection, or (7) are overweight.[25] Lower your risk with the following strategies:

- Become more fit
- Wear light, sweat-wicking clothing
- Exercise during cooler times of the day
- Avoid hazardous conditions
- Let your body gradually become accustomed to the environment
- Increase your workout slowly

If you suspect you are developing a heat-related illness, act immediately. For heat cramps, stop exercising, seek a cool environment, and drink water or sports drinks to restore your body's fluid and electrolyte balances. For heat exhaustion, rest in a cool environment, apply cold packs to your head and neck, drink water or a sports drink, and seek medical attention.

If you suspect heatstroke, seek medical attention immediately; untreated heatstroke is very serious and can be fatal. In heatstroke the body can no longer cool itself and ice-water immersion and IV fluids may be necessary right away. Because exercise increases your core body temperature, your risk of heat illness is greater when you are active, even in lower temperatures. Take extra precautions during difficult workouts to take breaks and drink fluids.

Prevent Cold-Related Illness Exercising in extreme cold is also risky. If you like to ski, hike in the mountains, swim in cold water, or just exercise in snowy, windy, rainy environments, take precautions to prevent **hypothermia**, in which the body's internal temperature drops so low that it can no longer warm itself back up. Untreated hypothermia is fatal. To avoid hypothermia:

heat exhaustion An elevated core body temperature, headache, fatigue, profuse sweating, nausea, and clammy skin brought on by sustained exertion in the heat with dehydration and electrolyte losses

heat stroke A core body temperature above 104°F, headache, nausea, vomiting, diarrhea, rapid pulse, cessation of sweating, and disorientation resulting from extreme exertion in very hot conditions

hypothermia A condition where the core temperature of the body drops below the level required for sustaining normal bodily functions

- Minimize heat loss by wearing a warm hat and clothing
- Keep yourself dry by wearing sweat-wicking clothing and change out of wet clothes as quickly as possible
- Exercise with a workout partner who can help recognize early warning signs of cold-related illness
- Avoid exercising in poor weather conditions
- Warm up thoroughly before exercising
- Drink fluids to stay hydrated
- If you start shivering, get out of the cold and warm up

Early warning signs of hypothermia include shivering, goose bumps, and fast, shallow breathing. The next stage involves violent shivering, loss of muscle coordination, mild confusion, pale skin, and potentially blue lips, ears, fingers, and toes. In the most dangerous and potentially fatal stage of hypothermia, shivering will stop and the person will have trouble thinking, speaking, walking, and using his or her hands. If you suspect you are at risk of hypothermia, get dry and warm as soon as possible. If you are in an advanced stage of hypothermia, you will need medical attention immediately.

Be Aware of the Impact of Air Quality Air pollution can irritate your air passageways and lungs, particularly if you have asthma, allergies, bronchitis, or other pulmonary disorders. If you experience a disruption in your breathing pattern, irritated eyes, or a headache, stop exercising and go indoors. Avoid exercising outdoors when the air quality is poor, particularly if you have a smog or air-quality alert in your city that day. If you exercise outside on a regular basis, take measures to reduce your intake of air pollution. Exercise in wilderness areas and parks, or on low-traffic streets. Try to exercise at times when the air quality is better, such as early in the morning and on weekends.

Watch for Hazards Watch for hazards in your environment that may cause you to trip and fall. When exercising indoors, seek out a space with a well-maintained floor where you can work out without obstructions. When exercising outdoors, seek out lower-impact surfaces such as a school track, running or bike path, or dirt trail. Use your common sense: Avoid slippery or muddy surfaces and areas with heavy vehicle traffic. If you exercise outdoors at night, wear reflective clothing and clip a light somewhere on your body so that drivers can easily see you.

Ensure Proper Hydration

If you sweat profusely and do not replace the lost fluid, you will become dehydrated. Your body needs a certain

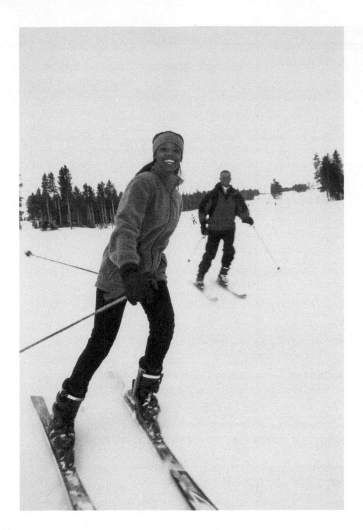

for a long period of time, over-hydrate your body, and lose salt through your sweat without replacing it with electrolytes in fluid or food. Since your body won't have enough electrolytes to run essential brain, heart, and nervous system functions, you'll end up feeling fatigued, sick, or, at worst, needing medical attention. Less fit individuals are at a higher risk of hyponatremia, so pay attention to your electrolyte replacement if you are new to longer exercise sessions.

Understand How to Prevent and Treat Common Injuries

The following are some of the most common exercise injuries, as well as guidelines for how to prevent and treat them. See **Table 3.4** for a summary of these and other common exercise injuries.

Delayed-Onset Muscle Soreness *Delayed-onset muscle soreness* (DOMS) is the muscle tightness and tenderness you may feel a day or two after a workout session. This soreness is due to microscopic tears in your muscle fibers and connective tissues; it occurs when the body sustains excessive overloads. Most people experience DOMS at one point or another and typically recover quickly. DOMS is a sign that you did too much too soon. If you experience DOMS, examine your program and find ways to decrease the time, intensity, resistance, or repetitions of the exercise.

Muscle and Tendon Strains A muscle or tendon strain is a soft-tissue injury that can be acute or chronic. An acute, sudden strain occurs due to a trauma or sudden movement/force that you are not accustomed to. A chronic, perpetual strain occurs from overstressed muscles that are worked in the same way over and over. Muscle strains involve damage to the muscle fibers; tendon strains involve damage to the tissue that connects muscles to bones. The primary symptoms of a strain are muscle pain, spasms, and weakness. In addition, there may be swelling, cramping, and difficulty moving the muscle involved. Commonly strained areas are the lower back and the back of the thighs (hamstrings).

Ligament and Joint Sprains A sudden movement or trauma can cause a sprain (damage to joint structures).

• A *mild* or *first-degree sprain* involves overstretching or slight tearing of the ligament(s), resulting in some pain and swelling but little or no decrease in joint stability.

amount of water in order to function. Loss of body water will decrease your blood volume and the blood flow to muscles, lowering exercise performance. Dehydration will also slow your sweat rate and significantly increase your susceptibility to heat-related illness.

According to the ACSM, you should lose no more than 2 percent of your body weight in fluid during an exercise session.[26] A loss of fluid equivalent to 1 percent of your body weight will cause you to feel thirsty; losses over 3 percent may start to affect your performance. Weigh yourself before and after exercise to determine how much water weight you have lost and adjust your fluid intake accordingly.

Water loss is an individual issue. Everyone sweats at different rates in response to exercise. To decrease water loss, start drinking additional fluid several hours before an exercise session and drink during exercise as well.

If you exercise for more than an hour, you may benefit from drinking fluid containing sugars and electrolytes (salts), such as a sports drink. This can be important to keep up your energy levels and reduce your risk of **hyponatremia**. Hyponatremia is a potentially life-threatening situation that can occur when you exercise

> **hyponatremia** A condition where the amount of salt in the blood is lower than normal

TABLE 3.4 Common Exercise Injuries, Treatments, and Prevention

Injury	Description	Treatment and Prevention
Delayed-Onset Muscle Soreness (DOMS)	Muscle tenderness and stiffness 24 to 48 hours after strenuous exercise	*Treatment:* Reduce exercise to light activity until the pain stops; gently stretch the area; heat and anti-inflammatory medications may help as well *Prevention:* Follow proper exercise programming guidelines
Back Pain	Sharp or dull pain and stiffness in the mid to lower back	*Treatment:* Reduce exercise until the acute pain stops; gently stretch the area; use ice, heat, anti-inflammatory medications; seek medical advice if the pain persists more than a few days *Prevention:* Strengthen abdominal and back muscles; stretch back and hip muscles; maintain a healthy body weight; have good posture and lifting techniques
Blisters	Red, fluid- or blood-filled pockets of skin, often on the feet after a long exercise session	*Treatment:* Change shoes that may have caused the blister; keep the area clean and cover if needed; do not deliberately pop blisters *Prevention:* Wear comfortable shoes that fit well and sweat-wicking socks (avoid all-cotton socks)
Muscle Cramps	Muscle pain, tightness, and uncontrollable spasms	*Treatment:* Stop activity; massage and stretch the affected area until the cramp releases *Prevention:* Follow warm-up, cool-down, and general exercise guidelines; stay fully hydrated for exercise
Muscle Strain	Damage to the muscle or tendon fibers due to injury or overtraining resulting in pain, swelling, and decreased function; varying levels of severity	*Treatment:* Reduce painful activity; use ice as needed; apply ice and/or heat after a few days; use anti-inflammatory medications if desired; stretch *Prevention:* Follow warm-up, cool-down, and general exercise guidelines; reduce or stop activity if muscles feel overly weak and fatigued
Joint Sprain	Damage to ligaments or joint structures; the result of an acute injury resulting in pain, swelling, and loss of function; varying levels of severity	*Treatment:* Stop activity; use ice, compression, and elevation; seek medical attention *Prevention:* Avoid high joint-stress activities; strengthen joint-supporting muscles; wear supportive bracing if necessary
Dislocation	Separation of bones in a joint causing structural alterations and potential ligament and nerve damage	*Treatment:* Stop activity; use ice and immobilization; seek medical treatment *Prevention:* Avoid high joint-stress activities; strengthen joint-supporting muscles; wear supportive bracing if necessary
Tendonitis	Chronic pain and swelling in tendons as a result of overuse	*Treatment:* Reduce exercise to light activity until the pain stops; apply ice and gently stretch the area; anti-inflammatory medications may help *Prevention:* Follow proper exercise programming guidelines; work for muscle balance in strength and flexibility
Plantar Fasciitis	Irritation, pain, and swelling of the fascia under the foot	*Treatment:* Reduce painful activities; gently stretch the area; for some people, ice, heat, and/or anti-inflammatory medications help *Prevention:* Wear good athletic shoes with adequate arch support and cushioning; warm up and stretch the plantar fascia prior to exercise
Runner's Knee	Patella-femoral pain syndrome where there is chronic pain behind or around the kneecap	*Treatment:* Reduce exercises that cause pain; use ice and anti-inflammatory medications if needed for pain and swelling *Prevention:* Work for balance in strength and flexibility in all of the knee-supporting muscles; wear good athletic shoes with support and foot control; exercise on softer surfaces; control weight
Shin Splints	Chronic pain in the front of the lower leg (the shins); can also occur as pain on the sides of the lower leg	*Treatment:* Reduce painful exercise; apply ice; gently stretch the area; switch to less weight-bearing activities *Prevention:* Work for balance in strength and flexibility in the lower-leg muscles; wear good athletic shoes with support and cushioning; exercise on softer surfaces

(Continued)

TABLE **3.4** (*Continued*)

Injury	Description	Treatment and Prevention
Stress Fracture	Small crack or breaks in the bone in overused areas of the body causing chronic pain; must be medically diagnosed via X-ray	*Treatment:* Perform non-weight-bearing exercise until the acute pain stops; seek medical attention; rest *Prevention:* Follow proper exercise programming guidelines to avoid overtraining; wear good athletic shoes with support and cushioning; exercise on softer surfaces

- In a *moderate* or *second-degree sprain,* ligaments are partially torn, and the area is painful, swollen, and bruised. Mobility is limited. Seek medical attention to determine the severity of the injury.

- A *severe* or *third-degree sprain* involves complete tearing or rupturing of the ligament or joint structures. Symptoms include excessive pain, swelling, bruising, and inability to move or put any weight on the joint. Immediate medical attention is necessary to determine whether any bones are broken.

The most common sprains occur in the ankle while landing from a jump, in the knee from a fall or a blow to the side, and in the wrist during a fall.

Overuse Injuries Overuse injuries are due to repetitive use. You are at an increased risk of an overuse injury if you are new to exercise, if you dramatically change your exercise routine, or if you do the same type of activity day in and day out.

Tendonitis is a typical overuse injury that can result from overusing the lower- or upper-body muscles. The repetitive contractions of skeletal muscles can cause pain and swelling in the tendons near joints. Common tendonitis locations are the elbow, ankle, and shoulder; these often result from tennis ("tennis elbow"), running, and weight-lifting, respectively.

A frequent overuse injury in runners and walkers is *plantar fasciitis,* or inflammation in the fascia on the underside of the foot. Pain in the arch and the heel of the foot, particularly when you are not warmed up (stepping out of bed in the morning), is the hallmark of plantar fasciitis.

Another injury common in runners is "runner's knee," or *patella-femoral pain syndrome.* Pain behind the kneecap (patella), inflammation, and tenderness can result from an imbalance in knee-stabilizing muscles that will cause the patella to get "off track" with your other knee joint structures. Women tend to have more

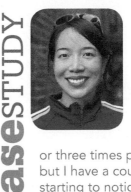

caseSTUDY

NAOMI

"A few weeks ago, I looked at running programs in my fitness book and online at RunnersWorld.com. Then I downloaded the MapMyFitness app to my phone to track my workouts. Since then, I've run two or three times per week. It's going pretty good, but I have a couple of problems. First, I am starting to notice a little pain on the front of my shins. I had this problem back in high school cross country, too. After reading my book, I think it is shin splints. I may need to get new shoes. Second, I can only do my runs after work and classes, so sometimes I run out of daylight. I don't want to get hit by a car, so I guess I should buy a reflective vest or something."

APPLY IT! What should Naomi consider when purchasing new running shoes? What else can she do during her twilight runs to increase her personal safety?

TRY IT! **Today,** list three things about your workout routine, your clothing/shoes, or your environment that might put you at risk for injury or illness. **This week,** for each risky item or behavior, list what steps you need to take to reduce your risk. **In two weeks,** implement at least three things that you need to do to increase your safety.

Hear It!
To listen to this case study online, visit the Study Area in MasteringHealth™.

problems with this syndrome than men due to the greater dynamic flexibility of their hips and knees.

Shin splints is the general term for any pain in the front or sides of the lower legs. It may be tendonitis, a muscle strain, connective tissue inflammation, or a stress fracture. In response to repetitive stresses on hard surfaces, the muscles, tendons, and connective tissues of your lower leg muscles become inflamed and painful. Shin splints are common in runners and high-mileage walkers. Over time, repeated stress to the lower leg can lead to a *stress fracture*, a small crack or break in a bone. If you think you have shin splints but the pain won't go away with rest, ice, and therapy, you should get medical attention to rule out a stress fracture.

Treating Injuries with RICE The **RICE** treatment for injuries involves *rest, ice, compression,* and *elevation.* After an injury, you should *rest* or stop using that body part and allow for treatment and recovery. Most injuries will require *ice* immediately to reduce blood flow, acute inflammation, and pain. Apply ice or an ice pack for 10 to 30 minutes at a time, three to five times a day until symptoms lessen. *Compression,* or applying pressure to the injury, can help injuries that are bleeding or swelling. An elastic bandage around the injury will reduce swelling but still allows adequate blood flow to the area. Tingling or discolored skin can be a sign that your wrapping is too tight. To promote blood flow back to the heart and lower the amount of swelling, *elevate* the injury above heart level.

The RICE treatment is a good start for most exercise and sports-related injuries. Seek medical attention if you are unsure how injured you are or if symptoms do not improve within a few hours.

Study Plan

MasteringHealth™

Build your knowledge—and wellness!—
in the Study Area of MasteringHealth
with a variety of study tools.

chapter summary

LO 3.1 How Does My Cardiorespiratory System Work?

- The **respiratory system** (also called the *pulmonary system*) consists of the air passageways and the lungs. Oxygen moves from the alveolar sacs in the lungs into the capillary blood, while carbon dioxide moves in the opposite direction.

- The **cardiovascular system** consists of the heart and blood vessels. One "beat" of your heart consists of a full heart cycle (systole and diastole).

- Your body breaks down stored and consumed nutrients to ATP via three **metabolic energy systems**: the *immediate, nonoxidative* (anaerobic), and *oxidative* (aerobic) systems. At **rest**, your body maintains homeostasis by breaking down fat via the oxidative energy system. In **exercise**, your body will use all three systems to supply ATP depending upon the intensity and duration of the activity.

LO 3.2 How Does Aerobic Training Condition My Cardiorespiratory System?

- Aerobic training increases the contraction strength and capacity of your heart, increasing your stroke volume.

LO 3.3 What Are the Benefits of Improving My Cardiorespiratory Fitness?

- Cardiorespiratory fitness decreases your risk of many diseases and improves self-esteem, mood, sleep, immune responses, sense of well-being, and overall physical functioning.

LO 3.4 How Can I Assess My Cardiorespiratory Fitness?

- Your VO_2max is the measure of your body's ability to deliver oxygen to the muscles and the muscles' ability to consume or use the oxygen during maximal exercise.

- Submaximal exercise test values are compared against norm charts or used to predict your maximal oxygen consumption.

LO 3.5 How Can I Create My Own Cardiorespiratory Fitness Program?

- Set cardiorespiratory fitness goals that follow the SMART goal-setting guidelines.

- Apply the FITT formula.

LO 3.6 How Can I Maintain My Cardiorespiratory Program?

- Understand the stages of progression when you are starting a new exercise program. Record, track, and reassess your progress.

LO 3.7 How Can I Avoid Injury during Cardiorespiratory Exercise?

- Design a personalized cardiorespiratory program.

- Wear appropriate clothing and footwear and take steps to prevent heat- and cold-related illnesses

- Ensure proper hydration.

- Understand how to prevent and treat common injuries.

review questions

LO 3.1 **1.** Which circulation system delivers blood to the lungs?
a. Pulmonary
b. Lymphatic
c. Hepatic
d. Cardiac

LO 3.1 **2.** Which energy system will provide most of the ATP during an hour-long bicycle ride?
a. The immediate energy system
b. The nonoxidative energy system
c. The creatine phosphate energy system
d. The oxidative energy system

LO 3.2 **3.** Which of the following will decrease with regular aerobic training?
a. Muscle cell size
b. Blood volume
c. Resting heart rate
d. Maximal cardiac output

review questions CONTINUED

LO 3.3 **4.** Regular cardiorespiratory fitness activities reduce your chance of developing
a. metabolic syndrome.
b. HIV.
c. athlete's foot.
d. dehydration.

LO 3.4 **5.** Which of the following would be the most accurate way to determine your cardiorespiratory fitness level?
a. VO$_2$max test
b. 1.5-mile run test
c. 3-minute step test
d. 1-mile walk test

LO 3.5 **6.** Which OMNI Scale of Perceived Exertion value is associated with training in your target heart rate range?
a. 1
b. 3
c. 7
d. 9

LO 3.6 **7.** Which of the following is the *best* way to safely plan for cardiorespiratory program progression?
a. Follow the 10 percent rule.
b. Increase your exercise duration every time you work out.

c. Test your cardiorespiratory fitness once a week.
d. Increase your exercise intensity each workout session.

LO 3.6 **8.** Which of the following is a good strategy to stay on track with your cardio fitness program?
a. Read articles online about fitness topics.
b. Post pictures around your house of being active.
c. Attend motivational talks about fitness and health.
d. Record your activities and track your progress over time.

LO 3.7 **9.** A dangerously low level of salt in the blood describes_____.
a. hyperthermia
b. hyponatremia
c. hypothermia
d. dehydration

LO 3.7 **10.** Pain in the heel and arch of the foot is the hallmark of this overuse injury:
a. tendonitis
b. shin splints
c. patella-femoral pain syndrome
d. plantar fasciitis

critical thinking questions

LO 3.3 **1.** Name three benefits of having a high level of cardiorespiratory fitness and explain how each impacts your overall health and wellness.

LO 3.5 **2.** What are the pros and cons of each method of intensity monitoring: target heart rate, perceived exertion, and the talk test?

check out these eResources

- **ACE Fit** Resources for workouts, podcasts, and finding a local trainer. Click on "Healthy Living," "Tools for Life," and "Fit Facts," and then you'll find the "Cardiovascular Exercise" link with cardio articles and workouts. **www.acefitness.org/acefit**
- **Couch to 5K** Combined walking/running program designed to get beginners ready for a 5K (3.1 miles) run in eight weeks. **www.c25kfree.com**
- **Map My Fitness** Track your activities, food, and gear with this app's easy-to-use interface and accurate tracking capabilities. **www.mapmyfitness.com**

- **Runner's World** Advice about shoes, nutrition, training plans, and more for beginners to seasoned runners. **www.runnersworld.com**
- **STRAVA** Popular app for bike enthusiasts to track rides by time, distance, and speed (it can track runs, too); plus challenges that connect cyclists who compete for things like climbing the highest or snapping the best photos mid-ride. **www.strava.com**

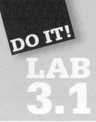

DO IT!

LEARN A SKILL

LAB
3.1

MONITORING
INTENSITY DURING
A WORKOUT

MasteringHealth™

Name: _____   Date: _____

Instructor: _____   Section: _____

Materials: Calculator and a stopwatch

Purpose: (1) To measure your resting heart rate (RHR); (2) to calculate your personal target heart rate range for exercise; and (3) to assess the intensity of your workout.

Section I: Counting Your Heart Rate

1. **Practice Taking Your Pulse** Take a *radial pulse* (a) by placing your middle and index fingers at the thumb side of your wrist. While the radial pulse is preferred, you can also gently press your middle and index fingers on the side of your throat to find your **carotid pulse** (b). Practice taking resting heart rate (RHR) measurement by counting your pulse for 60 seconds. Record below.
Resting Pulse (60 sec) _____ **1 full minute RHR**
Practice taking an exercise heart rate (EHR) measurement by jogging in place for two minutes and counting your pulse for 10 seconds. Record your 10-second count below and convert to a heart rate by multiplying by six.
Exercise Pulse (10 sec) _____ × 6 = _____ **Calculated 1-minute EHR**

(a)

SCAN TO SEE IT
ONLINE!

(b)

SCAN TO SEE IT
ONLINE!

2. **Determine Your True Resting Heart Rate** Take your pulse first thing in the morning on four different days. Record and average the results below. For an accurate resting heart rate, always count for a full minute. Ideally, you should take your pulse after a good night's rest and after waking up *without an alarm*.

	Resting Heart Rate (RHR)	Time of Day
Day 1		
Day 2		
Day 3		
Day 4		

Average RHR = _____

Section II: Calculate Your Target Heart Rate Range For Exercise

Calculate your personal target heart rate range for exercise using two methods: the maximum heart rate (HRmax) method and the heart rate reserve (HRR) method. Your target heart rate will provide a guideline for how many beats per minute (bpm) your heart should be beating during exercise, in order to improve cardiorespiratory fitness. Note that you must count your pulse within 15 seconds of stopping exercise in order for your heart rate to reflect the exercise rate. Thus, if you take five seconds to find your pulse and start counting, that leaves you 10 seconds to take an exercise heart rate.

Method #1: Maximum Heart Rate (HRmax)

1. Find your predicted HRmax = 220 − _____ = _____
                                                    (age)   (predicted HRmax)

2. Find your low HR target = _____ × .70 = _____ bpm ÷ 6 = _____
                                        (predicted HRmax)   *Low HR target*   *Low 10 sec target*

3. Find your high HR target = _____ × .90 = _____ bpm ÷ 6 = _____
                                        (predicted HRmax)   *High HR target*   *High 10 sec target*

Method #2: Heart Rate Reserve (HRR)

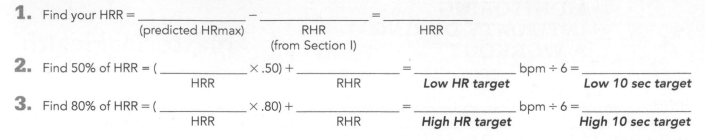

1. Find your HRR = _____ – _____ = _____
                (predicted HRmax)   RHR   HRR
                     (from Section I)

2. Find 50% of HRR = (_____ × .50) + _____ = _____ bpm ÷ 6 = _____
                   HRR   RHR   *Low HR target*   *Low 10 sec target*

3. Find 80% of HRR = (_____ × .80) + _____ = _____ bpm ÷ 6 = _____
                   HRR   RHR   *High HR target*   *High 10 sec target*

Section III: Monitor Your Workout Intensity Level

Practice monitoring your workout intensity during a 30-minute exercise session. You can choose any form of exercise that allows you to easily monitor your heart rate.

1. Calculate your estimated heart rate goal as a 10-second count for each time interval in the chart below.

2. Conduct your exercise session. Take your pulse and record your actual exercise heart rates.

3. In the last column of the chart, write your perceived exertion scores (1–10 OMNI Scale) 30 seconds before the end of the time period indicated on the workout schedule.

Time	Planned Intensity	Calculated HR 10 sec Count	Actual 10 sec HR	Perceived Exertion (1–10)
5 min warm-up	Slowly up to 55% HRmax	Predicted HRmax × .55 = _____ ÷ 6 = _____		
5 min	65% HRmax	Predicted HRmax × .65 = _____ ÷ 6 = _____		
4 min	75% HRmax	Predicted HRmax × .75 = _____ ÷ 6 = _____		
3 min	85% HRmax	Predicted HRmax × .85 = _____ ÷ 6 = _____		
4 min	75% HRmax	Predicted HRmax × .75 = _____ ÷ 6 = _____		
5 min	65% HRmax	Predicted HRmax × .65 = _____ ÷ 6 = _____		
4 min cool-down	55% HRmax	Predicted HRmax × .55 = _____ ÷ 6 = _____.		

Section IV: Reflection

1. How close were your calculated and actual heart rates during your 30-minute exercise session?

_____

_____

2. Did the intensity levels feel higher or lower than you thought they would at each percentage of HRmax?

_____

_____

DO IT!
LAB
3.2

ASSESS YOURSELF

ASSESSING YOUR
CARDIORESPIRATORY
FITNESS LEVEL

MasteringHealth™

Name: _____ Date: _____

Instructor: _____ Section: _____

Materials: Calculator, 16.25-inch step or bleacher bench, stopwatch, metronome

Purpose: To measure (1) recovery from physical activity, (2) walking speed, and (3) current level of cardiorespiratory fitness.

See It!
How do you keep your heart healthy? Watch the ABC Video "Exercise for Your Heart" at MasteringHealth™.

Section I: The Queen's College Step Test

For this test, you will be stepping on a 16.25-inch-high step bench for three minutes and then measuring your recovery pulse for 15 seconds.

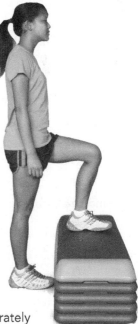

1. **Setup and preparation.** Set up a 16.25-inch-high step bench or bleacher bench (a typical gym bleacher bench is 16.25 inches high) in a place that will be safe to perform the test. Warm-up prior to the assessment with walking and range of motion exercises. Set the metronome to a pace of 96 beats per minute for men (24 steps/min) and 88 bpm for women (22 steps/min). Listen to the metronome and do a couple of practice steps to ensure that you can step with the right cadence ("up, up, down, down"). One foot will be stepping up or down with each beat of the metronome. Have a stopwatch available to time your three minutes on the step and your 15 second recovery heart rate (HR) afterward.

2. **Step up and down for three minutes.** Start the metronome and march in place to the beat. Start stepping up on the bench and down to the floor after starting the stopwatch. Maintain this exact pace for the entire three minutes.

3. **Stop and count your pulse for 15 seconds.** At the end of three minutes, stop stepping, turn off the metronome, and immediately find your carotid or radial pulse. Within five seconds of stopping the exercise, start counting your recovery pulse and count for 15 seconds.

4. **Record your results and calculate your estimated maximal oxygen consumption (VO_2max).** Record your 15-second recovery HR below and then use the appropriate formula (men or women) to calculate your estimated VO_2max. This number will more accurately reflect your fitness level if you followed the test instructions carefully.

5. **Find the cardiorespiratory fitness level that corresponds to your predicted VO_2max.** Use the chart at the end of Section III (page 97) to determine your cardiorespiratory fitness level, as determined by the Queen's College Step Test.

The Queen's College Step Test Results

15 Sec Recovery HR: _____ **(bpm)**

Estimated VO_2max: Plug in your HR from above, compute the number in parentheses first, and complete the calculation (based on your gender) to find your estimated VO_2max.

Men:

- VO_2max = $111.33 - [0.42 \times HR \text{ (bpm)}]$
- VO_2max = $111.33 - [0.42 \times$ _____ (bpm)]
- VO_2max = $111.33 -$ _____

VO_2max = _____ Fitness Rating: _____

Women:

- $VO_2max = 65.81 - [0.1847 \times HR\ (bpm)]$
- $VO_2max = 65.81 - [0.1847 \times \underline{\hspace{2cm}}\ (bpm)]$
- $VO_2max = 65.81 - \underline{\hspace{2cm}}$

VO_2max = _____ Fitness Rating: _____

Source: Based on W.D. McArdle et al., "Reliability and Interrelationships Between Maximal Oxygen Update, Physical Work Capacity and Step-Test Scores in College Women," Medicine and Science in Sports and Exercise 4, (1972): 182–6.

Section II: The One-Mile Walk Test

You will walk one mile and determine your heart rate response to the exercise immediately after. IMPORTANT REMINDERS: The accuracy of this test depends on four things: (1) Walk a measured, flat mile. (2) Walk during this test. Do not run. (3) Walk the mile as fast as you can. (4) Keep a steady pace throughout the mile. Do not "sprint" at the end.

1. **Preparation and warm-up.** Make sure that you have an accurate one-mile course to complete (four laps around a standard track) and a stopwatch. Warm up with three to five minutes of light walking and range-of-motion activities.

2. **Walk one full mile as fast as you can.** After completing the one mile, record your finish time (from your watch, stopwatch, or someone calling out the time) below. Convert the time from minutes and seconds to minutes with a decimal fraction.

3. **Immediately take an exercise heart rate and cool down.** Within five seconds of finishing the walk, find and count your pulse for 10 seconds. Multiply the number by 6 and record your HR below. After recording your finish time and your HR, cool down by walking slowly for another five minutes and doing some light stretching.

4. **Calculate your estimated maximal oxygen consumption (VO_2max).** Use the formula below to calculate your estimated VO_2max. This number will more accurately reflect your fitness level if you followed the test instructions carefully.

5. **Find the cardiorespiratory fitness level that corresponds to your predicted VO_2max.** Use the chart at the end of Section III to determine your cardiorespiratory fitness level, as determined by this one-mile walking test.

The One-Mile Walk Test Results

One-Mile Walk Time: _____ (min:sec); divide sec by 60 = _____ (min w/decimal)

Exercise HR: _____ (beats) × 6 = _____ (bpm)
(10 sec count)

Estimated VO_2max: Use the following equation to estimate VO_2max, where gender = 0 for female and 1 for male; time = walk time to the nearest hundredth of a minute; and HR = heart rate (bpm) at the end of the walking test. Plug in your weight and numbers from above and calculate the numbers in parentheses first. Complete the calculation to find your estimated VO_2max. See the chart on page 97 for your Walk Test VO_2max Fitness Rating.

- $VO_2max = 132.853 - [0.0769 \times body\ weight\ (lb)] - [0.3877 \times age\ (yr)] + [6.3150 \times gender] - [3.2649 \times time\ (min)] - [0.1565 \times HR\ (bpm)]$

- $VO_2max = 132.853 - [0.0769 \times \underline{\hspace{1.5cm}}\ (lb)] - [0.3877 \times \underline{\hspace{1.5cm}}\ (yr)] + [6.3150 \times \underline{\hspace{1.5cm}}$ (gender)$] - [3.2649 \times \underline{\hspace{1.5cm}}\ (min)] - [0.1565 \times \underline{\hspace{1.5cm}}\ (bpm)]$

- $VO_2max = 132.853 - \underline{\hspace{1.5cm}} - \underline{\hspace{1.5cm}} + \underline{\hspace{1.5cm}} - \underline{\hspace{1.5cm}} - \underline{\hspace{1.5cm}}$

- $VO_2max = \underline{\hspace{1.5cm}}\ (ml/kg \cdot min)$

Walk Test VO_2max Fitness Rating: _____

Section III: 1.5-Mile Run Test

1. **Preparation and warm-up.** Make sure that you have an accurate 1.5-mile course to complete (six laps around a standard track) and a stopwatch. Warm up with 5 to 10 minutes of walking/jogging and range-of-motion activities.

2. **Run (with walk breaks if needed) 1.5 miles as fast as you can.** After reaching 1.5 miles, mark your finish time (from your watch, stopwatch, or someone calling out the time) below. Convert the time from minutes and seconds to minutes with a decimal fraction.

3. **Cool down.** After recording your finish time, cool down by walking for five minutes and doing some light stretching.

4. **Calculate your estimated maximal oxygen consumption (VO$_2$max).** Use the formula below to calculate your estimated VO$_2$max.

5. **Find your cardiorespiratory fitness level that corresponds to your predicted VO$_2$max.** Use the chart at the end of this section to determine your cardiorespiratory fitness level, as determined by this 1.5-mile running test.

The 1.5-Mile Run Test Results

1.5-Mile Run Time: _____ (min:sec); divide sec by 60 = _____ (min w/decimal)

Estimated VO$_2$max: You will use the following equation to estimate VO$_2$max, where time = run time to the nearest hundredth of a minute. Plug in your time from above, compute the number in parentheses first, and complete the calculation to find your estimated VO$_2$max. See the chart below for your Run Test VO$_2$max Fitness Rating.

- VO$_2$max = [483 ÷ time (min)] + 3.5

- VO$_2$max = [483 ÷ _____ (min)] + 3.5

- VO$_2$max = _____ + 3.5

- VO$_2$max = _____ (ml/kg·min)

Run Test VO$_2$max Fitness Rating: _____

Estimated VO$_2$max Fitness Ratings (ml/kg-min)						
Men	**Superior**	**Excellent**	**Good**	**Fair**	**Poor**	**Very Poor**
18–29 yrs	>56.1	51.1–56.1	45.7–51.0	42.2–45.6	38.1–42.1	<38.1
30–39 yrs	>54.2	48.9–54.2	44.4–48.8	41.0–44.3	36.7–40.9	<36.7
40–49 yrs	>52.3	46.6–52.3	42.4–46.7	38.4–42.3	34.6–38.3	<34.6
50–59 yrs	>49.6	43.3–49.6	38.3–43.2	35.2–38.2	31.1–35.1	<31.1
60–69 yrs	>46.0	39.5–46.0	35.0–39.4	31.4–34.9	27.4–31.3	<27.4

Women	**Superior**	**Excellent**	**Good**	**Fair**	**Poor**	**Very Poor**
18–29 yrs	>50.1	44.0–50.1	39.5–43.9	35.5–39.4	31.6–35.4	<31.6
30–39 yrs	>46.8	41.0–46.8	36.8–40.9	33.8–36.7	29.9–33.7	<29.9
40–49 yrs	>45.1	38.9–45.1	35.1–38.8	31.6–35.0	28.0–31.5	<28.0
50–59 yrs	>39.8	35.2–39.8	31.4–35.1	28.7–31.3	25.5–28.6	<25.5
60–69 yrs	>36.8	32.3–36.8	29.1–32.2	26.6–29.0	23.7–26.5	<23.7

Reprinted with permission from the Cooper Institute, Dallas, Texas, from *Physical Fitness Assesment and norms for Adults and Law Enforcement*, Copyright ©2007, available online at www.CooperInstitute.org.

You may also use the chart below to estimate your fitness level using only your run time.

Estimated Run Time Ratings				
Men	**Excellent**	**Good**	**Fair**	**Poor**
Ages 20–29	<10:10	10:10–11:29	11:30–12:38	>12:38
Ages 30–39	<10:47	10:47–11:54	11:55–12:58	>12:58
Ages 40–49	<11:16	11:16–12:24	12:25–13:50	>13:50
Ages 50–59	<12:09	12:09–13:35	13:36–15:06	>15:06
Ages 60–69	<13:24	13:24–15:04	15:05–16:46	>16:46

Women	**Excellent**	**Good**	**Fair**	**Poor**
Ages 20–29	<11:59	11:59–13:24	13:25–14:50	>14:50
Ages 30–39	<12:25	12:25–14:08	14:09–15:43	>15:43
Ages 40–49	<13:24	13:24–14:53	14:54–16:31	>16:31
Ages 50–59	<14:35	14:35–16:35	16:36–18:18	>18:18
Ages 60–69	<16:34	16:34–18:27	18:28–20:16	>20:16

Reprinted with permission from The Cooper Insititute Dallas Texas from *Physical Fitness Aaaecements and Norms for Adults and Lew Enforcement*, Copyright © 2007, available online at www.CooparInutitutm.org.

Section IV: Reflection

1. Were you surprised by your fitness assessment results or were they in line with what you were expecting? Explain why or why not.

_____

_____

_____

_____

_____

_____

_____

Note: Your fitness level ratings should guide your choice of a cardiorespiratory fitness program. See Lab 3.3 and Programs 3.1 to 3.3 on pages 99 and 103–112 for more information.

DO IT!

LAB
3.3

PLAN FOR CHANGE

PLAN YOUR CARDIO-
RESPIRATORY FITNESS
GOALS AND PROGRAM

MasteringHealth™

Name: _____ **Date:** _____

Instructor: _____ **Section:** _____

Materials: Results from cardiorespiratory fitness assessments, calculator, lab pages.

Purpose: To learn how to set appropriate cardiorespiratory fitness goals and create a personal cardiorespiratory fitness program designed to meet those goals.

Section I: Short- and Long-Term Goals

Create short- and long-term goals for cardiorespiratory fitness. Be sure to use SMART goal-setting guidelines (specific, measurable, action-oriented, realistic, time-oriented). Select appropriate target dates and rewards for completing your goals.

Short-Term Goal (3 to 6 Months)

_____

_____

Target Date: _____

Reward: _____

Long-Term Goal (12+ Months)

_____

_____

Target Date: _____

Reward: _____

Section II: Cardiorespiratory Fitness Obstacles and Strategies

1. What barriers or obstacles might hinder your plan to improve your cardiorespiratory fitness? Indicate your top three obstacles below:

a. _____

b. _____

c. _____

2. Overcoming these barriers/obstacles will be an important step in reaching your goals. Write down three **strategies** for overcoming the obstacles listed above:

a. _____

b. _____

c. _____

Section III: Getting Support

1. List resources you will use to help you change your cardiorespiratory fitness:

Friend/partner/relative: _____

School-based resource: _____

Community-based resource: _____

Other: _____

2. How will you use these supportive resources to help you meet your cardiorespiratory fitness goals?

_____

_____

_____

_____

_____

_____

_____

Section IV: Cardiorespiratory Fitness Program Reflections

1. How realistic are the short- and long-term target dates you have set for achieving your cardiorespiratory fitness goals?

_____

_____

_____

2. How many days per week are you planning to work on your cardiorespiratory fitness program?

_____

3. What types of workouts are you planning to try?

_____

_____

_____

4. Do you have a workout partner? Do you plan to work with a workout partner, personal trainer, or instructor to help get you started?

_____

_____

_____

Section V: Cardiorespiratory Training Program Design

Plan a four-week cardiorespiratory training program, using resources available to you (facility, instructor, text). Complete the following training calendar (A = activity, I = intensity, T = time).

To get started: Review Programs 3.1 to 3.3 on pages 103–112 for running, cycling, and swimming. Choose a Beginning program if your Lab 3.2 fitness ratings are Fair or lower or the activity is new for you. Aim for an Intermediate program if your Lab 3.2 fitness ratings are Good, and try an Advanced program if your ratings are Excellent or above and you are used to this activity.

Four-Week Cardiorespiratory Training Program						
Sun	**Mon**	**Tues**	**Wed**	**Thurs**	**Fri**	**Sat**
Date: _____	Date: _____	Date: _____	Date: _____	Date: _____	Date: _____	Date: _____
A:	A:	A:	A:	A:	A:	A:
I:	I:	I:	I:	I:	I:	I:
T:	T:	T:	T:	T:	T:	T:
Date: _____	Date: _____	Date: _____	Date: _____	Date: _____	Date: _____	Date: _____
A:	A:	A:	A:	A:	A:	A:
I:	I:	I:	I:	I:	I:	I:
T:	T:	T:	T:	T:	T:	T:
Date: _____	Date: _____	Date: _____	Date: _____	Date: _____	Date: _____	Date: _____
A:	A:	A:	A:	A:	A:	A:
I:	I:	I:	I:	I:	I:	I:
T:	T:	T:	T:	T:	T:	T:
Date: _____	Date: _____	Date: _____	Date: _____	Date: _____	Date: _____	Date: _____
A:	A:	A:	A:	A:	A:	A:
I:	I:	I:	I:	I:	I:	I:
T:	T:	T:	T:	T:	T:	T:

Section VI: Tracking Your Program and Following Through

1. **Goal and Program Tracking:** Use the following chart or a web/app activity log to monitor your progress. Change the activity, intensity, or time of your workout plan to reflect your progress as needed.

2. **Goal and Program Follow-Up:** At the end of the course or at your short-term goal target date, reevaluate your cardiorespiratory fitness and ask yourself the following questions:

   a. Did you meet your short-term goal or your goal for the course? If so, what positive behavioral changes contributed to your success? If not, which obstacles blocked your success?

   _____

   b. Was your short-term goal realistic? What would you change about your goals or training plan?

   _____

	Dates	Activity	Times	Av. HR	RPE	Comments
Week 1						
Week 2						
Week 3						
Week 4						

Four-Week Cardiorespiratory Training Log

Activate, Motivate, & Advance YOUR FITNESS

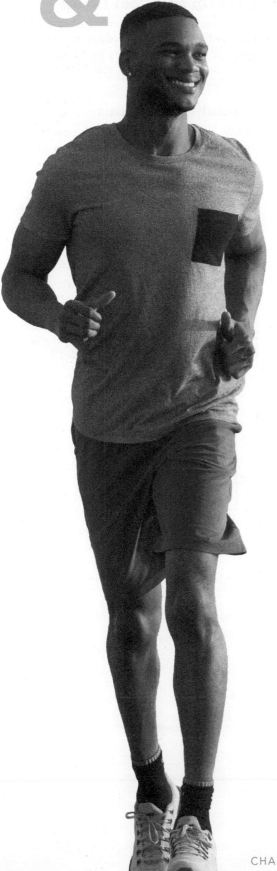

ACTIVATE!

New to running or just want to take your running to the next level? Either way, there is a running program for you! Going too far or too fast right away is the number-one cause of injury among new runners. Focus on the minutes instead of miles, and use these programs to gradually increase your run time.

What Do I Need for Running?

SHOES: Visit your local running store to find the most important item in your running toolbox, your shoes! The employees are generally experienced runners who can assist you in finding a good fit for your foot, running style, gait, running surface, and goals.

CLOTHING: Wear comfortable, supportive, and moisture-wicking clothing. In cold weather, wear layers. In the sun, wear sunscreen, sunglasses, and a hat or visor. At sunrise, dusk, or night, wear reflective clothing or a vest and lights.

How Do I Start a Running Program?

TECHNIQUE: Relax your shoulders and gently swing your arms (90-degree elbow) up to your chest and down to your hips. Keep hands loose and relaxed. Look forward, rather than down at the ground. Stay light on your feet and use shorter, quicker steps. Land on your mid-foot, roll to the ball of your foot and push off. Aim for a stride rate (your turnover) of 180 steps per minute. Count the number of times your right foot strikes the ground in a minute and multiply that by two.

ETIQUETTE: On a sidewalk or a multi-use path or trail, run on the right and pass on the left, after alerting others you are passing. Say, "On your left" as you approach. No matter where you run, never run more than two abreast. If you need to stop, step off to the right to allow others to get by.

Running Tips

ROAD RUNNING: Plan safe and interesting routes that consider both traffic and available running paths. Check with your local running store or club for routes and running partners. Let someone know where you are going and when you will return. Carry a cell phone, ID, a few dollars, and a water bottle. Pay attention to traffic signals/signs, and stay aware of your surroundings by wearing only one earphone. Run facing traffic when no path or sidewalk is available.

TRACK RUNNING: A track will give you a stable, soft, and well-lit running surface. As a bonus, you may have a rest room and a place to keep your belongings nearby. On a track, you can test pacing, adjust your run/walk ratios, and retest your cardiorespiratory fitness level regularly. Most tracks are 400 meters; four laps on the inner lane equal a mile. Use the outside lanes for most of your training and leave the inside lane (lane 1) for faster runners and sprinters and for timing yourself on a specific distance. If you are using the inside lane and a faster individual approaches behind you, move out to lane 2 or 3 to allow the person to pass. Finally, change your running direction every few runs to vary the stresses on your body.

TREADMILL RUNNING: Treadmills offer convenience, efficiency, and a safe, controlled environment. Familiarize yourself with the controls before starting. Maintain good posture and running form. Avoid using the handrails or drifting toward the back of the treadmill.

TRAIL RUNNING: Take a break from the asphalt jungle to run in nature. Ease into trail running by starting with flat, soft, easy-to-navigate trails and work your way up to more challenging ones. Take smaller steps, slow down, and constantly scan the trail to find the best footing. If possible, run with a buddy. On all trails, be sure that you know your route, take water, and tell someone of your location, start time, and anticipated end time.

Running Warm-Up and Cool-Down

Walk or jog at a slower pace for 5 to 10 minutes to warm up or cool down. After breaking a light sweat in your warm-up, add dynamic range-of-motion exercises. After you finish your cool-down, you can hold static stretches longer for improved flexibility.

Four-Week Running Programs

Adjust time, intensity, and training days to suit your personal fitness level and schedule.

BEGINNER RUNNING PROGRAM

Start here if: 1) you are new to running, 2) you are transitioning from walking to running, 3) you have taken a break from running for six months or more, or 4) your cardiorespiratory fitness level in Lab 3.2 was Fair or Poor.

GOAL: Transition from walking to running and build your run program gradually. Increase run minutes at a moderate intensity three to four days a week.

	Mon		Tue		Wed		Thurs		Fri		Sat		Sun	
	T	I	T	I	T	I	T	I	T	I	T	I	T	I
Week 1	20 1/4	L			20 1/4	L			20 1/4	L–M				
Week 2	24 1/5	L–M			24 1/5	M			24 1/5	M				
Week 3	32 1/7	M			32 1/7	M			32 1/7	M				
Week 4	24 2/10	M			24 2/10	M			24 2/10	M	24 2/10	M		

*T = Time. Total time is listed in minutes with the Walk/Run minute ratio below.
I = Intensity. Intensity is listed as Light/Lifestyle (L), Moderate (M), or Vigorous (V) (see Table 3.3 for the Cardiorespiratory Intensity Scales).
Workouts do not include warm-up or cool-down time.*

INTENSITY LEVEL | L | M | V |
Light Moderate Vigorous

Start here if you are already running 15 minutes continuously at least two days a week and/or if your cardiorespiratory fitness level in Lab 3.2 was Good or Fair.

GOAL: Run at a moderate to vigorous intensity level three to five days a week, complete a 30-minute continuous run, and incorporate vigorous interval training sessions.

	Mon		Tue		Wed		Thurs		Fri		Sat		Sun	
	T	I	T	I	T	I	T	I	T	I	T	I	T	I
Week 1	20	L–M	20	M	20	M			20	L–M				
Week 2	20	M			25	M			20	M	25	L–M		
Week 3	25	M			20	M	Interval	L–M–V			30	M		
Week 4	25	M	Interval	L–M–V	20	L–M	Interval	L–M–V			30	L–M		

T = Time. Total time is listed in minutes.
I = Intensity. Intensity is listed as Light/Lifestyle (L), Moderate (M), or Vigorous (V)
(see Table 3.3 for the Cardiorespiratory Intensity Scales).
Workouts do not include warm-up or cool-down time.

INTENSITY LEVEL | L | M | V |
Light Moderate Vigorous

Intermediate Program Interval Workout—Three Miles

800m (.5 mile) at 7 to 8 on the OMNI scale (V)
800m (.5 mile) recovery (easy jog or walk/jog) at 2 to 5 on the OMNI scale (L to M)
**REPEAT this 1:1 ratio two more times for a total of 4800m or 3 miles.

MOTIVATE!

Here are a few tips to keep you running:

MORNING WORKOUTS: Run first thing in the morning. That way, you can check it off your to-do list, and nothing can push your run off your schedule. Tip for success: Organize your running clothes, shoes, gear, water bottle, and breakfast the night before.

DON'T PUT AWAY YOUR GEAR: Place your workout log, shoes, workout clothes, water bottle, and stretching mat in plain sight, in your work bag, or your car. Visual cues can help you remember your goals and prioritize your run.

DO IT FOR CHARITY: Need a reason or just more support? Name your cause and chances are there is a local run or race to raise awareness and funds for it. Committing to run for worthy causes reminds you that you are fortunate to be healthy and able to run. Fuel your motivation by knowing you're doing good for more than just yourself.

ADVANCE!

Ready to challenge yourself? How about participating in your first 5K? If you've been there, done that, how about actually racing (picking up your pace to set a new personal record)? Follow the more advanced four-week program on the next page.

Start here if you are already running at a moderate pace for 25 minutes continuously and if your cardiorespiratory fitness level in Lab 3.2 was Excellent or above.

GOAL: Run 5K/3.1 miles!

	Mon		Tue		Wed		Thurs		Fri		Sat		Sun	
	T/D	I	T/D	I	T/D	I	T/D	I	T/D	I	T/D	I	T/D	I
Week 1	25	L–M	25	L–M			25	M	25	M				
Week 2	25	M			Interval	L–M–V			2 miles	M	30	M		
Week 3	25	M	Interval	L–M–V	2.5 miles	L–M	Interval	L–M–V	2.75 miles	M				
Week 4	30	M			35	L–M					Goal 5K Run!			

T/D = Time/Distance. Total time/distance is listed in minutes or miles.
I = Intensity. Intensity is listed as Light/Lifestyle (L), Moderate (M), or Vigorous (V)
(see Table 3.3 for the Cardiorespiratory Intensity Scales).
Workouts do not include warm-up or cool-down time.

INTENSITY LEVEL   L   M   V

Light   Moderate   Vigorous

Advanced Program Interval Workout

2 minutes at 85% HRmax or 7 to 8 on the OMNI scale (V)
2 minutes at <60% HRmax or 2 to 3 on the OMNI scale (L)
5 minutes at 65–84% HRmax or 5 to 6 on the OMNI scale (M)
****REPEAT twice more (total of three sets)

Activate, Motivate, & Advance YOUR FITNESS

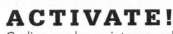

ACTIVATE!

Cycling can be an intense, calorie-burning workout, but it can also be a simple way to take care of errands, commute, meet up with friends, or just enjoy the great outdoors. Start with indoor or outdoor cycling, and as you get stronger, you can increase your mileage and speed.

What Do I Need for Cycling?

GEAR: Safe cycling requires quite a bit of equipment (helmet, padded cycling shorts, gloves, shoes, reflective gear, racks) and, of course, the bike. You can start on almost any style of bicycle, but most important, you need a bike that fits. Visit your local bike shop to get the right bike for you. If you are new to indoor cycling or unfamiliar with the bike, ask a trained instructor to assist you with proper bike setup.

How Do I Start a Cycling Program?

TECHNIQUE: Work on developing a smooth and efficient pedaling technique. Lighten up, pedal in a smooth circle, and pull through the back of the stroke. *Cadence* is pedaling speed in revolutions per minute (RPM). A cadence of 60 RPM means that one pedal makes a complete revolution 60 times in one minute. Monitor your cadence by counting the revolutions of one leg for 15 seconds and then multiply by four. The cadence range is 80 to 110 RPM for cycling on a flat road and 60 to 80 RPM for climbing hills.

ETIQUETTE: Participating in group rides will teach you the etiquette for road cycling and mountain biking. Inquire about weekly rides or a beginners' cycling group at your local bike shop.

Cycling Tips

INDOOR CYCLING: Weather, traffic, flat tires . . . with indoor cycling you won't have these excuses for missing your workout. Indoor cycling also allows you to precisely control your workout and mix periods of higher-intensity cycling with rest periods.

OUTDOOR CYCLING: Whether you choose streets, bike paths, or trails, plan safe routes that consider both traffic and terrain. Try using a mapping program or stop by your local bike shop to learn more about the routes and popular riding areas in your neighborhood. Safety tips: Brush up on your cycling skills, have proper reflective equipment, learn how to use a bike repair kit (fixing flat tires), and know local traffic laws and trail usage rules.

Cycling Warm-Up and Cool-Down

Cycle at a slower cadence for 5 to 15 minutes to warm up or cool down. After the cool-down portion of your ride, perform a few light stretches that focus on your low back muscles, hamstrings, quadriceps, and calves.

Four-Week Cycling Programs

Adjust time, intensity, and training days to suit your personal fitness level and schedule.

BEGINNER CYCLING PROGRAM

Start here if you are new to cycling, you are coming back after time off, or your cardiorespiratory fitness level in Lab 3.2 was Fair or Poor.

GOAL: Increase cycling minutes at a moderate intensity level three to four days a week, building to 100 total weekly minutes.

	Mon		Tue		Wed		Thurs		Fri		Sat		Sun	
	T	I	T	I	T	I	T	I	T	I	T	I	T	I
Week 1	20	L			20	L			20	L–M				
Week 2	25	M			25	M			25	M				
Week 3	20	M			25	M			15	M	30	L–M		
Week 4	25	M			25	M			25	M	25	L–M		

T = Time. Total time is listed in minutes.
I = Intensity. Intensity is listed as Light/Lifestyle (L), Moderate (M), or Vigorous (V) (see Table 3.3 for the Cardiorespiratory Intensity Scales). Workouts do not include warm-up or cool-down time.

INTENSITY LEVEL | L | M | V |
Light Moderate Vigorous

INTERMEDIATE CYCLING PROGRAM

Start here if you are already riding for 20 or more continuous minutes twice a week and your cardiorespiratory fitness level in Lab 3.2 was Good or Fair.

GOAL: Cycle at a moderate intensity level three to five days a week, build to a 40-minute ride, and incorporate vigorous interval training sessions each week.

	Mon		Tue		Wed		Thurs		Fri		Sat		Sun	
	T	I	T	I	T	I	T	I	T	I	T	I	T	I
Week 1	25	L–M			25	L–M			25	M	25	M		
Week 2	25	M			30	M			25	L–M	35	M		
Week 3	30	M	Interval	L–M–V	20	L–M	Interval	L–M–V	30	M				
Week 4	30	M	Interval	L–M–V	25	M	30	M			40	L–M		

T = Time. Total time is listed in minutes.
I = Intensity. Intensity is listed as Light/Lifestyle (L), Moderate (M), or Vigorous (V) (see Table 3.3 for the Cardiorespiratory Intensity Scales). Workouts do not include warm-up or cool-down time.

INTENSITY LEVEL | L | M | V |
Light Moderate Vigorous

Intermediate Program Interval Workout—25 Minutes

2 minutes of flat cycling (cadence 80 to 110 RPM) at 7 to 8 on the OMNI scale (V)
1 minute of recovery (pedal easy, below 80 RPM) at 3 on the OMNI scale (L)
**REPEAT this 2:1 ratio four more times for a total of 15 minutes
30 seconds of hill work (increase tension and drop cadence to 60 to 80 RPM) at 7 to 8 on the OMNI scale (V)
90 seconds of recovery (pedal easy, below 80 RPM with little or no resistance) at 3 on the OMNI scale (L)
**REPEAT this 1:3 ratio four more times for a total of 10 minutes

MOTIVATE!

Here are a few tips to keep you cycling:

RIDE FOR 10: If you lack energy or motivation for a spin, give yourself 10 minutes. Tell yourself that you can quit after 10 minutes if you still don't feel like riding. Chances are that once you start, you'll complete your workout. If not, at least you managed a solid 10 minutes and you can feel good about listening to your body and taking a rest day.

REWARD YOURSELF: Promise yourself a healthy treat or fun experience if you stick to your cycling program. Maybe a pedicure or a massage or a scoop of frozen yogurt?

INDOOR GROUP RIDE: Sometimes just knowing that others are expecting you is enough to help you show up for your workout. Try an indoor cycling class at your gym. You'll develop new friendships with other physically active people and increase your cardiorespiratory fitness. Win-win!

ADVANCE!

Ready to up your cycling game? Follow this more advanced four-week program.

ADVANCED CYCLING PROGRAM

Start here if you are already cycling at a moderate pace for 25 minutes continuously and your cardiorespiratory fitness level in Lab 3.2 was Excellent or above.

GOAL: Ride 20K/12.4 miles in ≤ 60 minutes (indoors or out)!

	Mon		Tue		Wed		Thurs		Fri		Sat		Sun	
	T/D	I	T/D	I	T/D	I	T/D	I	T/D	I	T/D	I	T/D	I
Week 1	25	L–M	25	M	30	L–M	30	M			35	M		
Week 2	30	M	20	V	6 miles	L–M	30	M			40	M		
Week 3	35	M	Interval	L–M–V			Interval	L–M–V	35	L–M	45	M		
Week 4	40	M	20	L–M	40	M	Interval	L–M–V			Goal 20k Ride!	M		

T/D = Time/Distance. Total time/distance is listed in minutes or miles.
I = Intensity. Intensity is listed as Light/Lifestyle (L), Moderate (M), or Vigorous (V) (see Table 3.3 for the Cardiorespiratory Intensity Scales).
Workouts do not include warm-up or cool-down time.

INTENSITY LEVEL | L | M | V |
Light   Moderate   Vigorous

Advanced Program Interval Workout—30 Minutes

3 minutes of flat cycling (cadence 80 to 110 RPM) at 85% HRmax or 7 to 8 on the OMNI scale (V)
1 minute of recovery (pedal easy, below 80 RPM) at 3 on the OMNI scale (L)
**REPEAT this 3:1 ratio four more times for a total of 20 minutes
1 minute of hill work (increase tension and drop cadence to 60 to 80 RPM) at 85% HRmax or 7 to 8 on the OMNI scale (V)
1 minute of recovery (pedal easy, below 80 RPM with little or no resistance) at 3 on the OMNI scale (L)
**REPEAT this 1:1 ratio four more times for a total of 10 minutes

Activate, Motivate, & Advance YOUR FITNESS

ACTIVATE

Low impact and fun, swimming is an excellent way to improve your overall fitness! Start and build slowly, focusing on minutes, not laps. As you gain strength, you will swim further and faster.

What Do I Need for Swimming?

GEAR: Look for a swimsuit that stays in place and moves with you, and be sure to try on goggles to ensure a good fit. You may want a swim cap to keep your hair out of your face. Many pools have equipment available that can improve technique and performance: kickboards, pull buoys, fins, and a pace clock. Lastly, don't forget your shatter proof water bottle and a towel!

How Do I Start a Swimming Program?

TECHNIQUE: Taking lessons is the best way to become more comfortable in the water and develop a more efficient technique. Inquire at your local college or American Red Cross chapter about adult swim classes or private swim coaches.

ETIQUETTE: Pools are busy at open swim times and you will rarely get a lane to yourself. Aim to share a lane with other swimmers close to your same speed. You will most likely encounter *circle swimming* (swimming in a counter-clockwise direction in the pool lane). Allow faster swimmers to take the lead, make sure there is a five-second gap between you and the person in front of you, and avoid swimming in the middle of the lane. If you need to take a break at the wall, keep to the side so that others can turn or rest as well.

Swimming Tips

OPEN WATER: Although it takes strong skills, open-water swimming can be exciting and invigorating! Check with your local swim store or a swim or triathlon club to find swim partners and learn more about safe open water swim areas. The water temperature is generally much cooler than a pool; many open-water swimmers wear neoprene wetsuits to stay warm. Practice "sighting" (looking up to see where you are in relation to land, buoys, docks) and swimming in a straight line before heading out.

Swimming Warm-Up and Cool-Down

A swimming warm-up and cool-down consists of slow water walking, water jogging, or swimming at a slow pace for 5 to 10 minutes. You can also warm up on deck with light, dynamic, full-range movements. After your cool-down, you can hold basic stretches for 10 to 30 seconds to improve flexibility.

Four-Week Swimming Programs

As you start a new swimming program, rest often, use resting swim strokes (elementary backstroke, sidestroke) as needed, and monitor your intensity periodically. Heart rates are typically 10 to 13 beats per minute lower when swimming than when performing exercise on land, so use perceived exertion instead of heart rate for your intensity targets (see Table 3.3). Adjust time, intensity, and days of the swims to suit your personal fitness level and schedule.

BEGINNER SWIMMING PROGRAM

Start here if swimming even one length of the pool is tiring for you. Focus on swim time, not distance or number of laps.

GOAL: Increase continuous swim minutes at a light- to moderate-intensity level three to four days a week, building to 100 total minutes by week four.

	Mon		Tue		Wed		Thurs		Fri		Sat		Sun	
	T	I	T	I	T	I	T	I	T	I	T	I	T	I
Week 1	15	L			20	L			20	M				
Week 2	20	M			25	M			25	M				
Week 3	25	M			20	M			15	M	25	M		
Week 4	25	M			25	M			25	M	25	M		

T = Time. Total time is listed in minutes.
I = Intensity. Intensity is listed as Light/Lifestyle (L), Moderate (M), or Vigorous (V)
(see Table 3.3 for the Cardiorespiratory Intensity Scales).
Workouts do not include warm-up or cool-down time.

INTENSITY LEVEL | L | M | V |
Light | Moderate | Vigorous

INTERMEDIATE SWIMMING PROGRAM

Start here if you swim comfortably at a moderate-intensity level for 25 minutes (continuously or with minimum rest) twice a week.

GOAL: Increase continuous swim minutes at a moderate-intensity level three to five days a week, build to a 40-minute swim, and incorporate vigorous interval training sessions each week.

	Mon		Tue		Wed		Thurs		Fri		Sat		Sun	
	T	I	T	I	T	I	T	I	T	I	T	I	T	I
Week 1	25	L–M			25	M			25	M	25	M		
Week 2	25	M			Intervals	L–M–V			25	M				
Week 3	30	L–M			25	M			25	M	35	L–M		
Week 4	35	M	Intervals	L–M–V	40	M			Intervals	L–M–V	30	M		

T = Time. Total time is listed in minutes.
I = Intensity. Intensity is listed as Light/Lifestyle (L), Moderate (M), or Vigorous (V)
(see Table 3.3 for the Cardiorespiratory Intensity Scales).
Workouts do not include warm-up or cool-down time.

INTENSITY LEVEL | L | M | V |
Light | Moderate | Vigorous

Intermediate Program Interval Workout—700 m/yds

3 × 100 m/yds with 60 seconds of rest between [100s at 7 to 8 on the OMNI scale (V) and rest at 0 to 2 (L)]
2 × 75 m/yds with 45 seconds of rest between [75s at 7 to 8 on the OMNI scale (V) and rest at 0 to 2 (L)]
3 × 50 m/yds with 30 seconds of rest between [50s at 7 to 8 on the OMNI scale (V) and rest at 0 to 2 (L)]
4 × 25 m/yds with 15 seconds of rest between [25s at 7 to 8 on the OMNI scale (V) and rest at 0 to 2 (L)]

MOTIVATE!

Here are a few tips to keep you swimming:

LEARN NEW SWIM SKILLS: Taking a lesson can help you develop confidence, which leads to more efficient swimming and increased enjoyment. The more you enjoy your workout, the better the results will be and the more likely you are to stick with it.

JOIN A TEAM: Lacking the support you need to swim regularly? Masters Swimming is a national program where adults 18 and older can swim in a team setting. You can swim at your own pace and be competitive or non-competitive—your choice! There are teams and clubs in communities across the country that offer swim practice/workout options and coaching; you will gain a new group of friends who will be expecting you at the pool!

TRY A WATER EXERCISE CLASS: Getting bored? Mix things up, make new friends, and take a break from swimming laps while still getting a great workout in the water. Most pools have different types of group water exercise classes; chances are one will be right for you.

ADVANCE!

Congratulations! You have established your swim fitness program. Are you ready to challenge yourself with a new goal? Below is a more advanced four-week program that you can follow.

ADVANCED SWIMMING PROGRAM

Start here if you swim at a moderate- to high-intensity level for 30 to 40 minutes three to four times a week.

GOAL: Swim a mile, continuous (or with minimum rest)! (1650 yards/1508 meters)

	Mon		Tue		Wed		Thurs		Fri		Sat		Sun	
	T/D	I	T/D	I	T/D	I	T/D	I	T/D	I	T/D	I	T/D	I
Week 1	25	L–M	700	M			700	M	25	M				
Week 2	30	M	1000	M	Interval	L–M–V			30	L–M				
Week 3	25	M	Interval	L–M–V	35	L–M	1200	L–M–V			40	M		
Week 4	Interval	L–M–V	1500	M	Interval	L–M–V	25	L–M			Goal Mile Swim!			

T/D = Time/Distance. Total time/distance is listed in minutes or yards/meters.
I = Intensity. Intensity is listed as Light/Lifestyle (L), Moderate (M), or Vigorous (V) (see Table 3.3 for the Cardiorespiratory Intensity Scales).
Workouts do not include warm-up or cool-down time.
Heart rates are typically 10 to 13 beats per minute lower when swimming than when performing exercise on land. Adjust heart rate targets accordingly.

INTENSITY LEVEL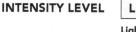

L	M	V
Light	Moderate	Vigorous

Advanced Program Interval Workout—1200 m/yds

3×100 m/yds with 60 seconds of rest between [100s at 65 to 84% HRmax, 5 to 6 on the OMNI scale (M), and rest at 0 to 2 (L)]
2×200 m/yds with 2 minutes of rest between [200s at 85% HRmax, 7 to 8 on the OMNI scale (V), and rest at 0 to 2 (L)]
1×500 m/yds [at 65 to 84% HRmax, 5 to 6 on the OMNI scale (M)]

Building Muscular Strength and Endurance

4

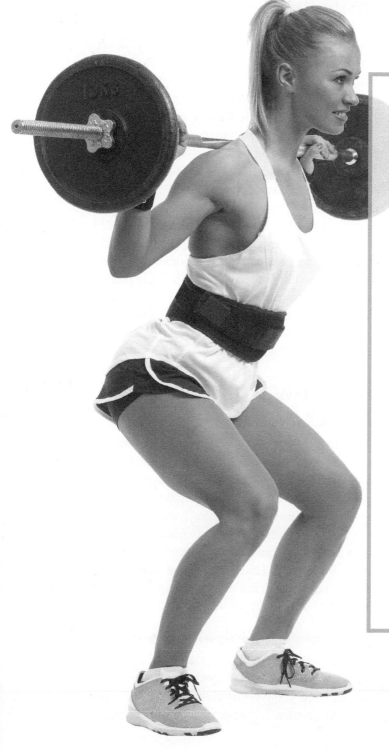

LEARNINGoutcomes

LO 4.1   Explain how resistance training is used to attain muscular fitness.

LO 4.2   Identify key skeletal muscle structures and explain how they work together to allow for basic muscle function.

LO 4.3   Articulate the fitness and wellness improvements you can make with regular resistance training.

LO 4.4   Evaluate your changes in muscle fitness over time by assessing your muscular strength and muscular endurance at regular intervals.

LO 4.5   Implement an effective resistance-training program compatible with your goals and lifestyle.

LO 4.6   Observe safety precautions when resistance training.

LO 4.7   Avoid the risks associated with supplement use and dramatic diet changes.

MasteringHealth™

Go online for chapter quizzes, interactive assessments, videos, and more!

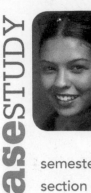
SIMONE

"Hi, I'm Simone. I'm from San Francisco and I'm a sophomore majoring in economics. I'm taking a fitness and wellness class this semester, and this week we're starting the section on muscular fitness. I'm curious about it because I've never lifted weights before! I like to go hiking and I take yoga classes from time to time, but I wouldn't call myself an athlete. Does it really make sense for someone like me to start a strength-training program?"

Hear It!
To listen to this case study online, visit the Study Area in MasteringHealth™.

W hether you're a beginner like Simone or an athlete interested in conditioning, this chapter answers common questions about muscular fitness, explains the benefits of resistance training, and gives you the tools for designing a program that is custom-made for you.

LO 4.1 What Is Muscular Fitness?

muscular fitness The ability of your musculoskeletal system to perform daily and recreational activities without undue fatigue and injury

muscular strength The ability of a muscle to contract with maximal force

muscular endurance The ability of a muscle to contract repeatedly over an extended period of time

resistance training Controlled and progressive stressing of the body's musculoskeletal system using resistance (i.e., weights, resistance bands, body weight) exercises to build and maintain muscular fitness

tendons The connective tissues attaching muscle to bone

Muscular fitness is the ability of your musculoskeletal system to perform daily and recreational activities without undue fatigue and injury. Muscular fitness involves having adequate muscular strength and endurance. **Muscular strength** is the ability of a muscle or group of muscles to contract with maximal force. It describes how strong a muscle is or how much force it can exert. Exercise professionals often measure muscular strength by determining the maximum weight a person can lift at one time. **Muscular endurance** is the ability of a muscle to contract repeatedly over an extended period of time. It describes how long you can sustain a given type of muscular exertion. One way to measure muscular endurance is to determine the maximum weight a person can lift 20 times consecutively.

You can build muscular strength and endurance through resistance training. **Resistance training** is also referred to as *weight training* or *strength training* and can be done with measured weights, body weight, or other resistive equipment (i.e., exercise bands). Resistance exercises stress the body's musculoskeletal system, which enlarges muscle fibers and improves neural control of muscle function, resulting in greater muscular strength and endurance. Resistance training offers such varied benefits that exercise professionals recommend it in nearly all fitness programs.

In 2013, 29.6 percent of adults over age 18 reported participating in muscle strengthening activities on two or more days of the week.[1] These numbers have increased over the years, which is great news! However, it still leaves 70 percent of the population not doing strengthening exercises at the recommended level.

If you are not participating, now is the perfect time to start. Facilities and classes are readily available at most colleges and universities and you may have a group of peers who wants to support one another in getting fit and healthy.

LO 4.2 How Do My Muscles Work?

The human body contains hundreds of muscles, each of which belongs to one of three basic types: (1) voluntary *skeletal muscle*, which moves the skeleton and generates body heat; (2) involuntary *cardiac muscle*, which exists only in the heart and pumps blood through the body; and (3) involuntary *smooth muscle*, which lines some internal organs and moves food through the stomach and intestines. Here we focus on skeletal muscles and the signals from the nervous system that coordinate and control their contraction.

An Overview of Skeletal Muscle

Each skeletal muscle is surrounded by a sheet of connective tissue that draws together at the ends of the muscle, forming the **tendons** (see **Figure 4.1**). Muscular contractions allow for skeletal movement because

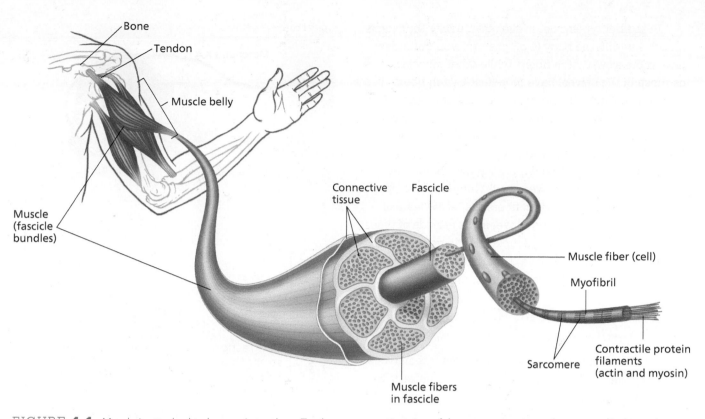

Labels on figure:
Bone
Tendon
Muscle belly
Muscle (fascicle bundles)
Connective tissue
Fascicle
Muscle fiber (cell)
Myofibril
Sarcomere
Contractile protein filaments (actin and myosin)
Muscle fibers in fascicle

FIGURE 4.1 Muscle is attached to bones via tendons. Tendons are a continuation of the connective tissue that surrounds the entire muscle as well as each muscle bundle (fascicle). A fascicle is made up of many muscle cells (muscle fibers). Within each muscle fiber, myofibril strands contain actin and myosin proteins.

muscles are attached to bones via tendons. These attached muscles pull the bones, which pivot at joints, creating a specific body movement.

Within each skeletal muscle are individual muscle cells called **muscle fibers**. Bundles of muscle fibers are called *fascicles*. Each muscle fiber extends the full length of the muscle. Within each muscle fiber are many **myofibrils**, each containing contractile protein filaments. These filaments are primarily made up of two kinds of protein—*actin* and *myosin*—which partially overlap at rest and give the whole cell a striped appearance. Actin and myosin filaments exist in repeating units called **sarcomeres**. A *sarcomere* is the smallest area in a muscle fiber where everything required for muscle contraction exists. Sarcomeres repeat along the length of the myofibril, and one muscle can contain more than 100,000 sarcomeres.

The microscopic structure and function of actin and myosin allow them to slide across each other, which shortens the sarcomere, myofibril, and muscle fiber. Simultaneous shortening of the many fibers within a whole muscle causes the pattern of muscular tension we call *contraction*. It is this whole-muscle contraction that moves bones and surrounding body parts.

Every muscle fiber can be categorized as *slow* or *fast,* depending on how quickly it can contract:

- **Slow-twitch muscle fibers** (Type I) depend on oxygen and contract slowly for longer periods of time without fatigue. In slow-twitch fibers, the energy for contraction primarily comes from the breakdown of fat in blood, muscle, and adipose tissue. Efficient fat breakdown requires oxygen and minimal levels of glucose.

- **Fast-twitch muscle fibers** (Type II) are not oxygen-dependent. They contract rapidly with a greater force, but also tire more quickly than slow-twitch fibers. In fast-twitch fibers, the energy for contraction primarily comes from creatine phosphate and glycogen in muscles, glycogen stores in the liver, and glucose in the blood.

muscle fibers The cells of the muscular system

myofibrils Thin strands within a single muscle fiber that bundle the skeletal muscle protein filaments and span the length of the fiber

sarcomeres Basic functional contractile units within skeletal and cardiac muscle that contain both thin actin and thick myosin protein filaments

slow-twitch muscle fibers Muscle fiber type that is oxygen-dependent and can contract over long periods of time

fast-twitch muscle fibers Muscle fiber type that contracts with greater force and speed but also fatigues quickly

Both fiber types exist in skeletal muscles, but some muscles within the body (e.g., postural trunk muscles) have more slow-twitch fibers, while other muscles (such as those in the calves) have more fast-twitch fibers. The proportion of muscle fiber types varies from person to person based on both genetics and training. Elite athletes have muscle fiber compositions that complement their sport. Marathoners, for instance, have higher levels of slow-twitch fibers that supply them with optimal muscular endurance. Power weight lifters, on the other hand, have more fast-twitch fibers that allow feats of enormous muscular strength over short periods of time. Sedentary individuals and people who do general resistance training typically have 50 percent slow-twitch and 50 percent fast-twitch fiber composition.

Muscle Contraction Requires Stimulation

For a voluntary skeletal muscle to contract, the nervous system must send a signal directly to the muscle. When you want to move any part of your body—for example, a finger on your right hand—your brain sends a signal down the spinal cord and through motor nerves to the skeletal muscles in that finger.

One motor nerve stimulates many skeletal muscle fibers, together creating a functional unit called a **motor unit** (**Figure 4.2**). A motor unit can be small or large, depending on the number of muscle fibers that the motor nerve stimulates. Motor units are made up of one type of muscle fiber, either slow-twitch or fast-twitch. Typically, small motor units have slow-twitch fibers and larger motor units have fast-twitch fibers.

The strength of a muscle contraction depends upon the intensity of the nervous system stimulus, the number and size of motor units activated, and the types of muscle fibers that are stimulated. For example, if you are getting ready to lift a heavy weight, your central nervous system sends a stronger signal. This activates a greater number of large, fast motor units, resulting in a more forceful muscle contraction than if you were merely picking up an apple.

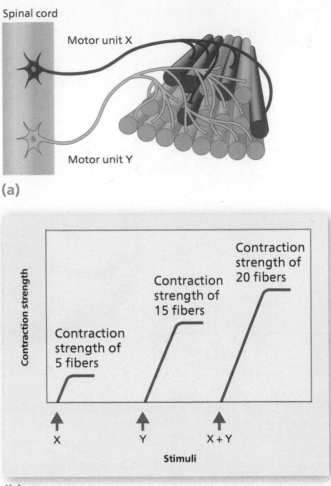

(a)

(b)

FIGURE **4.2** Motor units and muscle contraction strength. (a) Motor unit X is smaller (5 fibers) than motor unit Y (15 fibers). (b) The strength of a muscular contraction increases with increased fibers per motor unit (X vs. Y) and with more motor units activated (X + Y).

---

motor unit A motor nerve and all the muscle fibers it controls

isotonic A muscle contraction with relatively constant tension

isometric A muscle contraction with no change in muscle length

isokinetic A muscle contraction with a constant speed of contraction

---

Types of Muscle Contractions

All muscle contractions increase the tension or force within the muscle, but some contractions move body parts while others do not. There are three primary types of contractions: isotonic, isometric, and isokinetic. **Isotonic** contractions are characterized by consistent muscle tension as the contraction proceeds and a resulting movement of body parts (**Figure 4.3a**, page 117). An arm curl with a 10-pound hand weight involves isotonic contractions throughout your arm. **Isometric** contractions are characterized by a consistent muscle length throughout the contraction with no visible movement of body parts. An example of an isometric contraction occurs when you hold a hand weight at arm's length in front of you; your arm is not moving, but you feel tension in your arm muscles (**Figure 4.3b**). **Isokinetic** contractions are characterized by a consistent muscle contraction speed within a moving body part. In order to perform isokinetic contractions, you need specialized equipment that holds

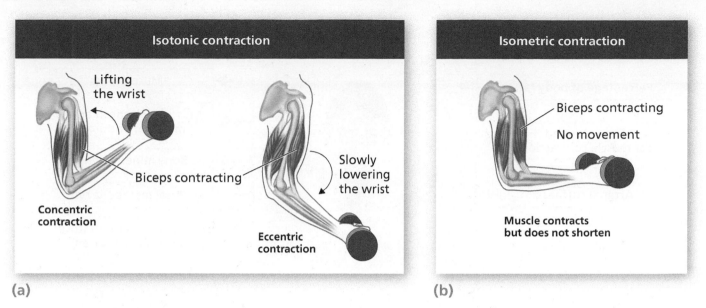

(a)

(b)

FIGURE **4.3** (a) Isotonic contractions include concentric (shortening) and eccentric (lengthening) contractions. (b) Isometric contractions produce force in the muscle with no movement.

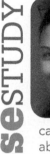

case STUDY

SIMONE

"I love to go on short hikes. There are some gorgeous trails in the San Francisco Bay Area. Some of them are hilly, but I don't mind—the views from the top are always worth it. My calves definitely get a workout! I'd like to be able to do longer hikes, but the truth is that I usually get tired after about three miles. I know there are some longer hikes with spectacular views, but I don't feel ready for them yet."

APPLY IT! Given what you've learned so far, what would you tell Simone about how resistance training can benefit her? Which type of muscle fibers would you guess that Simone has more of: slow-twitch fibers or fast-twitch fibers?

TRY IT! **Today,** go outside and enjoy a favorite activity. During the activity, name the muscle fiber types you are using most (slow-twitch or fast-twitch). **This week,** try isometric contractions by doing wall sits. Sit with your back against a wall, feet out in front of you, and your knees bent at 90 degrees or more (but not less than 90 degrees). Hold this position for 30 seconds to one minute. Repeat one to two more times. **In two weeks,** name the concentric and eccentric portions of each exercise you perform during a resistance-training session. Write this down in your workout log.

Hear It!

To listen to this case study online, visit the Study Area in MasteringHealth™.

the speed of movement constant as your arm, leg, or other muscles contract with varying forces.

Isotonic contractions are the most common in exercise programs. Lifting free weights, working on machines, and doing push-ups are all examples of isotonic contractions. Isotonic contractions can be either concentric or eccentric. **Concentric** contractions occur when force develops in the muscle as the muscle is shortening—for example, when you curl a free weight up toward your shoulder. In **eccentric** muscle contractions, force remains in the muscle while the muscle is lengthening. This occurs as you lower a free weight back to its original position. Figure 4.3a illustrates concentric and eccentric contractions in an arm curl exercise.

LO 4.3 How Can Regular Resistance Training Improve My Fitness and Wellness?

People used to think that weight lifting was only for improving body shape and producing bigger muscles. We now know that, in addition to improving physical appearance, resistance training can have significant fitness and wellness benefits.

Figure 4.4 summarizes these changes. We discuss the benefits of resistance training in detail in the following section.

concentric A muscle contraction with overall muscle shortening

eccentric A muscle contraction with overall muscle lengthening

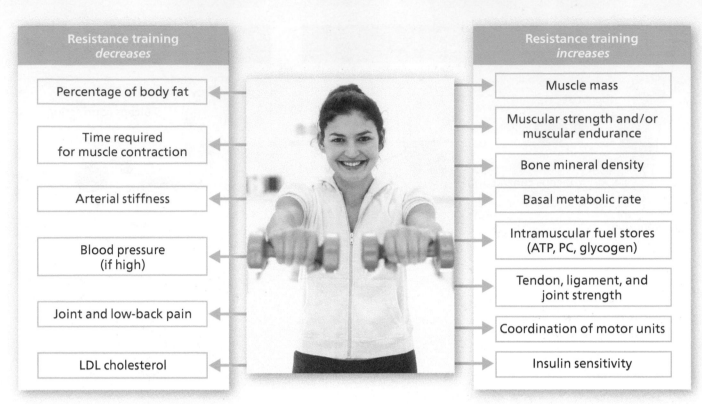

Resistance training *decreases*		Resistance training *increases*
Percentage of body fat		Muscle mass
Time required for muscle contraction		Muscular strength and/or muscular endurance
Arterial stiffness		Bone mineral density
Blood pressure (if high)		Basal metabolic rate
Joint and low-back pain		Intramuscular fuel stores (ATP, PC, glycogen)
LDL cholesterol		Tendon, ligament, and joint strength
		Coordination of motor units
		Insulin sensitivity

FIGURE **4.4** Physiological changes from resistance training.

Regular Resistance Training Increases Your Strength

Regular resistance training with an adequate load will increase muscle strength. Although men have larger muscles due to higher testosterone levels, men and women improve relative strength with resistance training at similar rates.[2] Stronger muscles benefit both men and women, since muscular strength is a strong predictor of mortality even after controlling for cardiorespiratory fitness and activity levels![3]

Neural Improvements When you start a resistance-training program, you will gain muscular strength before noticing any increase in muscle size. This is because internal adaptations to training take place before muscles enlarge. In the first few weeks or months of a resistance-training program, most of the adaptation involves increasing your ability to recruit motor units, which causes more muscle fibers to contract and results in stronger muscles for you!

hypertrophy An increase in muscle cross-sectional area

atrophy A decrease in muscle cross-sectional area

Increased Muscle Size With consistent resistance training, the amount of actin and myosin within your muscle

fibers increases. This results in **hypertrophy**, an increase in the size or cross-sectional area of the protein filaments. With more contractile proteins, a muscle can contract more forcefully; in other words, larger muscles are stronger muscles. While both slow- and fast-twitch muscles will enlarge with resistance training, greater increases in strength will result from hypertrophy of fast-twitch muscle fibers.

Muscle hypertrophy takes longer than neural improvements, but is the most important contributor to strength gains over time. The degree of hypertrophy or enlargement you can expect with weight training depends upon your gender, age, genetics, and training program design. Some individuals will develop larger muscles more quickly than others; some will experience only limited hypertrophy. In particular, women and men with smaller builds will realize less muscle development than those with larger builds, even with identical training programs (see the GetFitGraphic Pumping Up Women to Strength Train on the following page). Older individuals will have slower progress and overall less muscle development, but can still see significant improvements.

A program with heavier weights, longer durations, or more frequent training can produce greater muscle gains than a more standard program. People who stop resistance training will experience some degree of **atrophy** or a shrinking of the muscle. To avoid atrophy, you need to make a long-term commitment to resistance training and your fitness overall.

Regular Resistance Training Increases Your Muscular Endurance

Muscular endurance helps you perform both cardiorespiratory activities, such as hiking and running, and muscular fitness activities, such as circuit or sports training. In fact, just doing these activities will improve your muscular endurance. Muscular endurance activities trigger physiological adaptations that improve your ability to regenerate ATP efficiently and thus sustain muscular contractions for a longer period of time. The end result will be the ability to snowboard a long run instead of having to rest halfway down, to walk up three flights of stairs with ease, or to rake leaves vigorously for an hour without difficulty.

Regular Resistance Training Improves Your Body Composition, Weight Management, and Body Image

Improved body composition is an important outcome of resistance training: lean muscle tissue increases, fat tissue decreases, and thus the ratio of lean to fat improves. Research has demonstrated that such higher lean-to-fat ratios improve your overall health profile and reduce your risk of heart attack, diabetes, and death from cardiovascular diseases.[4] Fat does not turn into muscle or vice versa; the number of fat and muscle cells remains the same, with cells merely enlarging or shrinking depending on food intake and activity levels.

More muscle means a faster metabolic rate; pound for pound, muscle tissue expends more energy than fat tissue.[5] With more total calories being expended during the day, weight control becomes easier and more effective.[6] Resistance training should be combined with aerobic exercise for overall weight loss,[7] but resistance training during weight loss helps ensure that you will lose fat and not precious muscle tissue.[8] Your body can be lighter, stronger, and leaner (i.e., more toned) instead of just lighter (and potentially still flabby), as often happens with traditional diet-only weight-loss methods.

When you begin a resistance-training program, you may experience a slight initial weight gain as muscle tissue grows. If you focus only on the scale, this can be discouraging. Instead, focus on how much stronger and more toned your muscles feel. With a consistent fitness and nutrition program, fat loss will eventually "catch up" to muscle gain and will be reflected in weight loss as well. Since muscle tissue is more compact than fat

tissue, your body size will decrease over time as muscles become toned and fat tissues shrink. This, in turn, can improve your body image. In one study, college students realized measurable increases in overall body image or physical self-perception after 12 weeks of resistance training.[9]

Regular Resistance Training Reduces Your Cardiovascular Disease Risk

Regular resistance training can lower your risk of cardiovascular disease by improving heart and blood vessel functioning—increasing blood flow throughout your body. Research studies in numerous populations have shown that regular resistance training can lower blood pressure and blood cholesterol.[10] Long-term resistance training preserved cardiac function and decreased aortic stiffness in men compared to non-exercisers.[11] Being strong can even reduce your risk of dying from cardiovascular disease. In a recently published large study, grip strength (see Testing Your Muscular Strength below) was found to be a stronger predictor of cardiovascular disease mortality than blood pressure![12]

Regular Resistance Training Strengthens Your Bones and Protects Your Body from Injuries

Bone health is an important issue for everyone, from children to older adults. Osteoporosis-related fractures are common among older women and men and can dramatically impair mobility, independence, and quality of life. By putting stress and controlled-weight loads on the muscles, joint structures, and supporting bones, resistance training stimulates muscle tissue growth and the generation of harder, stronger bones,[13] thereby reducing the risk of fracture.

Building strong bones is especially important during childhood skeletal growth and development until about age 30. The "reservoir" of bone tissue you lay down in those years and then maintain throughout life will help prevent weak, brittle bones as you age. Even the bones of older individuals can benefit from strength training; in one study, eight months of resistance training positively affected hip bone density in older women, whereas no change occurred with moderate-impact aerobic exercise over the same time period.[14]

Whether you exercise for fun, fitness, or competition, preventing injuries is a key to continued participation. In any activity, strong muscles, bones, and connective tissues are the common denominator for preventing injury. Regular resistance training strengthens

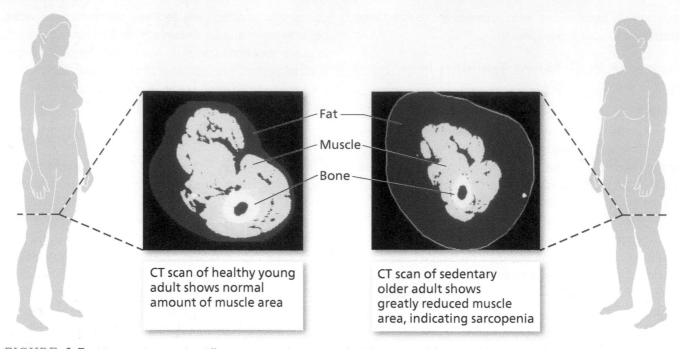

Fat

Muscle

Bone

CT scan of healthy young adult shows normal amount of muscle area

CT scan of sedentary older adult shows greatly reduced muscle area, indicating sarcopenia

FIGURE **4.5** CT scans showing the difference in muscle mass in a healthy young adult vs. an older adult with sarcopenia. Age-related muscle loss can be slowed down with resistance training.

not only muscles, but also the tendons, ligaments, and other supporting structures around each joint. As they grow stronger, they can better protect the joints themselves from injury. A stronger body can handle the physical stresses of everyday life (carrying heavy books or groceries, lifting laundry baskets, moving furniture, etc.) with less chance of injury. A strong, pain-free back and proper posture are crucial to daily functioning without injury. Individuals who participate in regular resistance-training exercise have stronger postural muscles and report less low-back pain.

Imbalanced muscles around a joint may alter joint alignment with subsequent pain or injury. A well-designed muscle fitness program will improve strength and muscle endurance in opposing muscular groups, promoting overall muscle balance, thereby reducing injury risk.

Regular Resistance Training Helps Maintain Your Physical Function with Aging

sarcopenia The degenerative loss of muscle mass and strength in aging

muscle power The ability of a muscle to quickly contract with high force

Between the ages of 25 and 30, men and women begin to lose muscle mass—eventually losing up to one-third of their muscle mass due to changes in

hormones, activity levels, and nutrition. Injury and chronic diseases can cause people to exercise less and accelerate typical muscle loss. **Sarcopenia**, literally "poverty of flesh," describes this age-related loss in skeletal muscle (see **Figure 4.5**). Sarcopenia reduces overall physical functioning by decreasing muscular strength and endurance and causing losses in **muscle power**, or the capacity to exert force rapidly.

Muscular strength declines more rapidly after age 40, and then after age 50, we lose approximately 15 percent of our strength per decade![15] While no one is immune from the aging process, resistance training throughout one's life can significantly slow natural muscle loss. In fact, older individuals who do resistance training can retain strength at or above that of untrained younger people.[16] Maintaining muscle mass as you age is associated with living longer[17] and the increase in muscular fitness and the improvements it brings to everyday physical functioning help individuals live independently for a longer portion of their lives.[18] See Chapter 15 for more information about sarcopenia and maintaining muscle fitness throughout your lifespan.

Regular Resistance Training Enhances Your Performance in Sports and Activities

A strong body that moves quickly, resists fatigue, and recovers easily from illness or injury is the aim for all types of athletes. These traits contribute to better

PUMPING UP WOMEN TO STRENGTH TRAIN

With fewer than 19% of college age American women meeting the CDC's strength training recommendations,[1] some women may need a boost to start strength training.

WHO DIDN'T PARTICIPATE IN ANY STRENGTH TRAINING OVER THE LAST WEEK?[2]

61% of undergraduate **WOMEN**

45% of undergraduate **MEN**

ARE THESE MYTHS STOPPING WOMEN FROM STRENGTH TRAINING?

MYTH	FACT
Women who **LIFT WEIGHTS** will develop bulky muscles.	It's **physiologically impossible** for most women to bulk up. Women don't have enough testosterone, the "muscle-bulking" hormone.
Women are **NOT AS STRONG** as men.	While technically true in most cases, it's because men (on average) have more muscle mass than women. Compared pound for pound, **women can be equally strong**.
Weight training will **REDUCE** your flexibility.	Resistance training can actually **enhance** your joint range of motion/flexibility.[3]
If you build muscle and then **STOP EXERCISING**, your muscle will turn to fat.	**Not possible!** Fat and muscle are two different substances; you can't turn one into the other.
The weight room is an **INTIMIDATING PLACE** full of men.	After an orientation to the gym, fellow exercisers and the gym equipment will be **familiar and welcoming**. Still intimidated? Try women-specific facilities and/or strength training classes.

STRENGTH TRAINING benefits women by

▶ **INCREASING** self-confidence and body image.

▶ **BUILDING BONES** to reduce the risk of osteoporosis.[4]

▶ **SLOWING** the 15% loss of muscle mass that women experience each decade after age 50.[5]

TO JUMP INTO Strength Training RIGHT NOW

- **LEARN** good technique to get the maximum benefit and to avoid injury.

- **START SLOWLY** with the number of repetitions, the amount of resistance, and the number of workouts per week.

- **USE THE PROPER** weight, where you can just barely finish the last 12-15 repetitions.

performances in sports and recreational activities. Resistance training is often the common denominator among sports training programs. Because of these benefits, physically active adults often incorporate some form of resistance training that builds strength and endurance in the muscle groups most crucial to their activity.

LO 4.4 How Can I Assess My Muscular Strength and Endurance?

Assessing your current muscular strength and endurance will allow you to compare the results to norm charts for your age and gender, or simply use them as a starting point for designing your resistance-training program. After you've followed your program for a while, follow-up assessments will help you evaluate your progress and make adjustments to stay on track.

Test Your Muscular Strength

Tests of muscular strength gauge the maximum amount of force you can generate in a muscle. People usually carry out these tests in a weight room where measured weights are readily available.

1 RM Tests One repetition maximum (1 RM) tests are the most common tool that personal trainers use to assess their clients' muscular strength. To participate in 1 RM tests safely, you must be medically cleared to lift weights, know weight-training guidelines, have some weight-training experience, follow test instructions, and identify qualified **spotters** to assist if necessary. If you are weight training on campus or at a gym, an instructor will be able to help you through these steps.

Performing a 1 RM test involves discovering the maximum amount of weight you can lift one time on a particular exercise. Aim to find your 1 RM within three to five trials so that muscle fatigue from repetitions does not change your result.

Individuals who are new to resistance training can predict their 1 RM

instead of actually attempting a maximum lift. To predict your 1 RM, you will lift, press, or pull a weight that will fully fatigue your upper- or lower-body muscles in 2 to 10 repetitions. You can then use a formula that converts actual weight lifted and real number of repetitions to predict your 1 RM for that exercise.

In **Lab 4.1** (at the end of this chapter), you will use chest-press and leg-press exercises to predict your 1 RM. You can perform these tests for any weight-training exercise and then convert to the predicted 1 RM value. Many weight-training programs use a percentage of your 1 RM or predicted 1 RM to determine a safe starting level for weight lifting.

Do It!
Access these labs at the end of the chapter or online at MasteringHealth™.

Grip Strength Test Another common test of muscle strength is the hand grip strength test using a piece of equipment called a *grip strength dynamometer.* As you squeeze the dynamometer (one hand at a time), it measures the isometric strength of your grip-squeezing muscles in pounds or kilograms (kg). If you have a grip strength dynamometer available, assess your grip strength with the online Alternate Lab: Assessing Grip Strength.

Test Your Muscular Endurance

Muscular endurance tests evaluate a muscle's ability to contract for an extended period of time. Some of these tests must be performed in a weight room, whereas others require only your body weight and can be performed anywhere.

20 RM Tests You can use any weight-training exercise to find your **20 repetition maximum (20 RM)**. This test determines the maximal amount of weight you can lift exactly 20 times in a row before the muscle becomes too fatigued to continue. The 20 RM tests are particularly useful for setting muscular endurance goals and tracking your progress. Identify your 20 RM within one to three tries to avoid fatiguing your muscles and altering your results. **Lab 4.2** at the end of this chapter 157 walks you through the steps of finding your 20 RM for the chest-press and leg-press exercises.

Do It!
Access these labs at the end of the chapter or online at MasteringHealth™.

Calisthenic or Body Weight Tests **Calisthenics** are conditioning exercises that use your body weight for resistance. Standardized calisthenic tests use sit-ups, curl-ups, pull-ups, push-ups, and flexed arm support/hang exercises to assess muscular endurance and compare your results to well-established physical fitness norms. The procedures for these tests vary but you can learn

---

one repetition maximum (1 RM) The maximum amount of weight you can lift one time

spotter A person who watches, encourages, and, if needed, assists a person who is performing a weight-training lift

20 repetition maximum (20 RM) The maximum amount of weight you can lift 20 times in a row

calisthenics A type of muscle fitness or flexibility exercise that employs simple movements without the use of resistance other than one's own body weight

how to perform the curl-up and push-up assessments in Lab 4.2. These assessments allow you to test yourself outside a weight-training facility and can be adapted for many fitness levels. In addition to standardized tests, some trainers will have you perform timed exercises (i.e., how many box jumps can you do in one minute) to assess how much your muscular strength, power, and/or endurance changes over time with training.

LO 4.5 How Can I Design My Own Resistance-Training Program?

Become your own personal trainer! Use the guidelines in this section to plan a safe and effective resistance-training program.

Set Appropriate Muscular Fitness Goals

Remember to use SMART goal-setting guidelines: *specific, measurable, action-oriented, realistic,* and with a *timeline.* Your goals may be appearance-based, function-based, or a combination of the two.

Appearance-Based Goals Many people have appearance-based goals for muscular fitness: They want larger muscles, or muscles that are more toned and less flabby. "Spot reduction" (i.e., trimming down just one area of the body) is another often-voiced goal. Researchers have proven spot reduction to be a myth—fat doesn't disappear through repeated exercise to one area.[19]

To judge your progress toward appearance-based goals, include some sort of measure in your resistance-training plan. For muscle size, measure the circumference of your biceps or calves, for example, and then set a goal to increase or decrease this number. For overall body size, your goal may be to increase lean tissue weight but decrease fat tissue and percentage of body fat. If your goal is to become more "toned," quantify this in some way. Look in the mirror and make notes about the way your body looks and moves. After you reach the target date for your plan, reread your notes, look in the mirror, and then reevaluate whether your muscle tone has improved.

Function-Based Goals Function-based goals focus on your muscular capabilities and include gaining better muscular strength, greater muscular endurance, or both. **Lab 4.3** will guide you in setting goals for realistic changes in muscle function and help you assess your improvements.

Do It!
Access these labs at the end of the chapter or online at MasteringHealth™.

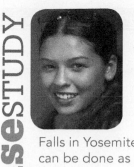

Explore Your Equipment Options

Should you use weight machines? Free weights? Other equipment? No equipment at all? These are important decisions that will be influenced by your goals, the type of equipment available to you, your experience with weight-training exercises, and your preferences.

Machines If you are new to resistance training, weight machines can be very useful. Systems such as Cybex®,

TABLE 4.1 Weight-Training Machines vs. Free Weights

Machine Weights	Free Weights
PROS	**PROS**
Safe and less intimidating for beginners	Can be tailored for individual workouts
Quicker to set up and use	Range of motion set by lifter, not machine
Spotters not typically needed	Some exercises can be done anywhere
Support of standing posture not needed	Standing and sitting postural muscles worked
Adaptable for those with limitations	Movements can transfer to daily activities
Variable resistance is possible	Good for strength and power building
Good isolation of specific muscle groups	Additional stabilizer muscles worked
Only good option for some muscle groups	Lower cost and more available for home use
CONS	**CONS**
Machine sets range of motion	More difficult to learn
May not fit every body size and type	A spotter may be needed
Some people lack access to weight machines	Incorrect form may lead to injuries
Posture-supporting muscles used less	More time may be needed to change weights
Limited number of exercises/machines	More training needed to create program

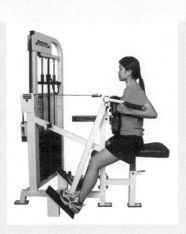
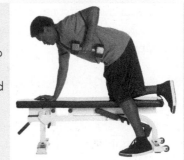

Nautilus®, Life Fitness®, and many others allow you to isolate and strengthen specific muscle groups as well as to train without a spotting partner.

Free Weights Exercise physiologists consider free-weight exercises to be a more advanced approach to weight training than machine-weight exercises. Free-weight exercises use **dumbbells**; **barbells**; incline, flat, or decline benches; squat racks; and related equipment. Free-weight exercises allow your body to move through its natural range of motion instead of the path predetermined by a weight machine. This both requires and promotes development of more muscle control. Some athletes prefer free-weight exercises because the balance and movement patterns are closer to their sport movement patterns, whether that be tossing a football, putting a shot, or doing the breaststroke.

Since workout facilities often have both free weights and weight machines, many people start their resistance-training program with machines and then progress to free weights within the first few months.

dumbbells Weights intended for use by one hand
barbells Long bars with weight plates on each end

Table 4.1 this page compares weight training with machines versus free weights.

Alternate Equipment You can increase resistance on your body with equipment other than machines or free weights. Resistance bands, stability balls, medicine balls, kettlebells, and battling ropes are popular types of alternate resistance equipment that people are using at home, in the gym, and in classes. See the Tools for Change Mix Up Your Resistance Tools box to Stay Motivated on page 125 to explore this equipment for yourself.

Body-Weight Training Listed as the number one worldwide fitness trend for 2015, body-weight training (also called *calisthenics* or *no-equipment training*) is hot![20] This type of training employs exercises, such as push-ups, pull-ups, lunges, squats, leg lifts, and curl-ups, that do not involve equipment but instead use your body weight to provide the resistance. Fitness classes and programs, such as yoga, Pilates, CrossFit, and boot camp, typically incorporate body weight exercises that help you increase your muscular fitness. As an added benefit, these exercises are perfect for maintaining muscular fitness while traveling.

Mix Up Your Resistance Tools to Stay Motivated

Are you tired of "lifting weights"? Do you want something more exciting than 3 sets of 10 push-ups? Try incorporating the following "tools" into your resistance training routine to spice it up and keep yourself motivated!

Resistance bands made of tubing or flat strips of rubber allow you to simultaneously increase resistance throughout a range of motion and to improve muscular endurance. This may be one of the most versatile and inexpensive pieces of resistance equipment you can own. You can perform many different exercises with these bands and they fold up and pack perfectly in a suitcase or gym bag for a portable workout. The bands or tubes come in varying resistance levels, so everyone can find the right level and you can progress your workout as you get stronger. Some of the exercises in **Figure 4.10** (pages 137–150) include resistance band exercises for the upper and lower body.

Stability balls (also called Swiss, fitness, or exercise balls) are 45, 55, or 65 cm diameter vinyl balls that have various uses for muscular fitness, endurance, and balance. Ball routines involve performing exercises while sitting, lying, and/or balancing on the ball. You must use core trunk muscles to counteract the natural instability of the ball, which enhances overall body function. See Figure 4.10 for a few stability ball exercise examples. In addition, you can use a stability ball in place of a chair or bench for dumbbell exercises to add an extra core and balance challenge.

Medicine balls are heavily weighted balls used either individually, with a partner, or in a group. You can hold a medicine ball while doing exercises or pass a ball from partner to partner for a functional increase in muscle endurance. Medicine balls typically range from 6 to 50 pounds and come in varying sizes. Most are designed to be lifted, tossed, thrown against a wall, or slammed down to the floor and will come in varying levels of "bounciness." Medicine balls are used in many fitness classes and found in sports and fitness facilities for individual use as well.

Kettlebells are weights with handles that can be used for traditional dumbbell exercises, controlled strength moves, or full body explosive exercises. Dating back to

18th century Russia, kettlebells are now used around the world for training and competitions. There are many options for kettlebell weights, sizes, and composition. Choose a lighter kettlebell for upper-body work and a heavier one for full- and lower-body exercises. Before performing the more complex explosive movements such as the kettlebell swing, clean, and the snatch, get qualified instruction in safe kettlebell use.

Battling ropes are long heavy ropes that are anchored at a fixed location. You manipulate the ropes to create waves in multiple directions and speeds. Heavier, longer ropes and larger, faster waves create higher levels of resistance and intensity. You can perform exercises with upper body movements only or incorporate the lower body for a total workout. Working with the ropes can increase heart rates for cardiorespiratory conditioning and increase muscular strength, endurance, and power. Due to the high-intensity nature of the rope exercises, you'll find battling ropes in workout classes and facilities that offer high-intensity interval training (HIIT).

TRY IT! **Today**, decide which of the above resistance tools sounds like the most fun. **This week**, try out one of them. You may have a ball or band in your home already or you can buy an inexpensive one. Alternatively, seek out a class or facility that utilizes this equipment. **In two weeks**, try out the new equipment as part of your workout routine and answer the following questions:

1. What type of alternate equipment did you try out?
   _____

2. How did you use it? _____
   _____

3. What did you like about it? _____
   _____

4. What was challenging? _____
   _____

5. Will you use the equipment again? Why or why not?
   _____

Source:
D. Sanforth et al., "Training Toys...Bells, Ropes, and Balls—Oh My!" *ACSM's Health & Fitness Journal* 19, no. 4 (2015): 5–11.

Understand the Different Types of Resistance-Training Programs

Try out a number of options for your resistance-training program. The right one for you will fit well with your goals, experience, and personal preferences.

Traditional Weight Training Traditional weight training takes place in a weight room and usually includes a combination of machine-weight, free-weight, and body-weight exercises. Individuals may work alone or with a partner and usually perform multiple **sets** and **repetitions** of a particular exercise before moving on to the next exercise. Exercises involve shortening (concentric) and lengthening (eccentric) muscle contractions, but some people advocate focusing more on lengthening contractions for enhanced benefits. See the Q&A box Can "Negatives" Help Me Get Strong Fast? on page 128 to see if eccentric resistance training is for you.

The next section provides guidelines for setting up your traditional weight-training program. See Lab 4.4 and Program 4.1 at the end of this chapter for sample weight-training programs.

Circuit Weight Training Circuit weight training is done in a specialized circuit-training room, a general workout room, or a weight room. Exercisers move from one station to another in a set pattern (the "circuit") after a certain amount of time at a station or after performing a certain number of repetitions of an exercise. Some circuits include only resistance-training exercises and focus on improving muscular fitness. Other circuits involve cardio equipment, such as stationary bicycles, mixed in with resistance exercises to improve both cardiorespiratory and muscular fitness.

Circuit exercises should be organized properly in order to ensure a safe and effective exercise session. For example, multi-joint exercises (bench press, leg press) are often performed before single-joint exercises (biceps curl, leg extension) and muscle groups worked are spread out to allow recovery between sets. Exercises that stress the core postural muscles are reserved for the end of the workout because these muscles provide important trunk support during seated and standing exercises.

Plyometrics and Sports Training Athletes use many of the weight-training exercises illustrated in this chapter, but they also perform exercises that specifically benefit their sports performance. Plyometrics, power lifts, and speed and agility drills are examples.

A **plyometric exercise** program incorporates explosive exercises that mimic the quick transition movements needed in many sports (e.g., basketball, wrestling, and gymnastics). These exercises are characterized by landing and slowing down the body followed immediately by rapid movement in the opposite direction (e.g., jumping down off a box and then immediately jumping back up as high as you can). Plyometrics is a highly specialized training method that should be performed under proper direction and by individuals who have achieved moderate muscular fitness levels.

Power lifts incorporate fast and forceful actions to improve strength and speed. Lifting for **power** stresses the nervous system to act quickly and the tendons, ligaments, and joint structures to become more stable. Sports that require high levels of explosive movement and power (football, wrestling, gymnastics, and track-and-field events) may require power-lifting training to build strength with speed. Power lifting is a competitive sport in itself. Competitive power lifts include the bench press, the squat, the dead lift, and the Olympic lifts (the clean and jerk and the snatch). Power lifting is best incorporated into your program after you have some weight-training experience and at least a moderate level of muscular fitness.

Speed and **agility** drills are making their way into mainstream sports training, boot camp-style classes, and even classes for older adults. Speed and agility drills improve muscle responsiveness, speed, footwork, and coordination. Typical drills include line sprints, high-knee runs, fast-foot-turnover running, and hopping quickly through varying foot patterns (using agility dots or other markers). Speed and agility drills can be performed by anyone who is physically fit enough to learn and perform the skills; however, instruction, modification, and monitoring are essential to prevent injuries.

Whole-Body Exercise Programs The increasing popularity of "functional" training—training that carries over to life activities—has given rise to exercise programs that focus on whole-body movements. These programs,

sets Single attempts at an exercise that include a fixed number of repetitions

repetitions The number of times an exercise is performed within one set

plyometric exercise An exercise where a rapid deceleration of the body is followed by a rapid acceleration in the opposite direction

power The ability to produce force quickly

speed The ability to rapidly accelerate

agility The ability to rapidly change body position or body direction without losing speed, balance, or body control

Studies have shown that participants in ECPs using kettlebells may increase their aerobic capacity[21] with reduced neck and lower back pain.[22] However, strength gains may not be as pronounced as in traditional strength training.[23]

If you are a beginning exerciser, you shouldn't start out with ECP, but you can certainly perform whole body exercises. For instance, instead of limiting yourself to stationary lunges, add a forward walking movement with a twist to the opposite side in every lunge step.

Apply the FITT Formula to Resistance Training

FITT stands for *frequency*, *intensity*, *time*, and *type*. The acronym represents a checklist for determining how often, how hard, and how long to exercise, and what types of exercise to choose at your current level of muscular fitness.

Frequency Your goals and your schedule determine how often you will train each week. At a minimum, you should work each muscle group twice per week. A full-body workout means two muscle fitness workouts per week. If you split your muscle workouts (e.g., into upper body and lower body), then you would go to the weight room four times per week. **Table 4.2** on page 129 presents American College of Sports Medicine (ACSM) guidelines for muscular fitness.

It is important to let each muscle group rest for 48 hours before taxing it again with resistance training. Especially when you are just beginning, schedule your workouts so they are at least two days apart. When you perform an intense weight-training session, micro-damage occurs within the muscle cells and rest time is needed for muscle repair and adaptation. Your muscles will adapt by constructing new actin and myosin contractile proteins and other supporting structures. Over time, this adaptation results in stronger, leaner, larger muscles. Intense workouts of the same muscle group on subsequent days will disrupt the repair and adaptation process. Rather than faster muscle development, this overtraining is likely to cause injuries, muscle fatigue, and weakening. An exception can be made for lower intensity muscular fitness classes or calisthenics, which can be done daily as long as they are not overly fatiguing.

Muscle soreness that sets in within a day or two is called delayed-onset muscle soreness (DOMS); it is a sign that your body was not ready for the amount of overload you applied. Contrary to popular belief, it is not

such as CrossFit, P90X, boot camp, and kettlebell, integrate various muscle groups into one exercise rather than isolating a single muscle group (see Chapter 3 for more information about CrossFit and HIIT training methods). The exercises aim to address three planes of movement (forward and back, side to side, and rotational) for increased crossover into daily activities and enhanced sports and recreation performance. Think of it as a combination of resistance, circuit, and HIIT training, performed with whole body movements. These programs are often called *extreme conditioning programs* (ECPs) because they employ multiple repetitions of challenging exercises in a short period of time.

Q&A   Can "Negatives" Help Me Get Strong Fast?

Recall that eccentric contractions, also called "negatives" or "heavy negatives," are lengthening contractions that help us slow down when we are going downhill or lowering a weight. Performing eccentric contractions quickly and forcefully is associated with delayed-onset muscle soreness (DOMS). However, there are many benefits as well.

Compared to shortening concentric contractions, our muscles are able to exert more force when lengthening. This means eccentric contractions allow you to perform exercises that require greater amounts of resistance and you'll gain more muscular strength as a result.[1] Not only that, low-intensity eccentric contractions will protect against muscle damage from high-intensity, maximal eccentric contractions—and the protective effect can last for a week.[2] So, low-intensity eccentric workouts during the week can prepare you to run, jump, and crawl faster through that weekend obstacle course race—and be less sore after!

Eccentric contractions cause less cardiovascular stress than concentric contractions. That means you'll likely perceive the workout as easier, even though you are getting stronger. When performed correctly, eccentric exercise training is safe and beneficial for beginning exercisers, older exercisers, and those with cardiorespiratory disease.[3] For those recovering from injuries, studies have shown improvements in joint pain and function with eccentric exercise.[4] You may even see your flexibility improve.[5]

When and how should you perform eccentric exercise training? Simply focus on the lowering or deceleration portion of a resistance training exercise. There are specialized machines that can be programmed to focus on the "negative" or lowering part of the lift. You can also use a partner to help give you more weight on the eccentric phase, or you can simply slow down the lengthening or lowering portion of the exercise to create more overload.

For instance, if you are struggling with push-ups, focus on lowering yourself down (the eccentric phase) until you've gained enough strength to consistently push yourself back up. If you have a goal to perform chin-ups, have a friend help you pull up and then slowly lower yourself down to focus on the eccentric contraction. Before long, you may be able to pull yourself back up again without help!

Since eccentric loading can cause more muscle damage, be sure to warm-up thoroughly. If you are incorporating quick or heavy eccentric contractions, limit the workouts to once per week to minimize damage and maximize recovery and adaptation. As with all resistance training, start slowly, focus on good form and posture, have a spotter for heavier lifts, and listen to your body. If you currently have joint pain, are recovering from an injury, or have a chronic disease, consult your physician before incorporating eccentric resistance training.

Sources:
1. M. O. Gois et al., "The Influence of Resistance Exercise with Emphasis on Specific Contractions (Concentric vs. Eccentric) on Muscle Strength and Post-Exercise Autonomic Modulation: A Randomized Clinical Trial," *Brazilian Journal of Physical Therapy* 18, no. 1 (2014): 30–37.
2. M. J. Lin et al., "Low-Intensity Eccentric Contractions of the Knee Extensors and Flexors Protect against Muscle Damage," *Applied Physiology, Nutrition, and Metabolism* 40, no. 10 (June 10, 2015): 1–8.
3. A. Gluchowski et al., "Chronic Eccentric Exercise and the Older Adult," *Sports Medicine* 45, no. 10 (August 14, 2015); R. Ellis et al., "Eccentric Exercise in Adults with Cardiorespiratory Disease: A Systematic Review," *Clinical Rehabilitation* 29, no. 12 (March 10, 2015).
4. M. F. Joseph and C. R. Denegar, "Treating Tendinopathy: Perspective on Anti-Inflammatory Intervention and Therapeutic Exercise," *Clinics in Sports Medicine* 34, no. 2 (2015): 363–74.
5. K. O'Sullivan, S. McAuliffe, and N. Deburca, "The Effects of Eccentric Training on Lower Limb Flexibility: A Systematic Review," *British Journal of Sports Medicine* 46, no. 12 (2012): 838–45.

lactic acid (lactate) that causes DOMS; as you learned in Chapter 3, accumulated lactic acid (lactate) is cleared from muscle cells within hours of exercise. If you choose weight amounts correctly, your muscles will sustain small amounts of micro-damage that does not result in soreness and that your body can repair within 48 hours after the workout.

Intensity The intensity of a weight-training program refers to the amount of **resistance** you apply through any given exercise. For each exercise, the intensity you choose will depend on your fitness goals for that particular muscle group or your body as a

> **resistance** The amount of effort or force required to complete the exercise

whole. The ACSM guidelines in Table 4.2 for muscular fitness can help you choose weight-training intensities (shown as a percentage of your 1 RM or percentage of predicted 1 RM).

The intensity or weight chosen for each exercise should be enough to overload the muscle group you are working—that means you should feel slight discomfort or muscle fatigue near the end of your exercise set. If you feel no fatigue during the entire set of repetitions and feel you could lift the weight another 3 to 10 times, the intensity is too low. Aim for muscle fatigue but not complete exhaustion.

Time: Sets and Repetitions Your fitness goals help determine the number of sets you will execute for each exercise, the number of repetitions within each set, and

TABLE 4.2 ACSM's Guidelines for Resistance Training in Healthy Adults

Goal	Level	Intensity (% 1 RM)	Repetitions	Sets	Rest (min between sets)[a]	Frequency (days/week)[b]	Number and Types of Exercises
Improve Muscular Fitness[c]	Beginner/ novice	40–70	8–12	1–3	2–3	2–3	8–10+ emphasizing multiple-joint exercises for opposing muscle groups in the lower body, upper body, and trunk; add single-joint exercises as needed for muscle balance
	Intermediate/ advanced	60–80	8–12	2–4	2–3	2–3	
Increase Muscular Endurance	All levels	<50	15–25	1–2	1–2	2–3	
Further Increase Muscular Strength	Intermediate	70–80	1–12	2–4	2–3	2–5	
	Advanced	>80	1–6	2–4	2–3	2–5	

[a]Decrease rest between sets for endurance and increase for strength; rest a particular muscle group 48 hours between workout sessions.
[b]2–3 days/week = total body workouts, 4–5 days/week = split routine to train each major muscle group twice per week.
[c]Muscular strength, mass, and to some extent, muscular endurance.

Data from American College of Sports Medicine, *ACSM's Guidelines for Exercise Testing and Prescription*, 9th ed. (Baltimore, MD: Lippincott Williams & Wilkins, 2014); N. A. Ratamess et al., "ACSM Position Stand: Progression Models in Resistance Training for Healthy Adults," *Medicine & Science in Sports & Exercise* 341, no. 3 (2009): 687–708; C. E. Garber et al., "American College of Sports Medicine Position Stand: Quantity and Quality of Exercise for Developing and Maintaining Cardiorespiratory, Musculoskeletal, and Neuromotor Fitness in Apparently Healthy Adults: Guidance for Prescribing Exercise," *Medicine & Science in Sports & Exercise* 43, no. 7 (2011): 1334–59, doi: 10.1249/MSS.0b013e318213fefb

the rest period between sets. Your weight-training experience and the time you have available to work out will affect your planning as well.

ACSM recommends that you perform two to four sets of each exercise during a given workout session (see Table 4.2), and in general, more sets will result in greater results.[24] However, if you are new to resistance training, you will see progress with just one set per muscle group. You can execute one, two, three, or four sets for all your exercises, or perform two sets of certain exercises, three of others, and so on. Keep in mind, however, that overtraining one particular muscle group can lead to muscle imbalance and injury.

Resting between sets affects your performance on subsequent exercises. Longer rest periods between sets are essential if you are lifting heavy weights for building strength, whereas, shorter rest periods are beneficial for enhancing muscular endurance.

Intensity and repetitions have an inverse relationship relative to muscular strength and endurance (see **Figure 4.6**). For muscular strength development, you will lift heavier weights and do fewer repetitions; for muscular endurance, you will lift lighter weights with more repetitions.

Type: Choosing Appropriate Exercises The final part of designing a muscular fitness program is choosing exercises that will help you achieve your goals and muscle balance. Create your own muscular fitness goals in Lab 4.3 and use **Figure 4.7** to start planning your resistance-training program. Next, complete **Lab 4.4** to plan a muscular fitness program

Do It!
Access these labs at the end of the chapter or online at MasteringHealth™.

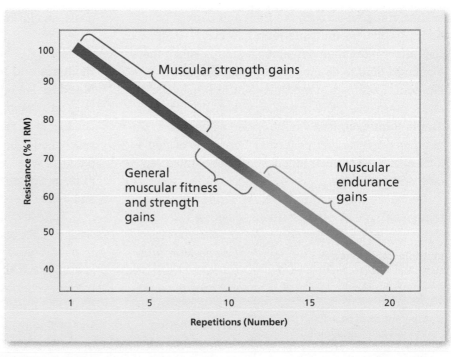

FIGURE **4.6** Fewer repetitions with higher resistance will produce gains in muscular strength. More repetitions with lower resistance will produce gains in muscular endurance.

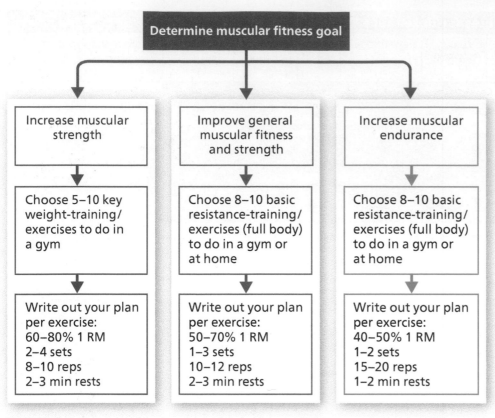

Determine muscular fitness goal

Increase muscular strength	Improve general muscular fitness and strength	Increase muscular endurance
Choose 5–10 key weight-training/ exercises to do in a gym	Choose 8–10 basic resistance-training/ exercises (full body) to do in a gym or at home	Choose 8–10 basic resistance-training/ exercises (full body) to do in a gym or at home
Write out your plan per exercise: 60–80% 1 RM 2–4 sets 8–10 reps 2–3 min rests	Write out your plan per exercise: 50–70% 1 RM 1–3 sets 10–12 reps 2–3 min rests	Write out your plan per exercise: 40–50% 1 RM 1–2 sets 15–20 reps 1–2 min rests

FIGURE **4.7** Use this flowchart as you design your muscular fitness program. Just starting? Begin at the lower end of all recommended ranges (for rest periods, begin at the upper end).

free weights, body-weight exercises, or a combination of all three. Most programs include all three and will be determined by your goals and the equipment available to you. See Program 4.1 (A Resistance-Training Program) at the end of this chapter for sample programs to get you started.

What If I Don't Reach My Goals?

You may find that your muscular development is not keeping up with your ambitions or that you cannot follow through consistently with training sessions. What other steps can you take to ensure success?

using **Figures 4.9** (page 135) and **4.10** (page 137) to help you select the best exercises.

Muscle balance requires a selection of exercises for the upper body, trunk, and lower body. Choose exercises from Figure 4.10 that work *opposing muscle groups,* muscles on both the front and back of your body. Emphasize **multiple-joint exercises**—exercises that affect more than one muscle group—since these exercises tend to be more functional and time-efficient. Examples of multiple-joint exercises include chest press, overhead press, leg press, and lunges. **Single-joint exercises** can be added as needed to target major muscle groups further. Examples of single-joint exercises include biceps curl, lateral raise, leg curl, and heel raise.

For a starting program, choose 8 to 10 exercises, remembering that each additional exercise will add time to your exercise session; with too many exercises, you may need to split your workout into alternating exercises on different days. Select weight machines,

multiple-joint exercises Exercises that involve multiple joints and muscle groups to achieve an overall movement

single-joint exercises Exercises that involve a single joint and typically focus on one muscle group

Track Your Progress Use a weight-training log, notebook, online program, or smart phone app to track your progress. Lab 4.4 provides you with a log that allows you to (1) see your week-to-week progress, (2) stay motivated, (3) detect problems with your program design or goals, and (4) know where to redesign your program if necessary.

Evaluate and Redesign Your Program as Needed Periodically reevaluate your muscular fitness program. Common times to reassess are at your target completion date, when you feel you aren't making progress, when your improvement rate is faster than anticipated, or when you feel overtraining fatigue or injury. First, retake the initial tests for muscular strength and endurance. Second, reassess your goals: accomplished or not? Third, evaluate your overall program and write out what you like and don't like about it. If you have met your goals and enjoy your program, continue but set more challenging goals based on FITT parameters. If you have not met your goals or don't like your program, rewrite the goals and target dates, redesigning to solve your issues. Get help from an exercise professional if needed.

Evaluating and redesigning should allow you, once again, to move toward your muscular fitness goals. Lab 4.4 provides practice at evaluation and redesign.

LO 4.6 What Precautions Should I Take to Avoid Resistance-Training Injuries?

Greater muscular fitness achieved through resistance training helps prevent general injury during sports or daily activity. However, weight training itself can cause injuries, such as muscle or tendon strains, ligament sprains, fractures, dislocations, and other joint problems. This is especially true if the lifter pushes for an unrealistic overload. You can prevent injuries by getting proper instruction and guidance and by heeding a few basic suggestions.

Follow Basic Weight-Training Guidelines

When starting your program, be conservative. Resist the temptation to begin with too many exercises or sets or with too much weight! Before increasing your intensity or duration, observe how your body responds to the training over a few weeks. After that, you can safely increase the number of repetitions and/or the amount of weight.

Follow the "10 percent rule." Limit increases in exercise frequency, intensity, or time to no more than 10 percent per week. Gentle increases will help prevent injury, overtraining, or soreness. Break this rule only if the initial intensity you selected was very low or a certified fitness professional instructs you to do otherwise.

Warm Up and Cool Down Properly

Weight-training guidelines include a warm-up and a cool-down before and after each session. A proper weight-training warm-up includes a *general warm-up* and a *specific warm-up*. The *general warm-up* consists of 5 to 10 minutes of cardiorespiratory exercises—walking, jogging (on or off a treadmill), biking, stationary biking, elliptical training, or any activity that increases body temperature (breaking a light sweat) and blood flow to muscles. The *specific warm-up* should include range-of-motion exercises that mimic (without weight added) the resistance exercises you'll be performing. Move your limbs through a full range of motion before using a given weight machine or lifting free weights. Then, do a warm-up set with very light resistance. Now you are ready to perform your serious sets.

Some people also like to stretch before weight training. If you want to add stretching to your warm-up, do your general warm-up first. Pre-exercise stretching should be light, and you should hold each stretch no more than 10 to 15 seconds. (See Chapter 5 for more about the timing of your stretches within the warm-up

and cool-down.) A proper cool-down for resistance training includes general range-of-motion exercises and stretches for the muscle groups you stressed during the weight-training session.

Know How to Train with Weights Safely

Guidelines for safe training include:

1. Get a proper introduction to weight training before you begin. Learn the safe way to sit, stand, move, and grip the equipment.

2. Learn the proper use of weights and weight machines. Understand the correct way to adjust machines for your height and use safety collars at the ends of weight bars.

3. When lifting heavy free weights, use a spotter to watch, guide, and assist if needed. Ask the spotter to ensure that you are lifting safely and can return the bar after the lift. Spotters may assist the lifter when the weight is near maximal and the lift requires body balance.

4. Wear gym shoes to protect your feet and provide a stable posture during standing lifts. Some lifters wear weight lifting gloves to improve grip and protect their hands.

5. Perform exercises in a slow and controlled manner, avoiding jerky or bouncy motions. Use a count of two up and four down to control the weight-lowering phase. Don't "drop" a weight to its starting position, whether lifting free weights or using a machine. The objective is to stay away from quick and heavy eccentric contractions that can lead to muscle strains.

6. Perform all exercises through a full range of motion. Figure out how to isolate some muscle groups and stabilize others.

7. Set up in a relaxed, balanced position and maintain that position throughout your lifts. Lifting while off balance creates strain on one side and can pull or tear a muscle. Balance your exercise program to build equal strength on both sides and from front to back.

8. Breathe continuously when performing resistive movements. Some weight lifters use the **Valsalva maneuver** (i.e., they exhale

> **Valsalva maneuver** The process of holding one's breath while lifting heavy weight; an increase in chest cavity pressure can result in light-headedness during the lift; excessively increased blood pressure can result after the lift and breath are released

forcibly with a closed throat so no air exits) as a way to stabilize the trunk during a lift. However, holding your breath this way can cause an unhealthy spike in blood pressure and slow blood flow to the heart, lungs, and brain. When lifting heavy weights, breathe out during the push or pull portion to avoid the Valsalva maneuver.

9. Use lighter weights when attempting new lifts. After taking time off from your routine, build back up by 3 to 5 percent per session (or 10 percent per week). Don't assume you can pick up where you left off!

10. Do not continue resistance training if you are in pain. Learn to differentiate the effort of lifting from the pain of an injury.

Get Advice from a Qualified Exercise Professional

A qualified trainer can help you learn the proper position for lifting each type of weight and design a program specific to your needs and goals. Seek out people qualified to provide accurate resistance-training information, especially if you are just getting started or before significantly changing aspects of your routine, such as amount of weight, number of repetitions, speed of movement, or body posture.

How can you recognize a qualified exercise professional? Ask questions such as:

• Are you certified as a personal trainer or fitness instructor by a reputable, nationally recognized organization? Look for certification by the ACSM, National Strength and Conditioning Association (NSCA), American Council on Exercise (ACE), or National Academy of Sports Medicine (NASM)?

• Do you have a certificate or degree in exercise science from an accredited two- or four-year college?

• What types of experience have you had as an instructor or personal trainer?

• How long have you been working in the field of fitness and wellness?

• What are your references from employers and past/present clients?

• How current are you with the changing guidelines and emerging trends in exercise and fitness, and how can you demonstrate this currency?

You'll want to look at practical details such as how much personal

ergogenic aids Any nutritional, physical, mechanical, psychological, or pharmacological procedure or aid used to improve athletic performance

trainers charge, whether they have liability insurance, and how well their schedule will accommodate yours. Intangibles are equally important: How well do you get along with them and how motivated do they help you feel?

Consider enrolling in a weight-training class at your school. Instructors in these classes are already screened for the qualifications listed here, and the cost will be significantly lower than hiring your own personal trainer.

Follow Individualized Guidelines If You Have Physical Limitations

Weight-training programs benefit virtually everyone, including people with some limitations or disabilities. Resistance training can decrease pain and increase mobility in people with joint issues and muscle disabilities. Older adults, obese individuals, and those with orthopedic conditions such as arthritis, multiple sclerosis, or osteoarthritis, will all benefit from regular resistance training.

For older adults ACSM recommends a minimum of 10 to 15 repetitions for 8 to 10 exercises twice per week. In addition, stair climbing or whole body strengthening exercises can be helpful.

Obese individuals face unique challenges when beginning a resistance training program. Some people will want to look for a class, trainer, or facility designed for overweight individuals. These instructors and facilities specialize in weight loss and foster an inclusive, welcoming atmosphere. If you don't have one of those facilities in your community, you may feel comfortable exercising in any local gym or choose to work out in your home.

Safety guidelines and appropriate exercises will vary and will be determined by each person's situation. Most people will need medical clearance before beginning a resistance-training program, and those with certain conditions and disorders may need specific recommendations from a physician. If your gym lacks specialized equipment, look for a trainer who can help you perform modified exercises on the available machines. Wheelchair exercisers can perform many seated resistance-training exercises in the gym or at home. Visit this book's website to view demonstrations of easily adaptable resistance-training exercises for people of all abilities.

LO 4.7 Is It Risky to Use Supplements or Change My Diet for Muscular Fitness?

Dietary supplements marketed as promoters of muscular fitness are called performance aids or dietary **ergogenic aids**. Some supplements are safe but ineffective; some are both unsafe and ineffective. Few, if any, are worth the risk and expense.

Manufacturers of nutritional supplements do not need to prove that their products are safe or effective. The Food and Drug Administration (FDA) may take unsafe products off the market, but this occurs only after the product is "tested" on the buying public. Research the risks of a supplement very carefully before considering its use.

Some ergogenic aids, such as anabolic steroids, are controlled substances. This means they require a prescription for legal use and should not be used for non-prescription purposes. Their use can get you banned from athletic competitions.

Anabolic Steroids

Anabolic steroids are synthetic drugs that are chemically related to the hormone testosterone. Physicians may prescribe small doses for people with muscle diseases, burns, some cancers, and pituitary disorders. Some athletes and recreational weight trainers take anabolic steroids—illegally, without a prescription, and for no valid medical reason—to increase muscle mass, strength, and power. However, their overwhelmingly negative side effects far outweigh any benefits. See **Figure 4.8** for the side effects of steroid use.

Besides being illegal, steroids promote heart disease, heart attacks, and strokes, even in athletes younger than 30. The drugs also cause blood-filled cysts in the liver that can burst and cause serious internal bleeding. Injecting steroids and sharing needles with other users can transmit dangerous infections. The disease risks include hepatitis, HIV, and endocarditis, a bacterial infection of the heart. Steroid use can also be habit forming, lead to other drug addictions, and even cause death.

Anabolic steroids can permanently disrupt normal development. A person's body and brain are still developing during adolescence and into the early twenties. Steroids interfere with the normal effects of sex hormones and most of these changes are irreversible. Steroid use can lead to behavioral changes, including irritability, hostility, aggression, and depression. These changes can continue even after the user stops using steroids.[25] Long-term anabolic steroid use can also cause cognitive deficits. In one study, greater lifetime exposure to steroids was related to greater losses in visual-spatial memory.[26] Lastly, because dramatically stronger muscles may exert more force than the body can handle, anabolic steroid use can also promote connective tissue and bone injuries.

Creatine

Creatine is a legal nutritional supplement containing amino acids. It is most often sold as creatine monohydrate in powder, tablet, capsule, or liquid form. The

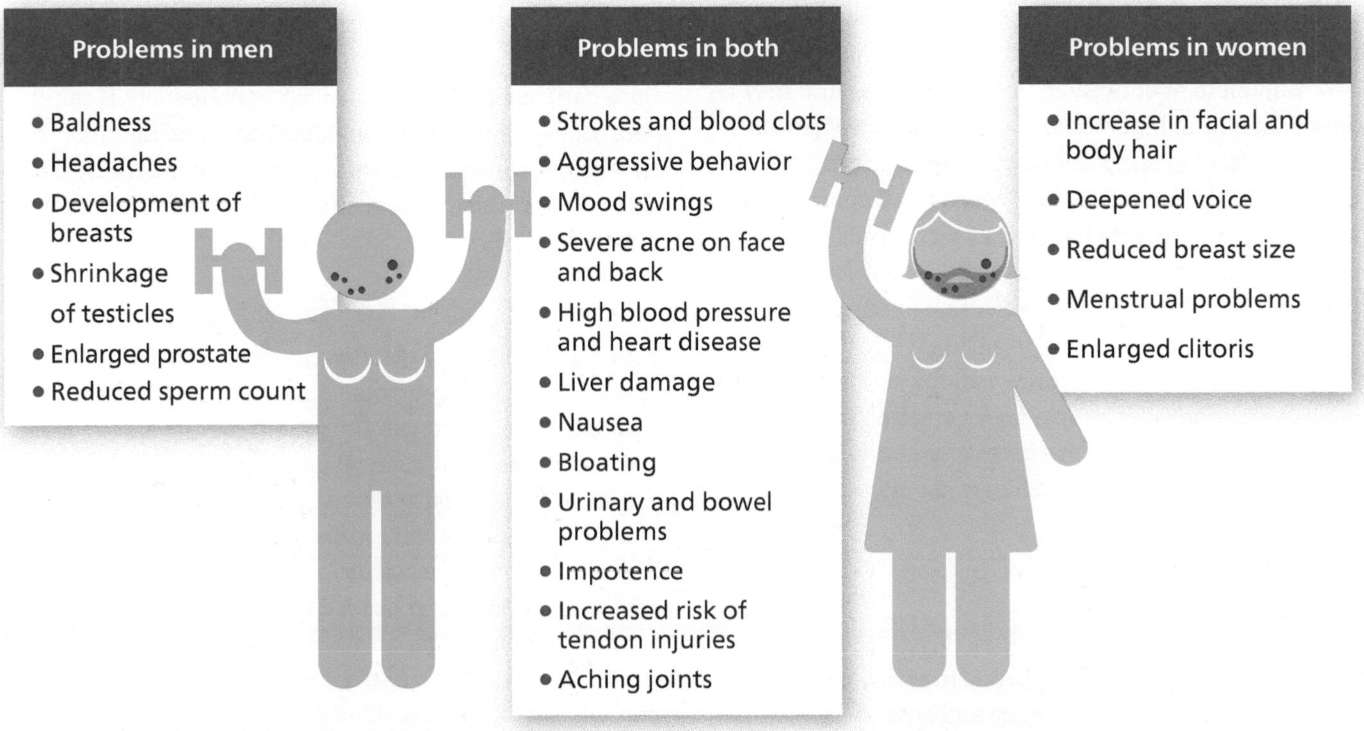

Problems in men	Problems in both	Problems in women
• Baldness	• Strokes and blood clots	• Increase in facial and body hair
• Headaches	• Aggressive behavior	• Deepened voice
• Development of breasts	• Mood swings	• Reduced breast size
• Shrinkage of testicles	• Severe acne on face and back	• Menstrual problems
• Enlarged prostate	• High blood pressure and heart disease	• Enlarged clitoris
• Reduced sperm count	• Liver damage	
	• Nausea	
	• Bloating	
	• Urinary and bowel problems	
	• Impotence	
	• Increased risk of tendon injuries	
	• Aching joints	

FIGURE **4.8** Side effects of steroid use in men and women.

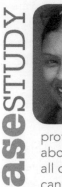
body's natural form of creatine (creatine phosphate) is generated by the kidneys and stored in muscle cells. You can also consume creatine in the diet by eating meat products.

Creatine taken at recommended levels can improve performance by temporarily increasing the body's normal muscle stores of creatine phosphate. Since this natural energy substance powers bursts of activity lasting less than 60 seconds, creatine users sometimes find they can train more effectively in power activities and may be able to maintain higher forces during lifting. This can increase training adaptations such as strength and muscle size.[27] Creatine intake also causes a temporary retention of water in muscle tissue that produces a small temporary increase in size, strength, and ability to generate power. Creatine has no effect on aerobic endurance.

So far, there have been few serious side effects reported in studies of people using creatine for up to four years. Since the long-term effects of creatine use are unknown, however, potential users should proceed with caution.

Adrenal Androgens (DHEA, Androstenedione)

Dehydroepiandrosterone (DHEA) is the body's most common hormone; it occurs naturally and acts as a weak steroid chemical messenger (it carries internal control signals and information). The US FDA banned DHEA in 1985 but brought it back in 1994 as an approved nutritional supplement. Manufacturers produce and sell it in a synthetic concentrated form despite the lack of definitive proof of its safety or effectiveness.[28] DHEA proponents claim that it increases muscle mass and strength, lowers body fat, alters natural hormone levels, slows down aging, and boosts immune functions. However, research studies have produced conflicting results on DHEA and overall do not provide strong evidence of a positive effect on muscle mass and strength or on body fat levels.[29]

Androstenedione (nicknamed "andro") is another naturally occurring steroid hormone with a structure related to both DHEA and testosterone. It is found naturally in meats and some plants. Even though manufacturers used to claim that "andro" increased testosterone levels, one pivotal study found that it actually lowered the body's natural production of testosterone, did not increase the body's adaptations to resistance training, and increased heart disease risk in men.[30]

Although the International Olympic Committee banned DHEA and androstenedione from athletic competitions in 1996 and 1997, respectively, only androstenedione was included in the Anabolic Steroids Control Act of 2004, prohibiting its sale without a prescription. It is now a "controlled substance," along with anabolic steroids. DHEA was given an exemption due to supporters advocating its purported "natural anti-aging" properties. Since the FDA took androstenedione off the market, its use is dwindling.

Both DHEA and androstenedione may lower your "good cholesterol" (HDL-C, high-density lipoprotein cholesterol), which increases cardiovascular disease risk. Both can increase your risk of estrogen-sensitive cancers (breast, ovarian, uterine), and could be dangerous for individuals with endocrine, liver, or mood disorders.[31] These serious side effects strongly argue against the use of DHEA or "andro."

Growth Hormone (GH)

Your body's pituitary gland produces human growth hormone (GH), which promotes bone and muscle growth and decreases fat stores. Drug manufacturers produce GH synthetically for medical use in children and young adults with abnormally slow or reduced growth and related disorders. Although the FDA regulates GH, athletes who want to gain an edge over their competitors sometimes obtain and use it illegally. Marketers claim that GH supplementation will counteract the muscle mass lost with disuse and aging, among other alleged benefits. However, GH side effects include irreversible bone growth (acromegaly/gigantism), increased risk of cardiovascular disease and diabetes, and decreased sexual desire, among others.

Anterior view (front)　　　　　**Posterior view (back)**

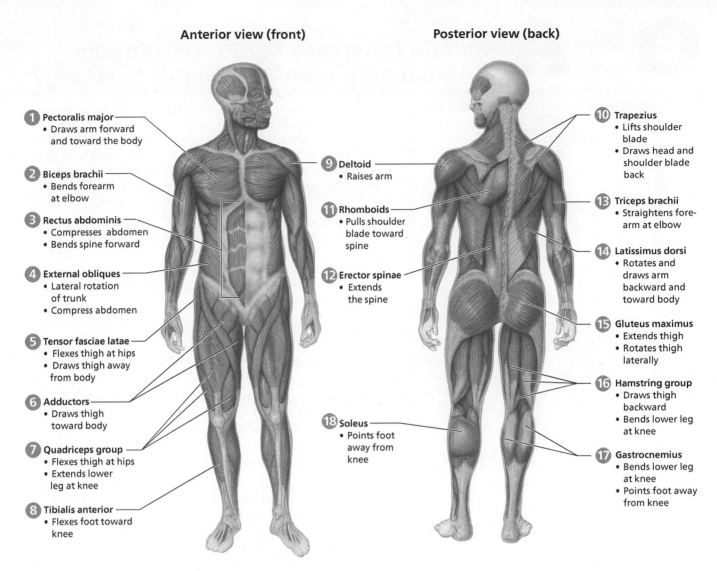

1. **Pectoralis major**
   - Draws arm forward and toward the body
2. **Biceps brachii**
   - Bends forearm at elbow
3. **Rectus abdominis**
   - Compresses abdomen
   - Bends spine forward
4. **External obliques**
   - Lateral rotation of trunk
   - Compress abdomen
5. **Tensor fasciae latae**
   - Flexes thigh at hips
   - Draws thigh away from body
6. **Adductors**
   - Draws thigh toward body
7. **Quadriceps group**
   - Flexes thigh at hips
   - Extends lower leg at knee
8. **Tibialis anterior**
   - Flexes foot toward knee

9. **Deltoid**
   - Raises arm
11. **Rhomboids**
    - Pulls shoulder blade toward spine
12. **Erector spinae**
    - Extends the spine
18. **Soleus**
    - Points foot away from knee

10. **Trapezius**
    - Lifts shoulder blade
    - Draws head and shoulder blade back
13. **Triceps brachii**
    - Straightens fore-arm at elbow
14. **Latissimus dorsi**
    - Rotates and draws arm backward and toward body
15. **Gluteus maximus**
    - Extends thigh
    - Rotates thigh laterally
16. **Hamstring group**
    - Draws thigh backward
    - Bends lower leg at knee
17. **Gastrocnemius**
    - Bends lower leg at knee
    - Points foot away from knee

FIGURE **4.9** These muscles or muscle groups are commonly used in resistance-training exercises. On pages 137–150, Figure 4.10 illustrates exercises you can use to work the muscle groups shown.

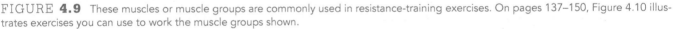

Marketers of oral GH supplements claim the same positive benefits to lean muscle mass and fat mass, but this is not borne out in tests or actual use. Oral GH, in fact, cannot even be absorbed from your digestive tract into your bloodstream! Exercise is a far better way to increase natural levels of GH. In particular, regular aerobic exercise can result in a two-fold increase in 24-hour GH release in young women.[32] Interestingly, one 30-minute session and three 10-minute sessions of exercise are both effective for stimulating GH increases.[33]

Amino Acid and Protein Supplements

Many bodybuilders and weight lifters take amino acid supplements because they believe that consuming protein or its building blocks (amino acids) will enhance muscle development. However, evidence is mixed that high intake of protein or protein-based supplements will improve training or exercise performance or build muscle mass beyond the levels achieved through normal dietary protein. When combined with resistance training, moderate increases in protein intake via supplements can increase lean muscle mass and strength beyond resistance training alone.[34] In contrast, supplementing with the building blocks of protein, amino acids (e.g., glutamine), seems to produce no benefit above and beyond resistance training itself.[35] Taking moderate doses of these supplements has no dramatic side effects, but large doses of either the supplements or protein itself can create amino acid imbalances, alter protein and bone metabolism, and increase risk of cardiovascular disease.[36] See the Q&A box Should I Increase My Protein Intake Immediately after Resistance Training? for more on protein supplements.

See It!
Watch "Sports Drinks Science: Is It Hype?" at MasteringHealth™.

Q&A

Should I Increase My Protein Intake Immediately after Resistance Training?

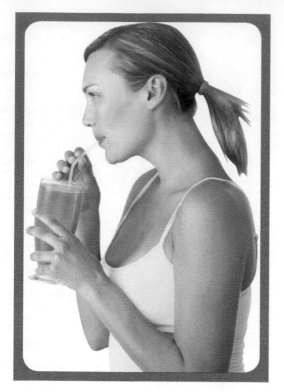

If you want to increase muscle strength and size, then definitely YES! Even if your goals are health and muscle maintenance, a balanced recovery meal or drink is beneficial.

After resistance training, the muscles you worked are depleted of nutrients and are in a state of muscle breakdown from the exercise. Providing nutrients and correcting protein imbalances helps repair breakdown damage and promotes recovery. Eating protein after exercise, particularly essential amino acids, promotes protein synthesis. Protein synthesis is even more pronounced if, in addition to protein, you consume easily digestible carbohydrates.[1] Carbohydrates increase the release of insulin into the blood, which in turn enhances protein storage in cells.

Timing is important. Immediately after resistance training the muscles are receptive to bringing protein into cells. That increased protein helps with repair and recovery and increases the strength and size of the muscle.[2] Increasing

your intake a little bit right *before* exercise can also help.[3] In one study, subjects who took protein supplements immediately before and after resistance training had 86 percent greater increase in lean tissue mass and 30 percent greater overall strength after 10 weeks of resistance training than those who took the same supplements in the morning and night (not close to the exercise session).[4]

How much protein should you take in? Recent evidence found that ingesting 20g of protein every three hours after resistance exercise stimulates protein synthesis better than smaller doses more frequently or larger doses less frequently.[5] Follow these tips for enhancing your post-resistance-training nutrition:

- Consume 100 to 500 calories—depending upon your body size, workout length and intensity, and goals.

- Consume something that is digested rapidly—a liquid source is great!

- Drink or eat something with essential amino acids—whey protein is a great source and you can get this in milk and chocolate milk.

- Make sure your snack is easily digested and has high-glycemic load carbohydrates—again, chocolate milk fills the bill!

- Consume about two parts carbohydrate to one part protein. Healthy fats can also be included.

- For the greatest effect, consume your post-exercise drink or snack within an hour, preferably within 30 minutes, after your exercise session.

- After an hour or later in the day, eat a full recovery meal with a balance of protein, carbohydrates, and healthy fats.

Sources:
1. M. Beelen et al., "Nutritional Strategies to Promote Post-Exercise Recovery," *International Journal of Sports Nutrition and Exercise Metabolism* 20, no. 6 (2010): 515–32.
2. T. A. Churchward-Venne et al., "Role of Protein and Amino Acids in Promoting Lean Mass Accretion with Resistance Exercise and Attenuating Lean Mass Loss during Energy Deficit in Humans," *Amino Acids* 45, no. 2 (2013).
3. C. Kerksick et al., "International Society of Sports Nutrition Position Stand: Nutrient Timing," *Journal of the International Society of Sports Nutrition* 5, no. 17 (2008), doi: 10.1186/1550-2783-5-17
4. P. J. Cribb and A. Hayes, "Effects of Supplement Timing and Resistance Exercise on Skeletal Muscle Hypertrophy," *Medicine & Science in Sports & Exercise* 38, no. 11 (2006): 1918–25.
5. J. L. Areta et al., "Timing and Distribution of Protein Ingestion during Prolonged Recovery from Resistance Exercise Alters Myofibrillar Protein Synthesis," *Journal of Physiology* 591, no. 9 (2013).

FIGURE 4.10 RESISTANCE-TRAINING EXERCISES

Videos for these exercises and more are available online in MasteringHealth.

LOWER-BODY EXERCISES

1 Squat

(a) **Free weight squat** and

(b) **Machine squat:** Place the barbell or pad on your upper back and shoulders. Stand with feet shoulder-width apart, toes pointing forward, hips and shoulders lined up, abdominals pulled in. Looking forward and keeping your chest open, bend your knees and press your hips back. Lower until the angle created between your thigh and calf is between 45 degrees and 90 degrees. Keep your knees behind the front of your toes. To return to the start position, contract your abdominals, press hips forward, and extend your legs until they are straight.

(c) **Ball squat:** Place the ball between your mid-back and a smooth wall. Your feet should be 6 to 12 inches in front of your hips, shoulder-width apart, and toes pointing forward. Contract your abdominals, look forward, and keep your shoulders and hips lined up as you lower your torso. Lower until the angle created between your thigh and calf is about 90 degrees. Your knees should be just above your toes (but not in front of them) or directly above your ankles depending on your starting position, strength, and ankle flexibility. If not, reposition your feet before the next repetition. Return to the starting position by contracting your legs and pushing the ball into and back up the wall.

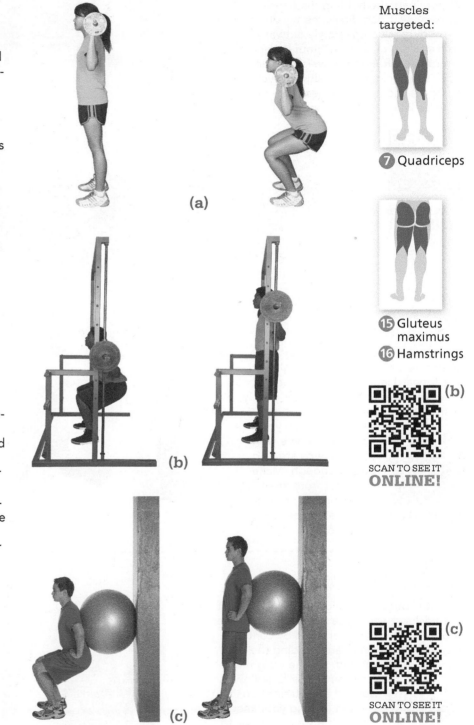

(a)

(b)

(c)

Muscles targeted:

7 Quadriceps

15 Gluteus maximus

16 Hamstrings

(b) SCAN TO SEE IT **ONLINE!**

(c) SCAN TO SEE IT **ONLINE!**

❷ Leg Press

Sit with your back straight or firmly against the backrest. Place your feet on the foot pads so your knees create a 60- to 90-degree angle. Stabilize your torso by contracting your abdominals and holding the hand grips or seat pad. Press the weight by extending your legs slowly outward to a straight position without locking your knees. Return the weight slowly back to your starting position. If your buttocks rise up off the seat pad, you may be lifting too much weight.

SCAN TO SEE IT
ONLINE!

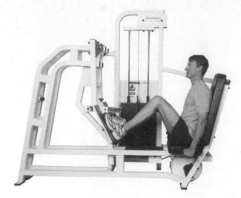

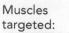

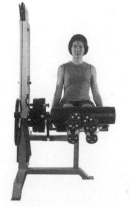

Muscles targeted:

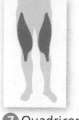

❼ Quadriceps

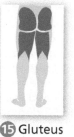

❶❺ Gluteus maximus
❶❻ Hamstrings

❸ Lunge

Stand with feet shoulder-width apart. Step forward and transfer weight to the forward leg. Lower your body straight down with your weight evenly distributed between your front and back legs. Keep your front knee in line with your ankle by striding out far enough. Make sure your front knee does not extend over your toes. Repeat with the other leg.

SCAN TO SEE IT
ONLINE!

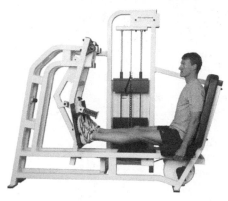

Muscles targeted:

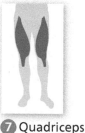

❼ Quadriceps

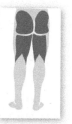

❶❺ Gluteus maximus
❶❻ Hamstrings

❹ Leg Extension

Sit with your back straight or firmly against the backrest and place your legs under the foot pad. Stabilize your torso by contracting your abdominals and holding the handgrips or seat pad. Lift the weight by extending your legs slowly upward to a straight position without locking your knees. Return the weight slowly to the starting position. If your buttocks rise up off the seat pad, you may be lifting too much weight.

SCAN TO SEE IT
ONLINE!

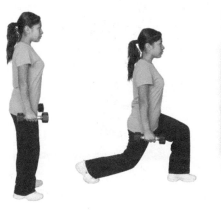

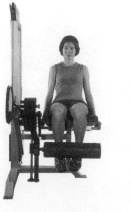

Muscles targeted:

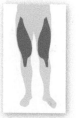

❼ Quadriceps

5 Leg Curl

(a) Machine: Lie on your stomach so your knees are placed at the machine's axis of rotation and the roller pad is just above your heels. Keep your head on the machine pad. Grasping the hand grips for support, lift the weight by contracting your hamstrings and pulling your heels toward your buttocks. Slowly lower the weight back to the start position.

(b) Calisthenics with ball: Lie on your stomach with knees bent and place the ball between your feet. Keep your head on the mat. Lower the ball to the ground and lift it back up by contracting your hamstrings and pulling your heels toward your buttocks.

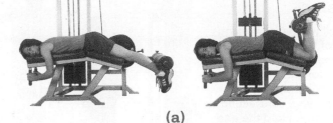

(a)

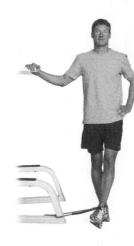 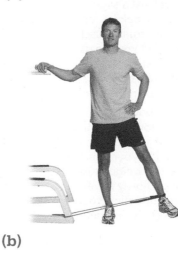

(b)

Muscles targeted:

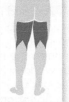

16 Hamstrings

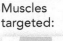

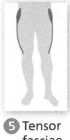 (b)

SCAN TO SEE IT
ONLINE!

6 Hip Abduction

(a) Machine: Sit with your back straight or firmly against the backrest and place your legs against the pads. Grasping the hand grips or seat pad for support, press your legs outward slowly by contracting your outer thighs or hip abductors. Be careful not to extend your legs further than your normal range of motion. Slowly lower the machine weight by bringing your legs back together.

(b) Calisthenics with resistance band: Connect the resistance band to a low point on a machine and attach the free end to your outside leg. Stand with good posture and hold onto a wall or machine for support. Contract your hip abductors and extend your leg out to the side of your body. Slowly release your outside leg back to the starting position beside or crossed slightly in front of your standing leg.

(a)

(b)

Muscles targeted:

5 Tensor fasciae latae

 (b)

SCAN TO SEE IT
ONLINE!

7 Hip Extension

(a) Machine: Stand tall with your working leg extended in front of you and connected to the cable machine. Support yourself by contracting your abdominals and holding on to the machine or handrails. Press your working leg behind you, contracting the gluteals and hamstrings. Hold the end position for one to three seconds before slowly returning to the starting position.

(b) Calisthenics with resistance band: Connect the resistance band to a low point on a machine and attach the free end to your lower leg. Stand with good posture and hold on to a wall or machine for support. Contract your gluteals and hamstrings and extend the working leg behind your body. Slowly release your leg back to the starting position slightly in front of your standing leg.

 **(a)**

SCAN TO SEE IT
ONLINE!

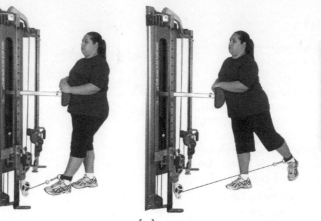

(a)

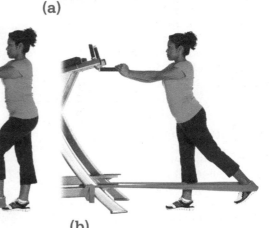

(b)

Muscles targeted:

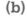

15 Gluteus maximus
16 Hamstrings

---

8 Heel Raise

(a) Straight-leg: Stand tall with good posture and place your heels lower than the toes. (You should feel just a slight stretch in the calf muscle.) Looking forward and contracting your trunk muscles for balance and support, lift your heels up by contracting your gastrocnemius muscle. Be sure to do a full range of motion and slow, controlled repetitions.

(b) Bent-leg: Place your body in the machine with your heels lower than the toes and the weight pad placed comfortably on your thighs. Lift your heels up slightly and release the weight support bar with your hand. Slowly lower and lift the weight by contracting your soleus calf muscle through its full range of motion.

 **(a)**

SCAN TO SEE IT
ONLINE!

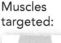

(a)

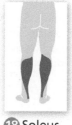

(b)

Muscles targeted:

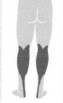

17 Gastrocnemius

18 Soleus

⑨ Hip Adduction

(a) **Machine:** Sit with your back straight or firmly against the backrest and place your legs against the pads set at a comfortable range of motion. Grasping the hand grips or seat pad for support, press your legs together slowly by contracting your inner thighs or hip adductors. Slowly return your legs to the starting position.

(b) **Calisthenics with resistance band:** Connect the resistance band to a low point on a machine and attach the free end to your inside leg. Stand with good posture and hold onto a wall or machine for support. Contract your hip adductors and cross your leg in front of your body to the opposite side of your body. Slowly release your leg back to the starting position beside or slightly to the side of your standing leg.

(c) **Calisthenics with ball:** Lie on your back with a ball pressed between your knees. Press your knees firmly together, squeezing the ball. Hold the squeeze for 3 to 10 seconds and release.

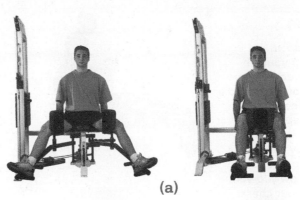

(a)

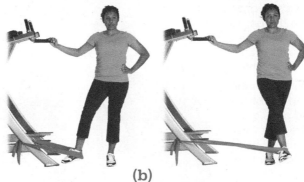

(b)

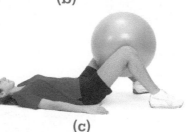

(c)

Muscles targeted:

❻ Adductors

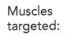 (b)

SCAN TO SEE IT
ONLINE!

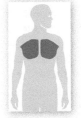 (c)

SCAN TO SEE IT
ONLINE!

UPPER-BODY EXERCISES

⑩ Push-Up

(a) **Full push-ups** and

(b) **Modified push-ups:** Support yourself in push-up position (from the knees or feet) by contracting your trunk muscles so that your neck, back, and hips are completely straight. Place hands slightly wider than shoulder-width apart. Slowly lower your body toward the floor, being careful to keep a straight body position. Your elbows will press out and back as you lower to a 90-degree elbow joint angle. Press yourself back up to the start position. Be careful not to let your trunk sag in the middle or your hips lift up during the exercise. Continually contract your abdominals to keep a strong, straight body position.

(a)

(b)

 (a)   (b)

SCAN TO SEE IT   SCAN TO SEE IT
ONLINE!   **ONLINE!**

Muscles targeted:

❶ Pectoralis major

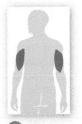

⑬ Triceps brachii

11 Chest Press

(a) Free weight: Lie down on the bench and position yourself with the weight bar directly above your chest. Stabilize your legs and back by placing your feet firmly on the ground and keeping your lower back flat. Grasp the bar with your hands slightly wider than shoulder-width apart and lift the bar off the rack. Slowly lower the bar to just above your chest. Press the weight up to a straight arm position and return the bar to the rack when your set of repetitions is complete. Use a spotter when lifting heavier free weights.

(b) Machine: Place yourself on the chest press machine and adjust the seat height so the hand grips are at chest height. Stabilize your torso by firmly pressing your upper back against the seat back and planting your feet on the ground or foot supports. Press the hand grips away from your body until your arms are straight. Slowly return your hands to the starting position.

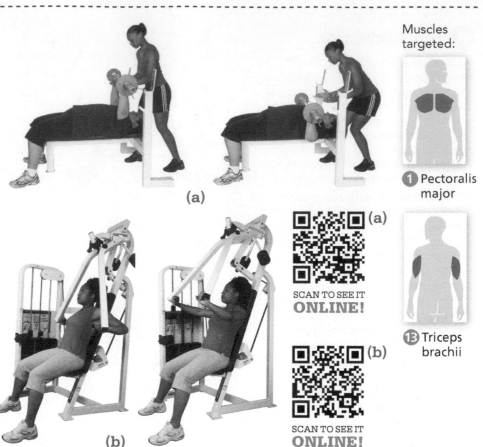

(a)

(b)

(a)

SCAN TO SEE IT
ONLINE!

(b)

SCAN TO SEE IT
ONLINE!

Muscles targeted:

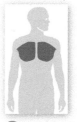

1 Pectoralis major

13 Triceps brachii

---

12 Chest Fly

(a) Machine: Sit with your back straight or firmly against the backrest, plant your feet on the ground or place on the foot pads, and grab the handles or place your arms behind the machine pads. Your arms should be directly to the side but not behind your body. Press your arms together slowly by contracting your chest and shoulder muscles. Slowly return your arms to the starting position.

(b) Bench chest flys: Lie down on the bench and position yourself with the dumbbells directly above your chest. Stabilize your legs and back by placing your feet firmly on the ground and keeping your lower back flat against the bench. Holding the dumbbells with a slight bend in your elbow joints, slowly lower them out to the side until your upper arms are parallel with the floor. Don't extend your arms beyond this position. Return your arms to the starting position by contracting your chest and shoulder muscles.

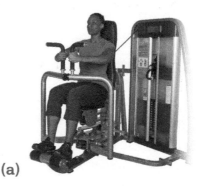

(a)

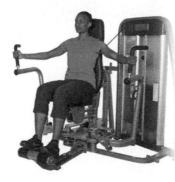

(b)

(a)

SCAN TO SEE IT
ONLINE!

(b)

SCAN TO SEE IT
ONLINE!

Muscles targeted:

1 Pectoralis major

13 Lat Pull-Down

(a) Machine: Position the seat and leg pad on the lat pull-down machine so your thighs are snug under the pad while your feet are flat on the ground. Grab the pull-down bar with a wide overhand grip on your way down to a seated position. Sitting directly under the cable, pull the bar down to your upper chest. Focus on contracting your mid-back first and then your arms by pulling your shoulder blades and elbows back and down. Slowly straighten your arms back to the starting position.

(b) Calisthenics with resistance band: Hold the resistance band above your head with your arms straight up and your hands shoulder-width apart. Pull down and outward with your hands. Focus on contracting the mid-back first and then the arms by pulling the shoulder blades and elbows back and down. End with the band at the top of your chest, hold for one to three seconds, then slowly straighten your arms back to the starting position.

 **(a)**

SCAN TO SEE IT
ONLINE!

 **(b)**

SCAN TO SEE IT
ONLINE!

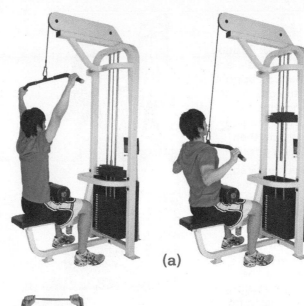

(a)

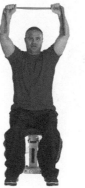

(b)

Muscles targeted:

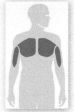

1 Pectoralis major
2 Biceps brachii

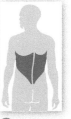

14 Latissimus dorsi

---

14 Assisted Pull-Up

Grab the pull-up bar with a wide overhead grip. Contract your back and arms to pull your body up until the bar is at chin height. Slowly straighten your arms back to the starting position.

SCAN TO SEE IT
ONLINE!

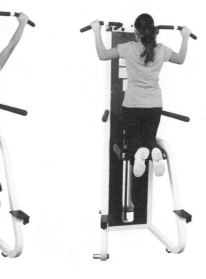

Muscles targeted:

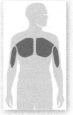

1 Pectoralis major
2 Biceps brachii

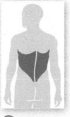

14 Latissimus dorsi

15 Row

(a) Machine compound row: Position the seat height until the handles are at the level of your shoulders. Sit upright and place your feet on the ground or foot pads. Grab the handgrips and pull your elbows back. Hold this position for one to three seconds, then slowly return to the starting position.

(b) Row on cable machine: Grab the cable machine handles, ropes, or bar. Make sure that you are seated so that your arms and shoulders are fully extended forward. Position your feet on foot pedals or firmly on the ground with your heels. Make sure there is a slight bend in your knees. Pull your shoulder blades and elbows back until your hands are just in front of your chest. Hold this position for one to three seconds, then slowly return to the starting position.

(c) Free weight dumbbell: Position your right hand and right knee on bench as shown. Keep your back flat and head in a straight line. Pull dumbbell up to the side of your chest with your left hand, contracting your mid-back and leading with your elbow. Return to starting position and repeat on other side.

(d) Calisthenics with resistance band: Wrap the resistance band low around a weight machine or around your feet in the seated position. Hold the resistance band with your arms straight out and initial tension on the band. Pull back with your hands, focusing on contracting the mid-back first. Pull your shoulder blades and elbows back until your hands are at your lower chest, hold for one to three seconds, then slowly straighten your arms back to the starting position.

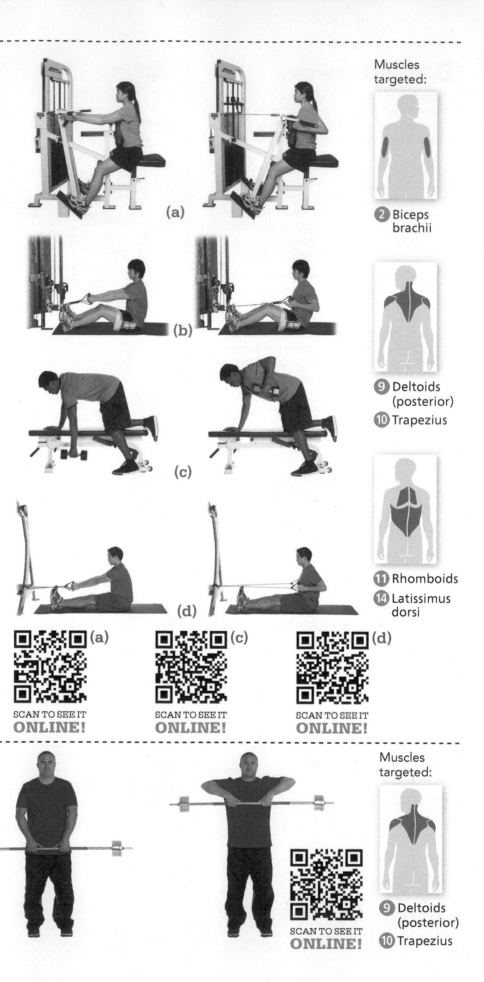

Muscles targeted:

❷ Biceps brachii

❾ Deltoids (posterior)
❿ Trapezius

⓫ Rhomboids
⓮ Latissimus dorsi

(a)

(b)

(c)

(d)

SCAN TO SEE IT **ONLINE!** (a)

SCAN TO SEE IT **ONLINE!** (c)

SCAN TO SEE IT **ONLINE!** (d)

16 Upright Row

Stand with your feet in a shoulder-width position. Keep your hips and shoulders aligned and your abdominals pulled in. Hold a barbell (or dumbbells) down in front of your body with straight arms and your hands positioned shoulder-width apart. Lift the weight to chest height keeping your elbows out, wrists straight, shoulders down. Return slowly to the starting position and repeat.

SCAN TO SEE IT **ONLINE!**

Muscles targeted:

❾ Deltoids (posterior)
❿ Trapezius

17 Overhead Press

(a) **Machine** and

(b) **Free weight dumbbell:** Sit with your back straight or firmly against the backrest, plant your feet firmly on the ground, and pull in your abdominals. Position your hands just wider than shoulder-width and just above the shoulders. Carefully press the weight over your head until your arms are straight but your elbows are not locked out. Slowly return the weight to the starting position and repeat.

 (a)

 (b)

SCAN TO SEE IT **ONLINE!**   SCAN TO SEE IT **ONLINE!**

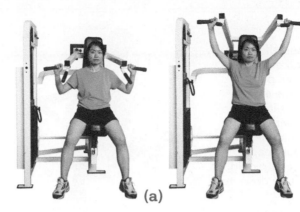

(a)

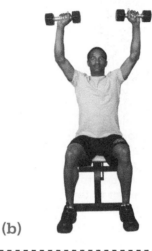

(b)

Muscles targeted:

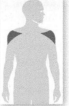

9 Deltoids (anterior and medial)

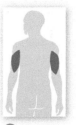

13 Triceps brachii

---

18 Lateral Raise

(a) **Machine:** Position yourself in the machine and sit with a tall, straight back. Contract your shoulders and lift your arms out to the side until they are parallel with the ground. Slowly lower your arms back down to your sides.

(b) **Free weight dumbbell:** Stand with your feet shoulder-width apart. Hold the dumbbells to your sides or slightly in front of you. Lift your arms out to the side until they are parallel with the ground. While lifting, your elbows should be slightly bent to avoid overextending the elbow joint. Keep the weights at the same height as your elbows and keep your shoulders down. Slowly return the dumbbells back down to the starting position.

 (a)

 (b)

SCAN TO SEE IT **ONLINE!**   SCAN TO SEE IT **ONLINE!**

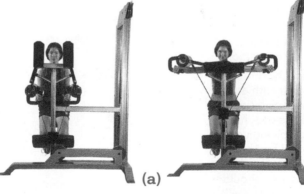

(a)

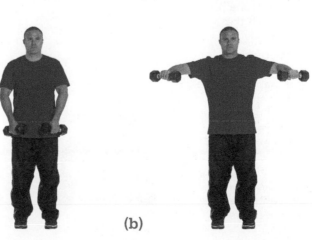

(b)

Muscles targeted:

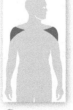

9 Deltoids (anterior and medial)

19 Biceps Curl

(a) Machine: Position yourself in the machine so your feet are on the ground and your elbows are placed at the axis of rotation for the exercise. Grasp the hand grips with an underhand grip and start with your arms straight but not overextended. Lift your hands toward your head until your biceps are fully contracted. Slowly lower the weight back down to the starting position.

(b) Free weight barbell: Stand with your feet either in a stride or a shoulder-width position and your knees slightly bent. Keep your hips and shoulders aligned and your abdominals pulled in. Hold a barbell down in front of your body with an underhand grip, straight arms, and your hands at shoulder-width. Lift the weight up to your shoulders while keeping your back straight and abdominal muscles tight. If you are leaning back to perform the lift, you may be lifting too much weight. Return the weight to the starting position slowly and repeat.

(c) Free weight dumbbell: For one-arm concentration curls, sit on a bench and hold a dumbbell in one hand. Start with your working arm extended toward the ground and your elbow pressed into your inner thigh. Lift the dumbbell up to your shoulder and return slowly to the starting position.

(d) Alternating free weight dumbbell: Sit on a bench or chair with a dumbbell in each hand. Sit with good posture (ears and shoulders over hips and abdominals contracted) and your feet planted on the ground for balance. Lift one dumbbell up to your shoulder turning your palm toward your shoulder as you lift. Slowly lower the dumbbell to the starting position as you lift the dumbbell in your other hand.

(e) Calisthenics with resistance band: Place the center of a resistance band under one foot and grab the free ends of the band with a straight arm on the same side. Stand tall with your feet either in a stride or side-to-side position and your knees soft. Keep your hips and shoulders aligned and your abdominals pulled in. Lift the resisted hand toward your shoulder until your biceps are fully contracted. Slowly lower your hand back to the starting position and repeat.

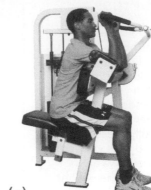
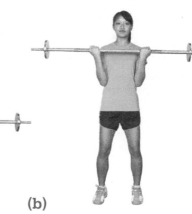

(a)

Muscles targeted:

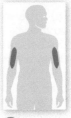

2 Biceps brachii

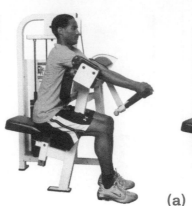

(b)

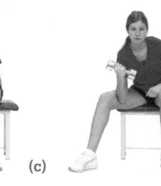

(c)

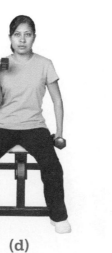

(d)

(e)

(a)

SCAN TO SEE IT
ONLINE!

(e)

SCAN TO SEE IT
ONLINE!

20 Pullover

(a) Free weight barbell: Lie on your back on a flat bench with your feet on the floor. Move the bar to the starting position with your upper arms just above your ears and your elbows slightly bent. Pull the weight back up and over the body without changing your elbow angle. Stop when the weight bar is directly over your chest.

(b) Machine: Adjust the seat so the machine pivots at your shoulder joints. Sit with your elbows against the pads and grasp the bar behind your head. Press forward and down with your arms until the bar is in front of your chest or abdomen. Slowly return to the starting position.

SCAN TO SEE IT **ONLINE!**

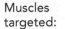

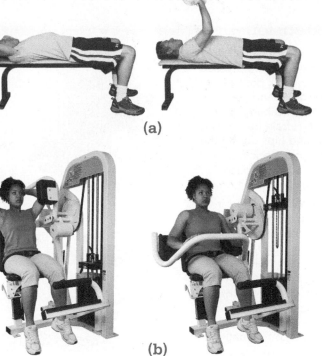

(a)

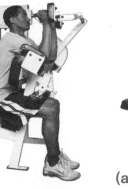 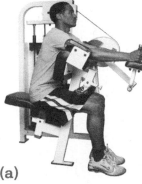

(b)

Muscles targeted:

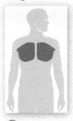

1 Pectoralis major

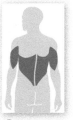

13 Triceps brachii
14 Latissimus dorsi

---

21 Triceps Extension

(a) Machine: Grab the hand grips and start with your arms bent to at least 90 degrees. Press your hands away and down until your elbows are straight but not locked out. Slowly release the weight back to the starting position.

(b) Free weight dumbbell: Start with the weight behind your head and your elbows lifted to the ceiling. Contract the triceps muscles to lift the weight over your head until your arms are straight. Slowly return to the starting position and repeat.

(c) Calisthenics with resistance band: Grasp the middle of a resistance band with one hand and the free ends with the other hand. Place one hand behind you and anchor the band at your hips or low back. Press the hand near your head upward by contracting your triceps muscle and extend your arm until straight. Slowly return the working arm to the starting position and repeat.

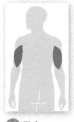

(a)

Muscles targeted:

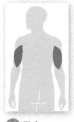

13 Triceps brachii

 (a)
 (b)
 (c)

SCAN TO SEE IT **ONLINE!**   SCAN TO SEE IT **ONLINE!**   SCAN TO SEE IT **ONLINE!**

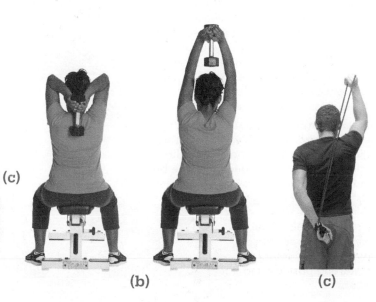

(b)   (c)

TRUNK EXERCISES

22 Back Extension

(a) Machine: Position yourself in the machine so that your hips are pressed all the way back, the back pad is on your mid to upper back, and your back is rounded over. Stabilize with your legs but try to refrain from pushing with your legs and hips during the exercise. Contract your back extensors and straighten out your back until you are in an upright position.

(b) Calisthenics on a mat: Start in a prone position with arms and legs extended and your forehead on the mat. Lift and further extend your arms and legs using your back and hip muscles. If you are free of low-back problems, you can lift a little further up for increased intensity. Hold the position for three to five seconds and then slowly lower to the mat.

(c) Calisthenics on a ball: Lie with your stomach over the ball, anchoring your feet and knees on the ground. Place your hands behind your head or extend your arms out straight for increased exercise intensity. Lift your head, shoulders, arms, and upper back until you have a slight curve in the back. Hold this position for three to five seconds and then lower to the ball.

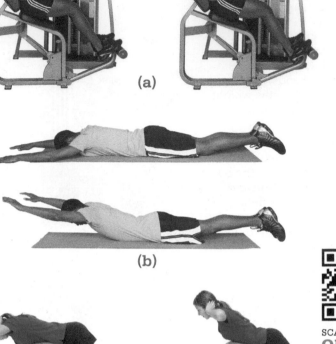

(a)

(b)

(c)

Muscles targeted:

12 Erector spinae

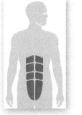

SCAN TO SEE IT **ONLINE!**

(c)

---

23 Abdominal Curl

(a) Machine: Place yourself in the sitting or lying abdominal machine according to the machine instructions. Place your feet on the ground or foot pads and grab the hand grips and/or place your arms or chest behind the machine pads. Contract your abdominals while flexing your upper torso forward. Slowly return to the starting position and repeat.

(b) Calisthenics on a ball: Lie back with the ball placed at your low- to mid-back region. Place your feet shoulder-width apart on the ground so that your knees are bent at about 90 degrees. Cross your hands at your chest or place them lightly behind your head. Contract your abdominals while flexing your upper torso forward. Slowly return to the starting position and repeat.

(a)

(b)

Muscles targeted:

3 Rectus abdominis

SCAN TO SEE IT **ONLINE!**

(a)

SCAN TO SEE IT **ONLINE!**

(b)

24 Reverse Curl

Lie on your back and place your hands near your hips. Lift your legs up so your body creates a 90-degree angle to the floor. Your knees may be bent or straight for this exercise. Contract your abdominals while lifting your hips up off the mat. Slowly return to the starting position and repeat. Be careful not to rock your hips and legs back and forth when doing this exercise; instead, perform a controlled lift of the hips upward.

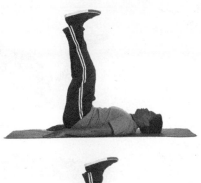

SCAN TO SEE IT
ONLINE!

Muscles targeted:

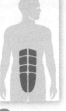

3 Rectus abdominis

---

25 Oblique Curl

Lie on your back with one foot on the mat and knee bent to 90 degrees. Rest the opposite ankle on your bent knee. With one arm providing support on the ground and the other hand behind your head, contract your oblique abdominals and lift your opposite shoulder toward the lifted knee (elbow stays out). Keep your supporting arm and elbow on the floor; do not pull on your head and neck with your hand. Return to the starting position slowly and repeat on the other side.

SCAN TO SEE IT
ONLINE!

Muscles targeted:

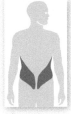

4 External obliques

---

26 Side Bridge

(a) **Modified side bridge** and

(b) **Forearm side bridge** and

(c) **Intermediate side bridge:** Lie on your side with your legs together and straight or bent behind you at 90 degrees. Support your body weight with your forearm or a straight arm. Lift your torso to a straight body position by contracting your abdominal and back muscles. Hold this position for a number of seconds or slowly drop the hip to the mat and lift back up for repeated repetitions.

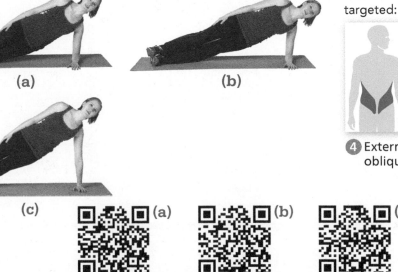

(a)

(b)

(c)

Muscles targeted:

4 External obliques

SCAN TO SEE IT (a)
ONLINE!

SCAN TO SEE IT (b)
ONLINE!

SCAN TO SEE IT (c)
ONLINE!

27 Plank

(a) **Modified plank** and

(b) **Forearm plank** and

(c) **Push-up position plank:** Lie on your stomach and support yourself in plank position (from the forearms or hands) by contracting your trunk muscles so that your neck, back, and hips are completely straight. Your forearms or hands should be under your chest and placed slightly wider than shoulder-width apart. Hold this position for 5 to 60 seconds, increasing duration as you gain muscular endurance.

 (b)

SCAN TO SEE IT
ONLINE!

 (c)

SCAN TO SEE IT
ONLINE!

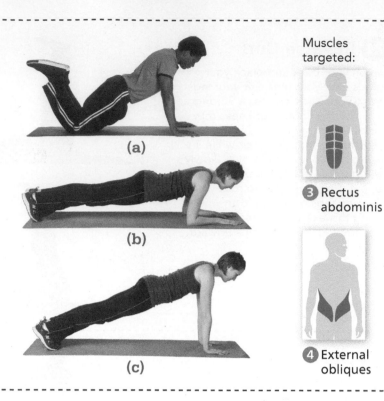

(a)

(b)

(c)

Muscles targeted:

3 Rectus abdominis

4 External obliques

Study Plan

MasteringHealth™

Build your knowledge—and wellness!—
in the Study Area of MasteringHealth
with a variety of study tools.

chapter summary

LO 4.1 What Is Muscular Fitness?

- **Muscular fitness** is the ability of your musculoskeletal system to perform activities without undue fatigue. **Muscular strength** is the ability to contract muscles with maximal force. **Muscular endurance** is the ability to contract muscles repeatedly over an extended period of time.

LO 4.2 How Do My Muscles Work?

- Skeletal muscle contractions pull on the bones via tendons, causing body movements at specific joints.
- Individual muscle cells (**muscle fibers**) are comprised of contractile protein filaments (actin and myosin) that exist in repeating units called **sarcomeres**.
- Muscle fibers are **slow-twitch** or **fast-twitch**.
- Muscle contractions increase force in the muscle and either move body parts (isotonic and isokinetic) or not (isometric).

LO 4.3 How Can Regular Resistance Training Improve My Fitness and Wellness?

- Regular resistance training increases muscular strength (neural adaptations and hypertrophy), muscular endurance, lean muscle tissue, and overall physical function. You might also reduce adipose tissue, lower disease risk, strengthen bones and joints, and improve sports and recreation performance.

LO 4.4 How Can I Assess My Muscular Strength and Endurance?

- Test your muscular strength via 1 repetition maximum (RM), estimated 1 RM, or grip strength assessments.
- Test your muscular endurance via 20 RM or calisthenic (body weight) assessments.

LO 4.5 How Can I Design My Own Resistance-Training Program?

- Set appearance-based, function-based, or combination SMART goals for muscular fitness.
- Apply the resistance training FITT formula to your selected exercises to reach your goals.

LO 4.6 What Precautions Should I Take to Avoid Resistance-Training Injuries?

- Follow weight-training guidelines to avoid injuries.
- Obtain medical clearance and professional guidance if you have limitations.

LO 4.7 Is It Risky to Use Supplements or Change My Diet for Muscular Fitness?

- Anabolic steroids are illegal without a prescription and have overwhelming side effects. Creatine monohydrate is legal and improves performance by temporarily increasing stored creatine phosphate. DHEA and androstenedione have significant side effects and are now banned in athletic competitions. Growth hormone supplementation may counteract muscle losses; however, oral forms are ineffective and side effects can be risky.

review questions

LO 4.1 1. Muscular strength is the ability to
   a. contract your muscles repeatedly over time.
   b. run a six-minute mile.
   c. look "toned" in a swimsuit.
   d. contract your muscle with maximal force.

LO 4.2 2. What is a single muscle cell called?
   a. Muscle fiber
   b. Muscle fascia
   c. Fascicle
   d. Contractile bundle

LO 4.2 3. Which of the following will result in a stronger muscle contraction?
   a. Eating more protein before your workout
   b. Activating slow, smaller motor units
   c. Taking DHEA before your workout
   d. Activating more motor units overall

LO 4.2 4. Sitting down in a chair and standing up again is an example of which type of exercise?
   a. Isotonic
   b. Isokinetic

c. Isometric

d. Isostatic

LO 4.3 **5.** Muscle strength improvements in the first few weeks of a program are due to

a. increased size of muscle fibers.

b. increased activation and coordination of motor units.

c. increased ability of muscles to move through a full range of motion.

d. increased blood flow to working muscles.

LO 4.3 **6.** Which of the following benefits of resistance training will reduce your risk of cardiovascular diseases?

a. Increased bone density

b. Increased muscle power

c. Reduced body fat levels

d. Better sports recovery

LO 4.4 **7.** A test of muscular endurance includes

a. a 1 RM test.

b. a grip-strength test.

c. a 20 RM test.

d. a sit-and-reach test.

LO 4.5 **8.** One disadvantage of using machines for resistance-training exercises is

a. it takes time to adjust the machine for your height and desired resistance level.

b. the machine does not promote the use of postural and stabilizing muscles during the exercise.

c. spotters are needed.

d. it can be hard to isolate specific muscle groups.

LO 4.6 **9.** Which of the following is part of the criteria you should use when selecting a personal trainer?

a. Certified by ACSM, NSCA, NASM, or ACE

b. Looks like someone who works out a lot

c. Recommended by a friend who was sore after a workout with the trainer

d. Able to provide dietary supplements at a reduced cost

LO 4.7 **10.** Which of the following supplements/drugs promotes irreversible bone growth, cardiovascular disease, diabetes, and decreased sexual desire?

a. Anabolic steroids

b. Creatine

c. Growth hormone

d. Androstenedione

critical thinking questions

LO 4.1 **1.** What is resistance training and how does it improve muscular strength and endurance?

LO 4.2 **2.** What is the predominant fiber type in the postural trunk muscles and why does this make sense?

LO 4.3 **3.** Discuss the role of resistance training in preventing injuries.

LO 4.3 **4.** Define sarcopenia and discuss how it can be reversed through exercise. How are sarcopenia and atrophy different?

LO 4.7 **5.** In your opinion, do any of the supplements discussed have benefits that outweigh the risks or side effects? Explain your answer.

check out these eResources

- **Active.com** Online resource with articles and advice about fitness, health, sports, and training. **www.active.com**
- **Consumer Lab** Information about supplement use, research, and reviews. **www.consumerlab.com**
- **FitStar Personal Trainer** Your own personal trainer: This interactive app asks you questions and customizes minimal equipment workouts for you (free basic or premium versions). **www.fitstar.com/personal-trainer**

- **National Strength and Conditioning Association (NSCA)** Website featuring articles, research, education, and hot topics in strength training. **www.nsca.com**
- **Sworkit** Simply-WORKIT, a free app for your smartphone or device with pre-designed or customizable body weight workouts. **www.sworkit.com**

DO IT!
LAB
4.1

ASSESS YOURSELF
ASSESSING YOUR MUSCULAR STRENGTH

MasteringHealth™

Name: _____ **Date:** _____

Instructor: _____ **Section:** _____

Materials: Calculator, leg press machine, chest press machine

Purpose: To assess your current level of muscular strength.

Note: Perform this lab with an instructor present to ensure proper form and safety.

SCAN TO SEE IT
ONLINE!

Section I: Muscular Strength Assessment
One Repetition Maximum (1 RM) Prediction Assessment

ACSM recommends measuring muscular strength by performing one repetition maximum (1 RM) or multiple RM assessments. Estimate your 1 RM for the chest press and leg press by finding the amount of weight you can maximally lift 2 to 10 times.

1. **Warm up.** Complete 3 to 10 minutes of light cardiorespiratory activity to warm the muscles. Perform range-of-motion exercises and light stretches for the joints and muscles that you will be using.

2. **Use proper form while executing the chest press and leg press exercises.** For the chest press, position yourself so the bar or handles are across the middle of your chest. Spread your hands slightly wider than shoulder-width. Bring the handles/bar to just above your chest and then press upward/outward until your arms are straight. For the leg press, position yourself so that your knees are at a 90-degree angle. Press the weight away from your body until your legs are straight.

3. **Perform one light warm-up set.** Set the machine at a very light weight and lift this weight about 10 times as a warm-up.

4. **Find the appropriate strength-assessment weight and number of repetitions.** Set a weight that you think you can lift at least 2 times but no more than 10 times. Perform the lift as many times as you can (to complete fatigue) up to 10 repetitions. If you can lift more than 10 repetitions, try again using heavier weight. Repeat until you find a weight you cannot lift more than 2 to 10 times. In order to prevent muscle fatigue from affecting your results, attempt this assessment no more than three times to find the proper weight and number of repetitions. If you experience muscle fatigue, rest and perform the test again on another day. Record your weight lifted and repetitions in the Muscular Strength Results section.

5. **Find your predicted 1 RM.** Predict your 1 RM based upon the number of repetitions you performed. If the weight you lifted was between 20 and 250 pounds, use the 1 RM Prediction Table on the next page to find your predicted 1 RM. If you lifted more than 250 pounds, use the Multiplication Factor Table on page 155 to find your predicted 1 RM. Record your predicted 1 RM in the Muscular Strength Results section.

6. **Find your strength-to-body weight ratio.** Divide your predicted 1 RM by your body weight for your strength-to-body-weight ratio (S/BW). Since heavier people often have more muscle, this is a better indicator of muscular strength than just the weight lifted alone. Record your S/BW in the Muscular Strength Results section.

7. **Find your muscle strength rating by using the Strength-to-Body Weight Ratio chart provided on the last page of this lab.** Finding your rating tells you how you compare to others who have completed this test in the past. Record your rating in the Muscular Strength Results section.

Muscular Strength Results

Chest Press: Weight lifted _____ Repetitions _____

_____ × _____ = _____
Weight lifted (lb)   Multiplication factor*   Predicted 1 RM (lb)

_____ ÷ _____ = _____
Predicted 1 RM (lb)   Body weight (lb)   S/BW ratio

Rating _____

Leg Press: Weight lifted _____ Repetitions _____

_____ × _____ = _____
Weight lifted (lb)   Multiplication factor*   Predicted 1 RM (lb)

_____ ÷ _____ = _____
Predicted 1 RM (lb)   Body weight (lb)   S/BW ratio

Rating _____

*Multiplication factor from the Multiplication Factor Table on page 155.

Section II: Reflection

1. Were your muscular strength results what you expected? Why or why not?

_____

_____

2. Based upon your strength assessment results, what is your basic plan to maintain or improve?

_____

_____

1 RM Prediction Table

Repetitions										
Wt (lb)	1	2	3	4	5	6	7	8	9	10
20	20	21	21	22	23	23	24	25	26	27
25	25	26	26	27	28	29	30	31	32	33
30	30	31	32	33	34	35	36	37	39	40
35	35	36	37	38	39	41	42	43	45	47
40	40	41	42	44	45	46	48	50	51	53
45	45	46	48	49	51	52	54	56	58	60
50	50	51	53	55	56	58	60	62	64	67
55	55	57	58	60	62	64	66	68	71	73
60	60	62	64	65	68	70	72	74	77	80
65	65	67	69	71	73	75	78	81	84	87
70	70	72	74	76	79	81	84	87	90	93
75	75	77	79	82	84	87	90	93	96	100

(Continued)

1 RM Prediction Table (Continued)

Wt (lb)	\multicolumn{10}{c}{Repetitions}									
	1	2	3	4	5	6	7	8	9	10
80	80	82	85	87	90	93	96	99	103	107
85	85	87	90	93	96	99	102	106	109	113
90	90	93	95	98	101	105	108	112	116	120
95	95	98	101	104	107	110	114	118	122	127
100	100	103	106	109	113	116	120	124	129	133
105	105	108	111	115	118	122	126	130	135	140
110	110	113	116	120	124	128	132	137	141	147
115	115	118	122	125	129	134	138	143	148	153
120	120	123	127	131	135	139	144	149	154	160
125	125	129	132	136	141	145	150	155	161	167
130	130	134	138	142	146	151	156	161	167	173
135	135	139	143	147	152	157	162	168	174	180
140	140	144	148	153	158	163	168	174	180	187
145	145	149	154	158	163	168	174	180	186	193
150	150	154	159	164	169	174	180	186	193	200
155	155	159	164	169	174	180	186	192	199	207
160	160	165	169	175	180	186	192	199	206	213
165	165	170	175	180	186	192	198	205	212	220
170	170	175	180	185	191	197	204	211	219	227
175	175	180	185	191	197	203	210	217	225	233
180	180	185	191	196	203	209	216	223	231	240
185	185	190	196	202	208	215	222	230	238	247
190	190	195	201	207	214	221	228	236	244	253
195	195	201	206	213	219	226	234	242	251	260
200	200	206	212	218	225	232	240	248	257	267
205	205	211	217	224	231	238	246	255	264	273
210	210	216	222	229	236	244	252	261	270	280
215	215	221	228	235	242	250	258	267	276	287
220	220	226	233	240	248	256	264	273	283	293
225	225	231	238	245	253	261	270	279	289	300
230	230	237	244	251	259	267	276	286	296	307
235	235	242	249	256	264	273	282	292	302	313
240	240	247	254	262	270	279	288	298	309	320
245	245	252	259	267	276	285	294	304	315	327
250	250	257	265	273	281	290	300	310	322	333

Multiplication Factor Table for Predicting 1 RM

Repetitions	1	2	3	4	5	6	7	8	9	10
Multiplication Factor	1.0	1.07	1.11	1.13	1.16	1.20	1.23	1.27	1.32	1.36

Table and multiplication factors generated using the Brzycki equation:

1 RM = weight (kg)/[1.0278−(0.0278 × repetitions)].

Source: Equation from M. Brzycki, "Strength Testing: Predicting a One-Rep Max from a Reps-to-Fatigue," *Journal of Physical Education, Recreation, and Dance* 64, no. 1 (1993): 88–90.

Strength-to-Body Weight Ratio Ratings

Chest Press						
Men	**Superior**	**Excellent**	**Good**	**Fair**	**Poor**	**Very Poor**
<20 yrs	1.75	1.34–1.75	1.19–1.33	1.06–1.18	0.89–1.05	0.89
20–29 yrs	1.62	1.32–1.62	1.14–1.31	0.99–1.13	0.88–0.98	0.88
30–39 yrs	1.34	1.12–1.34	0.98–1.11	0.88–0.97	0.78–0.87	0.78
40–49 yrs	1.19	1.00–1.19	0.88–0.99	0.80–0.87	0.72–0.79	0.72
50–59 yrs	1.04	0.90–1.04	0.79–0.89	0.71–0.78	0.63–0.70	0.63
>60 yrs	0.93	0.82–0.93	0.72–0.81	0.66–0.71	0.57–0.65	0.57
Women	**Superior**	**Excellent**	**Good**	**Fair**	**Poor**	**Very Poor**
<20 yrs	0.87	0.77–0.87	0.65–0.76	0.58–0.64	0.53–0.57	0.53
20–29 yrs	1.00	0.80–1.00	0.70–0.79	0.59–0.69	0.51–0.58	0.51
30–39 yrs	0.81	0.70–0.81	0.60–0.69	0.53–0.59	0.47–0.52	0.47
40–49 yrs	0.76	0.62–0.76	0.54–0.61	0.50–0.53	0.43–0.49	0.43
50–59 yrs	0.67	0.55–0.67	0.48–0.54	0.44–0.47	0.39–0.43	0.39
>60 yrs	0.71	0.54–0.71	0.47–0.53	0.43–0.46	0.38–0.42	0.38
Leg Press						
Men	**Superior**	**Excellent**	**Good**	**Fair**	**Poor**	**Very Poor**
<20 yrs	2.81	2.28–2.81	2.04–2.27	1.90–2.03	1.70–1.89	1.70
20–29 yrs	2.39	2.13–2.39	1.97–2.12	1.83–1.96	1.63–1.82	1.63
30–39 yrs	2.19	1.93–2.19	1.77–1.92	1.65–1.76	1.52–1.64	1.52
40–49 yrs	2.01	1.82–2.01	1.68–1.81	1.57–1.67	1.44–1.56	1.44
50–59 yrs	1.89	1.71–1.89	1.58–1.70	1.46–1.57	1.32–1.45	1.32
>60 yrs	1.79	1.62–1.79	1.49–1.61	1.38–1.48	1.25–1.37	1.25
Women	**Superior**	**Excellent**	**Good**	**Fair**	**Poor**	**Very Poor**
<20 yrs	1.87	1.71–1.87	1.59–1.70	1.38–1.58	1.22–1.37	1.22
20–29 yrs	1.97	1.68–1.97	1.50–1.67	1.37–1.49	1.22–1.36	1.22
30–39 yrs	1.67	1.47–1.67	1.33–1.46	1.21–1.32	1.09–1.20	1.09
40–49 yrs	1.56	1.37–1.56	1.23–1.36	1.13–1.22	1.02–1.12	1.02
50–59 yrs	1.42	1.25–1.42	1.10–1.24	0.99–1.09	0.88–0.98	0.88
>60 yrs	1.42	1.18–1.42	1.04–1.17	0.93–1.03	0.85–0.92	0.85

Source: Reprinted with permission from The Cooper Institute, Dallas, Texas from *Physical Fitness Assessments and Norms for Adults and Law Enforcement*, available online at www.cooperinstitute.org

ASSESSING YOUR MUSCULAR ENDURANCE

MasteringHealth™

Name: _____ Date: _____

Instructor: _____ Section: _____

Materials: Leg press machine, bench press machine, exercise mat, yardstick or ruler, tape, and metronome (or online metronome/app).

Purpose: To assess your current level of muscular endurance.

Note: Perform this lab with an instructor present to ensure proper form and safety.

Section I: Muscular Endurance Weight-Lifting Assessment
Twenty Repetition Maximum (20 RM) Assessment

The 20 RM assessment is a weight-lifting assessment of your muscular endurance. Perform the assessments before and after completing 8 to 12 weeks of muscular fitness exercises to measure your improvement.

1. Prepare for the muscle endurance assessments. If you have just completed the muscular strength assessments in Lab 4.1, you will already be warmed up. If not, follow the position, form, and warm-up instructions for bench press and leg press in Lab 4.1. Rest longer if you feel overly fatigued from your strength assessment.

2. Find your 20 RM for chest press and leg press. Set a weight that you think you can lift a maximum of 20 times. Perform the lift to see whether you were correct. If not, increase or decrease the weight and try again until you find your 20 RM. In order to be sure that muscle fatigue does not affect your results, try to find your 20 RM within three tries. If it takes longer, rest and perform the test again on another day. Record your results below.

Muscular Endurance Weight-Lifting Results

Chest Press: 20 RM weight lifted _____

Leg Press: 20 RM weight lifted _____

Section II: Muscular Endurance Calisthenic Assessment
Push-Up Assessment

SCAN TO SEE IT
ONLINE!

For this muscular endurance assessment, perform as many push-ups as you can. This test will assess the muscular endurance of your pectoralis major, anterior deltoid, and triceps brachii muscles. A partner is helpful to check your form and count your repetitions.

1. Get into the correct push-up position on an exercise mat. Support the body in a push-up position from the knees (women) or from the toes (men). The hands should be just outside the shoulders and the back and legs straight.

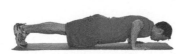
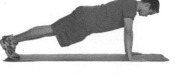

2. Start in the "down" position with your elbow joint at a 90-degree angle, your chest just above the floor, and your chin barely touching the mat. Push your body up until your arms are straight and then lower back to the starting position (count one repetition). Complete the push-ups in a slow and controlled manner.

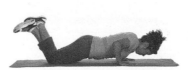
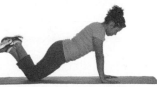

3. Complete as many correct-technique push-ups as you can without stopping. Record your results in the Muscular Endurance Calisthenic Results section below.

4. Find your muscle endurance rating for push-ups in the chart at the end of this lab and record your results.

Curl-Up Assessment

For this muscular endurance assessment, perform as many curl-ups as you can (up to 75). This test will assess the muscular endurance of your abdominal muscles.

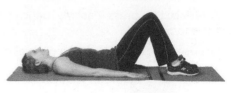

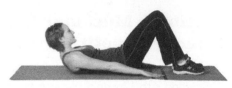

1. Lie on a mat with your arms by your sides, palms flat on the mat, elbows straight, and fingers extended. Bend your knees at a 90-degree angle. Have your partner mark your starting finger position for each hand with a piece of tape. Similarly, mark the ending position for each hand either 12 cm (under 45 years) or 8 cm (45 years or older) away from the first piece of tape. Your goal is to rise far enough on the curl-up to elevate your trunk by 30 degrees. Alternate methods include placing your hands across your chest and having your partner assess your 30-degree trunk elevation with each repetition or moving your hands from your thighs to the tops of your knees with each repetition.

2. Set a metronome to 40 beats/min and complete the curl-ups at this slow, controlled pace.

3. Curl your head and upper back upward, reaching your arms forward along the mat to touch the ending tape. Then curl back down so that your upper back and shoulders touch the floor. During the entire curl-up, your fingers, feet, and buttocks should stay on the mat. Your partner will count the number of correct repetitions you complete. Any curl-ups performed without touching the ending position tape should not be counted.

4. Perform as many curl-ups as you can without breaking cadence or pausing, to a maximum of 75. Record your score below. Determine your muscular endurance rating for curl-ups using the chart below and record your results.

**Alternative: One-minute timed curl-ups. Your instructor may choose to have you complete as many curl-ups as you can within one minute (without the metronome pacing). Using the same start and end positions, perform controlled repetitions of curl-ups for one minute and record your results below.

Muscular Endurance Calisthenic Results

Push-Ups: Repetitions_____   Rating_____

Curl-Ups: Repetitions_____   Rating_____

**Alternative: One-minute timed curl-ups: Repetitions _____

Section III: Reflection

1. What was surprising about your muscular endurance results, if anything?

_____

_____

2. How can you use your muscle endurance results to design your muscle fitness program?

_____

_____

Muscular Endurance Rating

Push-ups						
Men	**Superior**	**Excellent**	**Good**	**Fair**	**Poor**	**Very Poor**
20–29 yrs	>36	31–36	24–30	21–23	16–20	<16
30–39 yrs	>30	24–30	19–23	16–18	11–15	<11
40–49 yrs	>25	19–25	15–18	12–14	9–11	<9
50–59 yrs	>21	15–21	12–14	9–11	6–8	<6
60–69 yrs	>18	13–18	10–12	7–9	4–6	<4
Women	**Superior**	**Excellent**	**Good**	**Fair**	**Poor**	**Very Poor**
20–29 yrs	>30	22–30	16–21	14–15	9–13	<9
30–39 yrs	>27	21–27	14–20	12–14	7–11	<7
40–49 yrs	>24	16–24	12–15	10–11	4–9	<4
50–59 yrs	>21	12–21	8–11	6–8	1–5	<1
60–69 yrs	>17	13–17	6–12	4–6	1–3	<1
Curl-ups						
Men	**Superior**	**Excellent**	**Good**	**Fair**	**Poor**	**Very Poor**
20–29 yrs	≥75	56–74	31–55	24–30	13–23	<13
30–39 yrs	≥75	69–74	36–68	26–35	13–25	<13
40–49 yrs	≥75	67–74	51–66	31–50	21–30	<21
50–59 yrs	≥74	60–73	35–59	23–34	13–20	<13
60–69 yrs	≥53	33–52	19–32	9–18	1–8	<1
Women	**Superior**	**Excellent**	**Good**	**Fair**	**Poor**	**Very Poor**
20–29 yrs	≥70	45–69	32–44	21–31	12–20	<12
30–39 yrs	≥55	43–54	28–42	15–27	1–14	<1
40–49 yrs	≥55	42–54	28–41	20–27	5–19	<5
50–59 yrs	≥48	30–47	16–29	3–15	1–2	<1
60–69 yrs	≥50	30–49	19–29	9–18	1–8	<1

Source: Canadian Physical Activity, Fitness & Lifestyle Approach: CSEP—Health & Fitness Program's Appraisal and Counselling Strategy, 3rd edition, ©2003. Reprinted with permission from the Canadian Society for Exercise Physiology.

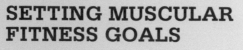
Name: _____ **Date:** _____

Instructor: _____ **Section:** _____

Purpose: To learn how to set appropriate muscular fitness goals (short- and long-term).

Section I: Short- and Long-Term Goals

Use the SMART (*Specific, Measurable, Action-Oriented, Realistic, Timed*) goal-setting guidelines to create short- and long-term goals for muscular strength and muscular endurance. Apply information discussed in the chapter and use your results from Labs 4.1 and 4.2. Remember that aiming to improve your assessment scores is a measurable way to set goals. Select appropriate target dates and rewards for completing your goals.

Short-Term Goals (3 to 6 months)

1. **Muscular Strength Goal:**

_____

Target Date: _____

Reward:

_____

2. **Muscular Endurance Goal:**

_____

Target Date: _____

Reward:

_____

Long-Term Goals (12+ months)

1. **Muscular Strength Goal:**

_____

Target Date: _____

Reward:

_____

2. **Muscular Endurance Goal:**

_____

Target Date: _____

Reward:

_____

Section II: Muscular Fitness Obstacles and Strategies

What barriers or obstacles might hinder your plan to improve your muscular fitness? Indicate your top three obstacles below and list strategies for overcoming each obstacle.

a. _____

b. _____

c. _____

Section III: Getting Support

1. List resources you will use to help change your muscular fitness:

Friend/partner/relative: _____   School-based resource: _____

Community-based resource: _____   Other: _____

Section IV: Reflection

1. How realistic are the short- and long-term target dates you have set for achieving your muscular fitness goals?

_____

_____

_____

_____

2. Are there any other strategies not listed above that could help you reach your goals?

_____

_____

_____

_____

3. Think about all of the opportunities that present themselves in your daily life to work toward muscular fitness. List as many of these as you can think of:

_____

_____

_____

_____

DO IT!

LAB
4.4

PLAN FOR CHANGE

YOUR RESISTANCE-TRAINING
WORKOUT PLAN

MasteringHealth™

Name: _____ Date: _____

Instructor: _____ Section: _____

Purpose: To create a basic, personal resistance-training workout plan. This lab includes forms for following up and tracking your muscular fitness program.

Directions: Complete the following sections.

Section I: Muscular Fitness Program Questions and Motivations

1. How many days per week are you planning to work on your muscular fitness program? _____

2. How experienced are you at resistance training? (select one below)

Novice　　　　　　　**Intermediate (training 1 to 2 years)**　　　　　　　**Advanced (training 3+ years)**

3. Which will you focus on first? (select one)　　　**Muscular strength**　　　**Muscular endurance**

4. The best muscular fitness programs work the entire body, but often people want to focus on some areas more than others. Which muscle groups do you want to focus on?

_____

5. Which type of equipment do you plan to use and why? (check all that apply)

☐ **Weight machines**

☐ **Free weights**

☐ **Body weight (calisthenic exercises)**

6. How much time do you plan for your resistance-training program on each workout day?

_____ Does this time estimate include your warm-up and cool-down? _____

7. Do you have a workout partner? Do you plan to work with a partner, trainer, or instructor to help you get started?

_____

*See **Program 4.1** on page 165 for a sample resistance-training program that will match your preferences and goals outlined above.

Section II: Resistance-Training Program Design

In the table on the following page, plan your resistance-training program using resources available to you (facility, instructor, text). If your muscular fitness rated as fair or below and/or you are new to resistance training, start with the Beginner Resistance-Training Program on page 166. If your muscular fitness rated as good or above and you have some resistance-training experience, start with the Intermediate Resistance-Training Program on page 166. If you have specific muscular endurance or muscular strength/mass goals and you have some resistance-training experience, start with the program on page 167 that best matches your goal. Complete one line for each exercise you have chosen to do in your program.

Exercise	Muscle(s) Worked	Frequency (days/week)	Intensity (weight in lb)	Sets (number)	Reps (number per set)	Rest (time between sets)
LOWER BODY						
1.						
2.						
3.						
4.						
5.						
6.						
7.						
8.						
UPPER BODY						
1.						
2.						
3.						
4.						
5.						
6.						
7.						
8.						
9.						
10.						
11.						
12.						
TRUNK						
1.						
2.						
3.						
4.						
5.						

Section III: Tracking your Program and Following Through

1. **Goal and program tracking:** Use a resistance-training chart (see next page) to monitor your progress. Change the amount of resistance, sets, or repetitions to ensure continuing progress toward your goals.

2. **Goal and program follow-up:** At the end of the course or at your short-term goal target date, reevaluate your muscular fitness and answer the following questions:

   a. Did you meet your short-term goal or your goal for the course? _____

   b. If so, what positive behavioral changes contributed to your success? If not, which obstacles blocked your success?

   _____

   _____

   c. Was your short-term goal realistic? After evaluating your progress during the course, what would you change about your goals or resistance-training plan?

   _____

   _____

DATE																					
EXERCISE	Wt.	Sets	Reps	Wt.	Sets	Reps	Wt.	Sets	Reps	Wt.	Sets	Reps	Wt.	Sets	Reps	Wt.	Sets	Reps	Wt.	Sets	Reps
1.																					
2.																					
3.																					
4.																					
5.																					
6.																					
7.																					
8.																					
9.																					
10.																					
11.																					
12.																					
13.																					
14.																					

Activate, Motivate, & Advance YOUR FITNESS

ACTIVATE!

With the long list of health, wellness, and fitness benefits associated with resistance training, there is no doubt you want to get started now! Don't make the common mistake of trying to do too much, too soon. Follow these programs to gradually increase your number of exercises, the weight/sets/repetitions, and the number of times you train each week.

What Do I Need for Resistance Training?

CLOTHING/SHOES: Wear comfortable, supportive clothing that allows for full range-of-motion movements. Weight-lifting gloves can increase your grip strength and prevent blisters and calluses. A pair of shoes with good traction and a non-slip sole will give you a stable base when you lift.

How Do I Start a Resistance-Training Program?

TECHNIQUE: Read through each exercise description carefully and learn the proper technique. If you need an exercise demonstration or assistance with a weight machine, ask your instructor or the fitness specialist at your facility. Perform each exercise in a slow and controlled manner through the full range of motion, taking care to avoid "locking out" your joints. If you are unable to maintain good form, decrease the weight or repetitions. Keep the weight balanced and use collars on weight bars to keep weights stable and secure. Exhale during the exertion phase (when the exercise is hardest). Finally, when lifting heavier free weights, it is always advisable to have a spotter. This is especially important for maximal efforts and for exercises that require the weight to pass over your head, face, or chest.

ETIQUETTE: Most facilities will have posted regulations for all patrons. Place weights, collars, and other equipment back on the rack when you finish using them. Wipe down machines, equipment, and benches after use. Most gyms supply wipes or spray bottles and paper towels—don't use your personal sweat towel. When you are resting between sets, let others use the machines or weights.

Resistance-Training Tips

AT THE GYM: Resistance training at a gym gives you access to a wide variety of equipment and free weights. Using essentials (machines and free weights) and the extras (balls, bands, etc.) provides variety, reduces boredom, and increases adherence.

AT HOME: There are dozens of exercises that use your body weight against gravity. Plus, you can always add a few pieces of equipment to your home gym as you progress. Items you might consider include bands or tubing, a stability ball, medicine balls, suspension training systems, kettlebells, and so on. For example, stability balls can help you improve core stability, static and dynamic balance, and functional performance.

Resistance-Training Warm-Up and Cool-Down

A resistance-training warm-up should include light cardiorespiratory exercises for 5 to 10 minutes before

adding dynamic movements of the muscles you'll be using. Then, complete a few repetitions with little or no weight to ensure proper form, posture, and body alignment. After resistance training, perform static stretches for muscles targeted in the workout.

Resistance-Training Programs

Adjust intensity, sets/reps, and training days to suit your personal fitness level and schedule.

BEGINNER RESISTANCE-TRAINING PROGRAM

Start here if you are new to resistance training or if you have taken a break of more than three months. This program will help you increase overall muscular fitness (both muscular endurance and strength) and help keep you injury free!

GOAL: Improve overall muscular fitness by performing eight exercises twice a week.

| Frequency | Intensity | Time | | | Number and Type of Exercises |
		Reps	Sets	Rest	
2 non-consecutive days a week	60% 1 RM	12	2	2 minutes between sets	8 multiple-joint exercises

Order of Exercises:
Leg Press

Heel Raises (can be performed through ankle plantar flexion while completing leg press)

Chest Press

Compound Row

Overhead Press

Lat Pull-Down

Abdominal Curl

Back Extension

INTERMEDIATE RESISTANCE-TRAINING PROGRAM

If you are already resistance training two days a week (full-body routine), then start here.

GOAL: Continue to improve muscular fitness by performing a split resistance-training program (upper/lower) four days of the week.

| Frequency | Intensity | Time | | | Number and Type of Exercises |
		Reps	Sets	Rest	
4 days a week: Upper body M/W Lower body T/Th	70% 1 RM	10	3	2.5 minutes between sets	Upper body: 7 multiple-joint exercises 1 single-joint exercise Lower body: 4 multiple-joint exercises 3 single-joint exercises

M/W Upper Body Order of Exercises:
Chest Press

Row

Chest Fly

Overhead Press

Lat Pull-Down

Upright Row

Biceps Curl

Triceps Extension

T/Th Lower Body Order of Exercises:
Squat

Lunge

Leg Extension

Leg Curl

Heel Raise

Abdominal Curl

Oblique Curl

Back Extension

MOTIVATE!

Track your resistance-training program—make note of days, actual exercises, sets, reps, load amounts, and rest intervals. Here are a few other tips to keep your training strong:

ADJUST YOUR TRAINING ROUTINE: Boredom is a motivation killer. Change your exercises regularly, incorporate different equipment, and/or change your training location from time to time.

MOTIVATE THROUGH MEDIA: Listen to music or podcasts during your rest intervals. In your downtime, try reading articles, blogs, or books about fitness, resistance training, healthy lifestyles, or your favorite sport.

STAY POSITIVE: Surround yourself with positive affirmations and training partners. Stay focused, review your goals, and acknowledge how much you have already accomplished.

JOIN A SOCIAL MEDIA SITE OR FITNESS MESSAGE BOARD: Check out the message boards of fitness websites for inspiration from others who have accomplished their goals or who are working toward goals similar to yours. Most message boards are designed to foster encouragement, discipline, and accountability.

MAKE A HEALTH CONTRACT WITH YOUR FAMILY: Everyone gets one private hour every day to exercise guilt-free. This will help establish your family's goal of a happy, healthy, and active lifestyle.

ADVANCE!

After establishing your resistance-training program, you may want to retake the estimated 1 RM (Lab 4.1) and 20 RM (Lab 4.2) tests and set new goals to take your training to the next level. Below are two resistance-training programs for specific goals.

MUSCULAR ENDURANCE PROGRAM

GOAL: Increase muscular endurance by performing 12 exercises three days a week.

Frequency	Intensity	Time			Number and Type of Exercises
		Reps	Sets	Rest	
3 non-consecutive days a week	50% 1 RM	15	3	45–60 seconds between sets	10 multiple-joint and 2 single-joint exercises

Order of Exercises:

Push-Up
Assisted Pull-Up
Squat
Lunge
Chest Fly
Row

Upright Row
Overhead Press
Biceps Curl
Pullover
Plank
Side Bridge (each side)

MUSCULAR STRENGTH AND MASS PROGRAM

GOAL: Build muscular strength and mass by performing a high-intensity split resistance-training program (upper/lower) four days of the week.

Frequency	Intensity	Time			Number and Type of Exercises
		Reps	Sets	Rest	
4 days a week: Upper body M/W Lower body T/Th	80% 1 RM	8	4	3 minutes between sets	Upper body: 7 multiple-joint exercises 1 single-joint exercise Lower body: 4 multiple-joint exercises 3 single-joint exercises

M/W Upper Body Order of Exercises:

Chest Press
Row
Overhead Press
Lat Pull-Down
Lateral Raise
Biceps Curl
Triceps Extension
Back Extension

T/Th Lower Body Order of Exercises:

Leg Press
Leg Extension
Leg Curl
Hip Abduction
Hip Adduction
Heel Raise
Abdominal Curl
Reverse Curl
Oblique Curl

5 Maintaining Flexibility and Back Health

LEARNINGoutcomes

LO 5.1 Articulate how regular stretching and being flexible can benefit your lifelong fitness and wellness.

LO 5.2 Identify the body structures, body systems, and individual factors that will determine your joint flexibility and back health over time.

LO 5.3 Use multiple assessment tools to evaluate your flexibility changes over time.

LO 5.4 Implement a stretching program that will maintain or improve your flexibility.

LO 5.5 Follow recommended fitness program guidelines to reduce your risk of stretching-related injuries.

LO 5.6 Evaluate your personal risk for the primary causes of lower-back pain.

LO 5.7 Incorporate strategies to reduce your risk for (or manage existing) lower-back pain.

MasteringHealth™

Go online for chapter quizzes, interactive assessments, videos, and more!

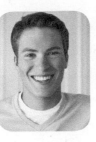

caseSTUDY

MARK

"Hi, I'm Mark. I live in Colorado Springs, at the foothills of the Rocky Mountains. I love the outdoors. I've been a backpacker, fisherman, and skier my whole life. My girlfriend has been telling me that I should really stretch more, but I'm skeptical. What's so important about stretching? Will it help me be a better hiker or skier? How do I figure out what kind of stretches I should do? And when and how often should I stretch?"

Hear It!

To listen to this case study online, visit the Study Area in MasteringHealth™.

Flexibility is the ability of joints to move through a full **range of motion**. Overall flexibility decreases as we get older, but declines can vary widely—depending upon how you use your body's joints.[1] A complete fitness program should include **stretching** and range-of-motion exercises to help you maintain flexibility and prevent joint problems.

In this chapter, we will cover how maintaining your flexibility can improve your mobility, keep your joints healthy, and help you relax. We will discuss the factors that determine how flexible a person is, present strategies for stretching safely and effectively, and provide guidelines for developing a personalized stretching program. We will also discuss the common problem of lower-back pain and offer strategies for incorporating a back-health component into your regular fitness plan.

LO 5.1 What Are the Benefits of Stretching and Flexibility?

Like Mark, many people are not in the habit of stretching and are not sure why stretching is important. Stretching offers many benefits, but the most compelling is simple: Being flexible will help you move freely, stay mobile, and complete activities you want to do with greater ease.

Improved Mobility, Posture, and Balance

One in five US adults reported having a disability in 2013. The most frequently reported disability was serious difficulty with walking or climbing stairs—or reduced mobility.[2] A regular stretching program helps you maintain mobility throughout your body. Your joints allow you to move—whether you are bending your knees to tie a shoelace, riding a bicycle around campus, or reaching for a bowl on the top shelf of a cupboard. Reduced flexibility can limit your ability to move about freely. Likewise, improved flexibility can result in greater freedom of movement. Keeping your body flexible and strong also helps you maintain your balance. Individuals who have better ankle strength and range of motion not only have better balance, but also greater functional ability—which means fewer falls and injuries.[3]

Regular stretching helps maintain a balance of muscle strength and muscle flexibility, which is important for proper joint alignment and posture. For example, if the muscles on the front of your hips get too tight, your pelvis can get pulled forward and cause a larger sway in your lower back. This will alter your posture and could even affect your balance. Good flexibility, developed through stretching, helps keep your joints and spine aligned and promotes overall body stability.

Healthy Joints and Pain Management

As many as 26 percent of all adults report pain or stiffness in joints. That number increases dramatically with age, and women are more likely to have those joint symptoms. Many adults have or will develop **arthritis**; 49 percent of people 75 years and older have been diagnosed with arthritis.[4] Regular exercise, including range-of-motion and flexibility exercises, is essential for people with arthritis to maintain function and manage joint pain.[5] Even in people without arthritis, stretching will improve joint function and decrease periodic joint pain.[6]

Possible Reduction of Future Lower-Back Pain

Flexibility may reduce your risk of lower-back pain in the future; however, research on the subject is inconclusive. While poor flexibility has been linked to lower-back pain in adolescents, these relationships are less

---

flexibility The ability of a joint (or joints) to move through a full range of motion

range of motion The movement limits of a specific joint or group of joints

stretching Exercises designed to improve or maintain flexibility

arthritis An umbrella-term for more than 100 conditions characterized by inflammation of a joint

clear in adults.[7, 8, 9, 10] Despite the mixed evidence, most experts agree that exercise to counteract the natural loss in muscle and connective tissue elasticity that occurs with aging can reduce your risk of lower-back pain.[11] We will discuss lower-back pain in more detail later in this chapter.

Muscle Relaxation and Stress Relief

After sitting for hours working on a term paper, doesn't it feel great to stand up and stretch? Staying in one position for too long, repetitive movement, and other stressors can result in stiff and "knotted" muscles. Gentle stretching and relaxation increases blood flow to tight muscles, stimulates the nervous system to decrease stress hormones, and ultimately helps relax areas of tension in your body.

LO 5.2 What Determines My Flexibility?

What makes one person a human pretzel, while others can barely touch their toes? Is flexibility attributed entirely to the amount of stretching that you do? Many factors affect your individual level of flexibility, including the structure and function of your joints, muscles, **tendons**, and nervous system, along with your age, gender, genetics, and activity level.

Flexibility can be classified as static or dynamic. **Static (passive) flexibility** is a measure of the limits of a joint's overall range of motion. **Dynamic (active) flexibility** is a measure of overall joint stiffness during movement (i.e., with muscular contraction).

Joint Structures, Muscles and Tendons, and the Nervous System

tendons Connective tissues that attach muscle to bone

static (passive) flexibility A joint's range-of-motion limits with an external force applied

dynamic (active) flexibility A joint's range-of-motion limits with muscular contraction applied

joint The articulation or point of contact between two or more bones

golgi tendon organs Muscle tension receptors located in tendons that are responsible for triggering muscle relaxation to relieve excessive muscle tension

Joint range of motion is determined by the joint structures, the muscles and tendons that cross over the joint, and the nervous system.

Joint Structures The individual components of a joint all affect the joint's mobility and stability (**Figure 5.1**). *Cartilage* is a strong, smooth tissue that cushions the ends of

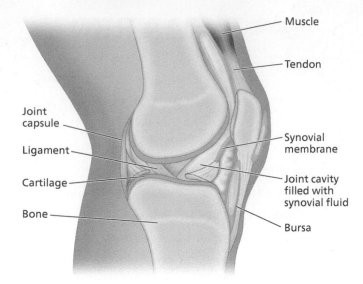

FIGURE 5.1 Joints are surrounded by a supportive joint capsule made of ligaments and synovial membranes. The joint cavity is filled with synovial fluid that (along with cartilage and bursa sacs) cushions and protects bones during movement. The stability of a joint is strengthened by muscle-tendon insertions surrounding the joint.

the bones, preventing them from rubbing directly against one another and providing impact protection. *Ligaments* are fibrous connective tissues that connect bone to bone. Some ligaments form the outer layer of the *joint capsule* to provide a reinforcing structure to the overall joint. Other ligaments provide further stability to the joint. The *synovial membrane* forms the inner layer of the joint capsule and secretes *synovial fluid* into the *joint cavity*. Synovial fluid lubricates and protects the joint. *Bursae (singular, bursa)* are small fluid-filled sacs that lubricate the movement of muscles over one another or muscles over bone.

Muscles and Tendons While joint structure accounts for 47 percent of the resistance to joint movement, individual *soft tissues* (muscles, connective tissue, ligaments, tendons, and skin) account for 53 percent of that resistance to movement![12] With regular activity, stretching, and increases in body temperature, muscles remain supple and are able to easily lengthen. With disuse and aging, soft tissues become stiffer, limiting flexibility.

The Nervous System Your nervous system stimulates muscle contractions and triggers muscle relaxation. Muscles and tendons contain nervous-system receptors that interpret information about the tension and length of muscles at any given moment. These receptors protect the muscles from damage caused by excessive force or by stretching too far. If there is too much tension or force within a muscle, receptors in the tendon (called **golgi tendon organs**) will trigger your muscle to relax.

DIVERSITY
Men, Women, and Flexibility

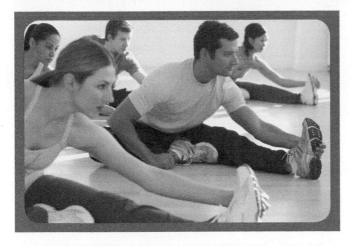

Women are more flexible than men, right? Not necessarily! This commonly held belief is not always true and may lull men into thinking that being inflexible is normal and okay.

Women generally are more flexible in the hip joint and hamstrings, which are the most common sites for flexibility testing.[1] Women may have greater flexibility in

these areas than males due to their wider hips, hormonal influences, and tendency to participate in activities that develop greater flexibility. In other joints and areas of the body, however, there is not a large difference between males and females. In fact, males may be more flexible in other areas, like the lumbar region of the spine.[2]

Interestingly, greater joint range of motion and flexibility can increase the chances of injury. Because women tend to have greater hip flexibility and internal rotation of the hip joint, they are more likely to have knee problems.[3] The bottom line is that both men and women can increase flexibility with stretching exercises,[4] and adequate range of motion should be a goal for everyone. Being able to move your body without restriction opens up activity options and makes life easier!

Sources:
1. J. T. Manire et al., "Diurnal Variation of Hamstring and Lumbar Flexibility," *Journal of Strength and Conditioning Research* 24, no. 6 (2010): 1464–71.
2. Ibid.
3. K. M. Sutton and J. M. Bullock, "Anterior Cruciate Ligament Rupture: Differences between Males and Females," *Journal of the American Academy of Orthopaedic Surgeons* 21, no. 1 (2013): 41–50.
4. D. J. Cipriani et al., "Effect of Stretch Frequency and Sex on the Rate of Gain and Rate of Loss in Muscle Flexibility during Hamstring-Stretching Program: A Randomized Single-Blind Longitudinal Study," *Journal of Strength and Conditioning Research* 26, no. 8 (2012): 2119–29.

If your muscle is stretching too far, receptors in the muscle fibers (called **stretch receptors** or **muscle spindles**) will trigger your muscle to contract. This reflexive contraction is called the **stretch reflex**. Have you ever had a doctor tap your knee and watch your leg kick out in response? The doctor was striking your *patellar tendon*. This rapidly stretches your quadriceps muscle, which triggers stretch receptors in the quadriceps to signal your nervous system. Your leg then kicks out because of a reflex contraction of your quadriceps muscle stimulated by the nervous system.

Reducing the stretch reflex and activating the golgi tendon organs allow your muscles to relax, elongate, and become more flexible.

Individual Factors

Individual factors such as genetics, gender, age, body type, and activity level also affect flexibility.

Genetics Most people are moderately flexible. They have flexible and less-flexible areas of their bodies and need to work to maintain their present level of flexibility. However, some people are naturally flexible, while others are extremely inflexible. Genetic differences in body

structure and elasticity of soft tissues accounts for some of that variation in flexibility.

Gender Although it is widely assumed that females are more flexible than males, this may only be true for specific joints, as discussed in the Diversity box Men, Women, and Flexibility on this page.

Age Flexibility changes throughout the lifespan. Flexible preschool children experience a decrease in joint range of motion until the preteen years, when flexibility increases again to its peak by 18 years of age.[13] In adulthood, flexibility decreases with age due to physical changes in muscles, joints, and connective tissues.[14] These changes are joint-specific and are primarily related to inactivity and disuse.

The good news is that with regular exercise, people of all ages can improve their flexibility. In a study of sedentary

> **stretch receptors (muscle spindles)** Muscle length receptors located within muscle fibers that trigger muscle contractions in response to rapid, excessive muscle lengthening
>
> **stretch reflex** The reflex contraction of a muscle triggered by stretch receptors (muscle spindles) in response to a rapid overextension of that muscle

adult women, researchers observed flexibility improvements when women participated in a 16-week strength training program.[15] The women who also stretched had slightly larger gains in flexibility. These results demonstrate that performing both strength and stretching exercises may lead to optimal improvements in flexibility.

Body Type Body type can affect flexibility but typically only at the extremes of body shape and size. Joint range of motion may be affected if an excessive amount of muscle or fat interferes with full joint movement. That said, genetics and training are far more influential factors in determining flexibility than is body type. For instance, there are people with stocky, muscular builds who are exceptionally flexible, including many gymnasts.

Activity Level Inactivity can reduce flexibility as muscles and connective tissues tighten and shorten with disuse. Overly repetitive physical activity can also result in muscle "stiffness." When done properly, stretching and regular physical activity can improve flexibility. We will introduce effective stretches and exercises later in this chapter.

Health Status Certain medical conditions can affect your joint health and range of motion. Diseases that affect your **collagen** and connective tissues can produce overly mobile or inflexible joints. Arthritis speeds up the destruction of collagen and cartilage, leading to joint inflexibility. Some genetic syndromes result in reduced or ineffective collagen causing hypermobility. Many pregnant women experience more flexible joints. An injury or scar tissue can impair your ability to move through your full range of motion.

LO 5.3 How Can I Assess My Flexibility?

Flexibility levels vary from joint to joint. As a result, most flexibility tests are designed to measure the flexibility of specific muscles and joints, not your body's overall level of flexibility. However, if you take a variety of flexibility tests, you can get a sense of how your body's overall level of mobility compares to recommended target ranges. This information will help you design a personalized program for developing flexibility.

Perform the "Sit-and-Reach" Test

One of the most common measures of flexibility is the "sit-and-reach" test. This test measures the flexibility of your lower back, hip, and hamstring muscles. These areas are often tight in individuals who are

collagen The primary protein of connective tissues throughout the body

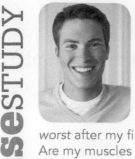
inactive. This muscular imbalance can negatively influence posture, balance, and risk of back pain. Lab 5.1 provides instructions for the sit-and-reach test.

Do It!
Access these labs at the end of the chapter or online at MasteringHealth™.

Perform Range-of-Motion Tests

Having an adequate range of motion in your joints and maintaining that range over time should be the primary goal of a flexibility fitness program. Lab 5.1 tells you how to perform range-of-motion tests on joints in your neck, shoulders, trunk, hips, and ankles. These tests will help you evaluate whether your joints are more flexible or less flexible than average.

LO 5.4 How Can I Plan a Good Stretching Program?

Regardless of whether you already stretch regularly, keep in mind the following guidelines to ensure a safe and effective program.

Set Appropriate Flexibility Goals

After completing the flexibility tests in Lab 5.1, decide what your goal is. Do you want to maintain your current level of flexibility or do you want to *improve* it?

Once you've decided, follow the SMART guidelines for setting specific goals. Recall that SMART stands for specific, measurable, action-oriented, realistic, and time-oriented. An example of a SMART goal designed to *maintain* your flexibility is, "My goal for the next year is to maintain the joint flexibility and range-of-motion levels recorded on my flexibility assessments by incorporating stretching into my workouts at least four times per week." An example of a SMART goal designed to *improve* your flexibility is, "My goal is to regularly stretch so that I can increase my lower-back, hip, and hamstring flexibility from 'poor' to 'good' on the sit-and-reach test by the end of the semester."

For most people, a primary goal is to be able to move their joints through a normal range of motion without pain. Achieving exceptionally high levels of flexibility may be desirable for some sports and activities but is not necessary for the average person.

Apply the FITT Formula to Your Stretching Program

Recall that FITT stands for frequency, intensity, time, and type. Use the FITT formula to design your own personalized stretching program. **Table 5.1** provides general guidelines from the American College of Sports Medicine (ACSM). Refer to this table as a starting point for designing your own program.

Frequency ACSM guidelines recommend stretching at least two to three days per week. If your current level of flexibility is already within "normal" ranges and you merely want to maintain that level, you should stretch two days per week. If your current level of flexibility needs improvement to reach a "normal" range, aim to stretch three or more days per week (daily is the most effective).

Should you stretch before a workout, after a workout, or both? The Q&A box When Should I Stretch? on page 174 explores these questions and others.

Intensity ACSM guidelines state that you should stretch "to the point of feeling tightness or slight discomfort." If you are feeling pain, you are stretching too far and risking injury. Pay close attention to your body whenever you stretch; your flexibility level may vary slightly from day to day.

Time Perform your stretching program for at least 10 minutes at a time and stretch all major muscle groups. Hold your stretches for 10 to 30 seconds each and repeat stretches two to four times. As soon as you start to stretch, your stretch reflex will activate. You can feel this as a slight increase in muscle tension when you move into a stretch position. By holding your stretches for at least 10 seconds, you are giving the stretch reflex time to lessen. You are also giving your golgi tendon organs time to activate, thus allowing your muscles to lengthen farther.

By repeating stretches multiple times, you enable your muscles to relax and lengthen a little bit more each time. If you are beginning a stretching program for the first time and feel uncomfortable with multiple repetitions, you can perform one repetition of each stretch and still obtain benefits. After a few weeks of stretching consistently, gradually increase the number of repetitions to the recommended two to four times per session. Aim to have your total stretching time for each exercise add up to 60 seconds.

Type There are numerous stretching techniques. The most common are highlighted below.

TABLE **5.1** ACSM's Flexibility Training Guidelines for Healthy Adults	
Frequency	2 to 3 days/week minimum; daily is most effective
Intensity	Stretch to the point of feeling tightness or slight discomfort
Time	10 to 30 seconds per static stretch repetition; 2 to 4 repetitions of each stretching exercise; aim for 60 seconds total time per exercise
Type	Static, dynamic, or PNF stretching of all major muscle groups*

*Ballistic stretching may be appropriate for some individuals in certain sports and recreational activities.

Source: Data from American College of Sports Medicine, *ACSM's Guidelines for Exercise Testing and Prescription*, 9th ed. (Baltimore, MD: Lippincott Williams & Wilkins, 2014).

Q&A   When Should I Stretch?

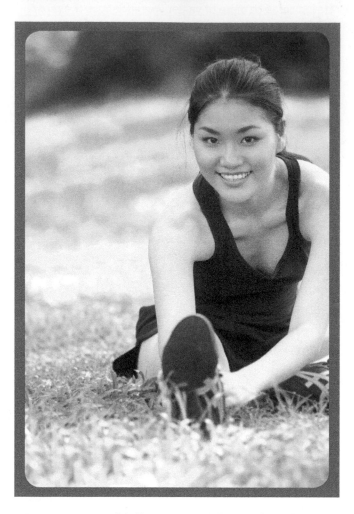

explosive performances for up to 24 hours![1] Conversely, dynamic stretching can improve sprint and explosive performance for up to 24 hours. The duration and timing of pre-event stretching is another consideration for competitive and recreational athletes. Even dynamic stretching impairs performance when it lasts too long (inducing fatigue) and is completed too close to the performance time.[2]

APPLY IT! It is now generally accepted that pre-exercise stretching does not reduce overuse injuries.[3] More research must be done, but flexibility recommendations now promote stretching to maintain joint mobility, but not to reduce injury during exercise. This is a surprise to many people, but it doesn't mean that you have to give up your favorite warm-up stretches:

- If you perform static stretches in your warm-up, stick to *light* static stretching (10 to 15 seconds). Performance detriments due to warm-up static stretching are primarily seen with stretches lasting 60 seconds or more.[4]

- If you want to stretch before a workout, be sure to warm up beforehand. Stretching cold muscles can result in injury.

- Emphasize dynamic stretches in your warm-up and make sure the movements are similar to your exercise, sport, or recreational activity.

- Avoid warming-up and stretching to the point of fatigue right before exercise or competition.

- Save most of your static stretching for after the workout—then you can really focus on increasing range of motion in tight areas!

Many people incorrectly think that they *have* to stretch before a workout. Actually, it is better to perform most of your static stretching *after* a workout, when your muscles are warm and your joint structures are more receptive to stretching.

For *most* individuals, light pre-exercise static stretches will not negatively affect exercise or recreational performance. If you are a power athlete, though, you may want to avoid too much static stretching before a competition or high-intensity workout. Extensive static stretching can reduce

Sources:
1. M. Haddad et al., "Static Stretching Can Impair Explosive Performance for at Least 24 Hours," *Journal of Strength and Conditioning Research* 28, no. 1 (2014): 140–46, doi: 10.1519/JSC.0b013e3182964836; H. Kallerud and N. Gleeson, "Effects of Stretching on Performances Involving Stretch-Shortening Cycles," *Sports Medicine* 43, no. 8 (2013): 733–50, doi: 10.1007/s40279-013-0053-x
2. O. Turki et al., "The Effect of Warm-Ups Incorporating Different Volumes of Dynamic Stretching on 10- and 20-m Sprint Performance in Highly Trained Male Athletes," *Journal of Strength and Conditioning* 26, no. 1 (2012): 63–72.
3. M. P. McHugh and C. H. Cosgrave, "To Stretch or Not to Stretch: The Role of Stretching in Injury Prevention and Performance," *Scandinavian Journal of Medicine & Science in Sports* 20, no. 2 (2010): 169–81.
4. A. D. Kay and A. J. Blazevich, "Effect of Acute Static Stretch on Maximal Muscle Performance: A Systematic Review," *Medicine and Science in Sports and Exercise* 44, no. 1 (2012): 154–64.

static stretching Stretching characterized by slow and sustained muscle lengthening

dynamic stretching Stretching characterized by controlled, full-range-of-motion movements that mimic exercise session movements

- **Static stretching** involves moving slowly into a stretch and holding. This simple and safe method is great for individuals who are just starting a stretching program. Static stretching is effective because the slow holds reduce the activation of stretch receptors. After a workout, static stretching assists with muscle recovery and helps you maintain or improve your flexibility.

- **Dynamic stretching** involves stretching through movement. During dynamic stretching, you mimic the motions of your workout or sports activity with slow,

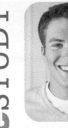
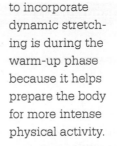

MARK

"The ski season just started. Out of curiosity, I asked a ski instructor for his opinions on stretching. He was surprised that I have been skiing my whole life but wasn't in the habit of stretching! He explained how stretching can help reduce muscle tension, improve my ability to make quick turns, and help prevent stiffness. He recommended quadriceps and hamstrings stretches and also suggested using a massage stick or foam roller. I'd like a simple stretching plan that I can follow, but I am not sure where to start or what's important."

APPLY IT! Are the quadriceps and hamstrings stretches in Figure 5.7 static or dynamic stretches? What is the difference? When should Mark perform these stretches, before or after skiing? Should Mark go out and buy a massage stick or foam roller?

TRY IT! Using Table 5.1, Figure 5.7, and Lab 5.3, write a simple stretching plan for Mark that addresses his goal to reduce stiffness after skiing.

Hear It!
To listen to this case study online, visit the Study Area in MasteringHealth™.

fluid movements. Dynamic stretching increases dynamic flexibility and can enhance muscle action during sports and recreational activities.[16] A good time to incorporate dynamic stretching is during the warm-up phase because it helps prepare the body for more intense physical activity.

- **Ballistic stretching** is characterized by bouncing, sometimes jerky, movements and high momentum. Ballistic stretching increases dynamic flexibility and can benefit trained athletes in sports requiring fast, explosive movements such as wrestling, gymnastics, tennis, and basketball. However, the bouncing movements in ballistic stretching rapidly activate the stretch receptors, making this method less effective at increasing static flexibility.

- **Proprioceptive neuromuscular facilitation (PNF)** uses the voluntary contraction of muscle groups to help facilitate relaxation and stretching in target muscles. In the most common method of PNF stretching, *contract-relax* PNF, the exerciser performs an isotonic or isometric contraction of the target muscle just prior to slow, passive stretching of that muscle. **Figure 5.2** shows an example of contract-relax PNF.

> **ballistic stretching** Stretching characterized by bouncing, jerky movements and momentum to increase range of motion
>
> **proprioceptive neuromuscular facilitation (PNF)** Stretching that is facilitated or enhanced by the voluntary contraction of the targeted muscle group or contraction of opposing muscles

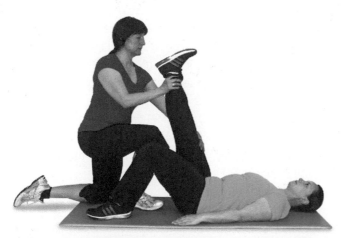

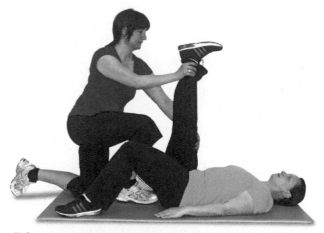

(a) Lie on your back with one leg bent and the other extended toward the ceiling. Have a partner hold your lifted leg as you try to press your leg to the ground for 6 seconds. Your partner can resist enough to allow no movement at all (isometric contraction) or just enough to allow gradual movement toward the ground (isotonic contraction). The contraction stimulates the golgi tendon organs to activate and promote muscle relaxation.

(b) Immediately following the 6-second contraction, relax your muscles and have your partner move your leg up and toward your chest into a passive stretch for the hips, hamstrings, and low back. Hold this stretch for 10 to 30 seconds and release.

FIGURE **5.2** An example of a contract-relax proprioceptive neuromuscular facilitation (PNF) partner exercise.

TABLE 5.2 Pros and Cons of Common Stretching Methods

Stretching Method	Pro	Con
Static	Safe, simple to use, effective at increasing static flexibility	Too much can reduce muscle power immediately after stretching, can be time-consuming
Dynamic	Increases dynamic flexibility, functional movements, enhances performance	Takes time to learn correct movement patterns
Ballistic	Can be beneficial for ballistic sports, increases dynamic flexibility	Not as effective at increasing overall flexibility, performing ballistic moves quickly can be unsafe
PNF	Effective at increasing static flexibility levels	Need a partner or equipment to perform, complicated method

Table 5.2 lists some of the pros and cons of each stretching method. For people starting a flexibility program on their own, static stretches are the safest option. **Figure 5.7** (starting on page 185) illustrates some common stretching exercises, and Program 5.1: A Flexibility Training Program (at the end of this chapter) offers options for sequencing and combining stretches. **Lab 5.3** (at the end of this chapter) walks you through the process of designing your own program.

Do It!
Access these labs at the end of the chapter or online at MasteringHealth™.

Consider Taking a Class

If you would like more structure and instruction in your stretching program, consider enrolling in a class. Yoga, tai chi, Pilates, dance, mobility, and martial arts classes can be fun, effective ways to improve your flexibility. For more information on these types of classes, see the Q&A box Can I Become Flexible without Stretching? on page 178.

Add Flexibility "Tools"

There are a number of flexibility tools that you can use in your own home and/or in a gym. These tools can increase the safety and effectiveness of your stretching, plus provide something new for variety and motivation!

Physical therapists and other health practitioners use **myofascial release therapy** to reduce muscle tightness, soft-tissue adhesions, and nervous-system over-activation. This increases joint and muscle extensibility, muscle balance, and overall function. In recent years, *self-myofascial release* has become popular with competitive and recreational athletes in many sports. Using a foam roller, massage

myofascial release therapy
Manual pressure and movement therapy that aims to decrease movement restrictions and pain in muscle tissue and the surrounding fascia

stick, tennis ball, or golf ball, you can perform these myofascial release techniques on yourself to improve your own muscle range of motion and reduce muscle fatigue.[17] Utilize this self-massage technique to loosen soft tissues before activity, after a workout to help muscles relax, and/or between workouts for pain relief and muscle balance.

You may have heard of *whole-body vibration* or seen one of these machines in your gym. Developed in the 1960s to help astronauts maintain muscle and bone mass in space, the whole-body vibration (WBV) machine transmits quick vibrations in one or more directions, stimulating muscle fiber contractions. The WBV machines are becoming more common because of the evidence supporting their use for increasing flexibility and muscle action. The evidence seems to be consistent for flexibility gains,[18] even over other potential benefits such as bone density, muscle strength and power, postural control, and balance. Static stretching during vibration on a WBV platform can help you retain the flexibility you gain.[19] If your gym has a WBV machine, talk with a trainer about designing a program for you. You can exercise while standing or lying on the platform. Work your way up to 20 to 30 minutes at a time. You can use the platform a few times per week or every day to increase your range of motion, and possibly your strength, balance, and bone density too!

See **Table 5.3** for an overview of several widely available flexibility tools.

See It!
Watch "The Do's and Don'ts of Stretching" at MasteringHealth™.

LO 5.5 How Can I Avoid Stretching-Related Injuries?

We used to think of stretching as a way to avoid injury, but we now know that stretching can actually *cause* injury if done improperly. To avoid a stretching-related injury, follow these guidelines.

TABLE 5.3 Flexibility Tools

Foam Roller or Massage Stick	Yoga Tools	Stretching Strap	Whole-Body Vibration
Foam cylinder or rolling stick used for myofascial release on tight body areas	Mat: a thin, long, non-slip mat Blocks: dense foam rectangular blocks Strap: strong cotton strap with a buckle	Long strap with multiple loops or yoga strap that can be used for various static, dynamic, and non-partner PNF stretches	Platform that vibrates and is used to enhance muscle action while exercising
Sized between 12 and 36 inches; density and design varies; choose a smaller version to use while traveling	Yoga mats are useful for all types of stretching; blocks and straps assist body positioning in poses and stretches	Several feet long, most of these straps have about 10 loops along the length for customizing your stretch position.	Make sure that the platform is large enough for the exercises you want to perform
Choose from a smooth surface or one with ridges for greater massage intensity	Look for a slip-resistant yoga mat that has adequate padding	Some straps come with instructional books or DVDs	Some platforms have a bar or handles for stabilization while working on standing exercises

Stretch Only Warm Muscles

An increase in body temperature prepares the joint fluid and structures for stretching, improves muscle elasticity, and allows for a greater range of motion. Increase your muscle temperature before stretching via *passive heat* (hot packs or a warm bath) or *active heat* (exercise). Both are effective to prepare you for stretching. However, if you are warming up your muscles prior to your main workout set, use active heat or exercise. After a workout, you can go right to static stretching because your muscles are already warm.

Perform Stretches Safely

One of the keys to safe and effective stretching is to avoid activating stretch receptors when you want a muscle to relax. Quick, bouncing movements can injure muscles because they are lengthening too far too quickly and the stretch reflex is creating tension at the same time. Avoid the stretch reflex by stretching slowly and holding your stretches for at least 10 seconds. This will allow the stretch receptors and golgi tendon organs to make nervous-system adjustments that allow muscles to relax and lengthen further.

Know Which Exercises Can Cause Injury

Figure 5.3 on page 179 shows common high-risk or **contraindicated** stretches with safer alternatives. Note that this figure is *not* all-inclusive. Choosing safe exercises is an individual process. Consider your personal limitations and health issues when deciding which exercises are best for your body.

contraindicated Not recommended

Q&A Can I Become Flexible without Stretching?

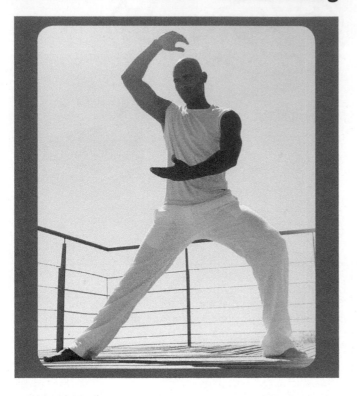

muscle endurance, flexibility, and coordination; they also reduce anxiety and stress.[4] Tai chi has become popular with many people, but older individuals in particular are drawn to this safe and effective way to exercise.

Other forms of martial arts can develop flexibility, as well. Look into classes for one of these popular martial arts: *capoeira, karate, jujitsu,* or *tae kwon do.*

Developed by Joseph Pilates in New York City in the 1920s, *Pilates* involves performing a sequence of exercises on a mat or specialized equipment. Pilates combines specific breathing patterns with stretching and resistance exercises to increase flexibility and muscle endurance, particularly in the core trunk-supporting muscles.

Dance is a fantastic and fun way to improve your flexibility and overall fitness. *Barre classes* are ballet dance-inspired fitness classes that are popular for people of all abilities and fitness levels. A ballet barre is used as a point of balance while working on isometric and dynamic muscle endurance, flexibility, and posture. Group movement classes, such as *aerobic dance* and *Zumba,* enhance flexibility through class movements and stretches in the cool-down phase.

Specific classes for increasing your *mobility* are popping up everywhere! The premise of these classes is that adequate joint mobility and moving well are the essential basics for success in all activities. Look for mobility classes at your local health club.

All of the activities described above require instruction by a trained professional, especially since some exercises can be risky for untrained or novice participants.

TRY IT! If a regular stretching routine doesn't appeal to you, try one of these classes to help you reach your flexibility goals:

Yoga originated in India about 5,000 years ago and has become popular in the United States. The forms of yoga most commonly practiced in the United States today require a combination of mental focus and physical effort while performing a variety of postures, or *asanas.* The physical aspect of yoga improves flexibility, posture, agility, balance, stamina, muscle endurance, coordination,[1] and risk factors for heart disease.[2] The mental aspect of yoga promotes attention, controlled breathing, relaxation, a union of mind and body, self-reported happiness, and an overall psychological sense of well-being.[3]

Tai chi is a martial art that was developed in ancient China by monks wanting to defend themselves. Tai chi practice involves a slow-moving, smooth, and continuous series of positions or forms. These exercises increase balance,

Sources:
1. B. L. Tracy and C. E. Hart, "Bikram Yoga Training and Physical Fitness in Healthy Young Adults," *Journal of Strength and Conditioning Research* 27, no. 3 (2013): 822–30.
2. P. Chu et al., "The Effectiveness of Yoga in Modifying Risk Factors for Cardiovascular Disease and Metabolic Syndrome: A Systematic Review and Meta-Analysis of Randomized Controlled Trials," *European Journal of Preventive Cardiology* (2014): December 15, pii: 2047487314562741
3. A Ross et al., "National Survey of Yoga Practitioners: Mental and Physical Health Benefits," *Complementary Therapies in Medicine* 21, no. 4 (2013): 313–23, doi: 10.1016/j.ctim.2013.04.001
4. M. Y. Chang et al., "Associations between Tai Chi Chung Program, Anxiety, and Cardiovascular Risk Factors," *American Journal of Health Promotion* 28, no. 1 (2013): 16–22, doi: 10.4278/ajhp.120720-QUAN-356; G. Zheng et al., "Effectiveness of Tai Chi on Physical and Psychological Health of College Students: Results of a Randomized Controlled Trial," *PLOS ONE* 10, no. 7 (2015): e0132605, doi: 10.1371/journal.pone.0132605

Be Cautious If You Are Hyperflexible or Inflexible

If you are really flexible, you may need to be more careful. Excessive hypermobility increases joint laxity or looseness, decreases joint stability, and can lead to permanent changes in connective tissue. Take precautions

to avoid overstretching, which may lead to injury or decreases in exercise performance.

On the other hand, if you have limited range of motion in one or more joints, avoid stretching beyond your abilities. Work gradually to improve your range of motion and overall flexibility. Inflexible people may be more susceptible to sudden acute injuries

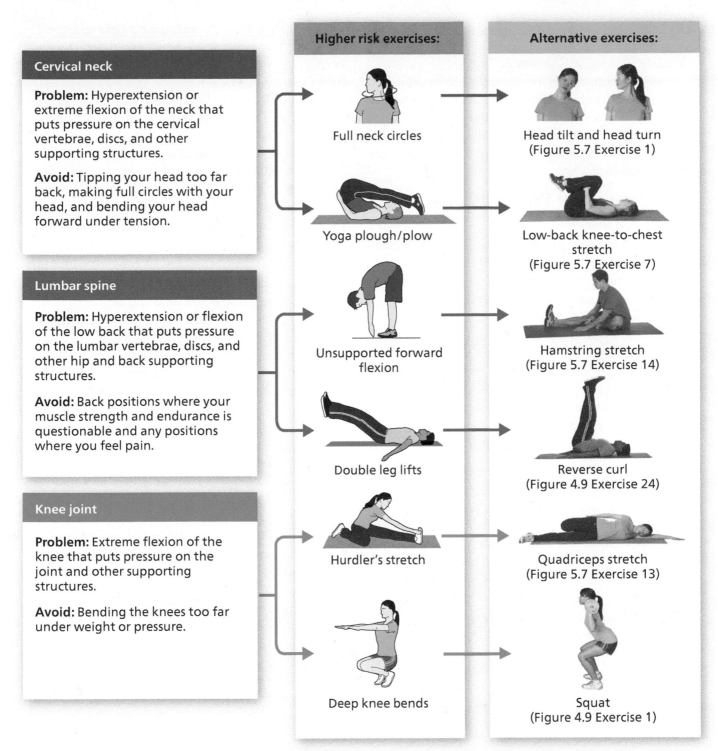

Higher risk exercises:	Alternative exercises:

Cervical neck

Problem: Hyperextension or extreme flexion of the neck that puts pressure on the cervical vertebrae, discs, and other supporting structures.

Avoid: Tipping your head too far back, making full circles with your head, and bending your head forward under tension.

Full neck circles

Head tilt and head turn
(Figure 5.7 Exercise 1)

Yoga plough/plow

Low-back knee-to-chest stretch
(Figure 5.7 Exercise 7)

Lumbar spine

Problem: Hyperextension or flexion of the low back that puts pressure on the lumbar vertebrae, discs, and other hip and back supporting structures.

Avoid: Back positions where your muscle strength and endurance is questionable and any positions where you feel pain.

Unsupported forward flexion

Hamstring stretch
(Figure 5.7 Exercise 14)

Double leg lifts

Reverse curl
(Figure 4.9 Exercise 24)

Knee joint

Problem: Extreme flexion of the knee that puts pressure on the joint and other supporting structures.

Avoid: Bending the knees too far under weight or pressure.

Hurdler's stretch

Quadriceps stretch
(Figure 5.7 Exercise 13)

Deep knee bends

Squat
(Figure 4.9 Exercise 1)

FIGURE **5.3** Choose safer alternatives to these common higher-risk exercises and stretches. Take into account your personal goals, experience, and limitations.

during sports and daily activities, and to lower-back injuries.

LO 5.6 Am I at Risk for Back Pain?

As we age, our mobility naturally decreases and our risk of back pain increases. In fact, 18 percent of college-age adults report already having low-back pain.[20] Among all US adults that number increases to 28.5 percent, with more women (30.2 percent) reporting low-back pain than men (26.4 percent).[21] This means that Americans spend a lot of money each year treating back pain symptoms—$86 billion and rising![22]

Since we know that college students are not immune to back-health issues, see the GetFitGraphic Back Pain and College Students (page 181) for tips on managing back pain and reducing your risk. Factors that increase your risk of lower-back pain include obesity, smoking, pregnancy, stress, inactivity, weak and inflexible muscles, and poor posture. In addition, a number of events can trigger back pain or cause a back injury, including accidents, sports injuries, repetitive movements, work trauma, and excessive sitting—especially if you already have other risk factors. Up next: A more detailed explanation of what causes back pain.

Understand the Primary Causes of Back Pain

You experience back pain when your movement causes a sprain, strain, or spasm in one of the muscles, tendons, or ligaments in the back. You may also feel pain when your spine structures become misaligned or injured and the spinal nerves become compressed or irritated. Back pain can also result from age- or disease-related degeneration of the bones and joints of the spine. Ultimately, most back pain is caused by a *sedentary lifestyle,* which results in muscle weakness (particularly in core trunk muscles), inflexibility, and imbalance. All of these conditions can lead to poor posture and body mechanics, and a higher risk of back pain and injury.

Muscular Weakness, Inflexibility, and Imbalance

The supporting musculature of the spine is important for maintaining healthy posture, mobility, and spine structures. Weakness and inflexibility in key muscles can lead to muscular imbalances that affect the alignment of your spine. Weak abdominals cause your pelvis to rock forward and increase the curvature in your lower back. This puts pressure on the spine and spine-supporting muscles, potentially leading to back pain. Inflexible, tight hip flexor muscles cause a forward tilt of the pelvis and this will also increase your lower back curvature.

Muscles become weak when they are not used regularly. Repetitive movements or long hours of sitting can also cause muscles to shorten and tighten up. If your spine-supporting musculature does not have a muscle balance that promotes good posture and body mechanics, you may have back pain or injury in the future.

Improper Posture and Body Mechanics Do you
have "text neck"? Looking at a phone or smart device for hours each day negatively affects your posture. While the human head weighs only about 10 to 12 pounds in an upright position, its weight can increase to 40 to 60 pounds when looking down.[23] That extra weight on the neck and spine means additional stress on the cervical spine, which could lead to early wear and tear, and possibly surgery. Since most Americans use a smartphone or device, this may mean an epidemic of neck and spine issues, especially among young adults who tend to spend more time on their devices.

Improper posture overall, like hunched shoulders and a protruding belly, can increase spinal pressure and promote back pain. Altered body mechanics resulting from improper posture puts you at risk for injury during all of your daily activities, but especially during exercise and sports.

Acute Trauma, Risky Occupations and Sports, and
Medical Issues Acute trauma to the back can happen to anyone at any age. Trauma could result from a car accident, falling, a sports-and-recreation injury, or any other accident that affects the spine. Avoiding risky activities and following basic safety precautions will reduce your chance of trauma.

Jobs that involve a lot of bending, twisting, and repeated lifting of heavy objects put workers at especially high risk of developing back pain. Occupations with a high incidence of back pain include truck driving, nursing, firefighting, construction, and some professional sports (e.g., football, power lifting, golf, and wrestling). Cycling in a bent-over position, running on hard pavement, or twisting while swinging a tennis racquet are examples of how even recreational sports can increase spinal stress and your risk of back pain.

Jobs that involve a great deal of sitting every day are considered high risk. So are occupations that are highly stressful and require long hours. Stress is a risk factor for back injury, and long hours at work reduce the time you have to exercise and relax, further increasing the risk of back pain.

Medical issues and individual health factors can play a significant role. For instance, smokers have an increased risk of low-back pain due to vascular damage, which facilitates disc degeneration.[24] Obesity and weight gain during pregnancy can increase lower-back pain due to greater loads on the spine, misalignment of the pelvis and low back, and muscular weakness.[25] Pain can also result from degenerative conditions such as arthritis or disc disease, osteoporosis or other bone diseases, congenital abnormalities, sciatica, infections, kidney stones, fibromyalgia, and general conditions that cause irritation or referred pain to the spine.[26]

BACK PAIN
AND COLLEGE STUDENTS

70% of Americans will experience lower-back pain at some point in their lives.

28% of Americans suffer from lower-back pain at any given moment.[1]

43% of college students report regular lower-back pain.[2]

Students who are sad, exhausted, overwhelmed and/or carrying heavy backpacks report the highest amounts of lower-back pain.[3]

WHAT CAN YOU DO TO PREVENT BACK PAIN?

▶ **Strengthen and stretch.** Add core strength and flexibility for back health.

▶ **Lose the backpack.** Carry backpacks no heavier than 10 to 15% of your weight.[4]

▶ **Study standing.** Try standing at a counter to study or walking around as you review for that midterm. Take frequent computer breaks.[5]

▶ **Get enough sleep and sleep smart.** Insufficient quantity and quality of sleep are associated with low back pain.[6] If you're sleeping on your back, put pillows under your knees to reduce pressure on your lower lumbar area. Even better, sleep on your side. Avoid sleeping on your stomach.

▶ **Quit smoking.** Smokers have higher rates of back pain than non-smokers.

▶ **Drop the extra pounds.** Extra weight puts a tremendous strain on your back.

▶ **Chill!** Feelings associated with stress increase the risk of back pain among college students.[7] Find ways to relax; your back will thank you!

DOES YOUR BACK ACHE?
TRY THESE OPTIONS FOR EASING BACK PAIN![8]

- Minimize bed rest (1 to 2 days max)
- Cold treatments (2 to 3 days)
- Heat treatments (as needed after acute pain has lessened)
- Light movement therapy (walking, swimming, stretching)
- Spine treatments with a chiropractor or physical therapist
- Alternative treatments (acupuncture, biofeedback, etc.)
- Medical advice/treatment after 3 days if pain persists
- Pain medications

LO 5.7 How Can I Prevent or Manage Back Pain?

After understanding your overall risk for back pain, it is important to know how the spine is structured and supported. This knowledge gives you the foundation to successfully incorporate strategies to reduce your risk of back pain. For those who already experience episodes of back pain, we will discuss ways to manage, resolve, and prevent future recurrences.

Understand How the Back Is Supported

The back comprises bones, muscles, and other tissues that form the back side of your trunk. The trunk contains most of your essential organs and bears the weight of your upper body. It is responsible for transmitting forces and movements from the upper limbs to the lower limbs, and vice versa. If something is amiss with your back or your trunk overall, any upper- or lower-body movement can be difficult. Your back and trunk are supported by the bony structures of the spine and by the core trunk muscles.

The Structure of the Spine The spine or *spinal column* (also called the *vertebral column*) is the series of bones called *vertebrae* that connect the upper-body and lower-body skeleton and protect the spinal cord. **Figure 5.4** shows the basic structure of the spine, with its four distinct regions and curvatures: *cervical, thoracic, lumbar,* and *sacral.* The normal curvatures are an essential part of the force-absorbing capabilities of the spine; however, too much curvature can be a risk factor for back pain.

Intervertebral discs are round, spongy pads of cartilage that act as shock absorbers. The discs have fibrous outer rings filled with gel and water-like substances that distend slightly when compressed. That distention acts to absorb shock. The discs ensure adequate space between the vertebrae. Changes in spinal alignment can damage these disc structures and cause pain.

If a disc bulges permanently out of its normal space, this is a **disc herniation**. The disc can bulge toward the spinal column or nerves and cause pain or numbness in the back or other areas of the body. Disc herniations most often occur in the lower lumbar region, where most of the body weight and forces are applied.

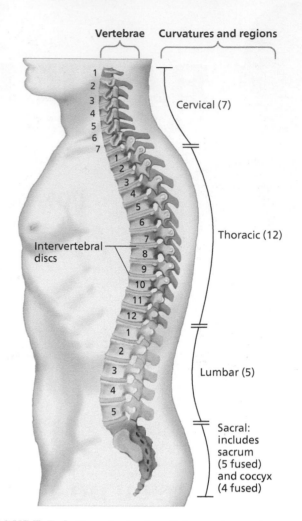

FIGURE **5.4** The spine has four distinct regions and curvatures (cervical, thoracic, lumbar, and sacral) made up of individual or fused vertebrae.

Trauma, aging, and physical inactivity can cause dehydration, hardening, or degeneration of intervertebral discs. Without adequate fluid content and elasticity, discs cannot perform their shock-absorber role very well. Physical inactivity, in particular, is associated with narrower intervertebral discs.[27] The resulting smaller joint space between vertebrae applies pressure to the spinal nerves. This can cause back, hip, or leg pain, and muscle weakness.

The Core Trunk Muscles The bones of the spinal column could not maintain our upright posture without supporting muscles. **Core muscles** include back, abdominal, hip, gluteal, pelvis, pelvic floor, and lateral trunk muscles. These muscles, located all around your body (**Figure 5.5**), are essential for supporting the spine and for performing sports, recreation, and everyday activities. The core trunk muscles work together to transmit forces between your upper and lower body. While weak core muscles can lead to back pain, strong core muscles can improve performance in all of your activities.

---

disc herniation A permanent bulging of an intervertebral disc out of its normal space

core muscles Musculature that supports the trunk (back, spine, abdomen, and hips)

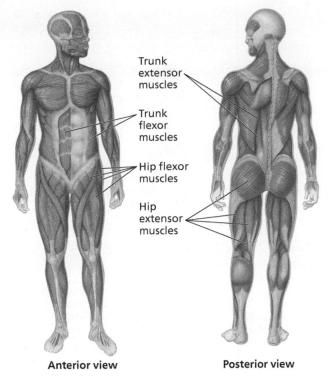

Trunk
extensor
muscles

Trunk
flexor
muscles

Hip flexor
muscles

Hip
extensor
muscles

Anterior view   **Posterior view**

FIGURE **5.5** Strengthening and stretching the spine-support-ing core muscles is essential for a healthy back. The core muscles include flexors and extensors of the trunk and hip.

Reduce Your Risk of Lower-Back Pain

You can reduce your risk of back pain by improving your body weight, muscle fitness, posture, and movement techniques. A review of multiple studies showed that exercise programs prevented back pain episodes in working-age adults, but other strategies, including shoe inserts and back supports, were not effective.[28]

Lose Weight The prevalence of lower-back pain rises with increases in body mass index or body weight and body fatness.[29] An increase in body weight puts extra strain and pressure on all the spinal structures. If the additional weight resides in the abdomen, the pelvis gets pulled forward and the resulting back curvature can cause back pain. Lowering your weight and body fat levels to recommended ranges will reduce your risk of lower-back pain.

Strengthen and Stretch Key Muscles[30] Most peo-ple's bodies have "weak" muscle areas, "tight" muscle areas, and areas that are both weak *and* tight.

- *Hip flexor muscles* tend to be tight in most people. This stems from extended sitting, resulting in short-ened and inactive muscles. If you have tight hip flexor muscles, add hip flexor stretches (see Figure 5.7 on pages 185–190) to your workout.

- *Hip extensor muscles* tend to be tight and weak, and most people will benefit from stretching and strength-ening them.

- *Trunk flexor muscles* (abdominals) are often weak in in-dividuals who are sedentary or overweight. Strengthen-ing your abdominal muscles will help protect your spine and back and improve your exercise performance.

- *Trunk extensor muscles* are responsible for keeping your spine upright while sitting, standing, and mov-ing. If you do a lot of hunched-over sitting, these mus-cles are probably weak, and you should add safe back extensor strengthening exercises to your program.

If you are predisposed to back pain, add specific back-health exercises to your current exercise routine. **Figure 5.8** (starting on page 191) illustrates back-health exercises that will help you stretch or strengthen key areas of the trunk and hips. Program 5.2: A Back-Health Exercise Program (at the end of this chapter) will help you get started.

Maintain Good Posture and Proper Body Mechanics If you have strong and flexible core trunk muscles, maintaining good posture and body mechanics

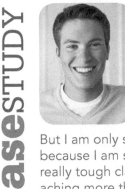

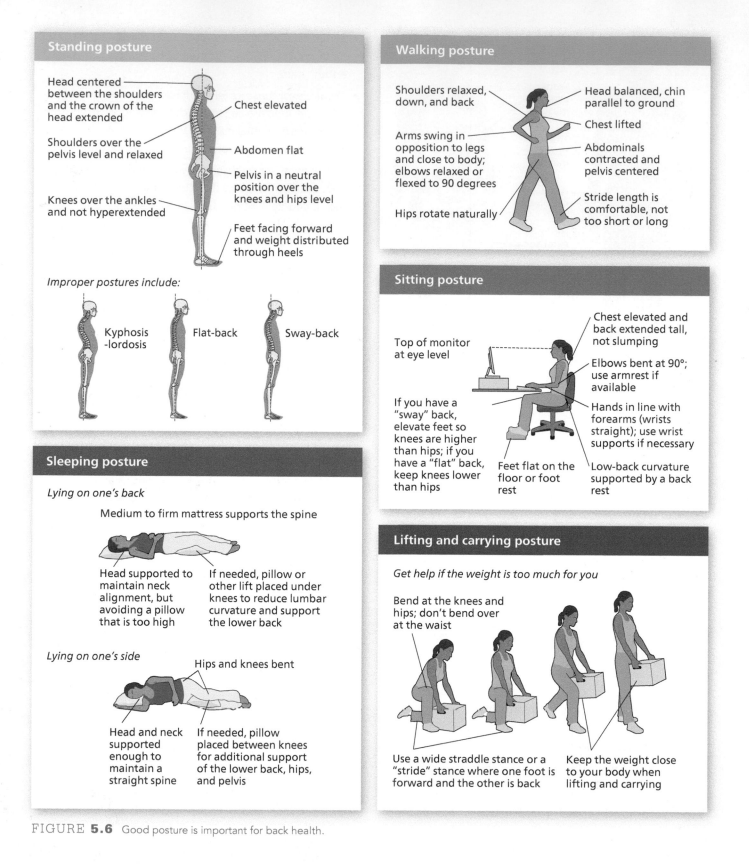

Standing posture

Head centered between the shoulders and the crown of the head extended

Shoulders over the pelvis level and relaxed

Knees over the ankles and not hyperextended

Chest elevated

Abdomen flat

Pelvis in a neutral position over the knees and hips level

Feet facing forward and weight distributed through heels

Improper postures include:

Kyphosis-lordosis

Flat-back

Sway-back

Walking posture

Shoulders relaxed, down, and back

Arms swing in opposition to legs and close to body; elbows relaxed or flexed to 90 degrees

Hips rotate naturally

Head balanced, chin parallel to ground

Chest lifted

Abdominals contracted and pelvis centered

Stride length is comfortable, not too short or long

Sitting posture

Top of monitor at eye level

If you have a "sway" back, elevate feet so knees are higher than hips; if you have a "flat" back, keep knees lower than hips

Chest elevated and back extended tall, not slumping

Elbows bent at 90°; use armrest if available

Hands in line with forearms (wrists straight); use wrist supports if necessary

Feet flat on the floor or foot rest

Low-back curvature supported by a back rest

Sleeping posture

Lying on one's back

Medium to firm mattress supports the spine

Head supported to maintain neck alignment, but avoiding a pillow that is too high

If needed, pillow or other lift placed under knees to reduce lumbar curvature and support the lower back

Lying on one's side

Hips and knees bent

Head and neck supported enough to maintain a straight spine

If needed, pillow placed between knees for additional support of the lower back, hips, and pelvis

Lifting and carrying posture

Get help if the weight is too much for you

Bend at the knees and hips; don't bend over at the waist

Use a wide straddle stance or a "stride" stance where one foot is forward and the other is back

Keep the weight close to your body when lifting and carrying

FIGURE **5.6** Good posture is important for back health.

is easier. The problem is that even with good muscular fitness, poor posture can become a habit. You might always hunch over at the computer and feel unnatural sitting up straight. Maybe you slouch when you are watching TV. Over time, poor posture can create back problems.

Poor posture and poor muscle fitness can also lead to improper body mechanics while you perform everyday activities. Poor body mechanics put you at risk of muscle strain and back pain. Lab 5.2 teaches you how to evaluate your posture, and **Figure 5.6** on this page illustrates proper postures for standing, walking, lifting, sitting, and lying down.

Properly Treat Lower-Back Pain

Do you already experience regular back pain? The GetFitGraphic Back Pain and College Students (page 181)

Do It!
Access these labs at the end of the chapter or online at MasteringHealth™.

lists some strategies for back-pain management. Incorporating your new fitness knowledge from this course will help you gain strength and stability in your key spine-supporting muscles, improve your posture, and help you maintain a healthy weight, thereby reducing your back pain or risk of back pain.

FIGURE 5.7

STRETCHES TO MAINTAIN OR INCREASE FLEXIBILITY

Perform all standing stretches from a good posture position (abs pulled in, feet facing forward, knees slightly bent). Perform all one-arm and one-leg stretches on both sides. Hold stretches for 10 to 30 seconds.

(Refer to Figure 4.8 on page 133 for the full-body muscle diagram.)

Videos for these exercises and more are available online in MasteringHealth.

UPPER-BODY STRETCHES

1 Neck Stretches

(a) Head turn: Gently turn your head to look over one shoulder, keeping both of your shoulders down.

(b) Head tilt: Keeping your chin level and your shoulders down, tilt your head to one side.

(a)
(b)

SCAN TO SEE IT
ONLINE!

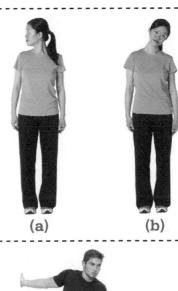

(a)   (b)

Muscles targeted:

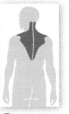

10 Trapezius

---

2 Pectoral and Biceps Stretch

Stand arm's length away from a wall. Reach your arm out to the side and place your palm flat on the wall. Turn your body away from the wall until you feel a comfortable stretch.

SCAN TO SEE IT
ONLINE!

Muscles targeted:

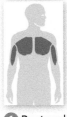

1 Pectoralis major

2 Biceps brachii

---

3 Upper-Back Stretch

Reach your arms out in front of you and clasp your hands while rounding out your back and lowering your head.

SCAN TO SEE IT
ONLINE!

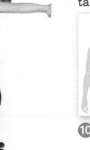

Muscles targeted:

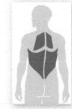

10 Trapezius   11 Rhomboids

14 Latissimus dorsi

4 Side Stretch

Reach one straight arm over your head and bend sideways at the waist. Focus on reaching up and over with your arm. The opposite hand can reach for the floor or be placed at your hip.

SCAN TO SEE IT
ONLINE!

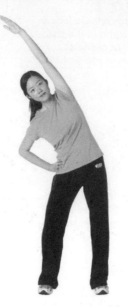

Muscles targeted:

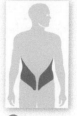

14 Latissimus dorsi

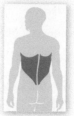

4 External obliques

5 Shoulder Stretch

Reach one arm across the chest and hold it above or below the elbow with the other hand. Keep both shoulders pressed down.

SCAN TO SEE IT
ONLINE!

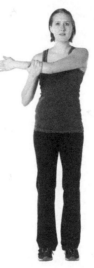

Muscles targeted:

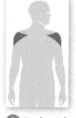

9 Deltoids

6 Triceps Stretch

Lift your arm overhead, reaching the elbow toward the ceiling and the hand down the back. Assist the stretch by using your other hand to either (a) press the arm back from the front or (b) reach over your head, grasp your arm just below the elbow, and pull back and toward your head.

 (a)

SCAN TO SEE IT
ONLINE!

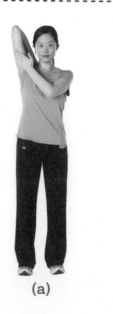

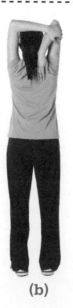

(a)   **(b)**

Muscles targeted:

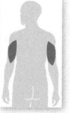

13 Triceps brachii

LOWER-BODY STRETCHES

7 Low-Back Knee-to-Chest Stretch

Lie on your back on a mat and lift either (a) one knee or (b) two knees toward the chest, grasping the leg(s) from behind for support.

(a)

SCAN TO SEE IT
ONLINE!

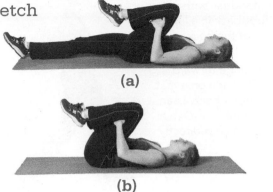

(a)

(b)

Muscles targeted:

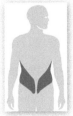

12 Erector spinae

8 Torso Twist and Hip Stretch

(a) Seated twist: Sit on a mat with your legs straight out in front of you. Bend one knee and cross that leg over your other leg. Turn your body toward the bent knee and twist your body to look behind you. Place the opposite arm on the bent leg to gently press into the stretch further.

(b) Lying cross-leg twist: While lying on your back, bend the knee and hip of one leg to 90 degrees. Keep the other leg straight and slowly move the bent leg across your body toward the floor. Keep your arms wide for balance and both shoulders down.

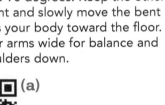

(a)

SCAN TO SEE IT
ONLINE!

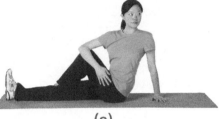

(a)

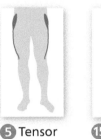

(b)

Muscles targeted:

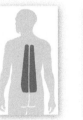

12 Erector spinae

4 External obliques

5 Tensor fasciae latae

15 Gluteus maximus

9 Gluteal Stretch

Lie on your back with one leg bent and the foot on the floor. Place the ankle of the other leg on your thigh just below the knee. Lift both legs toward the chest and support them with your hands clasped behind your thigh.

SCAN TO SEE IT
ONLINE!

Muscles targeted:

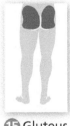

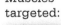

15 Gluteus maximus

10 Hip Flexor Stretch

(a) **Standing stretch:** Stand tall with one foot forward and one foot back in a lunge position. Lift up the heel of the back leg and press your hips forward.

(b) **Low-lunge stretch:** Lunge forward and gently place your back knee on a mat and release your foot to point back. Lean forward into the hip and thigh stretch but make sure that your front ankle is directly under your front knee.

 (b)

SCAN TO SEE IT
ONLINE!

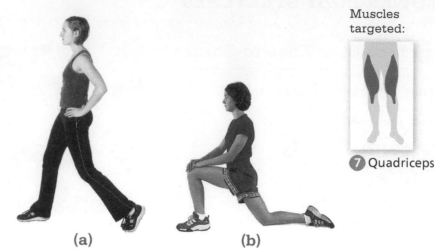

(a)   (b)

Muscles targeted:

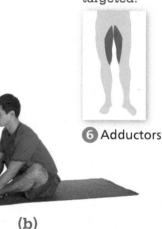

7 Quadriceps

---

11 Inner-Thigh Stretch

(a) **Side-lunge stretch:** With a wide stance, shift your weight onto one leg, bending that knee. Press your hips back to ensure that your bent knee does not extend beyond your ankle. Place your hands on your thigh, and keep your chest lifted and back straight.

(b) **Butterfly stretch:** Sitting on a mat, bring the bottoms of your feet together and pull your feet gently toward you. Actively contract your hip muscles to lower your knees closer to the ground. A slight lean forward will stretch the gluteal and low-back muscles as well.

 (b)

SCAN TO SEE IT
ONLINE!

(a)   (b)

Muscles targeted:

6 Adductors

---

12 Outer-Thigh Stretch

Stand at arm's length next to a wall. Place your outside foot on the floor closer to the wall, crossing over the inside leg. Lean your hip closer to the wall while you lean your upper body away from the wall for balance.

SCAN TO SEE IT
ONLINE!

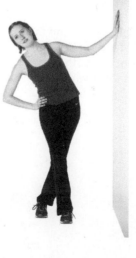

Muscles targeted:

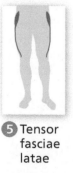

5 Tensor fasciae latae

13 Quadriceps Stretch

Grab your foot from behind and pull it back toward your rear until you feel a stretch in the front of your thighs. Maintain straight body alignment and keep your thighs parallel to one another. When (a) standing, assist your balance by holding a wall, a chair, or another form of support. The stretch can also be done from a (b) lying down position.

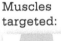 (a)

SCAN TO SEE IT
ONLINE!

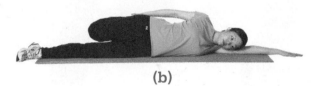

(a)

(b)

Muscles targeted:

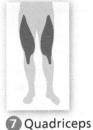

7 Quadriceps

14 Hamstrings Stretch

(a) **Modified hurdler stretch:** Sit with one leg extended and the other leg bent. The bent leg should have the knee facing sideways and the foot placed next to the extended leg near the calf, knee, or thigh. Keep your back straight and lean your body forward, moving your chest closer to your extended leg. Your hands can be placed on the floor next to your knee, calf, or ankle for support.

(b) **Supine lying:** Lying on your back, bend one knee and extend the other toward the ceiling. Support the stretch by placing your hands or a towel above or below the knee. As you become more flexible, bring your leg closer to your chest.

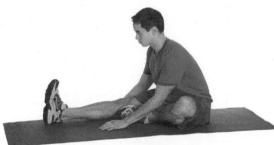

(a)

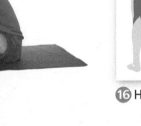

(b)

Muscles targeted:

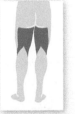

16 Hamstrings

15 Calf Stretches

(a) Gastrocnemius lunge: Lean into a wall in a lunge position, extending one leg straight behind you. Press the heel of your straight leg into the floor as you lean your body and hips into the wall.

(b) Gastrocnemius heel drop: Stand tall and place your toes on a raised surface (mat or step) that will not tip over. Balance by holding on to a wall for support as you lower your heels toward the floor.

(c) Soleus stretch: Starting in a lunge position (a), bend the back knee until you feel a stretch in the soleus muscle.

Muscles targeted:

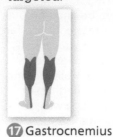 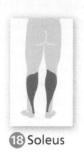

17 Gastrocnemius   **18** Soleus

 (a)

SCAN TO SEE IT
ONLINE!

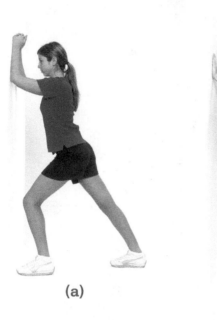

(a)   (b)   (c)

16 Shin Stretch

Reach one leg behind you and place the tips of your toes on the ground. Bend both knees and lower the body slightly as you press the top of your back foot toward the ground. Use a wall for support if needed.

SCAN TO SEE IT
ONLINE!

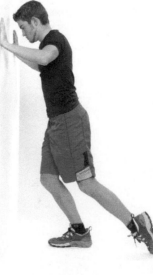

Muscles targeted:

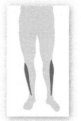

8 Tibialis anterior

FIGURE 5.8 **EXERCISES FOR A HEALTHY BACK**

Perform 3 to 10 repetitions of the back-health exercises, holding where appropriate for 10 to 30 seconds. (See Figure 4.8 on page 133 for a full-body muscle diagram.)

Videos for these exercises and more are available online in MasteringHealth.

---

1 Cat Stretch

Start on your hands and knees with a flat back. Looking at the ground, align your head with your spine. Drop your head and look back toward your knees while lifting your upper back toward the ceiling.

SCAN TO SEE IT
ONLINE!

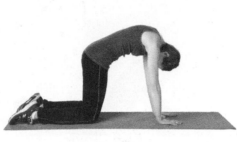

Muscles targeted:

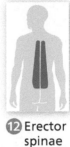

12 Erector spinae

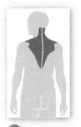

10 Trapezius; various neck muscles

---

2 Arm/Leg Extensions

Start on your hands and knees with a flat back. Looking at the ground, align your head with your spine. Extend your arm straight out in front of you while extending the opposite leg straight out behind you. Keep your arm and leg in a straight line with your spine.

SCAN TO SEE IT
ONLINE!

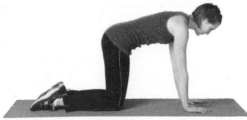

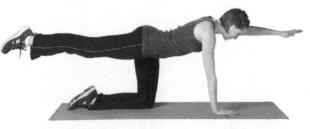

Muscles targeted:

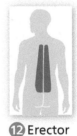

12 Erector spinae

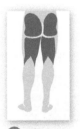

15 Gluteus maximus
16 Hamstrings

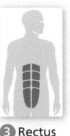

3 Rectus abdominis

③ Pelvic Tilt

Lie on your back with your knees bent and your feet flat on the floor. Relax and let the natural curve of your spine bring your lower back off the mat. Breathe out as you tilt the bottom of your pelvis toward the ceiling, pulling your abdominals in and pressing your lower back flat against the floor.

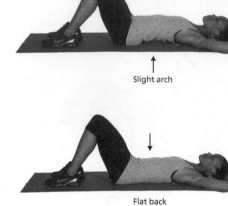

Slight arch

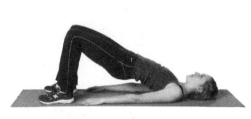

Flat back

Muscles targeted:

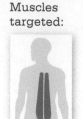 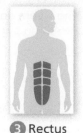

⑫ Erector spinae

③ Rectus abdominis; various hip/pelvis stabilizers

SCAN TO SEE IT
ONLINE!

④ Back Bridge

Lie on your back with your knees bent, your feet flat on the floor, and your arms extended straight along your sides. Lift your hips off the ground and press your pelvis toward the ceiling until your thighs and back are in a straight line. Avoid tucking your chin to your chest by looking at the ceiling and extending your neck.

Muscles targeted:

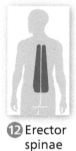 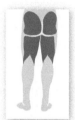

⑫ Erector spinae

⑮ Gluteus maximus
⑯ Hamstrings

SCAN TO SEE IT
ONLINE!

Other exercises that can help maintain back health include:

⑤ Plank (p. 150)

⑥ Side Bridge (p. 149)

⑦ Knee-to-Chest Stretch (p. 187)

⑧ Hamstring Stretch (p. 189)

⑨ Torso Twist and Hip Stretch (p. 187)

⑩ Hip Flexor Stretch (p. 188)

⑪ Abdominal Curl (p. 148)

⑫ Oblique Curl (p. 149)

Study Plan

chapter summary

LO 5.1 **What are the benefits of stretching and flexibility?**

- **Flexibility** is the ability of joints to move through a full **range of motion.**

- Stretching increases blood flow, enhances joint flexibility and function, decreases joint pain, lowers stress hormones, reduces your risk for lower-back pain, and helps you relax.

LO 5.2 **What determines my flexibility?**

- **Static** and **dynamic flexibility** in a particular **joint** are limited by the joint structures, the muscles and tendons that cross the joint, and the nervous system.

- Genetics, gender, age, body type, and activity level also affect flexibility.

LO 5.3 **How can I assess my flexibility?**

- Flexibility varies from joint to joint and a variety of flexibility tests are needed to assess your overall mobility.

- Joint-specific range-of-motion tests evaluate whether your joints are more or less flexible than average.

LO 5.4 **How can I plan a good stretching program?**

- Use SMART goal-setting guidelines for flexibility maintenance or improvement goals.

- Apply the FITT formula by stretching two to three days/week to the point of slight discomfort. Perform each stretch two to four times, holding 10 to 30 seconds each time.

- Choose static, dynamic, or PNF stretching techniques for all major muscle groups.

LO 5.5 **How can I avoid stretching-related injuries?**

- Increase muscle temperature via *passive* or *active heat* before stretching.

- Hold stretches for 10 seconds or more to allow receptors to make nervous-system adjustments.

- Replace contraindicated stretches with safer alternatives.

- Consider your personal limitations and health issues when selecting stretches.

LO 5.6 **Am I at risk for back pain?**

- Most back pain is caused by a *sedentary lifestyle,* and subsequent weakness and inflexibility in key muscles that affect your spine.

- Improper posture, trauma, risky sports and jobs, medical issues, and some individual health factors increase your risk.

LO 5.7 **How can I prevent or manage back pain?**

- The *spinal column* is a series of bones called *vertebrae.* *Intervertebral* discs are shock absorbers between the vertebrae, and the back, abdominal, hip, gluteal, pelvis, pelvic floor, and lateral trunk muscles all support the trunk.

- Reduce back pain by maintaining a healthy weight, improving strength and flexibility in key muscles, practicing good posture, and moving with good body mechanics.

review questions

LO 5.1 **1.** Keeping your _____ strong and flexible is associated with better balance and functional ability, plus fewer falls and injuries.
 a. hands
 b. shoulders
 c. knees
 d. ankles

LO 5.2 **2.** _____ is a measure of your overall joint stiffness during movement.
 a. Dynamic flexibility
 b. Static flexibility

 c. Passive flexibility
 d. Anatomical flexibility

LO 5.2 **3.** Which of the following triggers a muscle to relax when there is too much force or tension in the muscle?
 a. Muscle spindle
 b. Baroreceptor
 c. Golgi tendon organ
 d. Reflex receptor

LO 5.3 **4.** Since flexibility varies from joint to joint, which of the following will tell you the most about your overall body mobility?
a. The sit-and-reach test
b. Joint range-of-motion tests
c. The torso twist test
d. The back scratch test

LO 5.4 **5.** The intensity of each stretch should be stretching until you reach
a. your toes.
b. the point of tightness.
c. moderate burning pain.
d. your goal.

LO 5.4 **6.** Stretching that involves voluntary muscle contractions to facilitate relaxation describes
a. static stretching.
b. dynamic stretching.
c. ballistic stretching.
d. PNF stretching.

LO 5.5 **7.** Which of the following should you always do prior to stretching?
a. Drink 8 oz of water.
b. Run for 10 minutes.
c. Warm up your muscles with active or passive heat.
d. Take three to five deep breaths.

LO 5.6 **8.** Which of the following is the primary underlying cause of low-back pain?
a. Poor posture
b. Sedentary living
c. Muscle weakness
d. Poor flexibility

LO 5.7 **9.** What should you do first when attempting to lift or carry a heavy weight?
a. Keep the weight close to your body.
b. Bend at the knees and hips.
c. Use a straddle or stride stance.
d. Get help if the weight is too much for you.

LO 5.7 **10.** Which of the following acute back pain self-care treatments is not recommended?
a. Five days of bed rest
b. Light exercise
c. Pain relievers
d. Cold and hot treatments

critical thinking questions

LO 5.1 **1.** How does stretching contribute to muscle relaxation and stress relief?

LO 5.2 **2.** Explain how individual factors (genetics, gender, age, body type, activity level, and health status) affect flexibility levels.

LO 5.4 **3.** Have you ever done or been asked to do a contraindicated stretch? What would be an equally effective alternative?

LO 5.6 **4.** List three occupations that present high risk for low-back pain and explain why.

check out these eResources

- **Arthritis Foundation** Information for everyone seeking to relieve pain, prevent arthritis, or start exercise. Click on "Living with Arthritis," then "Exercise," and "Videos" or "Workouts" for stretching, yoga, and core workout ideas. **www.arthritis.org**
- **Harvard Health** Solid information about living a healthier life. Click on "Pain" and then select "Back Pain" for a collection of helpful articles and tips for back pain relief and prevention. **www.health.harvard.edu**
- **Sports Fitness Advisor** Click on "Flexibility Training" in the "Fitness Elements" section and then scroll down to articles about flexibility training, including self-myofascial release exercises. **www.sport-fitness-advisor.com**
- **Top End Sports** A collection of test protocols for assessing flexibility in the upper and lower body. **www.topendsports.com/testing/flex.htm**
- **Yoga Journal** Browse yoga poses by benefit to find "Yoga for Flexibility": pictures of yoga poses that enhance flexibility. **www.yogajournal.com**

DO IT!

LAB
5.1

ASSESS YOURSELF

ASSESS YOUR FLEXIBILITY

MasteringHealth™

Name: _____ **Date:** _____

Instructor: _____ **Section:** _____

Materials: Exercise mat, sit-and-reach box, a partner

Purpose: To assess your current level of lower-back, hip, and hamstring flexibility and your current level of joint mobility or range of motion.

Section I: The Sit-and-Reach Test

This test measures the general flexibility of your low back, hips, and hamstrings. The results are specific to those regions of your body and do not reflect your flexibility in other body areas.

1. **Warm-up.** Complete 3 to 10 minutes of light cardiorespiratory activity to warm up your body and then perform light range-of-motion exercises and stretches for the joints and muscles that you will be using.

2. **Prepare for the test:**

SCAN TO SEE IT
ONLINE!

Place the sit-and-reach box against a wall to prevent it from moving during the test. Sit without shoes behind the box, place your feet flat against the box at the 26 cm mark (the "zero" or foot mark for this test), and put your hands on top of the box.

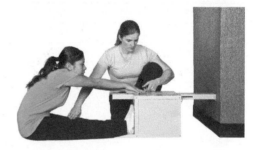

3. **Properly perform the test.** Place one hand on top of the other and keep the fingertips of both hands together. Keeping contact with the box, slowly bend forward, reach with your arms, and slide your fingertips out along the box as far as you can. Keep your legs straight, drop your head, and breathe out as you perform the test. Hold your ending position for at least two seconds. Your partner will watch to ensure that you have proper hand position and straight legs during the test.

4. **Find your reach distance.** Your *reach distance* is the most distant point reached with both fingertips. If you cannot keep your hands from separating, the most distant point reached by the fingertips of the *hand that is farthest back* should be considered the reach distance. Record the reach distance in centimeters. Perform the test twice and record your best reach distance of the two trials in the RESULTS section on the next page.

FLEXIBILITY RESULTS

Box Sit-and-Reach Test: Reach Distance (cm): _____   Rating: _____

5. **Find your flexibility rating by using the charts provided below.** Your rating tells you how you compare to others who have completed this test in the past. Record your rating in the RESULTS section above.

BOX Sit-and-Reach Test (centimeters)					
Men (age in years)	**Excellent**	**Very Good**	**Good**	**Fair**	**Needs Improvement**
15–19	≥39	34–38	29–33	24–28	≤23
20–29	≥40	34–39	30–33	25–29	≤24
30–39	≥38	33–37	28–32	23–27	≤22
40–49	≥35	29–34	24–28	18–23	≤17
50–59	≥35	28–34	24–27	16–23	≤15
60–69	≥33	25–32	20–24	15–19	≤14
Women (age in years)	**Excellent**	**Very Good**	**Good**	**Fair**	**Needs Improvement**
15–19	≥43	38–42	34–37	29–33	≤28
20–29	≥41	37–40	33–36	28–32	≤27
30–39	≥41	36–40	32–35	27–31	≤26
40–49	≥38	34–37	30–33	25–29	≤24
50–59	≥39	33–38	30–32	25–29	≤24
60–69	≥35	31–34	27–30	23–26	≤22

Source: *Canadian Physical Activity, Fitness & Lifestyle Approach: CSEP-Health & Fitness Program's Health-Related Appraisal & Counseling Strategy,* 3rd edition © 2003. Reprinted with permission from the Canadian Society for Exercise Physiology.

SCAN TO SEE IT ONLINE!

Section II: Joint Mobility—Range-of-Motion Tests

Range-of-motion tests assess your joints' ability to move through a normal range of motion. Follow the instructions for each of the tests shown below. Perform each test on both your right and left sides. Stop each movement when you feel resistance. To avoid injury, do not try to push past your normal range. Have a partner observe your movements, "eyeball" your estimated joint angle, and record your range-of-motion results on the next page.

1. Neck Lateral Flexion: Sit or stand with your head neutral and looking forward. Tilt your head to the side and drop your ear toward your shoulder.

Average range 0–45°
0°
45°

2. Shoulder Flexion: Starting with your arms at your sides, reach a straight arm forward and up toward your head.

180°
Average range 0–180°
0°

3. Shoulder Extension: With your arms at your sides, reach a straight arm behind you and up.

0°
50°
Average range 0–50°

4. Shoulder Abduction: Reach your straight arm out to the side and up to your head.

180°
Average range 0–180°
0°

5. Shoulder Adduction: Reach your straight arm down and across your body in front.

0°
50°
Average range 0–50°

6. Trunk Lateral Flexion: Standing upright with slightly bent knees and your arms at your sides, bend your torso sideways and reach your arm down your leg for support.

25°
0° Average range 0–25°

7. Hip Flexion: Lying on your back, lift a straight leg up into the air while keeping the other leg bent with the foot flat on the ground.

8. Hip Extension: Lying on your stomach with your head on the mat, reach your straight leg up behind you, keeping the other leg flat on the ground.

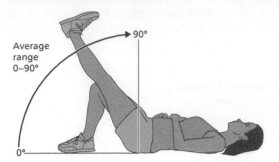

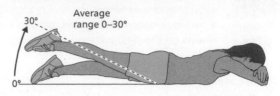

9. Hip Abduction: Standing upright with slightly bent knees, reach your straight leg out to the side.

10. Ankle Dorsiflexion: Sitting without shoes and your legs extended in front of you, flex your foot back toward your knee.

11. Ankle Plantar Flexion: Sitting without shoes and your legs extended in front of you, point your foot toward the floor.

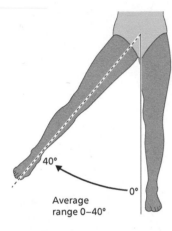

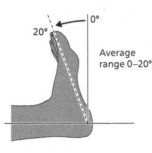

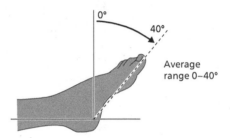

Joint Mobility RESULTS				
		Full Average Joint Range?		
Joint	**Movement and Average Range (degrees)**	**Right Side**		**Left Side**
1. Neck	Lateral Flexion 0–45	___ Yes ___ No		___ Yes ___ No
2. Shoulder	Flexion 0–180	___ Yes ___ No		___ Yes ___ No
3. Shoulder	Extension 0–50	___ Yes ___ No		___ Yes ___ No
4. Shoulder	Abduction 0–180	___ Yes ___ No		___ Yes ___ No
5. Shoulder	Adduction 0–50	___ Yes ___ No		___ Yes ___ No
6. Trunk	Lateral Flexion 0–25	___ Yes ___ No		___ Yes ___ No
7. Hip	Flexion 0–90	___ Yes ___ No		___ Yes ___ No
8. Hip	Extension 0–30	___ Yes ___ No		___ Yes ___ No
9. Hip	Abduction 0–40	___ Yes ___ No		___ Yes ___ No
10. Ankle	Dorsiflexion 0–20	___ Yes ___ No		___ Yes ___ No
11. Ankle	Plantar Flexion 0–40	___ Yes ___ No		___ Yes ___ No

Sources: Adapted from American College of Sports Medicine, *ACSM's Health-Related Physical Fitness Assessment Manual,* 4th ed. (Baltimore, MD: Lippincott Williams & Wilkins, 2014); American College of Sports Medicine, *ACSM's Resource Manual for Guidelines for Exercise Testing and Prescription,* 7th ed. (Baltimore, MD: Lippincott Williams & Wilkins, 2014).

*Note: Your flexibility ratings should help guide your flexibility program selections. See Lab 5.3 and Program 5.1: A Flexibility Training Program (at the end of this chapter) for more information.

Section III: Reflection

1. Were your flexibility and range-of-motion results what you expected? Why or why not?

_____

_____

_____

_____

_____

2. Based upon your flexibility assessment results, is your basic plan to maintain or improve flexibility?

_____

_____

_____

_____

_____

DO IT!

LAB
5.2

ASSESS YOURSELF

EVALUATE YOUR POSTURE

MasteringHealth™

Name: _____ **Date:** _____

Instructor: _____ **Section:** _____

Materials: Exercise mat, sit-and-reach box, a partner

Purpose: To evaluate your posture.

Section I: Posture Evaluation

Before you begin: Wear clothing that will not interfere with the assessment of your posture. If it is comfortable, men should wear shorts only, and women should wear shorts and a tank top. Remove your shoes. If you have long hair, pull it back into a ponytail for the assessment.

Stand against a wall and have a partner evaluate your posture using the chart on page 201. Your partner should assign you a score of 1 to 5 for each of the 10 areas of your body shown here.

SCAN TO SEE IT
ONLINE!

Posture Results	
Posture Score	*Posture Rating*
45 or higher	Excellent
40–44	Good
30–39	Average
20–29	Fair
19 or less	Poor

Source: Based on the Division of Physical Education and Research, State University of New York, *New York State Physical Fitness Test for Boys and Girls Grades 4–12. A Manual for Teachers of Physical Education* (Albany, NY: New York State Education Department, 1972).

*Note: Your posture ratings should help guide your program selections. For more information, see Program 5.2: A Back-Health Exercise Program at the end of this chapter.

Section II: Reflection

1. Did your partner find anything surprising to you about your posture? If so, why do you think you were not aware of it?

_____

_____

2. Based upon your posture evaluation results, is your basic plan to maintain or improve your posture?

_____

_____

	Good—5	Fair—3	Poor—1	Score
Head	Head erect, gravity passes directly through center	Head twisted or turned to one side slightly	Head twisted or turned to one side markedly	
Shoulders	Shoulders level horizontally	One shoulder slightly higher	One shoulder markedly higher	
Spine	Spine straight	Spine slightly curved	Spine markedly curved laterally	
Hips	Hips level horizontally	One hip slightly higher	One hip markedly higher	
Knees and Ankles	Feet pointed straight ahead, legs vertical	Feet pointed out, legs deviating outward at the knee	Feet pointed out markedly, legs deviated markedly	
Neck and Upper back	Neck erect, head in line with shoulders, rounded upper back	Neck slightly foward, chin out, slightly more rounded upper back	Neck markedly forward, chin markedly out, markedly rounded upper back	
Trunk	Trunk erect	Trunk inclined to rear slightly	Trunk inclined to rear markedly	
Abdomen	Abdomen flat	Abdomen protruding	Abdomen protruding and sagging	
Lower back	Lower back normally curved	Lower back slightly hollow	Lower back markedly hollow	
Legs	Legs straight	Knees slightly hyperextended	Knees markedly hyperextended	
			Total score	

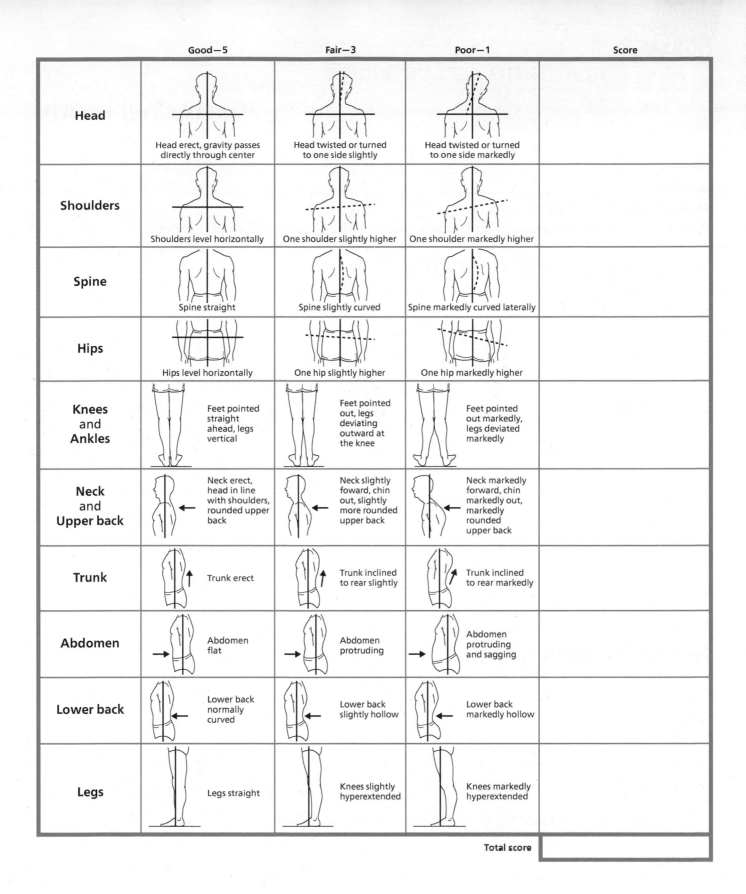

Name: _____ **Date:** _____

Instructor: _____ **Section:** _____

Materials: Results from Labs 5.1 and 5.2

Purpose: To learn how to set appropriate flexibility goals and create a personal flexibility program.

Section I: Short- and Long-Term Goals

Create short- and long-term goals for flexibility and back health. Be sure to use SMART goal-setting guidelines. Select appropriate target dates and rewards for completing your goals.

Short-Term Goal for Flexibility (3 to 6 months)

_____

_____

Target Date: _____

Reward: _____

Optional: Short-Term Goal for Back Health (3 to 6 months)

_____

_____

Target Date: _____

Reward: _____

Long-Term Goal for Flexibility (12+ months)

_____

_____

Target Date: _____

Reward: _____

Optional: Long-Term Goal for Back Health (12+ months)

_____

_____

Target Date: _____

Reward: _____

Section II: Flexibility Program Design

Complete one line for each exercise you have chosen to do in your program.

Review **Programs 5.1** and **5.2** (after this lab) for flexibility and back-health training.

Stretching Exercises	Frequency (days/week)	Time (sec)	Reps (number)	Total Time (sec)
LOWER BODY				
1.				
2.				
3.				
4.				
5.				
6.				
7.				
8.				
UPPER BODY				
1.				
2.				
3.				
4.				
5.				
6.				
7.				
8.				

Section III: Tracking Your Program and Following Through

1. **Goal and Program Tracking:** Use the following chart or a web/app activity log to monitor your progress. Change the frequency, time, sets, and reps frequently to ensure continuing progress toward your goals.

2. **Goal and Program Follow-up:** At the end of the course or at your short-term goal target date, re-evaluate your flexibility and answer the following questions:

a. Did you meet your short-term goal or your goal for the course? _____

b. If so, what positive behavioral changes contributed to your success? If not, which obstacles blocked your success?

_____

_____

c. Was your short-term goal realistic? After evaluating your progress during the course, what would you change about your goals or training plan?

_____

_____

Flexibility Training Log

Date	Stretches Completed (with time/reps)	Comments (e.g., stretches modified, stretches held longer, how you felt)

Activate, Motivate, & Advance YOUR FITNESS

ACTIVATE!

Looking to improve your posture, circulation, and joint mobility? Follow these programs to incorporate regular stretching into your weekly exercise routines.

What Do I Need for Flexibility Training?

GEAR: For flexibility training programs, you'll want a mat, towel, and something stable to hold onto for standing stretches. While you really don't need any other equipment, you may want to use a strap, foam roller, yoga block, or even a training partner.

CLOTHING: Wear comfortable clothing that allows for full range-of-motion movements.

How Do I Start a Flexibility Training Program?

TECHNIQUE: Ensure proper form, posture, and body alignment while stretching. Read through each exercise description for specific technique tips. If you need assistance, ask your instructor or a fitness specialist at your facility. Ease into the first repetition of each stretch exercise and hold at the point of tightness but not pain. Exhale with the stretch to help you relax and increase your flexibility.

ETIQUETTE: Most facilities have mats, equipment, and a designated stretching area for you to use. Wipe down your mat and any other equipment after use.

STRETCHING BEFORE A WORKOUT: Dynamic stretching performed during your warm-up can prepare your body for the upcoming more intense activity. Incorporate slow and controlled movements that mimic the motions of your workout.

STRETCHING AFTER A WORKOUT: After your workout, your muscles are warm and ready to be stretched. Static or PNF stretching performed at this time will result in the biggest gains in flexibility.

Flexibility Training Warm-Up and Cool-Down

Warming-up prior to stretching is crucial and should include gentle cardiorespiratory exercises for 3 to 10 minutes. After breaking a light sweat, add dynamic movements that increase your range of motion.

Flexibility Training Programs

Adjust intensity, volume, and training days to suit your personal fitness level and schedule.

Start here if your Lab 5.1 ratings were Fair or Needs Improvement, if you are new to flexibility training, or if you have not stretched for more than three months.

GOAL: Incorporate a full-body stretching routine into weekly schedule

Frequency	Intensity	Time	Number and Type of Stretches
2 non-consecutive days a week	Stretch to a point of mild tightness, not pain	Perform 2 to 3 repetitions of each stretch, holding for 10 to 20 seconds each time	8 static stretches

Order of Stretches

Side Stretch

Upper-Back Stretch

Pectoral and Biceps Stretch

Inner-Thigh Side Lunge

Quadriceps Stretch (Standing)

Hamstrings Stretch (Supine Lying)

Low-Back Knee-to-Chest Stretch (Two Knees)

Calf Stretch (Gastrocnemius Lunge)

INTERMEDIATE FLEXIBILITY PROGRAM

Start here if your Lab 5.1 ratings were Good or if you already stretch two days a week.

GOAL: Improve full-body range of motion and overall physical function

Frequency	Intensity	Time	Number and Type of Stretches
3 non-consecutive days a week	Stretch to a point of mild tightness, not pain	Perform 2 to 4 repetitions of each stretch, holding for 20 to 30 seconds each time	12 static stretches

Order of Stretches

Neck Stretches (Head Turn)

Side Stretch

Upper-Back Stretch

Shoulder Stretch

Pectoral and Biceps Stretch

Inner-Thigh Side Lunge

Outer-Thigh Stretch

Quadriceps Stretch (Lying)

Hamstrings Stretch (Supine Lying)

Low-Back Knee-to-Chest Stretch (Two Knees)

Gluteal Stretch

Calf Stretch (Heel Drop)

MOTIVATE!

It can be motivating to track your flexibility training program—make note of days, actual stretches, type of stretch, repetitions, and time held. Here are a few additional tips to keep you stretching:

FIND A PARTNER: With a stretching partner, you can keep each other accountable, help each other reach goals, and have greater options when incorporating PNF stretches, as well as a wider variety of both passive and active stretches. Bye-bye boredom!

TRY A NEW CLASS: Find classes near you specifically designed for stretching, foam rolling, core strength, and/or back health. You can also try a yoga or martial arts class that have flexibility exercises built right in! Learn something new, meet new people, and keep "reaching" toward your goals.

STRESS? WHAT STRESS? Take a deep breath. Exhale. Slowly move into your stretch. Hold for at least 10 seconds. Repeat three more times. Before you know it, you will feel refreshed and relaxed from head to toe. The simple act of performing your flexibility program can increase your circulation, decrease your blood pressure, and keep you calm and focused. Stretch more, stress less!

ADVANCE!

Are you training for a specific sport or activity? Here are flexibility programs specific for walkers/runners, cyclists, and swimmers. Once you've established your flexibility program and your Lab 5.1 ratings are Good, try out one of these sport-specific programs.

WALKING/RUNNING FLEXIBILITY PROGRAM

GOAL: Add stretches of specific use for walkers and runners

Frequency	Intensity	Time	Number and Type of Stretches
3 non-consecutive days a week	Stretch to a point of mild tightness, not pain	Perform 2 to 4 repetitions of each stretch, holding for 20 to 30 seconds each time	5 additional static stretches*

Perform after a walking/running cardiorespiratory workout, and in addition to the Intermediate Flexibility Program.

Stretches to Add
Hip Flexor Stretch (Standing for walkers and Low Lunge for runners)
Torso Twist and Hip Stretch (Seated Twist)

Hamstrings Stretch (Modified Hurdler)
Calf Stretch (Soleus Stretch)
Shin Stretch

CYCLING FLEXIBILITY PROGRAM

GOAL: Add stretches of specific use for cyclists

Frequency	Intensity	Time	Number and Type of Stretches
3 non-consecutive days a week	Stretch to a point of mild tightness, not pain	Perform 2 to 4 repetitions of each stretch, holding for 20 to 30 seconds each time	5 additional static stretches*

Perform after a cycling cardiorespiratory workout, and in addition to the Intermediate Flexibility Program.

Stretches to Add
Neck Stretches (Head Tilt)
Hip Flexor Stretch (Standing or Low Lunge)
Torso Twist and Hip Stretch (Seated Twist)

Calf Stretch (Soleus Stretch)
Shin Stretch

SWIMMING FLEXIBILITY PROGRAM

GOAL: Add stretches of specific use for swimmers

Frequency	Intensity	Time	Number and Type of Stretches
3 non-consecutive days a week	Stretch to a point of mild tightness, not pain	Perform 2 to 4 repetitions of each stretch, holding for 20 to 30 seconds each time	5 additional static stretches*

Perform after a swimming cardiorespiratory workout, and in addition to the Intermediate Flexibility Program.

Stretches to Add
Neck Stretches (Head Tilt)
Triceps Stretch
Hip Flexor Stretch (Standing)

Torso Twist and Hip Stretch (Seated Twist)
Shin Stretch

Activate, Motivate, & Advance **YOUR FITNESS**

Want to avoid back pain or manage pain you may already have? Try this program designed to help you strengthen your core trunk muscles and decrease tightness. Combine the Core Muscular Endurance and Core Flexibility programs for a complete back-health program. The exercises are designed to be incorporated into your current muscular fitness and flexibility programs.

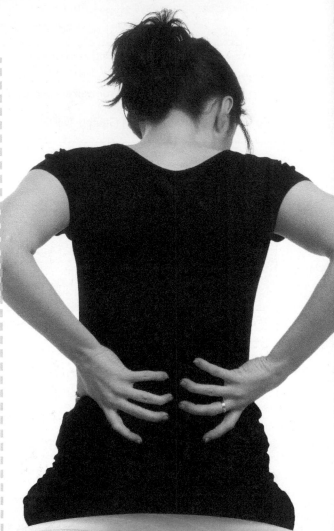

CORE MUSCULAR ENDURANCE PROGRAM FOR BACK HEALTH

GOAL: Increase core muscle endurance and strength

Frequency	Intensity	Time			Number and Type of Exercises
		Reps	*Sets*	*Rest*	
2 non-consecutive days a week	60% 1 RM	12	2	2 minutes between sets	8 core muscle exercises

Core Strength Exercises

Arm/Leg Extensions
Plank (hold each plank for 15 to 30 seconds and complete 2 to 4 repetitions)
Back Extension
Abdominal Curl

Reverse Curl
Oblique Curl
Pelvic Tilt
Side Bridge (hold each side bridge for 15 seconds and complete 4 repetitions)

CORE FLEXIBILITY PROGRAM FOR BACK HEALTH

GOAL: Decrease core muscle tightness

Frequency	Intensity	Time	Number and Type of Exercises
2 non-consecutive days a week	Stretch to a point of mild tightness, not pain	Perform 2 to 4 repetitions of each stretch, holding for 10 to 30 seconds each time	8 core stretch exercises

Core Stretches

Back Bridge
Low-Back Knee-to-Chest Stretch (Two Knees)
Gluteal Stretch
Hamstrings Stretch (Supine Lying)

Quadriceps Stretch (Lying)
Torso Twist and Hip Stretch (Seated Twist)
Cat Stretch
Hip Flexor Stretch (Low Lunge)

6 Understanding Body Composition

LEARNINGoutcomes

LO 6.1 Articulate the difference between body weight and body composition.

LO 6.2 Discuss how body composition is related to lifelong fitness and wellness.

LO 6.3 Evaluate your BMI, body circumferences, and body shape.

LO 6.4 Describe the tests used to assess body composition.

LO 6.5 Set and continually reevaluate goals to reach your healthy body fat percentage.

MasteringHealth™

Go online for chapter quizzes, interactive assessments, videos, and more!

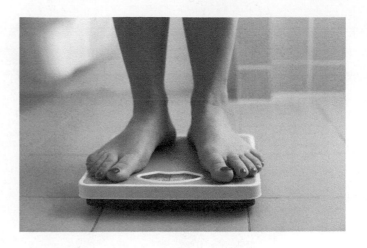

CASESTUDY

DANI

"Hi, I'm Dani. I started running and resistance training two months ago and feel great! I like the new muscle tone in my legs, and I've made a lot of friends from the running group I joined. The ironic thing is, I started working out mainly because I wanted to lose weight, but I actually weigh a little bit more right now than I did when I first started. It doesn't make any sense to me because my clothes fit better and I look more 'toned.' I've heard that muscle weighs more than fat, but that doesn't make any sense, either— doesn't a pound of muscle weigh the same as a pound of fat?"

Hear It!

To listen to this case study online, visit the Study Area in MasteringHealth™.

Do you know how much you weigh? Most people do. Do you know how much of your body is fat? Most people don't. In fact, it's impossible to get an exact answer to that question, but you can estimate it—and it's important. Using the scale as your only guide for body changes will limit your ability to set realistic weight loss goals.

In this chapter, you will learn about the components of body composition and why body size, shape, and composition are useful measurements of fitness and wellness. You'll also learn how each of these measurements is determined and how you can change or maintain your body composition. (In Chapter 8, you will combine your knowledge of physical activity, body composition, and diet to create your own weight-management plan.)

LO 6.1 How Do Body Weight and Body Composition Differ?

Using a scale to monitor your weight regularly is helpful, but don't focus on body weight exclusively. Knowing the amounts of lean and fat tissue that make up your overall body weight (your **body composition**) is an important tool for setting healthy body goals. A healthy body composition is an important determinant of overall health.

Estimating body composition involves determining your lean body mass, fat mass, and percent body fat. Your **lean body mass** is your body's total amount of lean or fat-free tissue (muscles, bones, skin, other organs, and body fluids). Your **fat mass** is body mass made up of fat (adipose) tissue. **Percent body fat** is the percentage of your total weight that is fat tissue—that is, the weight of fat divided by total body weight.

All fat tissue can be labeled as either essential fat or storage fat. **Essential fat** is necessary for normal body functioning; it includes fats in the brain, muscles, nerves, bones, lungs, heart, and digestive and reproductive systems. Men need a minimum of 3 to 5 percent essential body fat. Women need significantly more (12 percent essential body fat) because of reproductive system-related fat deposits in their breasts, uterus, and elsewhere (**Figure 6.1**, page 212). **Storage fat** is nonessential fat stored in tissue near the body's surface and around major body organs. Storage fat provides energy, insulation, and padding. Men and women have similar amounts of storage fat but may differ in the location of larger fat stores. Your individual amount of storage fat depends upon many factors, including your lifestyle and genetics.

---

body composition The relative amounts of fat and lean tissue in the body

lean body mass Body mass that is fat-free (muscle, skin, bone, organs, and body fluids)

fat mass Body mass that is fat tissue (adipose tissue)

percent body fat Percentage of total weight that is fat tissue

essential fat Body fat that is essential for normal physiological functioning

storage fat Body fat that is not essential but does provide energy, insulation, and padding

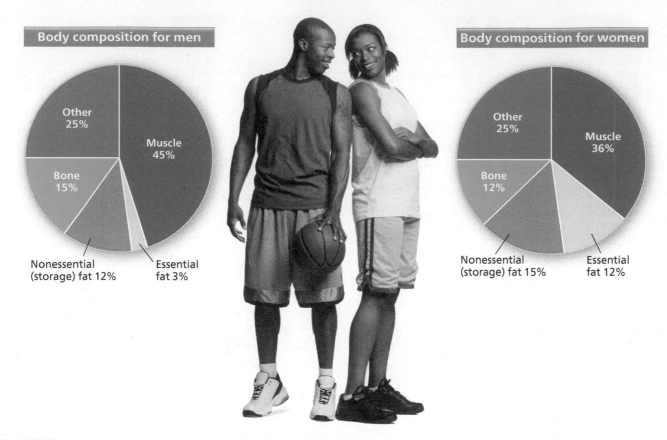

FIGURE **6.1** The body compositions of typical 20- to 24-year-old men and women vary primarily in the amounts of muscle and essential fat.

Data from: W. D. McArdle et al., *Exercise Physiology: Energy, Nutrition, and Human Performance*, 8th ed. (Baltimore, MD: Lippincott Williams & Wilkins, 2014).

LO 6.2 Why Do My Body Size, Shape, and Composition Matter?

Body size, shape, and composition encompass more than how you look. They are important components (and measurements) of your overall fitness and wellness.

Knowing Your Body Composition Can Help You Assess Your Health Risks

From the mid-1970s to 2012, the number of overweight children and adolescents increased from 5 to 15 percent of the US population![1] This is a problem because childhood obesity significantly increases your risk for cardiovascular disease and premature death and disability in adulthood.[2] Although research indicates that obesity rates have leveled off in recent years, current numbers of obese adults are extremely high, with more than 68 percent of US adults being overweight or obese. Of those, approximately 35 percent are classified as obese![3]

Studies of obesity often rely on measurements of total body weight rather than measurements of body composition. Total body weight is useful in studying large populations; however, it is less useful in assessing an individual's health risks and body changes. By knowing your percent body fat, you can more effectively determine your risks for chronic disease and decide just how much weight you should lose (or gain).

Evaluating Your Body Size and Shape Can Help Motivate Healthy Behavior Change

If you are just beginning an exercise program, it is often more useful to measure your progress by assessing changes in body size and shape, rather than weighing yourself daily on a bathroom scale. The reason: Healthy increases in muscle tissue (achieved by exercise) may cause you to temporarily gain weight even as your body size decreases, until the process of body fat loss catches up with muscle tissue gains. This is a *good* thing, but you would not know it if you relied solely on the scale to determine your progress. By monitoring improvements in your body size and shape instead, you can get a more realistic sense of your achievement and stay motivated to stick with an exercise program. The Q&A box What Is Muscle Tone and How Is It Related to Body Composition? on page 216 discusses muscle mass, body fat, and the term "muscle tone."

LO 6.3 How Can I Evaluate My Body Size and Shape?

How do you determine whether your body size and shape are "healthy"? There are three common methods: calculating your body mass index, measuring your body circumferences, and identifying the patterns of fat distribution on your body. (Evaluating your body composition is a somewhat more complicated process, which we discuss later in this chapter.)

Calculate Your Body Mass Index but Understand Its Limitations

Body mass index (BMI) is one of the most common measurements that doctors and researchers use to assess risk of weight-related disease, death, and disability.[4] BMI is a measurement based on your weight and height. You can calculate your BMI now, using the chart in **Figure 6.2**. As shown in **Figure 6.3** on page 214, very low and very high BMI scores are correlated with greater risk of death and disability.[5]

The limitation with using BMI scores to assess "fitness" or "fatness" is that they do not differentiate between fat mass and lean mass. BMI is solely determined by height and weight. While BMI measurements can be helpful for individuals of average muscle and bone density, they can be misleading for athletes, bodybuilders, children, older adults, and short or petite individuals. For instance, people who have exceptionally heavy skeletons and larger-than-average muscle mass may have BMI scores that classify them as "overweight," even if their percent body fat is in the "healthy" range. Because of BMI's limitations, consider other factors, such as percent body fat, when assessing your overall health and fitness. **Lab 6.1** at the end of this chapter walks you through how to calculate your own BMI.

Do It!
 Access these labs at the end of the chapter or online at MasteringHealth™.

Measure Your Body Circumferences

If you want to gain or lose weight, you can measure the circumference of your waist, hips, neck, upper arm, chest, thigh, and calf and then monitor changes in your body over time. You can also use waist and hip circumferences to assess disease risk.

> **body mass index (BMI)** A number calculated from a person's weight and height that is used to assess risk for health problems

Weight (pounds)

Height (feet and inches)	100	110	120	130	140	150	160	170	180	190	200	210	220	230	240	250	260
4'6"	24	27	29	31	34	36	39	41	43	46	48	51	53	55	58	60	63
4'8"	22	25	27	29	31	34	36	38	40	43	45	47	49	52	54	56	58
4'10"	21	23	25	27	29	31	33	36	38	40	42	44	46	48	50	52	54
5'0"	20	22	23	25	27	29	31	33	35	37	39	41	43	45	47	49	51
5'2"	18	20	22	24	26	27	29	31	33	35	37	38	40	42	44	46	48
5'4"	17	19	21	22	24	26	28	29	31	33	34	36	38	40	41	43	45
5'6"	16	18	19	21	23	24	26	27	29	31	32	34	36	37	39	40	42
5'8"	15	17	18	20	21	23	24	26	27	29	30	32	33	35	37	38	40
5'10"	14	16	17	19	20	22	23	24	26	27	29	30	32	33	34	36	37
6'0"	14	15	16	18	19	20	22	23	24	26	27	29	30	31	33	34	35
6'2"	13	14	15	17	18	19	21	22	23	24	26	27	28	30	31	32	33
6'4"	12	13	15	16	17	18	20	21	22	23	24	26	27	28	29	30	32
6'6"	12	13	14	15	16	17	19	20	21	22	23	24	25	27	28	29	30
6'8"	11	12	13	14	15	17	18	19	20	21	22	23	24	25	26	28	29
6'10"	11	12	13	14	15	16	17	18	19	20	21	22	23	24	25	26	27
7'0"	10	11	12	13	14	15	16	17	18	19	20	21	22	23	24	25	26

Key:
- Underweight (<18.5)
- Normal weight (18.5–24.9)
- Overweight (25.0–29.9)
- Obese: Class I (30.0–34.9)
- Obese: Class II (35.0–39.9)
- Obese: Class III (>40.0)

FIGURE **6.2** Estimate your BMI by finding where your weight and height intersect.

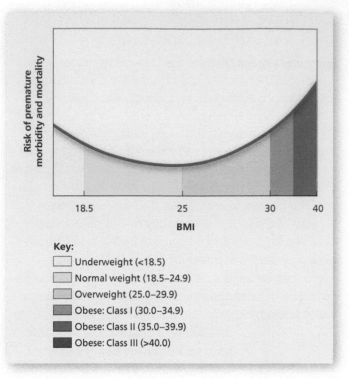

FIGURE **6.3** Extremely low or extremely high BMIs are associated with a greater risk of premature death and disability.

Data from: K. Flegal et al., "Excess Deaths Associated with Underweight, Overweight, and Obesity," *Journal of the American Medical Association* 293, no. 15 (2005): 1861–67.

Key:
- Underweight (<18.5)
- Normal weight (18.5–24.9)
- Overweight (25.0–29.9)
- Obese: Class I (30.0–34.9)
- Obese: Class II (35.0–39.9)
- Obese: Class III (>40.0)

As shown in **Table 6.1** on page 215, waist circumference (a marker of abdominal fat) can indicate greater risk of diabetes, high blood pressure, and heart disease if it is greater than 102 cm in males or 88 cm in females.[6] As the table also shows, the people at greatest risk are those with high waist circumferences *and* high BMIs.

waist-to-hip ratio (WHR) Waist circumference divided by hip circumference

android Body shape described as "apple-shaped," with excess body fat distributed primarily on the upper body and trunk

gynoid Body shape described as "pear-shaped," where excess body fat is distributed primarily on the lower body (hips and thighs)

subcutaneous fat Adipose tissue that is located just below the surface of the skin

visceral fat Adipose tissue that surrounds organs in the abdomen

You can also use waist and hip circumferences to determine your waist-to-hip ratio (WHR). **Waist-to-hip ratio** is your waist circumference divided by your hip circumference. Young men with a WHR of 0.94 or more and young women with a WHR of 0.82 or more fall into a high-risk category.[7] Although waist circumference and WHR are both

measures of disease risk, waist circumference is generally preferred because it is simpler, because of its relationship with abdominal fat, and because of its strong association to disease risk factors.[8] **Lab 6.2** (at the end of this chapter) will walk you through the process of measuring your body circumferences and determining your WHR.

Do It!
Access these labs at the end of the chapter or online at MasteringHealth™.

Identify Your Body's Patterns of Fat Distribution

Body fat distribution patterns are mostly genetically determined. You have probably noticed that people take after one parent in the way they "wear their fat." Some individuals tend to accumulate fat around their midsections; others collect it in the lower body or hips. These distributions contribute to an overall body shape that can be correlated to a higher or lower risk of disease.

The two most common body shapes are **android** ("apple-shaped") and **gynoid** ("pear-shaped") (**Figure 6.4**). A person with *android pattern obesity* has

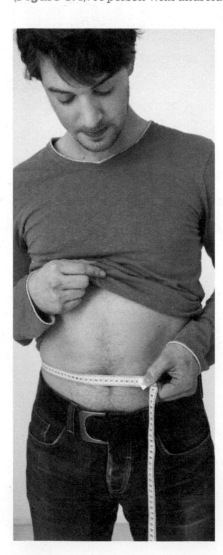

excess body fat on the upper body and trunk and has a greater risk of developing chronic disease than a person with *gynoid pattern obesity,* who carries excess body fat in the lower body. Higher waist circumferences due to excess abdominal fat are associated with higher levels of **subcutaneous fat** and **visceral fat**. Although both are associated with metabolic diseases, fat in the abdominal cavity (visceral fat) has a stronger relationship to disease risk.[9] The good news is that

TABLE 6.1 Waist Circumference, BMI, and Disease Risk

Weight Classification	BMI (kg/m^2)	Waist Circumference and Disease Risk*	
		Smaller Waist Men ≤102 cm (40 in) Women ≤88 cm (35 in)	Larger Waist Men >102 cm (40 in) Women >88 cm (35 in)
Underweight	<18.5	—	—
Normal weight	18.5–24.9	—	—
Overweight	25.0–29.9	Increased	High
Obese—I	30.0–34.9	High	Very high
Obese—II	35.0–39.9	Very high	Very high
Obese—III	>40.0	Extremely high	Extremely high

*Risk for type 2 diabetes, hypertension, and cardiovascular disease, relative to normal weight and waist circumference.

Source: Adapted from National Heart, Lung, and Blood Institute—Expert Panel on the Identification, Evaluation, and Treatment of Overweight in Adults, "Clinical Guidelines on the Identification, Evaluation, and Treatment of Overweight and Obesity in Adults: Executive Summary," *American Journal of Clinical Nutrition* 68 (1998): 899–917. Reprinted with permission.

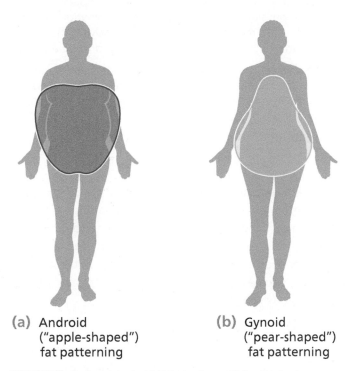

(a) Android ("apple-shaped") fat patterning

(b) Gynoid ("pear-shaped") fat patterning

FIGURE 6.4 (a) Android ("apple-shaped") fat distribution, associated with greater risk of heart disease and diabetes, is more common in men of all ages and postmenopausal women; (b) gynoid ("pear-shaped") fat distribution is more common in premenopausal women.

reducing total body fat will reduce subcutaneous fat, visceral fat, and disease risk.[10, 11] While men tend to store fat in the abdomen and women tend to store it in the lower body, there are exceptions, and fat distribution is strongly influenced by genetics. If you have an "apple-shaped" body, understanding the health risks can help motivate you to keep your "apple" from getting too large and round!

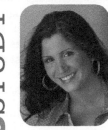

caseSTUDY

DANI

"My friend Emily explained to me that I probably gained weight after starting my exercise program because I was building muscle faster than I was losing fat and that I shouldn't worry about it. She suggested that I check my body measurements instead of getting on the scale. I like that idea, and she offered to help, but now I am not sure which ones to do. My problem areas have always been my hips and thighs. Should I measure those areas and call it good?"

APPLY IT! Why would body measurements/circumferences be a better way for Dani to measure her progress than body weight? Does her shape (gynoid or android) increase or decrease her risk for disease?

TRY IT! Today, write TWO specific short-term goals to help improve or maintain your current body size/shape (i.e., I will go to the gym three times next week):

1. _____

2. _____

In one week, did you meet your two goals? YES or NO

In two weeks, refine your short-term goals and add two longer-term body size/shape goals.

Hear It!
To listen to this case study online, visit the Study Area in MasteringHealth™.

Q&A What Is Muscle Tone and How Is It Related to Body Composition?

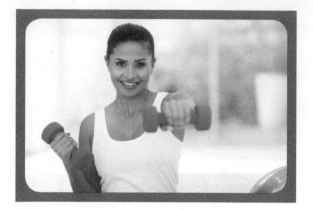

Muscle tone is an overused and misused term. The scientific definition of muscle tone is the residual tension or contraction of muscle. In other words, it is the unconscious low level of contraction in your muscles at rest. This definition is vastly different from how most people think about the term "tone." Generally, muscle tone is considered having muscles that appear defined and

feel firm and tight. Resistance training is the best way to achieve firmness and definition.

For years, women (and men) who wanted long, lean muscles were told to lift very light weights and perform lots of repetitions. This is a major exercise misconception. There is no evidence that using light weights and doing high repetitions (more than 20) results in more muscle tone over lifting heavier weights. In fact, heavier weights with fewer repetitions (8 to 12) are best for maximizing strength and muscle changes.

However, even the strongest muscle will not look toned if it is covered with layers of fat. Thus, to showcase your well-toned muscles, you may need to decrease your body fat percentage. This is best accomplished through dietary modifications and increasing your energy expenditure through physical activity. So it is the *combination* of exercised, trained muscles and low overall body fat that results in what most people consider good muscle tone.

A word of caution: Be wary of exercise infomercials that guarantee increased muscle tone. Since there is no way to measure muscle tone, companies don't have to prove that their products really work!

LO 6.4 What Methods Are Used to Assess Body Composition?

Unlike BMI and body circumference measurements, body composition (lean mass vs. fat mass) can only be estimated indirectly. A true, direct assessment of body composition requires dissection after death; in fact, researchers judge the accuracy of the indirect measures by comparing them with dissection results from cadavers.

Methods for estimating body composition range from assessments that trained fitness instructors can easily administer, such as skinfold measurements and bioelectrical impedance analysis, to sophisticated tests that must be conducted by clinicians in a lab or hospital setting. The most

accurate estimates of body composition are body scans such as an MRI (magnetic resonance imaging) or a CT (computed tomography) scan. These are used in medical settings to diagnose injury and illness but are not often used for body composition analysis alone. In the next section, we discuss methods that are commonly used to assess body composition.

Skinfold Measurements

Skinfold measurements are an easy, inexpensive way to estimate your percent body fat. **Calipers** are used to measure the thickness of a fold of skin and subcutaneous adipose tissue. Skinfold measurements at specific sites around the body are recorded and entered into an equation that predicts percent body fat. This prediction of percent body fat has an error range of 3 to 4 percent;[12] for example, if your body fat measurement is 16 percent, the true value could be anywhere from about 12 to 20 percent. Recent research has shown that current equations to predict body fat may result in additional over- or underestimates for ethnic, race, and age-diverse populations.[13] If you use this method to estimate your body fat, remember it is just that—an estimate!

skinfold A fold of skin and subcutaneous fat that is measured with calipers to determine the fatness of a specific body area

calipers A handheld and spring-loaded instrument with calibrated jaws and a meter that reads skinfold thickness in millimeters

Lab 6.3 (at the end of this chapter) provides instructions for skinfold measurements. Performing an accurate skinfold assessment takes education and practice, so ask a qualified fitness instructor to help you. Also, the difference between technicians can be a major source of error. Make sure the same technician performs the measurements if you are tracking body fat change over time.

Do It!
Access these labs at the end of the chapter or online at MasteringHealth™.

Dual-Energy X-Ray Absorptiometry

Dual-energy X-ray absorptiometry (DXA) is the "gold-standard" or criterion reference method for body composition assessment in clinical and research settings (**Figure 6.5**). In a DXA scan, low-radiation X-rays are used to distinguish fat, bone mineral, and bone-free lean components of the body. Measuring bone mineral (in addition to fat and lean mass) increases the accuracy of body fat estimates. In the medical setting, DXA scans are most often used to determine bone density for osteoporosis diagnosis. Body composition estimates can be obtained from whole body DXA scans that take less than three minutes. However, DXA tests are expensive, require a trained technician, and are not well designed to examine people who are extremely obese.

Hydrostatic Weighing

Hydrostatic weighing (also called *underwater weighing*) was widely used in research and college settings and prior to DXA was considered the criterion method of body composition assessment (**Figure 6.6**). In hydrostatic weighing, a person is first weighed outside a water tank and then weighed while completely submerged in the tank. Since fat is less dense than water, it

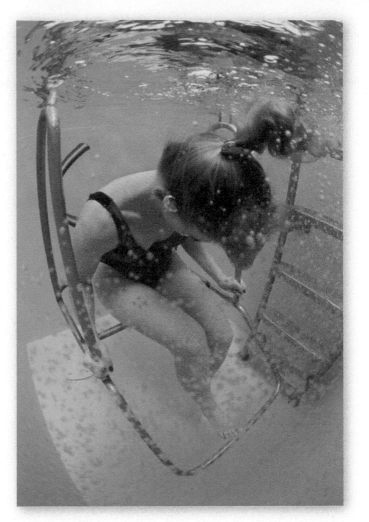

FIGURE **6.6** Hydrostatic (underwater) weighing uses total body water displacement to calculate estimated percent body fat.

will float, while lean body mass will sink because it is more dense than water. Therefore, a person with a high percent of body fat will weigh less in water compared to a leaner person of the same body weight. From this technique, body density can be calculated (density = mass/volume) and used to estimate percent body fat. The method is valid and reliable, but access to an equipped facility may be limited and not everyone is comfortable with being submerged.

Air Displacement (Bod Pod)

Air displacement plethysmography, commercially known

dual-energy X-ray absorptiometry (DXA) A technique using two low-radiation X-rays to scan bone and soft tissue (muscle, fat) to determine bone density and to estimate percent body fat

hydrostatic weighing A technique that uses water to determine total body volume, total body density, and percent body fat

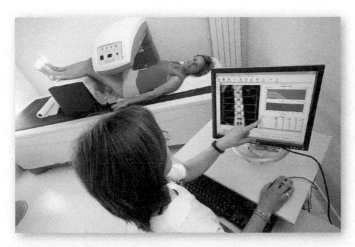

FIGURE **6.5** A DXA machine uses low-radiation X-rays to determine body composition.

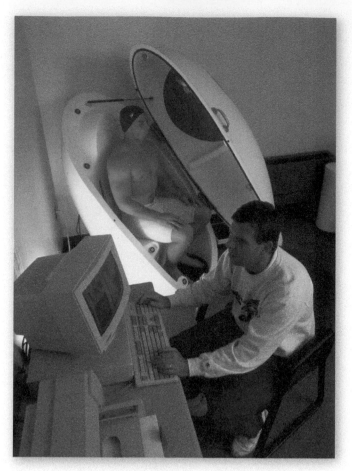

FIGURE **6.7** The Bod Pod uses total body air displacement to calculate estimated percent body fat.

as the **Bod Pod**, measures total body *air* displacement (**Figure 6.7**). The person being assessed puts on a swimsuit and cap, and then sits in the egg-shaped Bod Pod chamber while the air displacement is measured. The volume of air displaced is equal to the subject's body volume as he or she sits in the chamber. Similar to hydrostatic weighing, body density is calculated and converted to a body fat percentage. Bod Pod percent

body fat measurements are generally within 1 to 2 percent of hydrostatic- and DXA-measured levels of percent body fat.[14] Bod Pod measurements are available in many clinical and college settings, but availability in fitness settings is limited.

> **Bod Pod** An egg-shaped chamber that uses air displacement to determine total body volume, total body density, and percent body fat
>
> **bioelectrical impedance analysis (BIA)** A technique that distinguishes lean and fat mass by measuring the resistance of various body tissues to electrical currents

Bioelectrical Impedance Analysis

In **bioelectrical impedance analysis (BIA)**, a machine measures the resistance of various body tissues to electrical currents. BIA machines send small electrical currents through the body via the hands, feet, or both (**Figure 6.8**). Fat does not conduct electricity very well, so fat tissues will demonstrate a resistance to the currents. Fat-free tissues, namely muscle, have more body water and conduct electricity well; thus, fat-free tissues do not offer as much resistance to the currents. So, higher resistance indicates higher levels of overall body fat.

The error range of BIA is 3 to 4 percent, but accuracy depends upon the quality of the machine, the number and placement of the electrodes, and upon the subject's preparation, especially concerning water intake.[15] Higher or lower levels of body water will significantly alter a BIA machine's results, so it is important to hydrate normally.

The type of BIA machine will determine the body areas that are measured. Body fat scales (with foot electrodes) measure lower body and trunk resistances, whereas hand-held BIA machines (with hand electrodes) measure upper body and trunk resistances. Overall, BIA is an acceptable method of tracking body fat change if conditions are consistent (Lab 6.3).

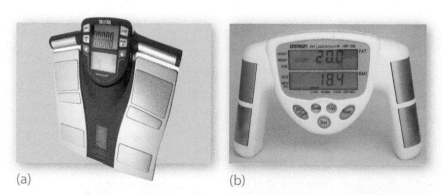

(a) (b)

FIGURE **6.8** Bioelectrical impedance analysis (BIA) machines measure the resistance of different body tissues to electrical currents. These measurements are then used to estimate percent body fat. On the left is a body fat scale; on the right is a hand-held BIA machine.

LO 6.5 How Can I Change My Body Composition?

After you assess your body size, shape, and composition, the next steps are evaluation, goal setting, and planning for maintenance or change.

TABLE **6.2** **Percent Body Fat Norms for Men and Women***

Body Fat Rating	Women (%)	Men (%)
Athletic/Low	14–20	6–13
Fitness	21–24	14–17
Acceptable	25–31	18–25
Obese	>32	>26

*Please note that there are no agreed-upon standards for recommended percent body fat; however, a range of 10 to 22 percent for men and 20 to 32 percent for women is considered healthy.

Source: From "Percent Body Fat Norms for Men and Women" in *ACE Lifestyle and Weight Management Coach Manual*, © 2013 American Council on Exercise. Reprinted with permission from the American Council on Exercise® (ACE®), www.acefitness.org.

Determine Whether Your Percent Body Fat Is within a Healthy Range

Because people accumulate fat very differently, not all fat is the same, and it changes as we age, it is difficult to specify the exact level of body fat that is "healthy" or "unhealthy." For instance, abdominal fat increases your risk for disease much more than fat on your calves does. Because of these differences, researchers do not agree upon desired body fat percentages for people of all ages, and you will find that research articles, books, and websites differ in their recommendations. **Table 6.2** provides percent body fat norms.

Set Reasonable Body Composition Goals

Real body composition changes take time. Quick weight loss is easier for those with more weight to lose, but most weight that is lost quickly consists of water and muscle—the very things you *don't* want to lose. To lose fat only, you have to be committed to exercise and slow, consistent weight loss. Aim for a body composition goal and a target weight that is healthy and that you can maintain for a lifetime. See Lab 6.3 for target weight calculations. See the GetFitGraphic on page 220 for more on spot reduction and the need for a whole-body approach to body composition.

Follow a Well-Designed Exercise and Nutrition Plan

True body changes come from sticking with a carefully planned and executed nutrition and exercise program. The fitness and nutrition chapters in this book will help you get started, but see Chapter 8 for weight and body management program ideas. For additional assistance, seek out qualified medical, nutrition, and fitness experts.

Monitor Your Body Size, Shape, and Composition Regularly

Stay motivated in your body change program by monitoring your progress regularly (use the labs in this chapter to guide your measurements). Here is a suggested schedule:

- Body size/shape (mirror and fit of clothes)—assess daily or weekly

caseSTUDY

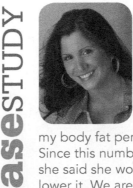

DANI

"A trainer at my gym gave me a skinfold test. I was amazed how much of my body is fat—50 pounds, wow! The trainer said that 50 pounds sounds like a lot, but my body fat percentage is actually 31 percent. Since this number is marginally high for my age, she said she would help me with a program to lower it. We are planning to retest my skinfolds in three months to see how all of my exercise is paying off!

APPLY IT! What other methods could Dani use to determine her body composition? What methods of assessing body composition are readily available to you? What percent body fat do you think Dani should aim for?

TRY IT! **Today**, estimate what you think your percent body fat is. **This week**, use one body composition measurement method to determine your percent body fat (see Lab 6.3). **In two weeks**, determine your body composition goal, your goal weight, and a target date for meeting your goals (see Lab 6.3 for goal weight calculations).

Hear It!
To listen to this case study online, visit the Study Area in MasteringHealth™.

CAN I GET RID OF **FAT** AND **CELLULITE** IN ONE AREA OF MY BODY?

Have you ever thought, "I don't need to work on my whole body. I just need to lose some fat off my hips (or thighs or abdomen)!"

METHODS PEOPLE USE TO TARGET **FAT** AND **CELLULITE** IN SPECIFIC AREAS

DO THEY WORK?

NO Ab-crunchers, thigh-slimmers, or arm-toners

These machines increase the strength, endurance, and firmness of the underlying muscles, but there's no change in fat in the target area without changes in overall caloric expenditure and consumption.

YES Laser therapy or liposuction

These procedures will take out and/or change fat cells, but in order to maintain such changes, you must adjust your diet and exercise.[1]

NOT REALLY
Skin creams

Skin creams may decrease the appearance of cellulite by causing the skin to swell, but the effect is minimal and non-lasting.

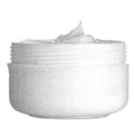

IS CELLULITE A SPECIAL TYPE OF FAT?

NO! Cellulite is **enlarged fat cells** that bulge out of their connective tissue compartments and **push into the skin, causing a bumpy appearance.**[2] More women than men have it due to greater irregularity in patterns of connective tissue.

Dimpling

Fat cells

Skin with Cellulite

Fibrous cords

Connective tissue

Skin without Cellulite

WHAT CAN I DO TO REDUCE CELLULITE **NATURALLY?**

EAT A HEALTHY DIET rich in fruits, vegetables, and fiber

STAY HYDRATED with plenty of fluids

EXERCISE REGULARLY to keep muscles firm and bones strong

MAINTAIN a healthy weight

DON'T smoke

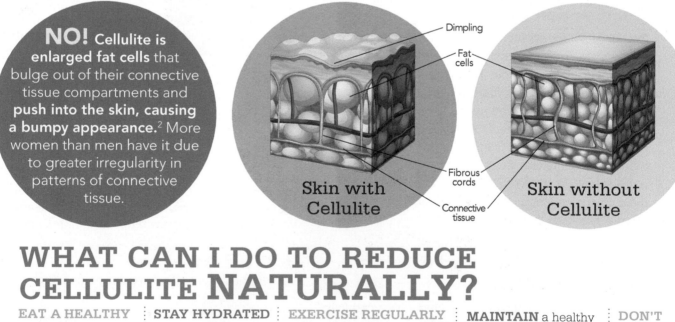
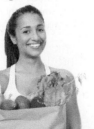

DIVERSITY
Self-Esteem and Unhealthy Body Composition Behaviors

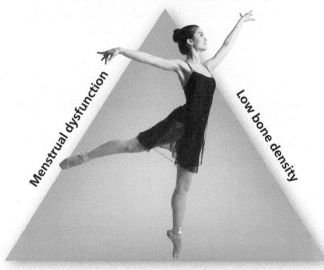

Low energy availability

Body composition can become a major problem for athletes in certain sports—not because they are too fat, but because they are too thin. This is true for both sexes, though the problem is more common in females, who are at risk of developing the female athlete triad (see figure). Men may also develop disordered eating habits, as well as a body composition disorder known as muscle dysmorphia, in which men who are of normal weight and even unusually muscular think that they are "puny." Some sports—gymnastics, figure skating, wrestling, ballet dancing, body-building—place a huge emphasis on appearance and having a light and lean body. The pressure to look lean and to weigh less can push athletes to cut back on what they eat and increase their workouts to the point where they lose too much weight.

An athlete's self-esteem can make a big difference. Lower self-esteem can lead to believing that life events are out of your control (external locus of control) and vice versa. One study has shown that if a female athlete has an internal locus of control (or belief that she has power or control over her body and training), she will be more immune to coach and social pressures that can lead to disordered eating.[1] This can help her avoid the female athlete triad, a triangle of three interrelated problems: menstrual dysfunction, low bone density, and low energy availability as a result of disordered eating or eating disorders. In the triad, too little caloric intake coupled with too much exercise can lead to hormonal changes and the stopping of menstruation.[2] Improper nutrition, including too little calcium and vitamin D, can lead to altered hormones and to bone loss and a risk of fractures. Such changes taking place in adolescence or early adulthood can permanently reduce the size of a woman's skeleton and increase her lifelong risk for osteoporosis. In dancers, one study has shown that the triad negatively affects cardiovascular health.[3]

Athletes with low self-esteem and at high risk for the female athlete triad should carefully monitor their body composition, menstrual health, eating habits, and perhaps bone density. If the triad is suspected, the athlete should eat more nutritious food and/or exercise less, and may need to seek treatment for an eating disorder.

See It!
Watch "Young Boys Exercising to Extremes" at MasteringHealth™.

Sources:
1. S. Scoffier, Y. Paquet, and F. d'Arripe-Longueville, "Effect of Locus of Control on Disordered Eating in Athletes: The Mediational Role of Self-Regulation of Eating Attitudes," *Eating Behaviors* 11, no. 3 (2010): 164–69.
2. A. M. McManus and N. Armstrong, "Physiology of Elite Young Female Athletes," *Medicine and Sport Science* 56 (2011): 23–46.
3. A. Z. Hoch et al., "Association between the Female Athlete Triad and Endothelial Dysfunction in Dancers," *Clinical Journal of Sport Medicine* 21, no. 2 (2011): 119–25.

- Weight—assess daily or weekly[16]
- Circumferences—measure monthly (or less frequently)
- BMI—measure monthly (or less frequently)
- Percent body fat—measure every other month (or less frequently)

Keep a separate log, journal, or notebook of your progress and how you're feeling, but do not feel burdened by it. Some people are more motivated by

journaling than others—find the monitoring system that works for you and use it consistently.

Remember, improving your body composition should help you feel good about yourself! The Diversity box Self-Esteem and Unhealthy Body Composition Behaviors talks about some problems to be watchful for.

See It!
Watch "Overweight and Healthy?" at MasteringHealth™.

Study Plan

chapter summary

LO 6.1 How Do Body Weight and Body Composition Differ?

- The amount of lean and fat tissue in your body is your body composition.

- Lean body mass is the total amount of fat-free tissue and percent body fat is the percentage of your total weight that is fat.

- Essential fat is the fat needed for healthy body systems. Storage fat is used for energy and insulation.

LO 6.2 Why Do My Body Size, Shape, and Composition Matter?

- More than 68 percent of US adults are overweight or obese.

- Knowing your body composition can help you determine your risks for chronic disease and decide how much weight to lose or gain.

LO 6.3 How Can I Evaluate My Body Size and Shape?

- Very low and very high BMI scores are correlated with greater risk of death and disability.

- Measure circumferences to monitor your body changes over time and assess risks for disease.

- Android obesity is associated with a greater risk of chronic disease than gynoid obesity.

LO 6.4 What Methods Are Used to Assess Body Composition?

- Skinfold measurement with calipers is an easy, inexpensive way to estimate your percent body fat.

- Dual-energy X-ray absorptiometry (DXA) uses low-radiation X-rays to distinguish fat, bone mineral, and bone-free lean mass.

- In hydrostatic weighing, a person's weight in water is used to obtain estimates of body density and percent fat.

- Air displacement plethysmography (the Bod Pod) measures total body air displacement to obtain body density and percent body fat estimates.

- Bioelectrical impedance analysis (BIA) uses electrical currents to measure resistance in the body and estimate body water and fat levels.

LO 6.5 How Can I Change My Body Composition?

- There are no universal recommended body fat percentages.

- Quick weight loss involves losing water and muscle. Carefully plan your program to lose fat only.

- Monitor your body regularly and assess changes daily, weekly, and monthly.

review questions

LO 6.1 **1.** The proportion of your total weight that is fat is called
a. body composition.
b. lean mass.
c. percent body fat.
d. BMI.

LO 6.1 **2.** Women have a greater amount of *essential fat* due to
a. larger calves and thighs.
b. their eating habits.
c. less physical activity.
d. reproduction-related fat deposits.

LO 6.2 **3.** _____ of the adults in the US are either overweight or obese!
a. Approximately 2/3
b. Approximately 1/2
c. Almost all
d. About 1/4

LO 6.3 **4.** Which of the following statements about BMI is true?
a. Your BMI is an estimate of your body fat percentage.
b. BMI differentiates between lean mass and fat mass.
c. Very low and very high BMI scores are associated with greater risk of mortality.
d. BMI stands for "Basic Measure Indices."

LO 6.3 **5.** Which of the following circumference measures indicates an increased risk of disease?
   a. A waist circumference over 100 cm for men and over 80 cm for women
   b. A waist circumference over 102 cm for men and over 88 cm for women
   c. A waist-to-hip ratio of 0.50 or higher
   d. A waist-to-hip ratio of 0.75 or higher

LO 6.3 **6.** Which of the following body shapes or body fat distribution patterns is associated with an increased risk of heart disease and diabetes?
   a. Bell-shaped
   b. Android pattern obesity
   c. Pear-shaped
   d. Gynoid pattern obesity

LO 6.4 **7.** Skinfold measurements are used to assess the amount of
   a. subcutaneous fat.
   b. visceral fat.
   c. essential fat.
   d. intramuscular fat.

LO 6.4 **8.** Which of the following body composition measurement methods uses air displacement to estimate total body volume, density, and percent body fat?
   a. Bioelectrical impedance analysis
   b. Hydrostatic weighing
   c. The Bod Pod
   d. Skinfold measurement

LO 6.4 **9.** Which body composition measurement method relies heavily on body water or hydration levels being normal (not too low or too high)?
   a. Bioelectrical impedance analysis
   b. Hydrostatic weighing
   c. The Bod Pod
   d. Skinfold measurement

LO 6.5 **10.** How often should you assess your percent body fat?
   a. daily
   b. weekly
   c. monthly
   d. every other month

critical thinking questions

LO 6.3 **1.** Explain the usefulness and limitations of using BMI to determine fitness goals.

LO 6.5 **2.** What factors should you consider when determining a healthy percent body fat range for yourself?

check out these eResources

- **About.com** Click on "Health" and then search for "Body Composition" for numerous articles about body composition definitions, assessment, and lifestyle change. **www.about.com**
- **FitDay** A free online diet and weight loss journal. Create a goal, track food, log activity, and see progress! **www.fitday.com**
- **National Institutes of Health** Search for "Body Composition" for basic information and research articles about body composition, health, and fitness. **www.nih.gov**

- **Spark People** Free powerful tools for your weight loss, fitness, and health goals: calorie counter, fitness programs integrated with wearable trackers, and connections to Spark People community members and experts. **www.sparkpeople.com**
- **YouTube** Search for "Body Composition" and look for informational and demonstration videos about body composition assessment methods. **www.youtube.com**

HOW TO CALCULATE YOUR BMI

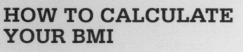

Name: _____   **Date:** _____

Instructor: _____   **Section:** _____

Purpose: To learn how to calculate your BMI.

Materials: Weight scale, measuring tape, calculator

Section I: Calculate your BMI

1. Record your weight and height below:

Weight _____ lb   Height _____ inches

2. Convert your weight and height to metric units:

Weight _____ lbs ÷ 2.2 = _____ kg

Height _____ inches × 2.54 = _____ cm ÷ 100 = _____ meters (m)

3. Calculate your BMI:

BMI = _____ ÷ [_____ × _____]

       (weight in kg)   (height in m)   (height in m)

BMI = _____ kg/m^2

Note: Square the height (multiply by itself) before dividing into weight.

4. Indicate your BMI rating in the table below:

Weight Classification	BMI (kg/m^2)	
Underweight	_____	< 18.5
Normal Weight	_____	18.5–24.9
Overweight	_____	25.0–29.9
Obese—I	_____	30.0–34.9
Obese—II	_____	35.0–39.9
Obese—III	_____	> 40.0

Section II: Reflection

1. Is your BMI category what you thought it would be?

_____

2. Remember that BMI categories can be misleading for individuals with above-average muscle mass. Do you fall into this category? _____

3. Monitoring changes to your BMI over time is one way to assess your progress with a fitness program. Within this course or on your own, recalculate your BMI two months after you begin a new exercise program. How has your BMI changed?

_____

DO IT!

LAB
6.2

ASSESS YOURSELF

MEASURE AND EVALUATE
YOUR BODY
CIRCUMFERENCES

MasteringHealth™

Name: _____ **Date:** _____

Instructor: _____ **Section:** _____

Purpose: To learn how to measure your body circumferences.

Materials: Measuring tape, partner

SCAN TO SEE IT
ONLINE!

Section I: Measuring Circumferences

Using a cloth or plastic tape measure, have a partner assist you with the following circumference measures. Be sure to mark your measurements (centimeters or inches) and record them to the nearest 0.5 cm or 0.25 inch. You can perform these measurements again to track how your body shape changes over time.

Site	Description	Measurement
Waist	For those with a visible waist, measure at the narrowest part of the torso; for those with a larger torso, measure at the navel.	
Hip	Measure with the legs slightly apart. Measure where the hip/buttock circumference is the greatest.	
Upper Arm	Measure midway between the shoulder and elbow.	Right: Left:
Forearm	Measure at the greatest circumference between the wrist and elbow.	Right: Left:
Thigh	Measure with your leg on a bench or chair (knee at 90 degrees). Measure halfway between the crease in your hip and your knee.	Right: Left:
Calf	Measure at the greatest circumference between the knee and ankle.	Right: Left:
Neck	Measure midway between the head and shoulders.	

Source: Based on American College of Sports Medicine, *ACSM's Guidelines for Exercise Testing and Prescription*, 9th ed. (Baltimore, MD: Lippincott Williams & Wilkins, 2014).

Section II: Evaluating Circumferences and Disease Risk

1. Calculate your waist-to-hip ratio (WHR):

WHR = _____ ÷ _____

        (waist circumference)   (hip circumference)

WHR = _____

2. Evaluate your WHR using the table below:

Disease Risk and WHR				
Age (years)	Low	Moderate	High	Very High
Men: 20–29	<0.83	0.83–0.88	0.89–0.94	>0.94
30–39	<0.84	0.84–0.91	0.92–0.96	>0.96
40–49	<0.88	0.88–0.95	0.96–1.00	>1.00
50–59	<0.90	0.90–0.96	0.97–1.02	>1.02
60–69	<0.91	0.91–0.98	0.99–1.03	>1.03
Women: 20–29	<0.71	0.71–0.77	0.78–0.82	>0.82
30–39	<0.72	0.72–0.78	0.79–0.84	>0.84
40–49	<0.73	0.73–0.79	0.80–0.87	>0.87
50–59	<0.74	0.74–0.81	0.82–0.88	>0.88
60–69	<0.76	0.76–0.83	0.84–0.90	>0.90

Source: Data from G. A. Bray and D. S. Gray, "Obesity. Part I—Pathogenesis," *Western Journal of Medicine* 149, no. 4 (1988): 429–41.

Evaluate your waist circumference using the table below:

Waist Circumference (WC)		
Disease Risk Category	Women	Men
Very Low	<70 cm (<28.5 in)	<80 cm (<31.5 in)
Low	70–89 cm (28.5–35.0 in)	80–99 cm (31.5–39.0 in)
High	90–109 cm (35.5–43.0 in)	100–120 cm (39.5–47.0 in)
Very High	>110 cm (>43.5 in)	>120 cm (>47.0 in)

Source: From G. A. Bray, "Don't Throw the Baby Out with the Bath Water," *American Journal of Clinical Nutrition* 70, no. 3 (2004): 347–49, by permission of the American Society for Nutrition.

3. Record your disease risk from WHR and waist circumference below:

Disease risk rating for WHR: _____

Disease risk category for WC: _____

Section III: Reflection

1. Do your ratings for disease risk based upon circumferences surprise you? _____

2. Which of your circumference measures are you most interested in changing and why?

_____

DO IT!

LAB
6.3

ASSESS YOURSELF

ESTIMATE YOUR PERCENT
BODY FAT (SKINFOLD TEST
AND BIA TEST)

MasteringHealth™

Name: _____ **Date:** _____

Instructor: _____ **Section:** _____

Materials: Skinfold calipers, BIA machine, appropriate clothing (shorts, tank top, sports bra for women)

Purpose: To assess your current percent body fat using either the skinfold procedure or a BIA machine or both.

Directions: Complete the sections below with a trained instructor.

SCAN TO SEE IT
ONLINE!

Section I: Skinfold Measurement

You will need an experienced, trained instructor to complete your measurements. Note the time of day of your measurements and perform any follow-up measurements at the same time of day.

1. Identify the correct skinfold locations. If you are male, locate the chest, abdomen, and thigh locations (see photos). If you are female, locate the triceps, suprailiac, and thigh locations (see photos). Your instructor should mark these locations on the right side of the body with a pen before using the caliper.

Chest	A diagonal fold measured midway between the shoulder/armpit crease and the nipple.	
Abdomen	A vertical fold measured one inch to the right of the navel.	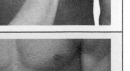

Thigh	A vertical fold measured midway between the crease in your hip and the top of your knee.	
Triceps	A vertical fold on the back of the upper arm midway between the shoulder and elbow.	
Suprailiac	A diagonal fold just above the hip bone, on the side of the body at the front edge of your relaxed arm.	

Source: Based on American College of Sports Medicine, *ACSM's Guidelines for Exercise Testing and Prescription*, 9th ed. (Baltimore, MD: Lippincott Williams & Wilkins, 2014).

2. Your instructor will measure each skinfold location using the technique below. Record the results below and then add the numbers for the three skinfold sites to obtain your overall skinfold sum.

Skinfold measurement technique: After locating the correct sites, grab a double fold of skin on both sides of the skinfold location. Open your fingers about three inches when lifting the fold (> than three inches is required for larger individuals). Holding the fold in place, pick up the calipers with your other hand. While still holding the fold, place the caliper jaws on the skinfold location, measuring halfway between the crest and the base of the fold. You should measure perpendicular to the fold and about one cm away from your fingers. Read the measurement two to three seconds after placing the calipers and record the skinfold numbers to the nearest 0.5 mm. For accuracy, measure each site three times and average the two closest numbers.

Men		Women	
Chest	_____ mm	Triceps	_____ mm
Abdomen	_____ mm	Suprailiac	_____ mm
Thigh	_____ mm	Thigh	_____ mm
Sum of 3 =	_____ mm	Sum of 3 =	_____ mm

3. Using the sum of three skinfolds, find your estimated percent body fat in the tables for women and men.

Sum of Skinfolds (mm)	Percent Body Fat Estimates for WOMEN (from triceps, suprailiac, and thigh skinfolds)								
	AGE (years)								
	Under 22	23–27	28–32	33–37	38–42	43–47	48–52	53–57	Over 57
23–25	9.7	9.9	10.2	10.4	10.7	10.9	11.2	11.4	11.7
26–28	11.0	11.2	11.5	11.7	12.0	12.3	12.5	12.7	13.0
29–31	12.3	12.5	12.8	13.0	13.3	13.5	13.8	14.0	14.3
32–34	13.6	13.8	14.0	14.3	14.5	14.8	15.0	15.3	15.5
35–37	14.8	15.0	15.3	15.5	15.8	16.0	16.3	16.5	16.8
38–40	16.0	16.3	16.5	16.7	17.0	17.2	17.5	17.7	18.0
41–43	17.2	17.4	17.7	17.9	18.2	18.4	18.7	18.9	19.2
44–46	18.3	18.6	18.8	19.1	19.3	19.6	19.8	20.1	20.3
47–49	19.5	19.7	20.0	20.2	20.5	20.7	21.0	21.2	21.5
50–52	20.6	20.8	21.1	21.3	21.6	21.8	22.1	22.3	22.6
53–55	21.7	21.9	22.1	22.4	22.6	22.9	23.1	23.4	23.6
56–58	22.7	23.0	23.2	23.4	23.7	23.9	24.2	24.4	24.7
59–61	23.7	24.0	24.2	24.5	24.7	25.0	25.2	25.5	25.7
62–64	24.7	25.0	25.2	25.5	25.7	26.0	26.2	26.4	26.7
65–67	25.7	25.9	26.2	26.4	26.7	26.9	27.2	27.4	27.7
68–70	26.6	26.9	27.1	27.4	27.6	27.9	28.1	28.4	28.6
71–73	27.5	27.8	28.0	28.3	28.5	28.8	29.0	29.3	29.5
74–76	28.4	28.7	28.9	29.2	29.4	29.7	29.9	30.2	30.4
77–79	29.3	29.5	29.8	30.0	30.3	30.5	30.8	31.0	31.3
80–82	30.1	30.4	30.6	30.9	31.1	31.4	31.6	31.9	32.1
83–85	30.9	31.2	31.4	31.7	31.9	32.2	32.4	32.7	32.9
86–88	31.7	32.0	32.2	32.5	32.7	32.9	33.2	33.4	33.7
89–91	32.5	32.7	33.0	33.2	33.5	33.7	33.9	34.2	34.4
92–94	33.2	33.4	33.7	33.9	34.2	34.4	34.7	34.9	35.2
95–97	33.9	34.1	34.4	34.6	34.9	35.1	35.4	35.6	35.9
98–100	34.6	34.8	35.1	35.3	35.5	35.8	36.0	36.3	36.5
101–103	35.3	35.4	35.7	35.9	36.2	36.4	36.7	36.9	37.2
104–106	35.8	36.1	36.3	36.6	36.8	37.1	37.3	37.5	37.8
107–109	36.4	36.7	36.9	37.1	37.4	37.6	37.9	38.1	38.4
110–112	37.0	37.2	37.5	37.7	38.0	38.2	38.5	38.7	38.9
113–115	37.5	37.8	38.0	38.2	38.5	38.7	39.0	39.2	39.5
116–118	38.0	38.3	38.5	38.8	39.0	39.3	39.5	39.7	40.0
119–121	38.5	38.7	39.0	39.2	39.5	39.7	40.0	40.2	40.5
122–124	39.0	39.2	39.4	39.7	39.9	40.2	40.4	40.7	40.9
125–127	39.4	39.6	39.9	40.1	40.4	40.6	40.9	41.1	41.4
128–130	39.8	40.0	40.3	40.5	40.8	41.0	41.3	41.5	41.8

Source: A. S. Jackson and M. L. Pollock, "Practical Assessment of Body Composition," *Physician and Sportsmedicine* 13, no. 5 (1985): 76–90. Copyright © 1985 JTE Multimedia, LLC. Used with permission.

Sum of Skinfolds (mm)	Percent Body Fat Estimates for MEN (from chest, abdomen, and thigh skinfolds)								
	AGE (years)								
	Under 22	23–27	28–32	33–37	38–42	43–47	48–52	53–57	Over 57
8–10	1.3	1.8	2.3	2.9	3.4	3.9	4.5	5.0	5.5
11–13	2.2	2.8	3.3	3.9	4.4	4.9	5.5	6.0	6.5
14–16	3.2	3.8	4.3	4.8	5.4	5.9	6.4	7.0	7.5
17–19	4.2	4.7	5.3	5.8	6.3	6.9	7.4	8.0	8.5
20–22	5.1	5.7	6.2	6.8	7.3	7.9	8.4	8.9	9.5
23–25	6.1	6.6	7.2	7.7	8.3	8.8	9.4	9.9	10.5
26–28	7.0	7.6	8.1	8.7	9.2	9.8	10.3	10.9	11.4
29–31	8.0	8.5	9.1	9.6	10.2	10.7	11.3	11.8	12.4
32–34	8.9	9.4	10.0	10.5	11.1	11.6	12.2	12.8	13.3
35–37	9.8	10.4	10.9	11.5	12.0	12.6	13.1	13.7	14.3
38–40	10.7	11.3	11.8	12.4	12.9	13.5	14.1	14.6	15.2
41–43	11.6	12.2	12.7	13.3	13.8	14.4	15.0	15.5	16.1
44–46	12.5	13.1	13.6	14.2	14.7	15.3	15.9	16.4	17.0
47–49	13.4	13.9	14.5	15.1	15.6	16.2	16.8	17.3	17.9
50–52	14.3	14.8	15.4	15.9	16.5	17.1	17.6	18.2	18.8
53–55	15.1	15.7	16.2	16.8	17.4	17.9	18.5	19.1	19.7
56–58	16.0	16.5	17.1	17.7	18.2	18.8	19.4	20.0	20.5
59–61	16.9	17.4	17.9	18.5	19.1	19.7	20.2	20.8	21.4
62–64	17.6	18.2	18.8	19.4	19.9	20.5	21.1	21.7	22.2
65–67	18.5	19.0	19.6	20.2	20.8	21.3	21.9	22.5	23.1
68–70	19.3	19.9	20.4	21.0	21.6	22.2	22.7	23.3	23.9
71–73	20.1	20.7	21.2	21.8	22.4	23.0	23.6	24.1	24.7
74–76	20.9	21.5	22.0	22.6	23.2	23.8	24.4	25.0	25.5
77–79	21.7	22.2	22.8	23.4	24.0	24.6	25.2	25.8	26.3
80–82	22.4	23.0	23.6	24.2	24.8	25.4	25.9	26.5	27.1
83–85	23.2	23.8	24.4	25.0	25.5	26.1	26.7	27.3	27.9
86–88	24.0	24.5	25.1	25.7	26.3	26.9	27.5	28.1	28.7
89–91	24.7	25.3	25.9	26.5	27.1	27.6	28.2	28.8	29.4
92–94	25.4	26.0	26.6	27.2	27.8	28.4	29.0	29.6	30.2
95–97	26.1	26.7	27.3	27.9	28.5	29.1	29.7	30.3	30.9
98–100	26.9	27.4	28.0	28.6	29.2	29.8	30.4	31.0	31.6
101–103	27.5	28.1	28.7	29.3	29.9	30.5	31.1	31.7	32.3
104–106	28.2	28.8	29.4	30.0	30.6	31.2	31.8	32.4	33.0
107–109	28.9	29.5	30.1	30.7	31.3	31.9	32.5	33.1	33.7
110–112	29.6	30.2	30.8	31.4	32.0	32.6	33.2	33.8	34.4
113–115	30.2	30.8	31.4	32.0	32.6	33.2	33.8	34.5	35.1
116–118	30.9	31.5	32.1	32.7	33.3	33.9	34.5	35.1	35.7
119–121	31.5	32.1	32.7	33.3	33.9	34.5	35.1	35.7	36.4
122–124	32.1	32.7	33.3	33.9	34.5	35.1	35.8	36.4	37.0
125–127	32.7	33.3	33.9	34.5	35.1	35.8	36.4	37.0	37.6

Source: A. S. Jackson and M. L. Pollock, "Practical Assessment of Body Composition," *Physician and Sportsmedicine* 13, no. 5 (1985): 76–90. Copyright © 1985 JTE Multimedia, LLC. Used with permission.

4. Record your estimated percent body fat.

% body fat = _____

Section II: BIA Measurement

1. Use a BIA machine to estimate your percent body fat. Hydrate normally for 24 hours before the test and use the machine before you exercise. Select the appropriate "athlete" versus "non-athlete" setting if it is available on your machine.

2. Record your estimated percent body fat.

% body fat = _____

Section III: Body Fat Rating

Based on your estimated percent body fat from the skinfold test and/or BIA test, indicate your body fat rating below:

Body Fat Rating	Women	Men
Athletic/Low	14–20%	6–13%
Fitness	21–24%	14–17%
Acceptable	25–31%	18–25%
Obese	>32%	>26%

Source: From "Percent Body Fat Norms for Men and Women" in *ACE Lifestyle and Weight Management Coach Manual*, © 2013 American Council on Exercise. Reprinted with permission from the American Council on Exercise® (ACE®), www.acefitness.org.

Body fat rating: Skinfold test = _____

Body fat rating: BIA test = _____

Section IV: Calculate your Goal Weight

If your body fat is higher than your goal, use the steps below to calculate your goal body weight. This calculation assumes that you are maintaining (not gaining or losing) lean body mass as you lose overall body weight. This takes a balanced program of exercise and healthy eating, and generally a maximal weight loss of 1 to 2 pounds per week.

Write your current % body fat as a decimal = _____ (move the decimal left two places).

Write your goal % body fat as a decimal = _____

a.   Fat Mass = _____ lbs (body weight) × _____ (decimal % fat) = _____ lbs.

b.   Lean Body Mass = _____ lbs (body weight) − _____ lbs (Fat Mass) = _____ lbs.

c.   Goal Body Weight = _____ lbs (Lean Body Mass)/1 − (decimal goal % fat) = _____ lbs.

Section V: Reflection

1. Did your estimated percent body fat or rating surprise you? _____

2. If you performed both tests, how does your percent body fat rating for the skinfold test compare to the BIA test? If the results differ greatly, can you identify possible sources of error (such as technique, hydration, type of machine, etc.)?

_____

_____

3. How does your percent body fat rating compare with your other disease risk ratings from Lab 6.2?

_____

_____

7 Improving Your Nutrition

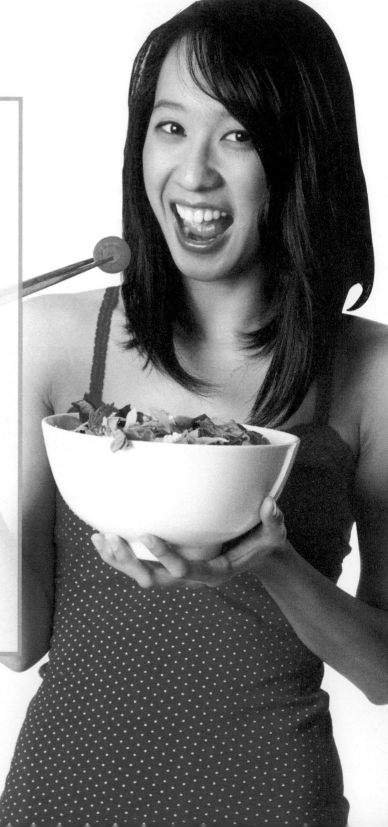

LEARNINGoutcomes

LO 7.1 Describe obstacles to a healthy diet during your college years along with a few ways to overcome the challenges.

LO 7.2 Identify the main nutrients in food and their roles in the body.

LO 7.3 Discuss the role of portion size, food labels, food groups, and whole foods in maintaining a balanced diet.

LO 7.4 Describe the special dietary needs of disparate groups, including elite athletes, everyday exercisers, women, children, teens, adults over 50, vegetarians, and those with diabetes.

LO 7.5 Explain food safety in terms of safe food-handling practices, organic foods versus non-organic, and food allergies and intolerances.

LO 7.6 Assess your current diet and create a behavior change plan for improved nutrition.

MasteringHealth™

Go online for chapter quizzes, interactive assessments, videos, and more!

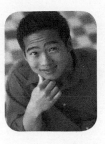

NICK

"Hi, I'm Nick. I'm a freshman and I live on campus in a dorm with my roommate, Tom. I moved here to Connecticut from Chicago. Living away from home for the first time has been quite an experience! I've been studying hard, taking a full load of classes, and trying to figure out if I want to major in history or political science. Plus, I'm in a few clubs and I'm playing a lot of soccer. I'm not on the team, but I like to play for fun. I'll jump into just about any pick-up game if I have time. I'm always rushing, though, and then I realize I'm starving! When I lived at home, there was always food around. My meal plan at the cafeteria covers 60 meals a month. For the others, I'm often scrambling at the last minute to grab something to eat."

Hear It!
To listen to this case study online, visit the Study Area in MasteringHealth™.

Hunger is one of our basic motivators. Eating—smelling, tasting, and consuming food—is one of life's great pleasures and supplies our bodies with energy and raw materials. Our challenge is to eat a healthy balance between the food our bodies *need* and the foods we enjoy or crave.

Food contains **nutrients**, chemical compounds that supply the energy and raw materials for survival. Our cells break down food molecules, releasing energy stored in their chemical bonds. The energy becomes available to drive the activities within our cells, tissues, and organs. Our cells also liberate raw materials as they break down food molecules and these supply our cellular repair, growth, and division.

Nutrition is the study of what we eat and how our bodies use the nutrients in food. Nutrition researchers study what we should be eating and how food affects our long-term health.

Unfortunately, nutritional findings are often contradictory. In addition, the media jump on each new claim, no matter how poorly substantiated. Understandably,

some people have grown confused and skeptical and have decided to eat whatever they want until the dust settles.[1] Sound familiar?

As in every area of science, new studies in nutrition occasionally invalidate older studies. Nevertheless, the field has made tremendous advances toward understanding our daily **diets**—the foods and drinks we select—as well as what we *should* be eating, what we should be *avoiding*, and why. The healthy diets we discuss in this chapter can help you stay fit and well. Keep in mind:

- A balanced diet helps sustain desirable body mass and weight and keeps your fat-to-lean ratios within a recommended range. This, in turn, can improve appearance and reduce your risk of disease.

- A good diet can help alleviate feelings of stress and depression, while a poor diet can contribute to them.

- A good diet can help prevent chronic diseases, frequent colds and infections, and the effects of vitamin deficiency. Conversely, poor diet is a major contributor to cardiovascular disease, diabetes, obesity, arthritis, osteoporosis, and several cancers.

If you are young and healthy, chronic diseases may seem remote. However, establishing good eating habits now can both improve your current fitness, wellness, and appearance, and diminish your later risk of chronic illness. This chapter helps you analyze and improve your nutrition to reap all of these benefits.

LO 7.1 Why Are My College Years a Nutritional Challenge?

If you are like most college students, you often reach for cheap snacks and fast food, and down them quickly, to save time and money. The typical student's diet resembles the typical American diet: More than one-half of total calories comes from added fats and oils; refined carbohydrates such as pizza crust, white rice, flour tortillas, and white bread buns; and added sweeteners such as sugar and corn syrup.[2] Among college students, the

nutrients Chemical compounds in food that are crucial to growth and function, including proteins, carbohydrates (starches and sugars), lipids (fats and oils), vitamins, and minerals

nutrition The study of how people consume and use the nutrients in food

diets The foods and drinks we select to consume

Less healthy eating habits	More healthy eating habits
Consuming sugary soft drinks with and between meals	Drinking water with and between meals
Skipping meals then gorging once or twice per day	Eating three meals plus one or two small, nutritious snacks at regular times
Eating large amounts of red meats, fatty meats, or fried meats	Choosing fish, lean poultry, tofu, or other proteins that are low in saturated fats
Choosing processed foods	Choosing whole foods such as fruits, vegetables, whole grains, nuts, seeds, and lean sources of protein
Hurriedly bolting down food on the run, in a car, or on a bike	Sitting down to eat a relaxed meal with friends or family
Finishing the large portions served at restaurants	Eating half of a large restaurant portion and taking the rest home
Snacking before bed	Eating earlier in the evening
Eating heartily to be social, regardless of appetite	If you're not very hungry, drinking a low-cal beverage or eating a piece of fruit to be social
Eating out of habit or boredom, for example, while watching TV	Sitting down at a table to eat only when hungry, finding another outlet for boredom
Reaching for food when feeling stressed or angry	Learning stress reduction techniques

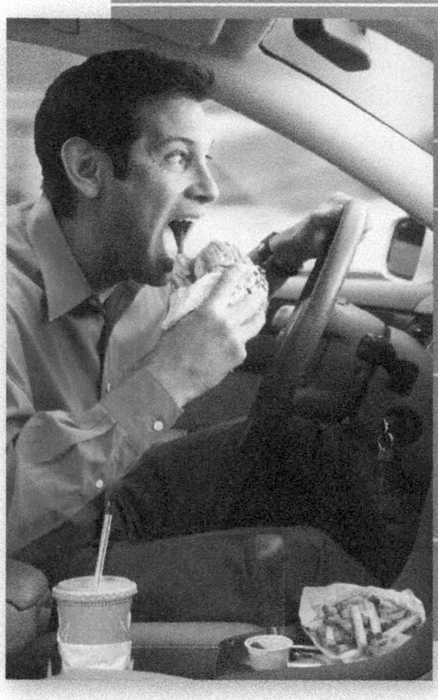

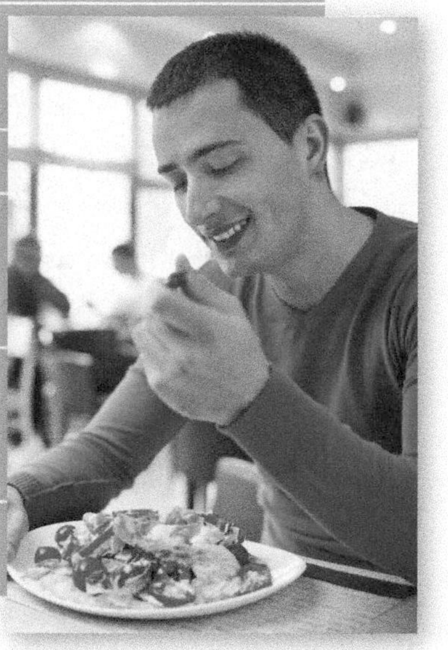

FIGURE **7.1** You can examine your own eating and snacking habits by comparing what, when, where, and how much you eat and drink to the sliding scale for each habit. You can also get ideas here for improving your daily diet.

Adapted from US Department of Health and Human Services and US Department of Agriculture, *Dietary Guidelines for Americans 2015–2020*, 8th ed., December 2015, www.health.gov

number-one takeout food is pizza, followed by Chinese food and burgers. Other favorites include fries, chicken wings, energy drinks, and cookies.[3] The most frequently eaten vegetables in America, on campus and off, are potatoes—more than 40 pounds per person per year.[4]

Most Students Have Less-Than-Optimal Eating Habits

Eating habits describe when, where, and how we eat; with whom we eat; what we choose to consume; and why we choose it. Like most Americans, college students, in general, have poor eating habits. Examples of poor eating habits

eating habits When, where, and how we eat; with whom we eat; what we choose to consume; and our reasons for choosing it

are eating fast food and eating while driving or watching television. Good eating habits include sitting down to a relaxed meal and consuming several servings of fresh fruits and vegetables every day. How are your eating habits? **Figure 7.1** can help you find out.

The GetFitGraphic Do Students Make the Grade When It Comes to Healthy Eating? on page 235 provides data on the typical student diet and how it stacks up. Most students, for example, eat half as many fruit and vegetable servings as the US Department of Agriculture (USDA) recommends; get one and a half to two times more sodium than they should in their salted and processed foods; and take in three times more refined sugar and saturated fat than the government deems healthy.[5] Compared to non-college young adults in the community, college students eat 70 percent more fast food.[6] This helps explain why the incoming international

DO STUDENTS MAKE THE GRADE WHEN IT COMES TO HEALTHY EATING?

The college student nutrition report card is in!

HOW DO STUDENTS' DIETS COMPARE TO THE USDA RECOMMENDATIONS?[1]

✓ Good   ✗ Bad

Nutrient	USDA Recommended Daily Consumption	Students' Average Daily Consumption	Grade
TOTAL PROTEIN	10–35% of calories	~16% of calories	✓
TOTAL CARBOHYDRATES	45–65% of calories	~53% of calories	✓
TOTAL FAT	20–35% of calories	~30% of calories	✓
SATURATED FAT & SUGARS	<10% of calories	~30% of calories	✗
CHOLESTEROL	<300 mg	~295 mg	✓
FIBER	~31 g	~19 g	✗
VITAMIN E	15 mg	~6.5 mg	✗
POTASSIUM	4,700 mg	~2695 mg	✗
SODIUM	1500–2300 mg	~3300 mg	✗
FOLATE	400 mcg	~390 mcg	✓
CALCIUM	1000 mg	~975 mg	✓
VITAMIN D	15 mcg	~4 mcg	✗
FRUITS & VEGETABLES	5–9 servings/day	~2.5 servings	✗

LET'S LOOK AT THREE NUTRIENT AREAS WHERE STUDENTS AREN'T MAKING THE GRADE: SODIUM, FATS, AND FRUITS & VEGETABLES.

SODIUM

Stop shaking the salt! Students consume an average of **1000 mg sodium** over the USDA recommendations. Where does all that salt come from?[3]

65% Foods from grocery stores

25% Foods eaten in restaurants

10% Foods cooked at home

FATS

75% of college freshman eat fried or high-fat fast foods at least three times a week

25% of college freshman eat fried or high-fat fast foods fewer than three times a week[4]

10 TROUBLEMAKERS

These ten foods supply 44% of the sodium in a typical college diet:[2]

1 Breads and rolls 2 Cold cuts and cured meats 3 Pizza 4 Poultry 5 Soups
6 Sandwiches 7 Cheese 8 Pasta dishes 9 Meat dishes 10 Snacks

FRUITS & VEGETABLES

Fill half your plate with fruits and veggies at every meal! The majority of students are getting only 1–2 servings of fruits and vegetables per day[5] instead of the U.S. government recommendations of 5 to 9 servings per day.[1]

0 servings = **5.6%**

1-2 servings = **65.7%**

3-4 servings = **24.1%**

5+ servings (USDA recommendation) = **4.6%**

students in a recent study gained an average of 9 pounds in their first semester at an American college.[7] These kinds of habits also help explain why most adult Americans, including college graduates, become heavier as the decades pass and why, among those over age 20, 37.7 percent of men and 40.4 percent of women are obese.[8] Understanding the information in this chapter and the next, on weight management, can make a measurable difference in your nutritional wellness.

College Life Presents Obstacles to Good Nutrition

Food is easy to find in the many vending machines, cafeterias, bars, restaurants, and markets on campus and off. But nutritious foods—low in saturated fat, salt, and sugars, for instance, and high in fiber and vitamin content—are harder to find on and near campus. Food choice is an important obstacle to student nutrition in addition to other obstacles: time and money pressures, lack of home-cooking facilities, personal habits and attitudes, and the emotional stresses that college can present.

Fast food and takeout solve both time and money issues, but most of the food at these restaurants provides poor nutrition. Even when students cook for themselves, however, nutritional misconceptions can still impede a healthy diet. For example, many people have better access to—and can better afford—canned and frozen fruits and vegetables, but avoid them. For all but leafy greens, however, the nutritional values are comparable and the lower prices make them a good bargain.[9]

If you do shop and cook, a few simple steps can help you achieve a balanced, affordable diet. Buy the fruits and vegetables you can afford. Watch for sales, use coupons. Make a shopping list and stick to it. Buy more plant proteins (e.g., beans and tofu), which cost less than meat, fish, or poultry. Double your recipes and freeze portions for later.

There are other obstacles to good nutrition, as well. One is our natural human craving for sweet, fatty, salty, and high-protein foods. We love those treats! And away from parental influence for the first time, many students regularly eat junk food, skip breakfast, snack frequently, and forget or avoid fruits and vegetables. Another obstacle is body dissatisfaction: Most students want to lose weight, while a sizeable minority want to gain weight or add muscle. They take various measures (details in Chapter 8) that do little except unbalance their nutrients, vitamins, and minerals.[10]

Additional contributors to poor diet are picky eating, stress eating, and social eating. Stress itself can cause people to eat more, especially high-calorie "comfort" foods and/or to drink more alcohol, with its load of empty calories. And socializing at parties and restaurants often paves a path of temptation. The Tools for Change box Tips for Ordering at Restaurants on page 237 helps you choose healthier menu items.

There are several keys to overcoming the food obstacles in college life:

- Learn about nutrition and what your body needs to maintain maximum wellness.
- Learn to distinguish good food choices from poor ones and good eating habits from bad ones.
- Frequent restaurants, stores, and cafeterias that offer a wide selection of healthy foods.
- Hang out with other students who care about nutritious eating.

||||||||||||||||||||||||||||||||||||||||||||||||||||||||||||||||||||||||||||||||

caseSTUDY

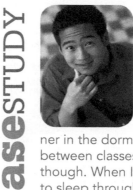

NICK

"I like the food in the dorm cafeteria most of the time, but I have to take care of about 30 meals on my own each month. The idea was that I'd eat breakfast and dinner in the dorm and grab lunch somewhere between classes. It hasn't worked out so far, though. When I don't have an early class, I tend to sleep through breakfast. Then, I've got to rush to my 11:00, so I usually chug down donuts and coffee from the campus store. Sometimes I get back to the dorm for lunch, but if I don't, I eat something on the run at the food court. The good thing is that my dorm has a late night café that accepts my meal plan. So if I'm up late studying, I can grab a pizza or bowl of cereal. I don't pay much attention to my diet or how many calories I'm eating. I figure at my age, it's more about getting enough calories than eating a 'balanced meal.' That's for older people, right?"

APPLY IT! What aspects of college life are influencing Nick's dietary choices? How do your own living situation and schedule affect your efforts to eat right?

TRY IT! Make a list of small lifestyle changes you could make to improve your diet and try to incorporate at least one in the coming week, another the following week.

Hear It!
To listen to this case study online, visit the Study Area in MasteringHealth™.

||||||||||||||||||||||||||||||||||||||||||||||||||||||||||||||||||||||||||||||||

Tips for Ordering at Restaurants

APPLY IT! No matter what type of cuisine you enjoy, there will always be healthy—and less healthy—options on the menu.

Cuisine	Lighter	Heavier	Tips
Italian	Spaghetti with marinara or tomato and meat sauce	Fettuccine Alfredo Fried calamari Lasagna	Avoid rich sauces. Try vegetarian pizza. Skip added parmesan.
Mexican	Plain bean burrito Chicken fajitas with lots of vegetables	Beef chimichanga Chile relleno (both are deep fried)	Skip fried tortillas, cheese, and sour cream. Choose fresh salsa, salads, grilled fish, or chicken.
Chinese	Hot-and-sour soup Stir-fried vegetables Szechuan shrimp	Kung pao chicken Moo shu pork Sweet-and-sour pork	Request brown rice instead of white. Avoid deep-fried dishes and added soy sauce. Choose steamed vegetables.
Japanese	Steamed rice and vegetables Tofu Broiled or steamed chicken and fish	Fried rice dishes Tempura (battered and deep-fried)	Avoid adding soy sauce. Avoid deep-fried dishes such as tempura. Ask for extra vegetables and less rice. Beware of food-borne illness from raw fish.
Thai	Clear broth soups Stir-fried chicken and vegetables Grilled meats Clear tea	Soups containing coconut milk Peanut sauces Deep-fried dishes	Avoid soups and curries high in saturated fat. Choose steamed brown rice over fried or white rice. Thai iced tea is loaded with sugar and fat.
American Breakfast	Hot or cold cereal with nonfat or 1 percent milk Pancakes with fruit and drizzled (not drowned) in syrup Scrambled eggs with whole wheat toast	Belgian waffle with whipped cream Sausage, eggs, biscuits and gravy Hash browns, catsup Three-egg omelet with cheese	Choose whole-grain cereals and low-fat or nonfat milk. Order omelets heavy on vegetables, light on cheese. Skip processed meats like bacon and sausage.
Sandwiches	Veggies and tofu Lean beef Turkey	Tuna salad Reuben 12" Submarine	Choose mustard, skip mayonnaise and cheese. Pile on dark green lettuce and sliced vegetables.
Seafood	Steamed, baked, grilled, or broiled fish or shell fish	Fried seafood platter Blackened catfish	Avoid fried or sautéed entrees. Squeeze on lemon instead of creamy and buttery sauces.
Fast Food	Grilled chicken sandwich Lean roast beef sandwich Entrée salad, dressing on the side Water, nonfat milk, unsweetened iced tea Fresh fruit and yogurt	Double-patty sandwiches Added cheese French fries and onion rings Deed fried chicken or fish Sugary soft drinks, shakes, or desserts	Skip mayo, sauces, and cheese. Choose oil and vinegar over creamy dressings. Order fresh fruit and vegetables. Read nutrition information to limit sugar, calories, saturated fat.
Coffeehouse	Latte or coffee with low-fat milk and no or low-cal sweetener Hot black, green, or herbal tea with low-fat milk and/or no or low-cal sweetener	Sweetened, flavored latte with whipped cream Chai with high-fat milk and sugar Hot chocolate or mocha with whipped cream	Avoid sugar and whipped cream. Request fat-free milk in blended drinks. Add flavor with a dash of cinnamon or nutmeg.

LO 7.2 What Are the Main Nutrients in Food?

Like all animals, humans need to "refuel": Our cells and bodies can't originate energy-containing raw materials for activity, growth, and repair, so we need to consume them each day. The nutrients we require are water, proteins, carbohydrates (starches and sugars), lipids (fats and oils), vitamins, and minerals. The three-dimensional shape of each kind of sugar molecule, fat molecule, and so on determines their chemical properties and, in turn, their roles in the body.

Some nutrients we must consume directly in foods; others our cells can "remodel" into the building blocks we need. Nutritionists use the term **essential nutrients** for those compounds we must get directly from foods.

Nutritionists can measure the energy stored in individual foods—the natural sugars and starches in an apple, for example, and the way our bodies release that stored energy during the digestion process. They measure the released energy in **calories**. One calorie (with a lowercase *c*) is the amount of energy required to raise the temperature of 1 gram of water 1 degree Celsius. Nutritionists usually apply the larger measure **kilocalories (kcal) or Calories (C)** when referring to food energy: 1 C equals 1,000 calories. A small apple, for example, the size of a tennis ball, might have about 50 or 60 C.

To avoid confusion, this book will use "calories" when referring to food energy in general as well as when designating the energy in a specific food. Active adults need about 2,000 to 2,500 calories of food energy per day. The more you exercise, the higher your calorie expenditure. Nutritionists used to believe that the body uses the calories in all nutrients equally and that you must simply balance total calories eaten and total calories

expended to prevent weight gain or loss. They no longer think that all calories are equal, however.[11] Chapter 8 explains in detail the role of calories from fats, proteins, and carbohydrates in weight maintenance.

Proteins Are Building Blocks of Structure and Function

Some people see proteins as the new elixir for wellness, weight loss, and bulking up. But what's the truth? The body of a 150-pound person has about 75 pounds of water (50 percent of body weight) and about 37.5 pounds of protein (25 percent), depending on muscle mass. **Proteins** are major structural components of nearly every cell and are especially important to the building and repairing of bone, muscle, skin, and blood cells. Proteins also make up the antibodies that protect us from disease, the enzymes that control all chemical reactions in the body, and the many types of hormones that regulate body activities. And proteins help transport oxygen, carbon dioxide, and various nutrients to body cells. When the body runs low on fats and carbohydrates as sources of ready energy, it can break down its own proteins and convert them to energy compounds. Protein supplies four calories of energy per gram.

Protein molecules are chains of subunits called *amino acids.* These "building blocks of life" contain carbon, hydrogen, oxygen, and nitrogen arrayed in particular ways. There are 20 different kinds of amino acids, each with a different three-dimensional shape. Your body uses the 20 types of amino acids to build tens of thousands of kinds of proteins. Many of these are *structural proteins* that make up parts of cells, tissues, and organs. Many kinds of structural proteins enable cells to move, to divide, and to transport materials around internally. Other structural proteins make up your hair strands, your fingernails and toenails, and the lenses of your eyes. A steady supply of amino acids in the diet allows your body to continuously build, repair, and replace its own structural proteins.

Proteins that perform crucial functions (rather than make up physical structures) are called *functional proteins.* They include **enzymes**, which facilitate thousands of kinds of chemical reactions within each body cell every second. The reactions that break down food, absorb nutrients, and build new cell parts require enzymes.

Proteins in the Diet Our bodies can manufacture only 11 of the 20 kinds of amino acids. Nutritionists call the other nine, which we must consume in food, the

---

essential nutrients Nutrients necessary for normal body functioning that must be obtained from food

calories A measure of the amount of chemical energy that foods provide. One calorie (lowercase *c*) can raise 1 gram of water 1 degree Celsius.

kilocalories (kcal) or Calories (C) A measure of energy equal to 1,000 calories, also designated kilocalorie (kcal); nutritionists use kcal or C when they refer to specific foods.

proteins Biological molecules composed of amino acids. Proteins serve as crucial structural and functional compounds in living organisms.

enzymes Proteins that facilitate chemical reactions but are not permanently altered in the process; biological catalysts

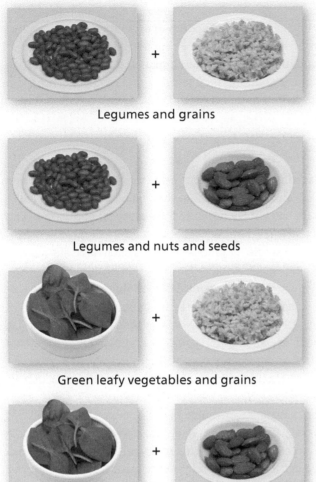

Legumes and grains

Legumes and nuts and seeds

Green leafy vegetables and grains

Green leafy vegetables and nuts and seeds

FIGURE **7.2** Combining plant foods from different groups (e.g., grains and legumes) on the same day can provide complementary proteins and all the necessary amino acids, even without eating meat or other animal foods.

essential amino acids. Dietary protein that supplies all the essential amino acids is called *complete protein,* or *high-quality protein.* Typically, protein from animal products is complete. *Incomplete proteins* lack some of the essential amino acids and therefore some of the building blocks we need to produce the full spectrum of body proteins. Plant proteins are often incomplete. Nevertheless, a vegetarian can easily combine plant foods to obtain *complementary proteins* from plant sources (**Figure 7.2**).

Daily Protein Needs More than a billion of the world's people face daily protein deficiency, but few Americans suffer it. The average American consumes between 60 and 100 grams (250 to 400 calories or more) of protein daily. For most adults, the recommended daily allowance for protein is 0.8 grams per kilogram of body weight per day; however, many experts now think this may be too low and that 1 to 1.2 g/kg is safe and healthy.[12] Consuming too much protein, on the other hand—particularly animal protein—can place added stress on the liver and kidneys and can cause a painful disease called *gout.* An overload of protein may also increase calcium excretion in urine, which can increase your risk of bone loss and bone fractures.[13]

Use **Figure 7.3** to calculate your daily protein needs. Here's an example: A healthy young woman weighing 132 pounds (60 kg) would need at least 48 grams (60 × 0.8). One gram is equal to 0.035 ounce; therefore, she would need about 1.68 ounces of

> **essential amino acids** Collectively, the 9 of the 20 types of amino acids, or building blocks, that our bodies cannot manufacture and that we must consume in our foods

Group	Daily protein requirement (g/kg body weight)	Calculating your daily protein requirement	Example (for average adult)
Most adults	0.8 g/kg	❶ Determine your body weight	❶ Weight = 132 lb
Recreational athletes	1.0–1.1 g/kg	❷ Convert pounds to kilograms: lb ÷ 2.21 lb/kg = kg	❷ 132 lb ÷ 2.21 lb/kg = about 60 kg
Elite athletes in training	1.2 –1.6 g/kg	❸ Multiply by 0.8 g/kg for average adult to get requirement in grams per day	❸ 60 kg × 0.8 g/kg = 48 g Result: A 132 lb adult would need 48 g of protein a day

FIGURE **7.3** Use these formulas to determine your daily protein requirements, depending on your activity level.

protein (0.035 × 48 = 1.68), which she could get, for example, by consuming one cup of skim milk, one-half cup of tofu, and one cup of cooked beans or 3 ounces of salmon. Experts think some protein at every meal is a healthy habit.[14]

In recent years, millions of people have tried the Atkins diet and similar diets that nearly eliminate carbohydrates and prescribe large quantities of protein. These diets *can* lead to weight loss (see Chapter 8). However, people with fluid imbalances, kidney or liver problems, or cardiovascular disease should avoid these diets altogether because they can further unbalance the body's fats, vitamins, and minerals and promote various chronic diseases. Others should limit the length of time they follow high-protein, low-carb diets.[15]

Protein and Fitness It is fairly common for athletes and fitness buffs to load up on animal protein under the misguided notion that eating more protein will cause them to build bigger muscles. But muscles grow in response to being worked: You must use them to grow them! The many vegetarian Olympic athletes are proof that training and effort—not mountains of animal protein—are the crucial ingredients. Research has also shown that 0.8 to 0.9 grams per kilogram of protein can suffice for a sedentary adult, but more—1.2 to 1.6 grams per kilogram per day—is needed for heavy endurance

and strength training.[16] Research suggests that along with exercise, 1 to 1.2 g/kg of protein per day may also help protect older adults from muscle wasting.[17] Extra protein can aid in cellular repair and replacement after surgery or during infections, and is required during pregnancy and breast-feeding.[18]

Carbohydrates Are Major Energy Suppliers

Carbohydrates, our most basic energy compounds, have ring- and chain-like three-dimensional structures that store and supply much of the energy for our normal daily activity. The **simple carbohydrates** or **sugars** are common in whole, unprocessed foods such as beets, sugarcane, carrots, other vegetables, and fruits such as grapes (**Figure 7.4a**). The **complex carbohydrates** include the starches found abundantly in grains (such as rice and wheat), cereals (such as oats), some fruits and vegetables (such as bananas and squash), and many root vegetables (such as potatoes, yams, and turnips) (**Figure 7.4b**).

Our cells can rapidly break down sugar molecules and release their stored chemical energy. For this reason, simple sugars such as glucose, sucrose (table sugar), and lactose (milk sugar) are a source of immediate fuel. Your muscle cells and your brain and nerve cells are particularly dependent on a steady supply of glucose, whether from fruits and vegetables or from the starches in grains. This dependence is the reason why low blood sugar, or *hypoglycemia,* can leave you feeling weak, shaky, and foggy-headed.

The US government's *Dietary Guidelines for Americans 2015–2020* urged people to consume more vegetables, fruits, and whole grains (for their complex carbohydrates). It recommended that we consume at least half of our grains as whole grains and that we eat

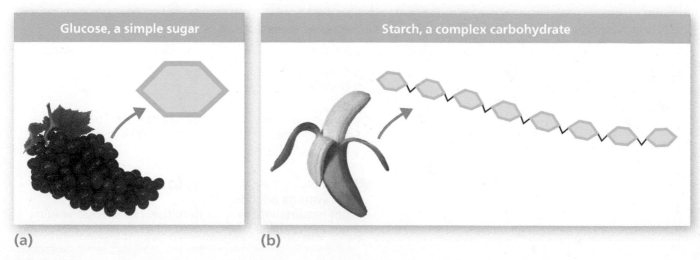

(a)   (b)

FIGURE **7.4** (a) Grapes are rich in glucose, a simple sugar. (b) Bananas contain starch, a complex carbohydrate.

TABLE 7.1 Whole Grains and Refined Grains

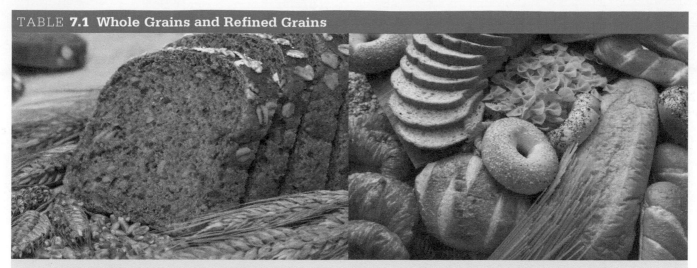

Whole grains—*Eat more of these*		Refined grains—*Eat fewer of these*	
brown rice	whole wheat bread	cornbread*	pitas*
buckwheat	whole wheat crackers	corn tortillas*	pretzels
bulgur (cracked wheat)	whole wheat pasta	couscous*	white bread
oatmeal	whole wheat sandwich buns	crackers*	white sandwich buns
popcorn	and rolls	flour tortillas*	and rolls
whole grain barley	whole wheat tortillas	grits	white rice
whole grain cornmeal	wild rice	noodles*	
whole rye	*Less common whole grains:*	pasta*	*Ready-to-eat breakfast cereals*
Ready-to-eat breakfast cereals:	amaranth		corn flakes
whole wheat cereal flakes	millet		
muesli	quinoa		
	sorghum		
	triticale		

*Most of these products are made from refined grains. Some are made from whole grains. Check the ingredient list for the words *whole grain* or *whole wheat* to decide whether they are made from a whole grain. Some foods are made from a mixture of whole and refined grains.

Source: United States Department of Agriculture ChooseMyPlate, "Food Groups: Grains," 2015, www.ChooseMyPlate.gov

half or fewer as refined grains (such as breads and cereals made with white flour). **Table 7.1** lists many whole and refined grains.

The guidelines also recommend eating fewer sugar-sweetened foods and beverages (to avoid an overload of simple sugars). Americans eat more than twice as many daily calories from sugar and other sweeteners as heart experts recommend: a maximum of 6 teaspoons (about 100 calories) for women and 9 teaspoons (about 150 calories) for men.[19] Sweeteners, "hidden" mostly in processed foods, promote tooth decay, supplant more nutritious foods, and appear to raise triglyceride levels in the blood and contribute to cardiovascular disease.[20]

See It!
Watch "Ditching Sugar" at MasteringHealth™.

Compared to sugars, starches and other complex carbohydrates (also called *polysaccharides,* meaning "many sugars") provide "timed release" energy. The body's cells must break most starch molecules down into sugar subunits before "mining" the stored energy. This slower breakdown makes most starches important as energy-storage compounds as well as structural building materials in plants and animals.

Fiber Americans eat too little fiber in their diets and find the whole subject confusing, in part because there are no clear rules for what a food manufacturer can call "whole grain."[21] While our domesticated horses and cows can derive energy from *cellulose* (a structural carbohydrate in the cell walls of plants), we humans lack that ability. Instead, cellulose acts for us as **fiber** or roughage—indigestible plant matter.

There are two types of fiber: insoluble and soluble. The cellulose in bran, whole grain breads and cereals, and in

fiber Indigestible carbohydrates in the diet that speed the passage of partially digested food through the digestive tract

Tips for Eating More Fiber

Most Americans should double their daily fiber intake. To increase the fiber in your diet, think "whole" instead of refined foods and choose more of these:

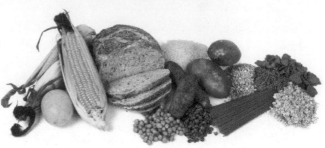

- Whole grains, including stone-ground wheat, bulgur wheat, wheat bran, wheat berries, whole barley, whole millet, whole quinoa, oatmeal, oat bran, popcorn, barley, cornmeal, whole rye, brown rice, and rice bran

- Peas, beans, nuts, and seeds

- Leafy greens such as baby spinach, endive, radicchio, arugula, mizuna, watercress, or dandelion greens

- Bran or flaxseed

- Fresh fruits and vegetables including, when edible, their cleanly scrubbed skins

- Plenty of liquids each day

  At the same time, choose fewer of these:

- White bread, buns, pizza dough, flour tortillas, and white rice

- Breakfast cereals that list "enriched" flour as the main ingredient

- Cookies, pastries, desserts, and candies

APPLY IT! What is your average daily intake of fiber?

TRY IT! **Today**, keep a food diary (or look at one you are already keeping) and, using food labels and other available information, calculate the total grams of fiber in your foods. You can find tips for using a food diary in Lab 7.2. **This week**, make a list of the fiber-containing foods you have eaten in the past week and next to each, write a food that you could swap for even more fiber. For example: "white rice→ brown rice," or "white bread bun→ whole wheat pita." **In two weeks**, keep a food diary for an entire day and again calculate the total number of fiber grams you consumed. Did you improve your fiber consumption? How does your new level compare with the USDA recommendation of 28 grams (females ages 19 to 30) and 34 grams (males ages 19 to 30)?

---

most fruits and vegetables acts as *insoluble fiber*: It speeds the passage of foods and reduces bile acids and certain bacterial enzymes. The roughage in oat bran; in some fruits (such as blueberries and apples); and in many beans, nuts, and seeds is s*oluble fiber*: It attracts and attaches to water molecules and forms a gel that can ferry cholesterol molecules out of the body. For this reason, soluble fiber appears to help lower blood cholesterol levels and risk of cardiovascular disease. Besides helping matter pass through the digestive tract (thus reducing constipation), both kinds of fiber help control appetite by creating a feeling of fullness without adding extra calories.

The daily recommended amount of fiber for an adult is 25 to 38 grams, but fewer than 5 percent of Americans—including most college students—consume that amount.[22] In addition, about 1 in 7 adults have high blood cholesterol levels that could be partially lowered by consuming more fiber.[23] The *Dietary Guidelines for Americans 2015–2020* recommends that we eat more whole, ground, cracked, or flaked grains (including whole oats, whole wheat, and brown rice), and decrease our consumption of refined carbohydrates such as white rice and white flour. The Tools for Change box Tips for Eating More Fiber can help you choose fiber-rich foods.

The Glycemic Index of Foods Nutritionists use a tool called the **glycemic index** to rank on a scale of 1 to 100 the rates at which different types of foods break down in the human digestive system and release glucose into the blood: the higher the number, the faster and greater the release of glucose. Plain white French bread has a glycemic index of 95; so does corn flakes; and white rice scores 89.

But nutritionists also impose a second measure called the glycemic load that brings a normal serving

glycemic index A measurement of the rate at which foods raise levels of glucose in the blood and, in turn, trigger the release of insulin and other blood-sugar regulators

size into the equation. For example, watermelon also has a fairly high glycemic index of 72/100, but because of the fruit's water and fiber content, you'd have to eat an enormous amount of it to get a big flood of blood glucose. The glycemic load of the fore-mentioned foods is French bread, 15; corn flakes, 23; white rice, 43; and watermelon 4. Eating foods with a high glycemic load causes both a flood of blood glucose and a corresponding release of insulin from the pancreas to handle the blood sugar. Over time, this kind of flooding and surging can lead to insulin resistance and can contribute to pre-diabetes and type 2 diabetes as well as to certain cancers; to overweight and obesity; and perhaps to heart disease.[24] A recent study attempting to measure people's blood sugar and fats while on high and low glycemic-load diets showed a confusing pattern that suggests the body's response is highly complex.[25]

The best advice is to eat a heart-healthy diet and not focus on glycemic index and load unless you have pre-diabetes or diabetes. This means eat lots of fruits, vegetables, whole grains, low-fat dairy, fish, chicken, legumes, nuts, and oils, and cut back on salt, sugary treats and beverages, and sources of saturated fat such as butter and red meat.[26] Those with diabetes or a high risk of it may benefit more directly from watching their glycemic load, as Chapter 11 explains.

"Low-Carb" Foods In recent years, food manufacturers have introduced thousands of "low-carb" foods, influenced, in part, by the popularity of high-protein weight loss diets. As we've seen, however, whole grain foods are packed with healthful nutrients and fiber. The culprit is not the "carbs" themselves but the quantity most people eat and the refining of the carbohydrates. Whole fruits and vegetables, and foods made with whole grains, seeds, and nuts, are nutrient-dense and retain the fibrous cellulose. Most "low-carb" foods are highly processed and contain substitute sugars such as mannitol, sorbitol, and dextrose. There is no solid evidence that "low-carb" products made with sweeteners protect you from diseases, and they cost much more than simple fruits, vegetables, whole grains, nuts, seeds, and beans.

Fats Are Concentrated Energy Storage

Preceding the "low-carb" diet craze was a "low-fat" craze that labeled all fats and oils as harmful. In fact, fats play vital roles in maintaining healthy skin and hair, padding the body organs against shock, promoting healthy cell function, insulating us against temperature extremes, and storing concentrated energy that can fuel

muscle activity when carbohydrates are in short supply. Although fats are widely misunderstood nutrients, they make foods taste better; they carry the fat-soluble vitamins A, D, E, and K to cells; and they provide certain essential compounds that we can't get from other foods or manufacture in our own cells.

Types of Fats *Fat* is a common term for **lipids**, a class of molecules that includes fats and oils. **Fats** such as butter, lard, and bacon grease, are solid at room temperature. **Oils** are usually liquid at room temperature; examples are corn and olive oils. Lipids also include *waxes,* such as beeswax, and *steroids,* such as steroid hormones, cholesterol, and certain vitamins.

Structurally, fats and oils are made up of long chains of carbon atoms called **fatty acids**. The fatty acids in most foods and in the body occur in the form of **triglycerides**, molecules that have a "head," which contains the compound glycerol, and three tails (**Figure 7.5a**, page 244). The "tails" are made up of fatty acid chains of various lengths. Chemical bonds between carbon atoms in the "tails" determine whether the chains remain straight and form solid fats (**Figure 7.5b**) or kink and form liquid oils (**Figure 7.5c**).

In a fatty acid tail where every available carbon bond is *saturated* or filled with hydrogen atoms, the fat itself is called a **saturated fat**. Saturated tails remain straight and can pack solidly against each other. This explains why butter, beef fat, and lard— all saturated fats— stay solid at room temperature.

In an oil, certain carbons in the tail lack hydrogen atoms (thus the label **unsaturated**) and the tails kink and bend. The bends prevent tight packing together, thus oils are slippery liquids rather than solids. Fatty acid tails with just one kinked (unsaturated) region are called

lipids A category of compounds, including fats, oils, and waxes, that do not dissolve in water

fats Lipids, such as butter, lard, and bacon grease, that are usually solid at room temperature

oils Lipids, such as corn and olive oil, that are usually liquid at room temperature

fatty acids The most basic units of triglycerides

triglycerides Lipid molecules made up of three fatty acid chains or "tails" attached to one glycerol "head" containing a three-carbon backbone; common form of fats in foods and in organisms

saturated fat A lipid, usually a solid fat such as butter, in which most of the chains of carbon atoms are loaded (or "saturated") with as many hydrogen atoms as the chain can carry

unsaturated fat A lipid, usually a liquid oil, in which most carbon chains lack the maximum load of hydrogen atoms

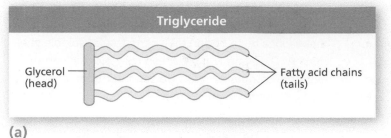

Triglyceride

Glycerol (head) → Fatty acid chains (tails)

(a)

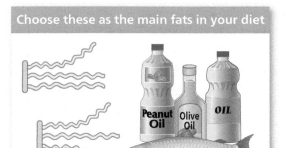

Reduce these fats in your diet

LARD Margarine Butter

Long-chain saturated fatty acids lack double bonds and have straight carbon chains. They pack together to make solid forms at room temperature.

(b)

Choose these as the main fats in your diet

Peanut Oil Olive Oil OIL

Mono- and polyunsaturated fatty acids can kink and bend at the double bond in the chain. Kinked chains slide past each other and act as liquid oils.

(c)

FIGURE **7.5** (a) Structure of triglyceride. The chemical makeup of fatty acid chains in fats and oils helps explain their structure: Lard and butter (b), which contain high levels of saturated fats, are usually solid. Olive, peanut, and most other oils (c), which contain high levels of mono- and polyunsaturated fats, are usually liquid.

Figure from *Nutrition: An Applied Approach*, 4th Edition, by Janice Thompson and Melinda Manore. Copyright ©2014 Pearson Education. Reprinted and Electronically reproduced by permission of Pearson Education, Inc., Upper Saddle River, New Jersey.

monounsaturated fatty acids (**MUFAs**; *mono* means "one"). Olive oil, canola oil, and cashew oil are all rich in monounsaturated fatty acids. Tails containing two or more linked regions are called **polyunsaturated fatty acids** (**PUFAs**; *poly* means "many"). Corn oil, safflower oil, and soy oil are all rich in polyunsaturated fatty acids.

Food manufacturers sometimes alter oils by pumping hydrogen atoms into liquid oils, a process called hydrogenation. This results in partially hydrogenated oils that can contain some *trans* fatty acids or **trans fats**. These have cooking properties of solid fats. Some types of margarine and shortening and many kinds of processed foods contain *trans* fats. Dairy products and meat naturally contain small amounts of *trans* fats, as well. The federal *Dietary Guidelines for Americans 2015–2020* recommend that we avoid or greatly decrease the intake of foods containing *trans* fats. We will discuss the health consequences of eating *trans* fats later.

All of our food sources of fats and oils contain both saturated and unsaturated fats, in different ratios (**Figure 7.6**, page 245). For example, a tablespoon of safflower oil contains 0.8 gram of saturated fat, 10.2 grams of monounsaturated fat, and 2 grams of polyunsaturated fat. A tablespoon of butter typically contains 7.2 grams of saturated fat, 3.3 of grams monounsaturated fat, and a trace of polyunsaturated fat.

Most nutritionists think that lipids high in saturated fats are unhealthy for you, especially if you eat them frequently. Animals tend to make saturated fats, and plants tend to make unsaturated fats. Some plants, however, generate oils that are very high in saturated fats. Cocoa butter, palm kernel oil, and coconut oil contain more saturated fat per tablespoon than butter, beef fat, or lard! Since lipids high in mono- and polyunsaturated fats are healthier for you than those high in saturated fat, it pays to learn about and choose oils wisely. In Figure 7.6, the oils containing the widest purple and red bands (depicting mono- and polyunsaturated fatty acids) are the healthiest. The fats and oils with the widest blue bands (saturated fatty acids) are the least healthy.

Omega-3 and Omega-6 Fatty Acids Our cells cannot synthesize certain acids and therefore we must consume each of them in our diet. These fatty acids are called **essential fatty acids**. They include *linoleic acid,* an omega-6 fatty acid, and *linolenic acid,* an omega-3 fatty acid.

monounsaturated fatty acids (MUFAs) Lipids whose fatty acid chains have just one kinked (unsaturated) region

polyunsaturated fatty acids (PUFAs) Lipids whose fatty acid chains have two or more kinked (unsaturated) regions

trans fats Unsaturated lipids or oils with hydrogen atoms added to cause more complete saturation and make the oil function as a solid

essential fatty acids Lipid components, including linolenic acid, EPA, DHA, and linoleic acid, that the body cannot manufacture and which we must obtain in polyunsaturated oils

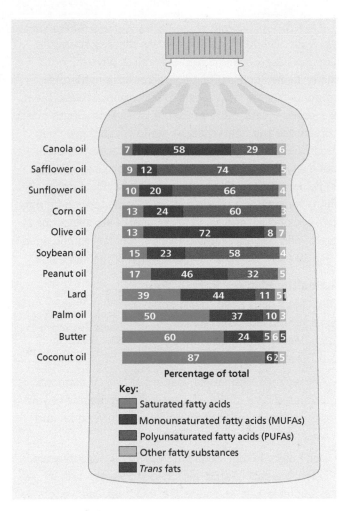

Canola oil	7	58	29	6
Safflower oil	9	12	74	5
Sunflower oil	10	20	66	4
Corn oil	13	24	60	3
Olive oil	13	72	8	7
Soybean oil	15	23	58	4
Peanut oil	17	46	32	5
Lard	39	44	11	51
Palm oil	50	37	10	3
Butter	60	24	5	65
Coconut oil	87	6	25	

Percentage of total

Key:
- Saturated fatty acids
- Monounsaturated fatty acids (MUFAs)
- Polyunsaturated fatty acids (PUFAs)
- Other fatty substances
- *Trans* fats

FIGURE **7.6** Common fats and oils have varying percentages of saturated and unsaturated fats, making them more or less healthful in the diet.

An **omega-6 fatty acid** is polyunsaturated and kinks at two sites, one being the sixth carbon along the "tail." An **omega-3 fatty acid** kinks at three sites, one being the third carbon along the tail. Other omega-3 fatty acids include EPA and DHA, which the human body can modify into linolenic acid. Polyunsaturated oils such as canola oil, corn oil, soybean oil, and sunflower oil all contain high levels of omega-6 fatty acids. Polyunsaturated oils such as flaxseed oil, walnut oil, and, to a lesser degree, certain fish oils, canola oil, and soybean oil contain relatively high percentages of omega-3 fatty acids.

The body can modify omega fatty acids into various fats we need for blood clotting, building cell membranes in the brain, contributing to healthy blood vessel walls, and counteracting inflammation. As a result, they lower the risks for heart disease and Alzheimer's disease, and help prevent inflammatory and autoimmune diseases, such as ulcerative colitis and rheumatoid arthritis.[27] Recent studies have shown that eating foods rich in omega-3s such as flaxseed, walnuts, and the flesh of oily fish (sardines, mackerel, salmon) is more protective than simply taking supplements (pills) containing the oil.[28]

Dietary Fats and Your Health As your body breaks down the fats and oils in a food, it packages the lipids into particles called **lipoproteins** that can move along easily in the bloodstream. Lipoproteins contain lipid and protein portions, and carry both triglycerides and **cholesterol**, the most common steroid in the body (recall that steroids are one structural class of fats). Our cells need and make cholesterol to keep membranes pliable and to form raw materials for steroid hormones and other substances. In common usage, lipoproteins carrying cholesterol are simply called *cholesterol.* When we consume more calories than we need, the body makes extra triglycerides and stores them as body fat.

Eating saturated fat and *trans* fat raises the level of both triglycerides and so-called bad cholesterol or **low-density lipoproteins (LDLs)** in your bloodstream. Over time, elevated levels of LDLs can lead to plaque deposits inside the blood vessels. These plaques can constrict blood flow, raise blood pressure, and lead to heart disease, heart attacks, and strokes (details in Chapter 10). Eating saturated fat also raises the level of so-called good cholesterol or **high-density lipoproteins (HDLs)** in the blood, but to a lesser degree. Eating polyunsaturated oils raises HDL levels to a much greater degree. HDLs prevent and reduce plaque deposits in the blood vessels and therefore

omega-6 fatty acid A polyunsaturated fatty acid that has double-bonded carbons at two sites, including one at the sixth carbon along the chain

omega-3 fatty acid A polyunsaturated fatty acid that has double-bonded carbons at three sites, including one at the third carbon along the chain

lipoproteins Lipid-plus-protein transport particles that can move along easily in the bloodstream; carry triglycerides or cholesterol

cholesterol A waxy lipid in the steroid class that is an important component of cell membranes and is transported in the blood by carriers called *LDL* and *HDL*

low-density lipoproteins (LDLs) A form of lipoprotein sometimes called "bad cholesterol"; LDL levels rise in response to saturated fats in the diet and can contribute to plaque deposits inside blood vessels

high-density lipoproteins (HDLs) A form of lipoprotein sometimes called "good cholesterol"; HDL levels rise in response to polyunsaturated fats and prevent and reduce plaque deposits in the blood vessels

help protect against cardiovascular disease, strokes, and heart attacks. That's the main reason why both the federal dietary guidelines and the American Heart Association urge us to choose oils over saturated fats.

The bottom line remains: Eating saturated fat regularly or in large quantities is a bad idea. The World Health Organization even places fatty processed meats such as bacon, hot dogs, and sausages in the same category of cancer risk as smoking and exposure to asbestos particles.[29] This is partly due to the meat's fat content, partly to preservatives, and partly to dangerous compounds formed when red or processed meats are fried or grilled at high heat.

Nutritionists once warned people to avoid eating cholesterol, especially in eggs. Recent studies have confirmed, however, that most people can eat up to 300 milligrams of cholesterol per day (one egg yolk contains 210 mg) without raising their blood cholesterol or their risk of heart disease.[30] Those with diagnosed diabetes or cardiovascular disease, though, should seek medical advice on eating cholesterol.[31]

Researchers continue trying to untangle the interconnections between lipids, body fat, and disease. In the meantime, the USDA, US Food and Drug Administration (FDA), American Heart Association, and other advisory groups recommend that you cut back on fatty meats, egg yolks (beyond one per day), high-fat dairy products, and other sources of saturated fats, cholesterol, and *trans* fats.

The picture is much clearer for *trans* fatty acids: There is consensus that hydrogenated oils are more damaging than saturated fats and more closely linked to stroke, heart attack, and diabetes.[32] *Trans* fats increase LDLs and simultaneously lower HDLs, a doubly negative effect. *Trans* fats also raise triglyceride levels. After a meal, the liver takes cholesterol and triglycerides that we don't use immediately, packages them into HDLs and LDLs, and sends them through the blood for storage in fat cells.[33] In 2013, the FDA deemed them no longer "generally regarded as safe" to eat and gave food manufacturers until 2018 to phase them out.[34] The *trans* fat content of foods is now indicated on food labels. If you look closely at ingredient lists, you can still find "partially hydrogenated oil" in some brands of stick margarine, coffee creamer, canned frosting, microwave popcorn, refrigerated dough, and baked goods.[35]

In contrast to trans fats, consuming mono- and polyunsaturated oils has a doubly positive effect: These fats lower LDLs and raise HDLs. As Figure 7.6 shows, most—although not all—cooking oils are high in mono- and polyunsaturated fats and low in saturated fats.

Many nutritionists encourage people to consume more oils. The Mediterranean-style diets in countries like Italy, Greece, and Spain are rich in olive oil, nuts, seeds, beans, fish, fruits, vegetables, and moderate amounts of wine with meals, but contain little red meat, processed meats, dairy products, or sweets. Death rates from stroke and heart disease are lower in these countries, and Americans who follow Mediterranean diets can cut their incidence of stroke or heart attack by 30 percent.[36] The USDA www.ChooseMyPlate.gov website recommends a combined daily consumption (in nuts, fish, cooking oil, and salad dressings) of six teaspoons of mono- and polyunsaturated oils per day for women aged 19 to 30 and seven teaspoons for men of the same age.

A Healthy Plan for Fats in Your Diet Most of us need to cut down on saturated fats while getting more heart-healthy fats into our diet. Here are some ideas:

> **Live It!**
> Complete Worksheet 24 Cutting Out the Fat at MasteringHealth™.

- Always read food labels, looking at both the amount of saturated fat and the percentage it represents of your daily recommended maximum for saturated fat and total fat.

- Don't assume that foods are healthy because they are labeled "low-fat." Watch out for added sugars, refined carbohydrates, salt, and *trans* fats (disguised as "vegetable shortening" or "partially hydrogenated vegetable oil").

- Choose oils such as canola, soy, olive, and safflower that contain high levels of mono- and polyunsaturated fats.

- For topping bread and crackers, alternatives to butter include buttery spreads (without *trans* fats), all-fruit jams (without added sugars), fat-free cream cheese, salsa, hummus, olive oil, or low-fat salad dressing.

- For protein, choose beans, nuts, seeds, tofu, lean meats, fish, or poultry and cut down or eliminate fatty meats such as bacon, sausages, hot dogs, bologna, pepperoni, or organ meats. Even for fish and chicken, remove skin. For all meats, avoid frying. Drain off fat after cooking.

- Choose dairy products such as skim milk, nonfat yogurt, and fat-free cottage cheese, which contain 0 percent fat. Whenever possible, avoid reduced-fat dairy products containing 2 percent fat and whole-milk dairy products containing 4 percent fat. Also choose nonfat or low-fat frozen yogurt or sorbet rather than ice cream. And cut back on cheese: Cheese is a major source of saturated fat and cholesterol (as well as sodium) in the American diet.

- Cook with chicken broth, wine, vinegar, low-calorie salad dressings, or unsaturated oils (mono- and polyunsaturated) rather than butter, margarine, sour cream, mayonnaise, and creamy salad dressings.

- To increase omega-3s, eat walnuts, flaxseed, tofu, beans, winter squash, and fatty fish (i.e., salmon, tuna, bluefish, herring, or sardines). The USDA recommends two servings of fatty fish per week. Note that salmon, canned tuna, North Atlantic mackerel, and catfish can contain high levels of mercury, so 12 ounces (two servings) is a limit. Other fish such as King mackerel, tilefish, swordfish, and shark can have higher levels of mercury—so high, in fact, that reproductive-age women and children should avoid them completely and others should eat them with caution.[37]

- Add green leafy vegetables, walnuts, walnut oil, and milled flaxseed to your diet.

- Limit processed and convenience foods. These often contain sugars and other refined carbohydrates and high levels of sodium in addition to *trans* fats.

Don't demand daily nutritional perfection from yourself or concentrate on individual nutrients. Try to balance your intake of different foods over a few meals and a couple of days at a time. If you have a high-fat breakfast or lunch, balance it with a low-fat dinner. If you forget to eat at least five servings of fruits and vegetables today, eat extra servings tomorrow.

Vitamins Are Vital Micronutrients

Vitamins are organic compounds that we need in tiny amounts to promote growth and help maintain vitality and wellness. Vitamins take part in the minute-by-minute cellular reactions that help maintain our nerves and skin, contribute to the production of blood cells, help us build bones and teeth, assist in wound healing, and help cells harvest food energy to fuel their activity. Some vitamins are toxic in high doses, and for many vitamins, time spent on the shelf, heat from cooking, and certain other environmental conditions can diminish their potency in foods.

Some vitamins can dissolve only in water and some only in fat. *Water-soluble vitamins,* including vitamin C and the B vitamins, dissolve easily in water and can be absorbed directly into the bloodstream.[38] The body usually excretes excess water-soluble vitamins in the urine, thus they seldom build up and cause toxicity problems. Because we don't store them in our tissues, we must consume water-soluble vitamins on a regular basis in foods. By contrast, *fat-soluble vitamins* (vitamins A, D, E, and K) must be associated with tiny fat globules for our intestines to absorb them. The liver and fat tissue store

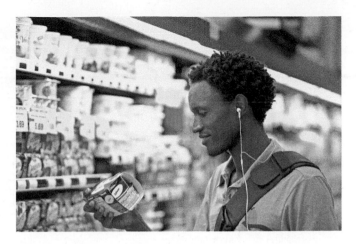

excess, unused quantities of the fat-soluble vitamins, so high levels can accumulate in the liver and eventually damage bones and/or kidneys, raise blood pressure, and interfere with blood clotting. Vitamin vendors often make various claims about the benefits of taking vitamin supplements. Few Americans, however, suffer from true vitamin deficiencies, and taking very high levels of vitamins can lead to a toxic condition, *hypervitaminosis*.

Table 7.2 on page 248 lists 13 vitamins, their primary functions in the body, recommended intake, and reliable food sources.

Most of us can get the vitamins and minerals we need from a healthy diet. Certain groups—including children, aging adults, elite athletes, vegetarians, pregnant and nursing mothers, and those with particular medical conditions—do need extra vitamins and minerals. Our section on special nutritional needs will explain these extra requirements and the best ways to fulfill them.

Minerals Are Elemental Micronutrients

The micronutrients called **minerals** allow our nerves to transmit impulses, our hearts to beat, oxygen to reach our tissue cells, and our digestive tracts to absorb vitamins from food. They are usually not toxic, and we excrete excess quantities of most minerals from the body. The **major minerals** (also called

vitamins Organic compounds in foods that we need in tiny amounts to promote growth and help maintain life and health

minerals Elements such as calcium or sodium that allow vital physiological processes, including nerve transmission, heartbeat, oxygen delivery, and absorption of vitamins

major minerals Elements needed in relatively large amounts, including sodium, calcium, phosphorus, magnesium, potassium, and chloride

TABLE 7.2 Guide to Vitamins

Vitamin Name	Primary Functions	Recommended Intake	Reliable Food Sources
Thiamin	Carbohydrate and protein metabolism	Men: 1.2 mg/day Women: 1.1 mg/day	Pork, fortified cereals, enriched rice and pasta, peas, tuna, legumes
Riboflavin	Carbohydrate and fat metabolism	Men: 1.3 mg/day Women: 1.1 mg/day	Beef liver, shrimp, dairy foods, fortified cereals, enriched breads and grains
Niacin	Carbohydrate and fat metabolism	Men: 16 mg/day Women: 14 mg/day	Meat/fish/poultry, fortified cereals, enriched breads and grains, canned tomato products
Vitamin B_6	Carbohydrate and amino acid metabolism	Men and women aged 19–50: 1.3 mg/day	Garbanzo beans, meat/fish/poultry, fortified cereals, white potatoes
Folate	Amino acid metabolism and DNA synthesis	Men: 400 µg/day Women: 400 µg/day	Fortified cereals, enriched breads and grains, spinach, legumes, spinach, liver
Vitamin B_{12}	Formation of blood cells and nervous system	Men: 2.4 µg/day Women: 2.4 µg/day	Shellfish, all cuts of meat/fish/poultry, dairy foods, fortified cereals
Pantothenic acid	Fat metabolism	Men: 5 mg/day Women: 5 mg/day	Meat/fish/poultry, shiitake mushrooms, fortified cereals, egg yolks
Biotin	Carbohydrate, fat, and protein metabolism	Men: 30 µg/day Women: 30 µg/day	Nuts, egg yolks
Vitamin C	Collagen synthesis; iron absorption, and promotes healing	Men: 90 mg/day Women: 75 mg/day Smokers: 35 mg more per day than RDA	Sweet peppers, citrus fruits and juices, broccoli, strawberries, kiwi
Vitamin A	Immune function, maintains epithelial cells, healthy bones, and vision	Men: 900 µg Women: 700 µg	Beef and chicken liver, egg yolks, milk Carotenoids found in spinach, carrots, mango, apricots, cantaloupe, pumpkin, yams
Vitamin D	Promotes calcium absorption and healthy bones	Adult aged 19–70: 15 µg/day (600 IU/day)	Canned salmon and mackerel, milk, fortified cereals
Vitamin E	Protects cells membranes, and acts as a powerful antioxidant	Men: 15 mg/day Women: 15 mg/day	Sunflower seeds, almonds, vegetable oils, fortified cereals
Vitamin K	Blood coagulation and bone metabolism	Men: 120 µg/day Women: 90 µg/day	Kale, spinach, turnip greens, Brussels sprouts

macrominerals) are elements that the body needs in relatively large amounts. We need smaller amounts of the **trace minerals** (also called *microminerals*). **Table 7.3** on page 249 lists most of the major and trace minerals, their functions, recommended intake, and food sources. We discuss three minerals—sodium, calcium, and iron—in more detail because of their crucial roles in the body and their excesses or deficiencies in diets. These three are so important, in fact, that nutrition labels list their amounts in each serving of food we eat.

trace minerals Elements that the body needs in very tiny amounts; includes iron, zinc, copper, iodine, selenium, fluoride, and chromium

Sodium We need sodium, the Na in sodium chloride (NaCl), or table salt, to regulate the water contents of blood

and body fluids; to help transmit nerve impulses; to aid muscle contraction, including the heartbeat; and to allow several metabolic functions inside cells. Most of us, however, consume much more sodium than we need.[39] Nutritionists estimate that the average American consumes around 3,300 milligrams per day, mostly from salted snacks and processed foods.[40] The average adult at rest and not sweating profusely needs only 180 to 500 milligrams of sodium (about one-quarter teaspoon) per day for normal body functioning.[41] The *Dietary Guidelines for Americans 2015–2020* recommends that everyone restrict sodium to less than 2,300 milligrams (less than 1 teaspoon) per day. Certain groups (those over 51 years old, African Americans, and people with hypertension, diabetes, or chronic kidney disease) should reduce their sodium consumption to below 1,500 milligrams per day. Pickles, salty snack

TABLE 7.3 Guide to Minerals

Mineral Name	Primary Functions	Recommended Intake	Reliable Food Sources
Sodium	Fluid and acid-base balance; nerve impulses and muscle contraction	Adults: 1.5 g/day (1,500 mg/day)	Table salt, pickles, most canned soups, snack foods, lunch meats, tomato products
Potassium	Fluid balance; nerve impulses and muscle contraction	Adults: 4.7 g/day (4,700 mg/day)	Most fresh fruits and vegetables: potato, banana, tomato juice, orange juice, melon
Phosphorus	Energy compounds, fluid balance and bone formation	Adults: 700 mg/day	Milk/cheese/yogurt, soy milk and tofu, legumes nuts, poultry
Selenium	Regulates thyroid hormones and reduces oxidative stress	Adults: 55 µg/day	Seafood, milk, whole grains, and eggs
Calcium	Part of bone; muscle contraction, acid-base balance, and nerve transmission	Adults: 1,000 mg/day	Milk/yogurt/cheese, sardines, collard greens and spinach, calcium-fortified juices
Magnesium	Part of bone; muscle contraction	Men: 400 mg/day Women: 310 mg/day	Spinach, kale, collard greens, whole grains, seeds, nuts, legumes
Iodine	Synthesis of thyroid hormones	Adults: 150 µg/day	Iodized salt, saltwater seafood
Iron	Part of hemoglobin and myoglobin	Men: 8 mg/day Women: 18 mg/day	Meat/fish/poultry, fortified cereals, legumes
Zinc	Immune system function; growth and sexual maturation	Men: 11 mg/day Women: 8 mg/day	Meat/fish/poultry, fortified cereals, legumes

foods, processed cheeses, many breads and bakery products, and smoked meats and sausages often contain several hundred milligrams of sodium per serving. Many fast-food entrées and convenience entrées pack huge amounts of sodium. For example, a 4-ounce McDonald's cheeseburger contains 680 mg of sodium and a Quarter Pounder with cheese contains 1,110![42]

Many experts believe that there is a link between excessive sodium intake and hypertension (high blood pressure).[43] Researchers began recommending several years ago that people with hypertension cut back on sodium to reduce their risk of cardiovascular disorders.[44]

You can shake your own salt habit by choosing low-sodium or salt-free food products. For example, buy salt-free tortilla chips; your salsa dip probably has more than 200 mg of sodium per serving. Order popcorn without salt. Switch to kosher salt—an equivalent measure has less sodium than regular table salt. Instead of adding salt to food you prepare, try using fresh or prepackaged herb blends to season foods. These small changes can add up to a significant reduction in unneeded sodium. They could even save your life someday: An enormous multinational study of sodium consumption projected that 88 percent of the world's adults eat at least 50 percent more salt each day than the World Health Organization recommends. In the study year 2010, the authors calculate that *this over-consumption itself* caused about one-tenth of all the mortality from heart disease or about 1.65 million deaths.[45]

Calcium High sodium intake has another major downside: It also increases calcium loss in urine, which can increase your risk for debilitating fractures as you age.[46] The element calcium (Ca) is crucial for the development and maintenance of bones and teeth, blood clotting, muscle contraction, nerve transmission, and fluid balance between the cell's interior and its environment. Nevertheless, 40 percent of Americans consume less than the 1,000 to 1,300 milligrams of calcium per day recommended by government guidelines.[47]

Chapter 11 discusses a common result of too little calcium: **osteoporosis**, a disease of thinning, weakened, porous bones that affects more than 54 million Americans or half of the women and about one-quarter of the men over age 50.[48] Getting enough calcium in childhood and adolescence and then sustaining adequate levels throughout adulthood can help you prevent osteoporosis later.[49]

Dairy products are among the richest dietary sources of calcium, but calcium-fortified orange juice, almond milk, or soy milk are also good sources, as are leafy green vegetables and many other foods (see Table 7.3). Be aware that too much sodium can cause you to excrete calcium and thus

osteoporosis A disease of thinning, weakened, porous bones during which too little calcium is deposited or retained in the bones

deplete it from your bones, as can the phosphoric acid (phosphate) added to carbonated colas and certain other soft drinks.[50] Calcium/phosphorus imbalance may lead to kidney stones and bone spurs and to the deposits or plaques inside blood vessels that contribute to cardiovascular diseases.

Vitamin D improves absorption of calcium; that's why dairies are required by law to add it to milk. In some studies, deficiencies of Vitamin D also appear linked to the risks for heart disease, cancer, arthritis, and Alzheimer's disease.[51]

Sunlight shining on your skin also increases your body's own manufacture of vitamin D, so a moderate amount of sunlight helps improve calcium absorption. The best way to obtain calcium with vitamin D is to consume calcium-rich foods such as low-fat or fat-free dairy products, fortified soy and almond milk, salmon, tuna, eggs, and fortified cereals as part of a balanced diet. Some people do need extra calcium, including children, teens, pregnant and nursing mothers, and adults over 60.

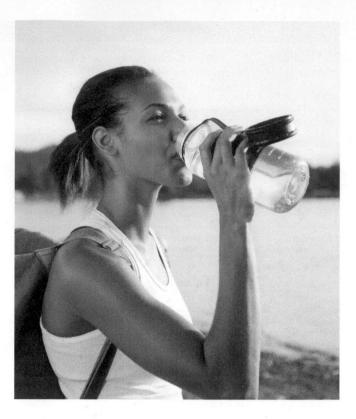

Iron Each of us needs the element iron (Fe) for producing healthy blood, for muscle function, and for normal cell division. Women aged 19 to 50 need about 18 milligrams per day; men aged 19 to 50 need about 8 milligrams per day. Worldwide, iron deficiency is the most common nutrient deficiency, affecting more than 2 billion people.[52] In many developing countries, more than 40 percent of the young children and women of childbearing age suffer from **iron-deficiency anemia**. In this condition, the body fails to produce enough of the red hemoglobin pigment in the blood, leading to unusually low oxygen levels and unusually high carbon dioxide levels. The result is usually mental and physical fatigue. In developing countries, most of the iron deficiency is due to poor diet and/or parasites. In high-income countries, the condition is less common and is usually caused by vegetarian diets or medical conditions.[53] In the United States, about 10 percent of toddlers, adolescent girls, and women of childbearing age show iron-deficiency anemia.[54] Mexican American and non-Hispanic black women under 50 have rates that are 20 to 50 percent higher.[55] Table 7.3 on page 249 lists good dietary sources of iron.

Researchers have linked iron deficiency to a host of problems, including poor immune system functioning and a propensity toward certain cancers. Some research has also suggested a link between too much iron in the diet

> **iron-deficiency anemia** A disease in which the body takes in too little iron and makes too little oxygen-carrying hemoglobin

and/or stored in the body and a higher risk for cardiovascular disease, cancer, and Alzheimer's and other brain diseases.[56]

Acute iron toxicity due to ingesting too many iron-containing supplements remains the leading cause of accidental poisoning in small children in the United States. Dozens of children have died from overdoses of as few as five iron tablets.[57]

Water Is Our Most Fundamental Nutrient

Imagine you are stranded on a desert island for a reality TV show and you can take along just one provision. Would you choose food, water, or a cell phone? We hope you said water!

Humans are mostly water—close to 60 percent. Watery fluids bathe each of our internal cells. They help maintain a proper balance of salts within our blood and tissues, help maintain pH balance, and help facilitate the transport of substances throughout the body. Human blood plasma (the fluid portion of blood exclusive of red and white blood cells and other solid components) is approximately 92 percent water.[58] This proportion must remain fairly constant for blood to efficiently carry oxygen and nutrients to the cells and carry away carbon dioxide and other wastes.

Even under the most severe conditions, the average person can live for weeks on the energy stored in body fat. You can also get along without certain vitamins and minerals from foods for an equal amount of time before experiencing serious deficiency symptoms. Without water, however, you would become **dehydrated**, or depleted of normal levels of body fluids, within hours. Within one day without drinking water, you would probably begin to feel sluggish, dizzy, and nauseated, and would experience headaches, muscle cramps, or weakness. After a few days without water, your tongue would be parched and swollen, your heart would be racing, and you'd very likely go into shock and die.

A person's need for water varies dramatically based on age, size, diet, exercise, overall health, and environmental temperature and humidity levels. Most of us get enough water through foods and beverages just by satisfying our thirst.[59] People with certain diseases such as diabetes or cystic fibrosis, however, excrete extra fluid and must generally take in a higher volume. On a hot day, especially if exercising, you need to consciously replace fluids lost to sweat and exhalation. It is possible, though, to take in too much water and become nauseated, confused, or weak or even to lose consciousness from excess hydration leading to *hyponatremia* (sometimes called water intoxication). In this condition, salt concentrations in the blood drop too far. Heavy perspiration can contribute to the salt imbalance. If you are drinking despite not feeling thirsty, or you actually gain water weight during an active exercise session, you may be imbibing more than you need. Thirst is a good indicator for most people during all but the most extreme exercise. Children and seniors may need to consume water on a schedule while exercising.[60]

Commercial energy drinks can help exercisers replenish water lost through sweat and to restore salt and sugar. Many people dilute them with water, however, to prevent taking in more salt and sugar than they actually lose during exercise. Drinking water and eating part of a banana every 15 minutes during a 2- to 3-hour bicycle race provides a similar benefit to consuming a sports drink but supplies more vitamins and fiber.[61] Some energy drinks include ingredients that are ineffectual or that can be harmful in large quantities. For example, researchers have failed to confirm any health benefit for ingredients such as taurine, bee pollen, and ginkgo biloba.[62] High concentrations of added sugars can boost energy in the short term but can create sluggishness later. Added vitamins C and B are unnecessary in a balanced diet, and in fact, vitamin water drinks, along with unnecessary supplements can lead to imbalances and toxicities.[63]

LO 7.3 How Can I Achieve a Balanced Diet?

The average American adult consumes about 1,000 calories more per day than the average citizen worldwide and yet still gets unbalanced nutrition. To counter this trend, the US government:

- Sets guidelines for minimum and recommended levels of nutrients, vitamins, and minerals;

- Requires standardized nutrition labels on most packaged and processed foods;

- Determines appropriate portion sizes;

- Publishes an interactive website, www. ChooseMyPlate. gov, to help individuals manage their daily nutrition, including

dehydrated Depleted of normal, necessary levels of body fluids

calorie counting and energy expenditure through exercise; and

- Regulates the safety of our food supply.

The many tools the USDA, FDA, National Academy of Sciences, and other governmental agencies provide can help you achieve a better diet, maintain a healthy weight, and help prevent several chronic diseases.

Follow Guidelines for Good Nutrition

There are so many parts to the government's nutritional advice to the public that they publish an overview—think of it as a cheat sheet for nutrition—called the *Dietary Guidelines for Americans*. We discuss the government's nutritional guidelines for specific sex, age, and ethnic groups later in this chapter. Here, we summarize the major recommendations in the latest (2015–2020) version:

- **Eat a Healthy Diet throughout Life.** People of all ages should eat an appropriate amount of calories to maintain healthy body weight, get enough nutrients, and cut the risks for chronic disease. A healthy diet emphasizes fruits and vegetables; at least half of daily grains as whole grains; fat-free or low-fat dairy products and/or soy beverages fortified with calcium and vitamin D; lean protein foods; and oils. People should also limit sugar, saturated fat, sodium, and alcohol.

- **Focus on Variety, Nutrient Density, and Amount of Food.** People should pay attention to choosing foods from all food groups, maximizing nutrients, and controlling calories. This means learning about the nutrients in foods, proper portion sizes, and limiting your intake to healthy calorie levels based on size, age, build, and activity level.

- **Limit Calories from Added Sugars and Saturated Fat, and Reduce Sodium Intake.** Healthy eating means consuming a balance of foods and beverages that are low in added sugars and saturated fats. Most Americans also need to reduce their intake of sodium to reach a desired level of 2,300 mg per day or less. Alcoholic beverages contain sugars. If you drink, the government recommends that you limit yourself to no more than one drink per day for women and up to two for men—and only if of legal age.

- **Shift to Healthier Food and Beverage Choices.** Learning about and focusing on healthier patterns is just the start: Every day you should consume varied, nutrient-dense, calorie-appropriate foods, limit harmful foods, and maintain these wellness choices throughout life.

- **Support Healthy Eating Patterns for All.** Exercise your right to make healthy choices and support healthy patterns for everyone at home, at school, in the workplace, and in communities.

Understand Your Recommended Nutrient Intakes

Fulfilling your daily nutritional needs is easier because several government scientific advisory boards serve up an "alphabet soup" of specific recommended daily minimum and maximum intakes for each type of nutrient (fat, carbohydrates, proteins), and for the various types of vitamins and minerals:

- **Dietary Reference Intake (DRI)** is a listing of 26 nutrients essential to maintaining health. The DRI listing identifies recommended and maximum safe intake levels of the nutrients for healthy people, and identifies minimum levels needed to prevent deficiencies and diseases. DRIs are an umbrella category for several older classifications. The National Academy of Sciences Food and Nutrition Board publishes DRIs.

- **Recommended Dietary Allowances (RDAs)** are a listing of the average daily nutrient intake levels of vitamins and minerals that meet most people's daily needs.

- **Reference Daily Intakes (RDIs)** are a listing of needed daily nutrients based on the RDAs. Tables 7.2 (page 248) and 7.3 (page 249) list the current RDIs for various vitamins and minerals.

- **Daily Reference Values (DRVs)** cover some nutrients the RDIs left out that proved to be important for daily dietary monitoring. They cover fat (including saturated fat and cholesterol), carbohydrates (including fiber), protein, sodium, and potassium. **Table 7.4** on page 253 lists the current DRVs for these nutrients.

Dietary References Intakes (DRIs) A listing of 26 nutrients essential to maintaining health, including recommended and maximum safe intake levels of the nutrients for healthy people and minimum levels needed to prevent deficiencies and diseases

Recommended Dietary Allowances (RDAs) A listing of the average daily nutrient intake level for a list of vitamins and minerals that meets most people's daily needs

Reference Daily Intakes (RDIs) A listing of needed daily nutrients based on the RDAs. The National Academy of Sciences introduced RDAs in 1941 and updates the list periodically.

Daily Reference Values (DRVs) Set of general intake guidelines of total fat, saturated fat, cholesterol, carbohydrates, protein, fiber, sodium, and potassium

TABLE 7.4 Daily Reference Values (DRVs)

Food Component	DRV
Fat	65 grams (g)
Saturated Fatty Acids	20 g
Cholesterol	300 milligrams (mg)
Total Carbohydrate	300 g
Dietary Fiber	25 g
Protein*	50 g
Sodium	2,400 milligrams (mg)
Potassium	3,500 mg

(Based on 2,000 calories a day for adults and children over 4 only)

*DRV for protein does not apply to certain populations; Reference Daily Intake (RDI) for protein has been established for these groups: children 1 to 4 years: 16 g; infants under 1 year: 14 g; pregnant women: 60 g; nursing mothers: 65 g.

Adapted from US Food and Drug Administration, "FDA Food Labeling Guide," updated August 2015, www.fda.gov

- **Daily Values (DVs)** are the RDIs and the DRVs as printed on food labels. American consumers need to know what's in their food and what they should be eating without sorting through a bunch of confusing acronyms. Therefore, the FDA invented a simpler term, DV, for all the important nutrients from the RDI and DRV lists to include on food labels. If you look on any food label, you will see a column labeled "% Daily Value."

Read Food Labels

You can tell what you are buying and eating because the US government requires nutrition labels on the pack-

Daily Values (DVs) A listing of all the important nutrients from two less-inclusive government lists—the RDIs and the DRVs; DVs are printed on all nutrition labels

ages of most food products. Reading and understanding these labels can help you judge appropriate portion sizes and the nutritional merits of the foods you eat. By law, every food package must:

- Prominently identify the product, such as "multigrain cereal" or "fat-free milk";
- State the quantity of food by weight, volume, or number of pieces so you can judge the value of what you're buying;
- List all the ingredients by common name in order of amount from most to least by weight;
- Give contact information for the food company in case you want more information; and
- Supply nutritional information in a standardized panel so you can compare and judge the dietary merits of the product before you buy it.

The Nutrition Facts panel (**Figure 7.7**) provides the greatest concentration of information; it identifies a

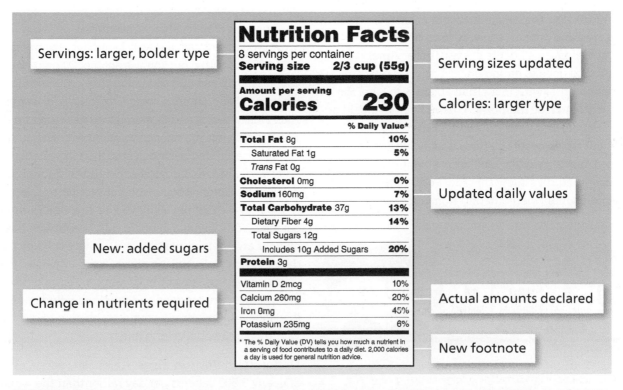

FIGURE **7.7** An important part of improving personal nutrition is reading food labels and understanding the information they provide. In 2015, the US FDA revised the Nutrition Facts panels on food packages to help consumers find significant items such as calories, added sugars, and the amounts of nutrients for which many Americans are deficient.

serving size and how many servings you'll get in a package. The panel tells you in bold letters and numbers how many calories each 1-cup serving provides. It lists DVs for nutrients that people should watch carefully in their diets. Revised in 2015, the panel now compares each food serving to the DVs for total saturated fat and saturated fat. It lists *trans* fats (but there is no DV for it since we should avoid this ingredient). The label provides the percentage of DV for cholesterol, total carbs, and fiber. It lists vitamin D and calcium, as before. But it now includes iron and potassium, and makes listing vitamins A and C simply voluntary for food manufacturers.

The new label lists protein and both natural and added sugars, although there are no DVs for sugar. The "added sugars" category is particularly significant because collectively, the corn syrup, fructose, dextrose, mannitol, brown sugar, and so on in a processed food can represent the *most common ingredients*.

The "Facts Up Front" Nutrition Keys on food packages act as a kind of "CliffsNotes" for quickly judging a food's content (**Figure 7.8**). A package of cookies, for example, might include calories, grams of saturated fat and sugar, and milligrams of sodium per serving in big type. Keep in mind, though, that presently, these front panels are voluntary and a manufacturer is unlikely to lists the Facts Up Front on truly unhealthy food. If that panel is missing, look even more closely at the mandatory Nutrition Facts on the side or back of the package!

The FDA now requires nutritional information for foods served and consumed away from home. This is significant because 43 cents of every dollar Americans spend on food goes to eating out.[64] The rules require chain restaurants (with more than 20 sites) to label the calorie content on all menus and menu boards (including drive-throughs) and have printed information available to hand out on request. The rules also include vending machines, movie theaters, and amusement parks.[65] Significantly, studies show that most consumers do use the calorie counts when ordering from a menu and

reduce an average of 150 calories over what they might have ordered without this information.[66]

The US government can make nutritional information available—but it's up to you to read the labels, understand the issues, and make good choices.

Determine Your Calorie Needs If you read the fine print near the bottom of any nutrition label, you will see that the lists of nutrients are based on diets of either 2,000 or 2,500 calories per day. The government based its daily values of 65 grams of fat, 300 grams of carbohydrates, and 50 grams of protein on a 2,000-calorie diet. Does that make 2,000 the right number for an active teenager, a professional basketball player, and an older woman who is 4'11" tall? Obviously, no.

A round number like 2,000 calories makes it easy to extrapolate your actual calorie needs and serving sizes. It is also a maintenance level of energy input for a medium-sized person—about 150 pounds—who expends a medium amount of energy such as 30 minutes of moderate activity a few times per week. Food labels usually also provide a second level—2,500 calories—as a calculation base for larger or more active people. Determine your personal calorie needs based on your size, age, gender, activity level, and medical conditions as well as your basal metabolic rate (BMR), which is partly inborn and partly activity-based.

Your BMR, the amount of energy your body uses in a given time period while resting or sleeping, accounts for 50 to 70 percent of your calorie consumption each day and allows you to maintain a steady heartbeat, a temperature of about 98.6°F, and so on. You use another 20 percent of your calories moving around and doing physical work such as walking, talking, carrying things, running, or sweeping the floor. Finally, eating and digesting food itself uses up about 5 to 10 percent of the calories you burn each day.

In determining calorie needs, the big variables are body size, BMR, and energy expenditure through physical activity. Larger people, more muscular people, and those who do hard physical work or exercise burn extra calories. You can get a specific calorie estimate based on your own height, weight, and activity level by using diet analysis tools such as www.ChooseMyPlate.gov. (We'll revisit this subject in Chapter 8). To calculate appropriate serving sizes and numbers when reading food labels and planning your diet, be sure to calculate your own individual calorie needs.

Understand Portion Sizes Americans eat an average of nearly 3,500 calories per day rather than the world average of 2,400 to 2,600. Why? One reason is that our food portions are too big.

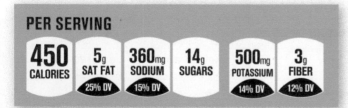

PER SERVING

| 450 CALORIES | 5g SAT FAT 25% DV | 360mg SODIUM 15% DV | 14g SUGARS | 500mg POTASSIUM 14% DV | 3g FIBER 12% DV |

FIGURE **7.8** Nutrition Keys: One serving of this imaginary product has a whopping 450 calories, contains one-quarter of a day's saturated fat, one-sixth of a day's sodium, and the gram equivalent of three teaspoons of sugar. It does, however, also provide some potassium and fiber.

The US government recommends that each of us eat a certain number of servings each day from each food group based on standard serving sizes. Most Americans, however, don't know how to recognize standard portions. It helps to have some visual aids for estimating proper serving sizes and recognizing the right amount of food. **Figure 7.9** illustrates various foods, healthy serving sizes in cups and ounces, and visual devices for remembering proper portions. For example, one serving of cooked whole-wheat pasta or brown rice is half a cup, about the size of half a baseball. This figure puts into

startling perspective the mountains of pasta, thick wedges of pie, stacks of plate-sized pancakes, bucket-sized soft drinks, and other servings we accept as normal, especially at restaurants.

Use Food Guides The USDA has issued Food Guides since the 1940s to help Americans select healthy diets.[67] The plate icon introduced a few years ago uses segments of certain colors and sizes to symbolize the kinds and relative amounts of foods and nutrients consumers should select each day (half the plate are fruits and vegetables; a little more than one-quarter of the plate are grains; less than one-quarter is protein; and a small amount is dairy) (see **Figure 7.10** on this page). The supporting website (www.ChooseMyPlate.gov) provides personalized diet, nutrition, and exercise recommendations based on your sex, age, size, and activity level.

Acquire Skills to Improve Your Nutrition

Do you know the nutritional value of your own diet? Do you know how to find out? A few simple skills will help you analyze and improve your diet. Developing a habit of quickly checking eight items from the typical food label can greatly improve your daily nutrition. **Lab 7.1** will

Do It!

Access these labs at the end of the chapter or online at MasteringHealth™.

1 Serving Looks Like . . .	1 Serving Looks Like . . .
Grain Products	**Vegetables and Fruit**
1 cup of cereal flakes = fist	1 cup of salad greens = baseball
1 pancake = compact disc	1 baked potato = fist
½ cup of cooked rice, pasta, or potato = ½ baseball	1 medium fruit = baseball
1 slice of bread = cassette tape	½ cup of fresh fruit = ½ baseball
1 piece of cornbread = bar of soap	¼ cup of raisins = large egg
1 Serving Looks Like . . .	**1 Serving Looks Like . . .**
Dairy and Cheese	**Meat and Alternatives**
1½ oz cheese = 4 stacked dice or 2 cheese slices	3 oz meat, fish, and poultry = deck of cards
½ cup of ice cream = ½ baseball	3 oz grilled or baked fish = checkbook
Fats	2 tbsp peanut butter = ping-pong ball
1 tsp margarine or spreads = 1 die	

FIGURE **7.9** One of the challenges of following a healthy diet is judging how big a portion size should be and how many servings you are really eating. The comparisons on this card can help you recall what a standard food serving looks like. For easy reference, photocopy or cut out this card, fold on the dotted line, and keep it in your wallet. You can even laminate it for long-term use.

Source: National Heart, Lung, and Blood Institute, "Serving Size Card," accessed November 2015, www.nhlbi.nih.gov/health/educational/wecan/downloads/servingcard7

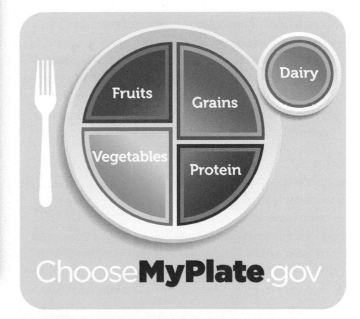

FIGURE **7.10** The ChooseMyPlate.gov icon shows the proper proportion of each food group in a healthy diet. The supporting website provides each visitor with an individualized recommendation for daily servings and portion sizes of each food type.

Source: US Department of Agriculture, "ChooseMyPlate," 2015, www.ChooseMyPlate.gov

walk you through this process. Here are the eight items you should look for regularly:

- *What is the main ingredient?* If it is water, corn syrup, or enriched (translation, "white") flour, are you getting your money's worth—and good nutrition?

- *How do the total fats and saturated fats compare to the listed DV?* Just one tablespoon of butter, for example, will provide one-third of your DV for saturated fat. Do you really want to consume that much fat in one pat?

- *What is the trans fat content?* Reduce or eliminate *trans* fats because of their potentially negative health consequences.

- *How does the sodium compare to the % DV?* People diagnosed with high blood pressure, diabetes, kidney disease, and certain other conditions must limit sodium levels. Others should limit sodium to recommended levels.

- *Does the food provide any fiber?* If not, could you substitute something that does—for example, baby spinach leaves instead of iceberg lettuce in a salad, or a fresh apple instead of canned pineapple, or brown rice instead of white?

- *Finally, what percentage of calories come from added sugars?* Technically, there is no DV for sugars or other sweeteners, but you can now see the grams of added sugars listed on food labels. Sugars are common in cereals, sauces, and other processed foods and add empty calories that you could devote to more filling and nutritious foods. For example, instead of eating a cup of raisin bran with 19 grams of sugar and 188 calories of food energy, try choosing one cup of bran flakes with only 5 grams of sugar and 122 calories, and then adding a cup of sliced, fresh strawberries (high in volume, flavor, vitamin C, and fiber and containing only 55 calories).

Keep a Food Diary To get an accurate idea of whether your diet is nutrient rich or poor, try to record snacks and meals for a few days. This is best done immediately after eating, not hours later when you have discarded wrappers with nutrient labels or lost count of serving sizes. For those

Live It!
Complete Worksheet 19 Food Log at MasteringHealth™.

working to manage their weight, keeping track of food, calorie, and nutrient intake doubles the amount of weight lost.[68]

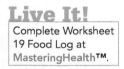

whole foods Dietary items produced and consumed with the minimum of processing (refining, adding preservatives, or altering form for quick preparation)

Keeping a food diary helps you learn to judge serving sizes. It requires you to read and apply the information on nutrition labels, learn the value of your typical foods, and substitute healthier items for the foods you usually choose. Many free food diary apps are now available for downloading to smart phones and tablets (see eResources on page 269).

Use Diet Analysis Software An online program such as www.ChooseMyPlate.gov is a powerful tool for keeping track of what you eat, analyzing its nutrient content, and making needed changes to your diet. It is just one of several such programs that can streamline your efforts to achieve better nutrition.

To use this USDA website and its personalized features, visit www.ChooseMyPlate.gov. Find the box "I want to. . .," and select "Get a Personalized Plan." Enter your age, sex, weight, height, and general activity level. From there you can learn your recommended daily calorie consumption, the number of servings you should eat from the five main food groups, and other helpful pointers.

Do It!
Access these labs at the end of the chapter or online at MasteringHealth™.

The site also provides a meal tracking worksheet and a tracker to help you assess the nutrients in specific foods. **Lab 7.2** gives you practice in using www.ChooseMyPlate.gov to analyze and record your food needs, nutrients, physical activity levels, and other helpful information.

Choose the method—online or on paper—that works best for you because that's the one you'll stick with. Creating your own nutrition plan (see page 267) will also help you practice with the new tools.

Adopt the Whole Foods Habit

Make each bite you take more nutritious by choosing primarily **whole foods**, or dietary items produced with the minimum of refining, preservatives, or processing for quick preparation.

See It!
Watch "Grain Labels Do Not Reflect the 'Whole' Truth" at MasteringHealth™.

A century ago, virtually all food was "whole." Many packaged foods today, however, have long lists of additives that reduce the cost of ingredients, extend shelf life, intensify flavor, and make food preparation easier. People have learned to like the taste and convenience of processed foods, but these products tend to contain hidden fats and sugars, relatively large amounts of sodium, and various additives and preservatives. They also tend to have less naturally occurring fiber and fewer vitamins.

For example, for $2 to $3, you could buy a roughly 2-ounce bag of processed, preserved, and dried apple "chips." The one-serving package holds pieces from two or more peeled apples and contains about 200 calories, up to 50 grams of carbohydrates, and more than 40 grams of sugars, some of them added. The "chips" also contain preservatives such as sulfur to keep them from turning brown and additives to enhance the flavor. For the same $2 to $3, you could buy several fresh apples, each containing only about 95 calories, 17 grams of carbohydrates, no added sugars, and no preservatives or additives. The peel is full of cancer-fighting compounds; and the skin provides twice as much fiber as in the processed chips. Slice the fresh apple and sprinkle on cinnamon to double its anti-cancer and anti-inflammatory benefits.

Live It!
Complete Worksheet 18 Grocery Shopping List at MasteringHealth™.

Clearly, shifting from processed foods to whole foods doesn't mean you have to sacrifice good taste or feel hungry. Besides the healthful nutrients in the cinnamon-sprinkled apple, its volume is also higher and thus it keeps you full longer. The same is true for virtually all whole foods whether snacks, breads, cereals, entrees, or fruits and vegetables.

Choose Nutrient-Dense Foods You may have heard people talk about "empty calories." What they mean is that some foods and beverages provide calories without other healthful nutrients. By contrast, **nutrient-dense foods** provide rich sources of vitamins, minerals, antioxidants, and fiber and minimize saturated fat, added sugars, sodium, and refined carbohydrates. Choosing nutrient-dense foods means striving to maximize the food value of every meal and snack you consume.

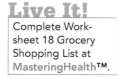

Let's do another comparison: a glass of cola and a hot dog versus a glass of low-fat milk and a small serving of salmon. The cola provides 105 calories, all from added sugars. In about the same number of calories, the milk provides 8 grams of protein along with vitamin D and calcium. The cola is nutrient-poor; the milk is nutrient-dense.

Now compare the hot dog and salmon. A hot dog on a white-bread bun supplies 420 calories. It contains more saturated fat than the DV for a whole day. It provides 9 grams of protein, along with most of a day's allotted sodium and refined white flour in the bun, lacking much fiber. The World Health Organization also calls processed meats such as hot dogs "human carcinogens."[69] In contrast, a serving of salmon provides fewer than half the calories (200 compared to 420), 10 grams of heart-healthy omega-3 fatty acids, twice as much protein, and a small fraction of the sodium. The cola and hot dog meal is a nutritional loser; the salmon and glass of milk are nutrient-dense and with some added vegetables or fruit, would be a winning meal.

Reaching for nutrient-dense foods every time you get hungry will greatly benefit your lifelong fitness and wellness. If your diet consists primarily of processed foods such as pastries, coffee drinks, pizza, hamburgers, and cola, you may not even know what wellness feels like! Why should you care about eating too many calories, too much saturated fat, too many refined carbohydrates, and too much sodium? Because dietary excesses can affect your appearance, social life, brain power, energy level, athletic performance, ability to fight off infections, and overall sense of well-being.[70] Try shifting toward nutrient-dense foods, and watch for positive changes in those short-term measures. Focus on establishing habits that keep you looking and feeling vibrantly well today and your lifelong wellness will improve, too.

Choose High-Volume, Low-Calorie Foods We eat for many reasons, but the primary one is *satiety*: a feeling of fullness and the physical and emotional pleasure it brings. Nutrition researchers have discovered that each of us has a characteristic weight of food that we eat in a day. You can eat that weight of food in candy bars, potato chips, steak, and ice cream, but you will be getting too few nutrients and too many calories and you probably wouldn't feel full for very long. You could eat that same weight of food in celery, iceberg lettuce, and wheat bran and still get too few nutrients, but the volume would help keep you full. The proper goal is a filling, calorie-appropriate diet that also emphasizes nutrient density. Classic

nutrient-dense foods Foods or beverages that provide a high level of nutrients and thus maximize the nutritional value of each meal and snack consumed

antioxidants Compounds in foods that help protect the body against the damaging effects of oxygen derivatives called *free radicals*

nutritional research has shown that eating nutritious foods with more volume due to higher air or water content can help people feel full and satisfied longer.[71] This is especially helpful for people who want to maintain their weight.

Foods with high contents of water, fiber, or protein tend to keep you full and satisfied longer, while those with high contents of fat, sugar, or refined carbohydrates leave you feeling hungry sooner. However, the water must be in the food (as in soups, fruits, and vegetables) and not just in a glass accompanying your meal. Apparently, your brain's satiety center knows the difference and isn't fooled by drinking water coupled with a candy bar. **Figure 7.11** compares two sandwiches with approximately the same number of calories, but very different ingredients and ability to keep you feeling full longer. **Table 7.5** lists familiar foods by calorie density.

Select High-Fiber Foods Fiber adds bulk and a chewy quality to food. Both help satisfy hunger better and for longer periods. Soluble fiber such as that in oats, barley, and apples, for example, lowers LDL cholesterol. Grains that are intact (such as brown rice or bulgur wheat) instead of finely ground (as in whole wheat flour)

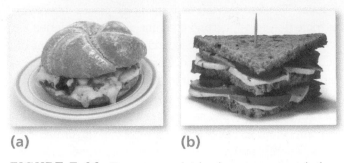

(a)   (b)

FIGURE **7.11** These two sandwiches have approximately the same number of calories (300), but one (a) is small and filled with saturated fat. It contains mayonnaise, butter, cheese, and bacon on a white roll. The other sandwich (b) is large, high-volume, and rich in fiber and vitamins. It contains whole wheat bread, tomato, lettuce, green and red peppers, and cheese.

have a lower glycemic index. High-fiber foods also improve the passage of digested material through the digestive tract, helping to prevent constipation.

Choose Antioxidant-Rich Foods *Free radicals* are molecules with unpaired electrons that the body produces in excess when it is overly stressed. Free radicals can damage or kill healthy cells, cell proteins, or genetic material in cells. Many biologists have theorized that free radicals are one cause of aging. **Antioxidant** compounds stimulate the production of enzymes that scavenge free radicals, slow their formation, and actually repair the damage from oxidative stress. Thus, the theory goes that if you consume lots of antioxidant

TABLE **7.5** Comparing Calorie Density in Common Foods

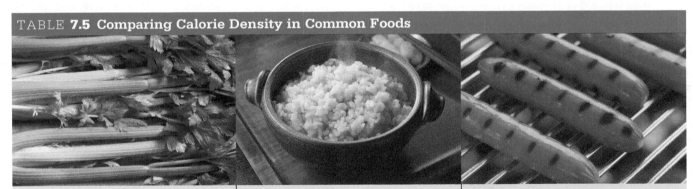

Examples of Foods with Low Calorie Density—*Consume a variety of these daily*	Examples of Foods with Medium Calorie Density—*Consume a few of these daily*	Examples of Foods with High Calorie Density—*Reduce consumption of these daily*
Raw celery (1250 g = 200 calories)	Brown rice, cooked (179 g = 200 calories)	Hot dog, Oscar Meyer beef (61 g = 200 calories)
Watermelon (666 g = 200 calories)	Enriched spaghetti, cooked (126 g = 200 calories)	French fries, McDonald's (59 g = 200 calories)
Raw broccoli (588 g = 200 calories)	Chicken breast, roasted (121 g = 200 calories)	Potato chips, plain salted (37 g = 200 calories)
Red or green grapes (290 g = 200 calories)	Salmon, cooked, Alaskan wild (110 g = 200 calories)	Peanut butter, smooth salted (34 g = 200 calories)

Data from Nutrient Data Laboratory Home Page U.S. Department of Agriculture, "USDA National Nutrient Database for Standard Reference Release 28," Agricultural Research Service, 2015.

compounds, you will greatly reduce the negative effects of oxidative stress, including aging, cancer, heart disease, diabetes, Alzheimer's disease, and other medical conditions. Among the nutrients touted for their protective effects are vitamin C, vitamin E, beta-carotene and other carotenoids, and the mineral selenium.

Large studies over long periods of time support the hypothesis that we get antioxidants from eating fruits and vegetables. As **Table 7.6** shows, fruits and vegetables *do* help protect us against cancer, heart disease, brain disorders, and other medical conditions. They also benefit physical training and performance.[72] Antioxidant supplements, on the other hand, have proven disappointing or even harmful. The Q&A box Should You Take Supplements? on page 261 explains the research in more detail.

Here's a brief summary. The recent thinking on antioxidants includes two interesting—and somewhat surprising—points. First, it is true that free radicals can sometimes damage certain cells and tissues. But the unpaired electrons are probably instrumental in the body's own defense mechanisms, triggering gene activity that brings about cellular repair.[73] In other words, even if we could mop up all of the body's free radicals with massive doses of antioxidants, we shouldn't do it. Second, antioxidants are plant compounds that evolved primarily as chemical defenses against plant-eating insects and other predators. The small quantities of antioxidants that we humans consume in fruits and vegetables probably inflict a very mild form of stress on our body cells and the responses they trigger (as we just saw) bring about beneficial cell growth and repair.[74] Biologists call this process *hormesis*. And because of hormesis, our cells' response to mild stress protects them from greater stress. On the other hand, swallowing

TABLE 7.6

Color	Nutrients	Health Benefits	Types
Red	Vitamin A, C, manganese antioxidants (quercetin, lycopene)	Reduce risk of cancer and heart disease, decrease inflammation, increase immunity, eye/skin/hair health	Tomatoes, peppers, beets, radishes, red apples, red potatoes, grapefruit, cherries, raspberries, strawberries, watermelon
Green	Vitamin K, B-Vitamins, folate, potassium, antioxidants (chlorophyll, carotenoids, lutein)	Promote eye health, lung health, liver function, healthy cell production, reduce risk of cancer, increase blood clotting, lower blood pressure	Broccoli, cabbage, brussel sprouts, cucumbers, green peppers, dark leafy greens, peas, asparagus, green beans, zucchini, avocados, kiwi, green apples, green grapes, pears
Orange/Yellow	Vitamin C, A, B6, potassium, folate, antioxidants (beta-carotene, lutein, alpha-carotene)	Reduce risk of cancer and heart disease, promote eye/skin/hair health, increase immunity, decrease inflammation	Carrots, orange/yellow peppers, squash, sweet potatoes, pumpkin, oranges, bananas, apricots, cantaloupe, nectarines, peaches, pineapple
Blue/Purple	B-vitamins, antioxidants (anthocyanins, resveratrol, flavonoids)	Reduce risk of cancer and heart disease, protect cells from damage, improve memory, prevent aging	Eggplant, red onions, purple cabbage, purple cabbage, purple potatoes, blueberries, blackberries, plums
White	Vitamins C, K, folate, potassium, antioxidants (allicin, quercetin, quercetin, anthoxanthins)	Lower cholesterol, reduce risk of cancer and heart disease, protect cells from damage, increase immunity, promote eye/skin/bone health	Cauliflower, garlic, jicama, mushrooms, onions, parsnips, turnips, potatoes, rutabagas

large quantities of Vitamins C, E, or other antioxidant supplements actually *interferes* with normal hormesis; it derails our natural defenses, and leaves us less healthy.[75] It's not even clear that a daily multivitamin is beneficial.

When it comes to nutritional supplements, many Americans believe "What can it hurt?" and "If some is good, more is better." The emerging picture, however, seems to be "Supplements *can* hurt," and "Less is better than more."

Unless you have special dietary needs (see our next section), follow the advice in ChooseMyPlate: You can get all the healthful vitamins you need by filling half of your plate at every meal with colorful fruits and vegetables.

Phytochemicals Antioxidants are just one class of plant compounds collectively called *phytochemicals* (literally "plant chemicals"). Fruit, flowers, and plant leaves form a bright rainbow of colors, in part because plants can generate pigment molecules with antioxidant properties. We've already mentioned *beta-carotene* (which is an orange pigment). Other carotenoids include *lycopene,* which gives red pigment to tomatoes and watermelon, and *lutein* and *zeaxanthin*, found in various green and yellow foods (see Table 7.6) The familiar green chlorophyll pigments are also dietary antioxidants.

Other phytochemicals include:

- Sulphorophane, found in broccoli and other cruciferous vegetables (including kale, Brussels sprouts, cauliflower, cabbage, collard greens, and bok choy)

- Caffeine, polyphenols, flavonoids, and catechins in tea and coffee

- Capsaicin in hot peppers

- Curcumin in turmeric

- Resveratrol in grapes

- Phenols, quercetin, and anthocyanin in plums, blueberries, and other blue or purple plant parts

- Sterols and stanols in nuts and seeds

- Ergosterol in mushrooms[76]

Again, filling half of your plate with plant foods at each meal will provide you with a cornucopia of phytochemicals that boost your immunity, lower your blood pressure, help protect you from cancer, and more.

---

folate A form of vitamin B that is vital for spinal cord development and helps break down homocysteine as the body digests proteins

Foods Containing Folate **Folate** (also called *folic acid* or vitamin B_9) is a form of vitamin B that plays a role in the development of the spinal cord. Folate also helps break down the compound homocysteine, which is produced as the body digests meat and other high-protein foods. By helping break down homocysteine, folate may also protect against cardiovascular disease, heart attacks, and strokes.[77] Foods rich in folate include sunflower seeds, dark leafy greens, bean sprouts, cooked beans, asparagus, and peanuts. Many people, including reproductive-age women, consume low levels of folate in their diet. For this reason and to help prevent developmental defects such as spina bifida, the FDA requires food manufacturers to fortify with folate all bread, cereal, rice, and macaroni products sold in the United States.

LO 7.4 Do I Have Special Dietary Needs?

The *Dietary Guidelines for Americans 2015–2020* highlights several groups with special nutritional needs and concerns, including children, teens, adults over 50, vegetarians, and diabetics. To this we add, and begin our discussion with, elite and everyday exercisers because many college students want nutritional advantages in fitness and competition.

Most Exercisers Can Follow General Nutritional Guidelines

Sports physiologists and nutritionists have conducted hundreds of studies of recreational, collegiate, and professional athletes, trying to determine optimal energy and nutrient levels for peak performance. Their findings may surprise and disappoint many fitness enthusiasts: They closely follow general nutritional guidelines with only a few minor adjustments, and they emphasize the same "food first" philosophy (rather than supplements) that athletic trainers are adopting in greater and greater numbers.[78]

Carbohydrates The best source of energy before and during exercise is complex carbohydrates—bread, pasta, cereals, grains, vegetables, and fruits. They should provide up to about 5 to 7 g/kg body weight/day for general training or about 55 to 65 percent of daily calories.[79] Restricting carbohydrates can impede your fitness efforts by leaving you energy-deprived. Sugars can give a little energy boost but can also cause a rise in insulin and a drop in blood sugar that produces fatigue.

Proteins For moderate strengthening and endurance exercise, 0.8 to about 1.0 gram of protein per kilogram of

Q&A Should You Take Supplements?

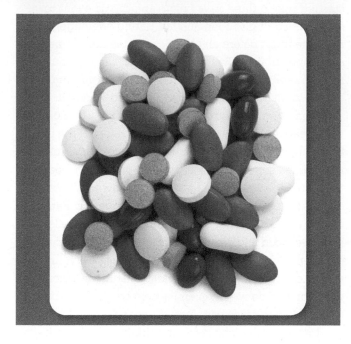

Manufacturers sell $32 billion worth of supplements each year in the United States.[107] Nearly 40 percent of all Americans take multivitamins and 88 percent of college athletes take one or more nutritional supplements.[108] Before you reach for a supplement, however, consider two significant points: (1) Supplements, especially those claiming to enhance athletic performance, can be dangerous. (2) Research has shown that vitamin and mineral supplements offer few if any benefits for preventing chronic diseases and, especially in high doses, may actually increase the risk of chronic disease.

Many people assume that the FDA or other government agency tests the safety, purity, and efficacy of supplements before they go on the market. In fact, no agency is responsible for safeguarding the public from supplements. The FDA can recall products only after consumers, watchdog groups, or medical experts show that they are harmful. What's more, the recall process is slow and enforcement is spotty.[109] A group of researchers, for example, went looking for 274 supplement products that the FDA had banned because they contained steroids, stimulants, heavy metals, or other ingredients that were causing illness, hospitalizations, and even deaths. The group found that three years after the FDA recalls, 10 percent of the banned supplements were still being sold—and most still contained the same harmful compounds![110]

Millions of people take vitamin and mineral supplements in the hopes of warding off heart disease, cancer, Alzheimer's, and other chronic illnesses. A growing body of research evidence, however, suggests that quite often, the pills provide little if any benefit and in high doses, can increase mortality rates from various causes.[111] There are notable exceptions. Folic acid supplements, for example, do reduce the incidence of stroke in patients at high risk of having one.[112]

Some nutrition experts still believe in taking supplements. They point out that the majority of Americans eat a suboptimal diet and have deficiencies that they could fill with low-dose vitamin and mineral supplements.[113] Some experts also point to the special nutritional requirements of certain medical patients (such as those at risk for stroke) and subsets of the public (children, teens, women under 50, adults over 60, and so on), arguing that people are poor at eating highly nutritious corrective diets.[114]

APPLY IT! The questions surrounding supplement use remain unresolved, but you can nevertheless take commonsense steps for your own nutritional wellness:

- Beware of supplements that claim to enhance athletic performance, and look for ways to improve your diet, instead. The National Athletic Trainers' Association, for instance, has taken the position that coaches should help college and other athletes achieve better performance through diet. They call this a "food-first philosophy."[115]

- Also beware of flooding your body with high levels of vitamins, minerals, antioxidants, and phytochemicals that could stress your cellular functions more than they assist them (see page 260). Again, concentrate on fixing your diet unless you have a special nutritional need. If you do, seek medical advice and supervision.

---

body weight can suffice. Protein does not in itself help build muscle. Only activity, including weight training, adds new muscle. Lower-fat protein sources that minimize saturated fat are better than fatty meats or full-fat dairy products. Both carbohydrates and proteins should be part of a varied and balanced diet of whole, nutrient-dense foods.

Elite Athletes Have Extra Nutritional Needs

Elite athletes—those with the potential for intercollegiate, Olympic, or professional sports—do need to modify their eating patterns for better training and performance.

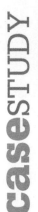

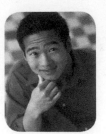

NICK

"I'm not an 'athlete,' but I do like sports. I've never worried too much about supplementing my diet with extras. I figure as long as I eat enough to feel satisfied, my body's getting what it needs. Some of my friends—like Tom, who's a cross-country runner—are always drinking sports drinks and eating energy bars. I've also noticed Tom often has a pasta dinner two days before a big run, and then he will eat a lighter meal the night before the race. He also takes a bunch of supplements from a nutrition store. I wonder if I should be doing some of that stuff?"

APPLY IT! How do Nick's and Tom's nutritional needs differ? Should Nick begin taking supplements? Why would Tom eat pasta two nights before a big run, instead of the night before?

TRY IT! **Today**, analyze your own physical activity. Could you benefit from consuming more or fewer calories? **This week**, calculate your calorie expenditures during physical activity each day for three days in a row. **In two weeks**, add or subtract some calories depending on what you discover.

Hear It!
To listen to this case study online, visit the Study Area in MasteringHealth™.

Calories People in regular training for competitive sports need extra calories. Athletes often have greater muscle mass than the average person, and muscle tissue consumes more calories than fat tissue, even at rest. A tall young man training with a football or basketball team, for example, could require 5,000 calories or more daily. High activity levels sustained for long periods— running during a soccer match, for example—also require extra fuel.

Carbohydrates and Protein About 55 to 70 percent of that extra athletic fuel should come from complex carbohydrates.[80] Some nutritionists recommend the upper end of the range for sustained high-level activities. This amounts to 7 to 10 g/kg body weight/day of complex carbohydrates. Those participating in heavy endurance and strength training also need extra protein for muscle building and tissue repair: 1.2 to 1.6 grams per kilogram per day.[81]

Pre- and Post-Event Meals Endurance events requiring heavy exertion for more than 90 minutes use two types of internal body fuels, glycogen and fat. Your muscles can store about 90 minutes' worth of glycogen, and additional storage in your liver can fuel a few more minutes of exercise. After that, your body uses its own fat to fuel activity. Endurance athletes such as marathon runners, swimmers, and soccer players often consume 60 or 70 percent of their diet in complex carbohydrates starting two to three days before an athletic event to store sufficient glycogen and fat. Eating one huge starch meal the night before an athletic event is neither necessary nor desirable. This kind of gorging can cause the body to retain water, making muscles feel stiff the next day and making the athlete feel slow and sluggish.

Many trainers instruct athletes to drink plenty of water; eat complex carbohydrates on the day of the event, three or four hours before it starts; and avoid proteins, fats, refined sugars, caffeine, and gas-producing foods in the pregame meal. Protein is relatively slow to digest and can lead to increased urination and dehydration. Fats and oils are also slow to digest. Sugar induces a surge of insulin in the blood and can cause an energy dip later, during the event. A small amount of caffeine can boost your energy during the event, but a large amount can increase urination and dehydration and accelerate the heartbeat. Gas-producing foods can upset digestion.

Many athletes choose sports drinks diluted with water. You can read more about hydration in Chapter 2.

Selecting foods to eat post-performance is part of *meal timing*—taking in nutrients when your body is most primed to use them. Trainers sometimes use the term "metabolic window" to refer to the best time to help restore the muscles' energy supply.[82] Soon after a training or performance session you should eat some protein as well as some simple and complex carbohydrates. A good target for elite exercisers is 20 grams of protein to help your muscles build and recover from an exercise session.[83] Good suggestions include cereal with fat-free dairy, soy, or almond milk; whole-wheat crackers or pretzels and hummus; or part of a turkey sandwich with lots of veggies.[84]

Research shows that meal timing has a significant effect on your appetite. Skipping meals, getting ravenously hungry, then "gorging" most of your day's calories at dinner is far more likely to cause fat accumulation than "grazing" on five or six small meals throughout the day. Sumo wrestlers deliberately apply this principle to put on hundreds of pounds of fat. If they spread their daily 6,000 calories into five or six meals instead of two, they would weigh up to 25 percent less![85]

Vitamins and Minerals The body's energy production and use requires B vitamins; bone- and blood-building require iron and calcium; sweating causes the loss of sodium and potassium that must be replenished during or after events. A balanced diet provides most athletes with enough vitamins and minerals to meet recommended intakes.

Vegetarians Must Monitor Their Nutrient Intake

Between 5 and 15 percent of all Americans claim to be one of the following, arranged in order from the strictest and most exclusive of animal products to the least: Strict *vegetarians* (also called *vegans*) avoid all foods of animal origin, including dairy products and eggs; *lacto-vegetarians* avoid animal flesh but eat dairy products; *ovo-vegetarians* avoid animal flesh and dairy products but eat eggs; *lacto-ovo-vegetarians* consume both dairy products and eggs; and *semi-vegetarians* consume fish and/or poultry but no red meat. About 90 percent of self-identified vegetarians consume dairy products on a given day and 65 percent eat eggs.[86] Vegetarians eat considerably more legumes, nuts, seeds, algae-based products, and quinoa and other whole grains than do non-vegetarians.[87]

Vegetarian diets have certain benefits.[88] Most people who follow a balanced vegetarian diet weigh less than non-vegetarians of similar height. Most also have healthier cholesterol levels, less constipation and diarrhea, and a lower risk of dying from heart disease or cancer than those who eat red meat.[89] Vegetarians consume less saturated fat, and this, in addition to lifestyle factors such as avoiding tobacco and exercising more, helps lower their mortality risk. Based on these benefits as well as the environmental concerns of additional greenhouse gases released during the production of meat and other animal foods, many universities are initiating "Meatless Monday Dinners" in campus dining halls.[90]

Despite their benefits, vegetarian diets can have deficiencies. However, with careful food choices, vegetarians can avoid them. Semi-vegetarians who eat dairy products and small amounts of chicken or fish are seldom nutrient-deficient. Vegans can get enough essential amino acids through complementary combinations of plant products (review Figure 7.2 on page 239). Lacto-vegetarians usually get enough vitamins D and B_{12} from dairy products, but strict vegans can develop deficiencies. Fortified products such as soy or almond milk can usually provide enough of these vitamins. Vegans are sometimes deficient in vitamin B_2 (riboflavin) since it is found mainly in meat, eggs, and dairy products. They can get enough B_2, however, by eating generous amounts of broccoli, asparagus, almonds, and fortified cereals. Because meat is rich in iron and dairy products are rich in calcium, vegans who avoid both can develop deficiencies of these minerals. Solutions include choosing mineral-rich plant foods (see Table 7.3)

and/or taking supplements with the advice of a nutritionist or physician.

In general, vegetarians can stay in excellent health by eating a broad variety of grains, legumes, fruits, vegetables, and seeds each day (**Figure 7.12**). The USDA website www.ChooseMyPlate.gov has more nutritional information and meal planning tips for healthy vegetarian diets.

Pregnancy Widens the Range of Nutritional Needs

Research shows that a mother's good nutrition during pregnancy can head off certain diseases for her baby even decades into his or her life, including heart disease, diabetes, and chronically high cholesterol.[91] Proper nutrition during pregnancy can also prevent later problems for the mother herself. One-third of American women are obese during their childbearing years, and the typical 30- to 40-pound weight gain during pregnancy can contribute to a range of medical issues including gestational hypertension and diabetes.[92] Retaining too much weight after pregnancy can increase a mother's risk of developing permanent type 2 diabetes. On the other hand, dieting and exercising obsessively to stay slim throughout pregnancy (so-called "pregorexia") can also be harmful. Based on our modern scientific knowledge of nutritional needs and toxic exposures, pregnant and nursing women now walk a delicate line. They must get enough folic acid, iron, iodine, calcium, vitamins A and D, and macronutrients (especially protein), and yet avoid smoking, alcohol, too much caffeine, food-borne bacteria, high mercury levels in seafood, and the toxoplasmosis parasite (common in housecats and harmful to the fetus)![93] Obstetricians are usually very helpful in providing nutritional information and guidance.

Nutrition throughout the Life Cycle

At times throughout the life cycle, we all have special dietary needs. Children and teens have special nutritional needs, as do women under 50, men and women over 60, and members of particular ethnic groups. Here are some highlights:

- Women of reproductive age who could become pregnant need 400 micrograms of folate per day to prevent potential neurological defects in a developing fetus. Pregnant women need 600 micrograms per day.

- Premenopausal women, especially those with heavy menstrual bleeding, need 18 milligrams of iron per day in foods or in total from foods and a multivitamin. They must also get enough vitamin C to help them absorb iron from foods.

Breakfast

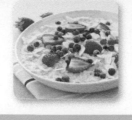

1 cup cooked oatmeal with 1 cup of mixed berries
½ banana
1 cup non-fat soy, rice, almond, or cow's milk

Lunch

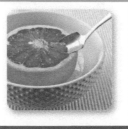

1 whole wheat wrap, filled with:
 1 tablespoon nonfat cream cheese, hummus, and/or salsa
 ½ cup chopped vegetables (such as red peppers,
  green onions, avocado)
 1 cup mixed leafy greens
 ½ to 1 cup black or kidney beans
 2 tablespoons grated soy cheese or non-fat cow's milk cheese
Sliced apple sprinkled with cinnamon
Iced tea or club soda with a lemon slice

Snack

1 ounce roasted unsalted almonds or ½ cup baby
 carrots with 2 tablespoons hummus
An orange or grapefruit

Dinner

Grilled veggie burger on whole wheat bun with condiments
 (lettuce, ketchup, mustard, salsa, pickles)
Side salad with oil and vinegar dressing and chopped veggies
 (such as tomatoes, cucumbers, celery, carrots)
1 cup steamed broccoli with 1 teaspoon whipped butter or
 butter-like spread
½ cup lemon sorbet with sliced strawberries and
 two small cookies
Water or tea

FIGURE **7.12** Vegetarians can plan healthy meals by making careful food choices for breakfast, lunch, snack, and dinner that contribute vital nutrients in each meal. Here's one example of a daily vegetarian diet that includes protein, calcium, B vitamins, and other nutrients.

Based on information from the US Department of Agriculture and www.ChooseMyPlate.gov.

- Older adults need sufficient potassium for normal muscle contraction and nerve transmission and sodium within a healthy range to supply cellular needs but lower the risk of high blood pressure.

- Older adults, dark-skinned individuals, and people who do not get regular exposure to sunlight have a special need for vitamin D. The government currently recommends that people under 50 consume 200 IU (International Units) of vitamin D per day, people between 50 and 70 consume 400 IU per day, and people over 70 consume 600 IU per day.

- People over 50 naturally produce less stomach acid and absorb less vitamin B_{12} from foods. Older adults should be careful to get at least 2.4 micrograms of B_{12} per day or more, especially if they take stomach acid blockers.

- Research suggests that along with exercise, 1 to 1.2 g/kg of protein per day may also help protect older adults from muscle wasting.[94] Extra protein can also aid in cellular repair and replacement after surgery or during infections.

- Cigarette smoking decreases bone density and interferes with the body's normal use of vitamin C. Smokers therefore need to consume more calcium (1,200 mg/day) and vitamin C (110 mg in women, 125 mg/day in men) compared to 90 milligrams for non-smoking adults.

- Men and postmenopausal women need 10 milligrams of iron per day but should be careful not to get too much.

- Most adults under 50 need 1,000 milligrams of calcium. Pregnant women, nursing mothers, teens, and older adults need extra calcium (1,200 to 1,500 mg/day) for the development and maintenance of bones and to lower the risk of osteoporosis.

- People with diseases that disrupt normal metabolism or nutrient absorption (e.g., diabetes and certain cancers) can develop vitamin or mineral deficiencies. Physicians often recommend special diets or multivitamins as part of their treatment.[95]

- The USDA dietary guidelines provide specific pointers to help kids and teens get the balance of nutrients they need to support their growth and development (see Tables 7.2 and 7.3).

Those with Diabetes Must Reduce Carbohydrates

Anyone diagnosed with type 1 or type 2 diabetes will receive specific information from medical providers about both drug treatments and dietary changes. Because diabetes is a disorder of blood-sugar regulation, patients usually must cut back on sweets and desserts, both to reduce surges of sugar in the blood and to control obesity, which can lead to and intensify diabetes. Choosing foods with a lower rather than higher glycemic index (see page 241) is also beneficial, and this usually means whole rather than processed foods and reduced fat content overall. The American Diabetes Association advises diabetics to eats lots of non-starchy vegetables and fruits, choose whole grains over processed grain products, include beans and lentils in the diet, eat fish two to three times per week, choose lean meats and nonfat dairy products, drink water and diet drinks instead of sugary drinks, avoid saturated fats and *trans* fats during cooking, and watch portion sizes.[96]

LO 7.5 Food Safety for Everyone

Food: Handle with Care

Sometimes people think they have the flu when it is actually "food poisoning." Food-borne illnesses usually cause diarrhea, nausea, cramping, and vomiting. They usually occur five to eight hours after eating and last only a day or two. For healthy people, food poisoning is unpleasant and inconvenient. For the very young, the elderly, or people with severe illnesses, it can be fatal. The Centers for Disease Control and Prevention estimates that every year 48 million Americans are sickened, 128,000 are hospitalized, and 3,000 die from foodborne illnesses.[97]

See It!
Watch "FDA Proposes New Food Safety Rules" at MasteringHealth™.

A rise in imported fruits and vegetables, as well as increased urbanization, industrialization, travel, and restaurant dining, raises the risk of unsafe food handling and results in illness.

To avoid foodborne illness, be aware of cleanliness in stores and restaurants. When purchasing food, pay attention to expiration dates.

Use proper techniques for storing and handling food at home: Keep your hands and all cooking surfaces clean. Separate raw foods from cooked foods during storage and cooking. Scrub and thoroughly rinse produce before eating it. Heat foods to high enough temperatures

to kill germs. Refrigerate perishable foods. And finally, use special care when you handle raw eggs, meat, poultry, and fish; unwashed or outdated bean or alfalfa sprouts; and unpasteurized milk and juices—they are the items most likely to cause food poisoning.

Organic and GMO Foods

For many years, the market for organic foods has been rising faster than food sales in general. Today, 81 percent of US families buy organic foods, at least occasionally.[98]

Researchers are divided on whether organic food is more nutritious.[99] But there is little doubt that pesticide residues remain on non-organic produce, and that in high enough doses, food pesticides can lead to cancer, nerve damage, birth defects, and other medical problems.[100] Many people support the "locavore" movement that advocates buying locally grown produce at farmer's markets and through direct arrangements with local growers in an effort to get fresher produce that may have a shorter shelf life but also carry fewer pesticides.

See It!
Watch "Organic Produce" at MasteringHealth™.

Some people have concerns about the safety of foods produced with the use of genetically modified organisms or their products, or foods that are irradiated to kill micro-organisms and prolong shelf life. Both the World Health Organization and the American Association for the Advancement of Science report no additional risks or adverse health effects compared to consuming crops modified through conventional plant genetics.[101] You can learn more about these issues by visiting the online resources at the end of this chapter.

Food Sensitivities, Allergies, and Intolerances

A food allergy or hypersensitivity is an abnormal immune response to a food component—usually a protein. The reaction can range from mild tingling or swelling in the mouth or throat to skin hives, vomiting, abdominal cramps, diarrhea, or trouble breathing. More than 150 foods can cause allergic reactions, but eight foods account for 90 percent of all food allergies in the United States: milk, eggs, peanuts, wheat, soy, tree nuts (such as walnuts, pecans, cashews, and pistachios), fish, and shellfish.[102]

About 30 percent of people think they have a food allergy. In fact, only 5 percent of children and 4 percent of adults actually do.[103] Even though they remain rare, however, some allergies—such as peanut allergies in children—have increased three-fold in recent years.[104]

Food intolerance usually involves a milder digestive upset due to enzyme deficiencies or other non-immune causes. Examples include lactose intolerance (which affects 1 in 10 American adults), gluten intolerance, and reaction to sulfites, certain food dyes, or MSG (monosodium glutamate).[105] There is considerable confusion and misinformation about food intolerance, especially involving gluten. If you have recurrent symptoms, it's important to get a legitimate diagnosis of food allergy or intolerance through the campus health clinic or your off-campus physician, as well as to learn about and follow safe-eating guidelines.

LO 7.6 How Can I Create a Behavior Change Plan for Nutrition?

You've no doubt heard the famous phrase, "You are what you eat." But did you know that its origin was a book written in 1825 by Anthelme Brillat-Savain—a French lawyer who loved eating above all else? What he actually wrote was, "Tell me what you eat and I shall tell you what you are." We could modify that slightly to make it perfectly relevant to this book and to you, the reader: Tell us what you eat and we'll tell you how fit and well you're likely to be—now and in the future!

Assess Your Current Diet

Would you benefit from changes to your current diet? The most successful way to change long-ingrained eating habits is to break the task into steps and keep track of your progress.

Record What You Eat If you completed Lab 7.2, you are on your way to a better diet. Self-awareness is the necessary starting point for change, followed by your own actions for self-improvement.[106]

> **Live It!**
> Complete Worksheet 20 Your Eating Habits at MasteringHealth™.

You should get a pretty clear idea of how many calories your daily diet provides and whether it meets, exceeds, or falls short of the daily recommendations for carbohydrates, fats, proteins, fiber, vitamins, minerals, and fruits and vegetables. If there are gaps in your food diary, keep track of your hour-by-hour food consumption for another day or two so you have a clear picture of your typical nutritional profile.

Identify Your Patterns Go through your food diary and analyze your reasons for eating each meal and snack. Was it primarily hunger? Socializing? Boredom? If it is hunger, are you satisfying that need with nutrient-dense foods? If it is primarily socializing, are you even hungry at the time? Does peer pressure persuade you to eat an after-dinner snack of pizza and frozen yogurt when you could be happy with a salad or an apple? If you are eating out of boredom or stress—snacking on chips and cola while studying, for example—could you find a more nutritious alternative such as carrot sticks, whole-wheat crackers, unsalted peanuts, popcorn, or grapes?

By reflecting on and identifying your own reasons for food preferences and eating habits, you can start to understand your patterns and perhaps change them for the better. It is seldom easy or automatic to improve your diet because it means breaking long-standing habits. But new behaviors become simpler if you realize when and why you reach for certain foods and that the resistance to change may come from within yourself or your family and friends.

Review Your Behavior Change Skills

Examining your current eating patterns is just one part of applying behavior change skills to improve your nutrition. Here are some other ways you can incorporate the behavior change model:

- *Look at your motivation.* Do you really want a different and better diet? What do you see as the immediate benefits? What do you expect over the long term? Solidifying your motivation can help you get ready for change.

- *Identify barriers to a better diet.* What are some of the difficulties you foresee in achieving better nutrition? Time? Money? Eating in less-than-optimal ways with friends and family? Naming some of those barriers and coming up with alternatives can help you on the path to change. If you have trouble brainstorming solutions, the student health service or counseling center may be able to help you.

- *Make a commitment to learning about better nutrition.* List ways in which an improved diet will benefit your life. What could eating more whole grain fiber do for you? How about consuming more fruits and vegetables? Listing these will help you stick with your plan for change.

- *Choose a target behavior by identifying your biggest nutritional concern.* What is the most pressing issue with your current diet? Review your food diary. If you see that you're getting too few fruits and vegetables each day but too much saturated fat, outline an approach for eating more produce and getting less saturated fat in your meals and snacks. If you discover that fried meats and cheese are pushing up your daily fat total, think of nutrient-dense whole food alternatives.

- *Note where you stand in the typical stages of change.* Are you contemplating change? If so, gathering more information or talking more with friends and family might help. Are you planning for change and getting ready to take action?

- *Have you noticed any helpful role models?* Do you know people with good eating habits and a nutritious diet? Observing their food choices and talking to them about your nutritional issues may help you learn to counter your current habits with others based on better food choices, more successful eating patterns, and solid nutritional information.

Get Set to Apply Nutritional Skills

With this chapter, you've already begun to learn and apply nutritional skills. Review your use of them and look for ways to improve those skills and call upon them daily.

Examine food guides to compare your daily servings of various food groups with the amounts that nutritionists recommend from governmental agencies or from academic institutions. Read food labels more often and watch for those nutrients you've identified as problematic in your own diet. For example, watch for hidden fats and sugars and look for opportunities to increase fiber.

Recognize proper portion sizes and note when the helping you are served in a restaurant or cafeteria is way too big (e.g., three cups of pasta instead of half a cup) or way too small (e.g., a side salad the size of a golf ball instead of a softball). Use www.ChooseMyPlate.gov or other kinds of diet software to get an individual analysis of the daily calories and nutrients you consume and how they compare with the recommended daily intakes of each and to keep track of what you eat.

See It!
Watch "Menu Calorie Counts: How Accurate Are They?" at MasteringHealth™.

Both behavior-change skills and nutritional tools can help you plan your own program for improved nutrition. Working on this plan can give you practice at recognizing nutrient-dense foods. You can start to choose high-volume, low-density alternatives to high-density, high-calorie foods. You may find that you now prefer whole grains to refined ones. And you may start to savor the colors, flavors, and textures of fruits and/or vegetables.

Your plan may be your first deliberate application of nutritional tools and behavioral-change skills for nutrition. In time, however, it should become a continual and automatic part of each day. The goal is to balance nutrients and control calories naturally as part of your long-term efforts for fitness and wellness and your ongoing management of body mass and weight.

Create a Nutrition Plan

Begin planning your own program by using **Lab 7.3**. As you work through the lab, write down your own notes and observations and swap them with others in your class, perhaps during a class discussion or in a small discussion group.

Do It!
Access these labs at the end of the chapter or online at MasteringHealth™.

Keep track of calories for your new plan. Are you on track? Where could you cut or add without increasing saturated fats, sugars, or refined carbohydrates?

After two weeks, discuss the plan and your results with your fitness/health instructor, and revise if necessary. Again, if possible, discuss your experiences with others in your class to exchange successful ideas and get support for your efforts.

For several weeks, continue tracking your daily diet, either manually or using www.ChooseMyPlate.gov —at least track the number of servings of the main food groups. This helps you eat sufficient amounts of the foods you need to increase (e.g., whole grains, fruits, vegetables, beans, nuts) and helps you cut back on those that are already overrepresented (e.g., saturated fat or sugars and refined carbohydrates). Continue applying nutritional skills such as reading labels and comparing serving sizes to the portions in Figure 7.9 on page 255.

Don't try for perfection! Approach your diet in sets of two or three days at a time. When you have a day with too few fruits and vegetables, increase them the next day. When you have a day with too little protein, have more the next day. If you get too much protein one day, eat less the next or eat less-concentrated protein foods such as tofu, beans, or skim milk. See Program 7.1 at the end of this chapter for further guidance in planning your diet.

Study Plan

chapter summary

LO 7.1 Why Are My College Years a Nutritional Challenge?

- Most students eat on the run and have mediocre to poor eating habits.
- Healthful foods are sometimes harder to find on and near college campuses.

LO 7.2 What Are the Main Nutrients in Food?

- Proteins, carbohydrates, and fats are our major nutrients.
- We also need several water- and fat-soluble vitamins along with specific minerals and water itself.

LO 7.3 How Can I Achieve a Balanced Diet?

- The US government publishes comprehensive guidelines for needed nutrient levels and those that Americans should increase and decrease in their diets.
- Skills for improving your nutrition include controlling portion size, keeping food diaries, and eating whole foods that are nutrient-dense.

LO 7.4 Do I Have Special Dietary Needs?

- Regular and elite exercisers must monitor their pre- and post-exercise meals for adequate protein and other nutrients.

- Vegetarians must insure adequate levels of several nutrients that are harder to consume from plants.
- Pregnant women must get enough nutrients for themselves and the fetus without gaining too much or too little weight.
- Each of us has special nutritional needs between infancy and old age. People of certain ethnicities and/or those with medical conditions may have additional needs.

LO 7.5 Food Safety for Everyone

- Good food handling practices can decrease the risk of food-borne illness.
- Many consumers choose organic foods and look for GMO-free foods.
- Food allergies are rare but sensitivities and food intolerances are more common and should be diagnosed.

LO 7.6 How Can I Create a Behavior Change Plan for Nutrition?

- Assess your current diet, record daily intake to reveal patterns, and apply behavior change skills and nutritional tools to fashion more nutritious food plans.

review questions

LO 7.1 1. All of these are obstacles to a healthy diet while in college except:
  a. Fast food tends to be cheap and easy to get on campus.
  b. Students have distractions such as cell phones, computer screens, and commuting to class or work while eating.
  c. Students can't afford fruits and vegetables.
  d. Students come to college with pre-existing preferences for junk food.

LO 7.2 2. Essential amino acids are
  a. found only in animal proteins.
  b. found only in plant proteins.
  c. best taken as supplements.
  d. protein building blocks your body can't produce.

LO 7.2 3. Simple carbohydrates
  a. are important amino acid compounds.
  b. act as structural compounds in plants.
  c. provide fiber in the diet.
  d. deliver energy in a quickly usable form.

LO 7.2 4. Using the glycemic index, you can determine
  a. the percentage of glucose in a food.
  b. the percentage of glycine in a food.
  c. how quickly a food will boost your blood sugar levels.
  d. the caloric content of a food.

LO 7.2 5. What do nutritionists sometimes call "bad cholesterol"?
  a. Saturated fat
  b. Butter
  c. HDLs
  d. LDLs

review questions CONTINUED

LO 7.2 6. Calcium can
  a. cause osteoporosis (brittle bones).
  b. delay blood clotting.
  c. prevent proper nerve impulse transmission.
  d. play an important role in muscle contraction.

LO 7.3 7. Which of the following would be considered a healthy, nutrient-dense food?
  a. Cheddar cheese
  b. Soft drink
  c. Potato chips
  d. Fat-free milk

LO 7.3 8. An example of an antioxidant would be
  a. vitamin C.
  b. vitamin B_{12}.
  c. sodium.
  d. iron.

LO 7.3 9. By law, a food label must
  a. tell the exact number of items in the package.
  b. give the manufacturer's business address.
  c. calculate the percentage of calories from fat.
  d. provide a recommended serving size.

LO 7.4 10. Which of the following is true?
  a. Exercisers need to double or triple their protein consumption.
  b. People should take a daily multivitamin as insurance against poor diet.
  c. Because they are proportionately smaller, children need less calcium than adults.
  d. Vegans who plan meals carefully are still likely to have nutrient deficiencies.

LO 7.5 11. For proper food handling and safety
  a. use all produce straight from the garden or market without washing.
  b. avoid pasteurized milk and juices.
  c. observe expiration dates on food packaging.
  d. store raw and cooked foods together in airtight containers.

LO 7.6 12. One of these will help you plan and achieve better nutrition:
  a. Eliminating certain food groups.
  b. Avoiding nutrient density.
  c. Keeping a food log.
  d. Perfecting your daily effort.

critical thinking questions

LO 7.1, LO 7.3, LO 7.6 1. Write out a healthy menu for yourself for one breakfast, one lunch, and one dinner, including portion sizes for each type of food you select.

LO 7.2 2. Excluding water, what are the major types of nutrients in food? What are the main roles of each?

LO 7.2 3. Name several protective functions of dietary fiber.

LO 7.2 4. Differentiate *trans* fat and saturated fat. Name two dietary sources of each. Which is worse, and why?

LO 7.3 5. How do antioxidants protect the body against the damaging effects of free radicals?

LO 7.4 6. Describe the requirements for calcium and vitamin D in children, women of childbearing age, and people over 50.

check out these eResources

- **Healthline Review** Find reviews of calorie counting apps for your cell phone. **www.healthline.com**
- **LiveScience Review** Find reviews of health-related apps. **www.livescience.com**
- **Mayo Clinic** Check out alternative food pyramids for Mediterranean, Asian, Indian, Latin, and vegetarian diets. **www.mayoclinic.org**

- **Office of Disease Prevention and Health Promotion** Read the federal dietary guidelines for more in-depth information on nutrition. **www.health.gov**
- **US Food and Drug Administration** Get information on a long list of current topics including food allergies, food safety, dietary supplements, sodium, nutrition, gluten, and many more. **www.fda.gov**

DO IT!

LAB
7.1

LEARN A SKILL

**READING A FOOD
LABEL**

MasteringHealth™

Name: _____ **Date:** _____

Instructor: _____ **Section:** _____

Purpose: To learn how to read food labels and analyze the nutritional content of a packaged food.

Directions: Select any packaged food item from your kitchen or from a grocery store. Find the "Nutrition Facts" panel on the package and answer the following questions.

1. What is the name of the packaged food you are examining?

_____

2. What is the "serving size" stated on the Nutrition Facts panel?

_____

Does this "serving size" match the portion you typically consume of this food in one sitting? Is it bigger or smaller than the amount that you typically consume?

_____

3. Examine the ingredients. What are the main ingredients (i.e., which items are listed first)?

_____

Does this list of main ingredients surprise you? How nutritious are the main ingredients?

_____

4. Complete the following table for your chosen food, listing amounts and % Daily Value (% DV) for various nutrients:

Calories (per serving)	Total Fat	Saturated Fat	*Trans Fat*	Sodium	Dietary Fiber	Sugars	Vitamins/ Minerals
	Amount:	Amount:	Amount:	Amount:	Amount:	Amount:	Amount:
	% DV:	% DV:	% DV:	% DV:	% DV:		% DV:

Examine your data. Is this food excessively high in fat, saturated fat, *trans* fat, or sodium? Does it provide any dietary fiber? How much added sugar is in this food? Does this food supply any vitamins and minerals?

_____

_____

5. What is your overall assessment of the nutritional value of the packaged food you have examined? How does the particular food you examined compare to other typical foods in your daily diet?

_____

_____

6. Healthy eaters make regular label reading a part of every shopping trip. What can you add to your behavior-change contract for nutrition that will help you develop a life-long food-label-reading habit?

_____

_____

DO IT!

LAB
7.2

ASSESS YOURSELF

KEEPING A FOOD DIARY AND
ANALYZING YOUR DAILY
NUTRITION

MasteringHealth™

Name: _____ **Date:** _____

Instructor: _____ **Section:** _____

Purpose: To get an initial assessment of your current nutrition and identify areas to be improved.

Directions: Follow the instructions below. You will need Internet access to complete this lab.

1. Log on to www.supertracker.usda.gov/foodtracker.aspx (or use one of the food tracking apps listed under eResources on page 269).

2. Click "CREATE PROFILE" in the upper right-hand corner of the page if you are accessing this site for the first time. Click "LOG IN" if you are returning.

3. Click on "Track Food & Activity" at the top of the page and select "Food Tracker." Enter all of the food items you have eaten today. (It's best to complete this at the end of the day when you have finished all of your meals.) Enter each food individually by entering the name of the food in the search field and clicking "Go." If you cannot find the exact food you are looking for, select the food that is the most similar. After you have located a food, it should show up on the left side of the screen. Select a serving size from the drop-down menu and enter the number of servings you consumed. Choose a meal time and click "Add" to save the food in your tracker. Repeat until you have entered all of the foods you consumed today. (Don't forget to include any snacks and beverages!)

4. Click on the "My Reports" tab, and select "Food Groups & Calories." Select a date range and click "Create Report." How does your food intake compare to the recommendations for food groups and calories?

   _____

   _____

   _____

   _____

5. Click on "Nutrients Reports" at the top of the screen. Select a date range and click "Create Report." This report will illustrate how your intake of specific nutrients compares to the recommendations.

   a. Does your intake of any nutrient fall short of the recommendations? If so, which nutrient(s)?

   _____

   _____

   b. Does your intake of any nutrient exceed the recommendations? If so, which nutrient(s)?

   _____

   _____

Note: For more accurate results, record your intake for at least three consecutive days, and then analyze your data again.

IMPROVING YOUR NUTRITION

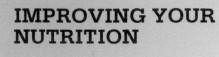

MasteringHealth™

Name: _____ Date: _____

Instructor: _____ Section: _____

Purpose: To create a detailed plan for improving your personal nutrition.

Materials: Results from Lab 7.2.

Section I: Planning Changes to Your Diet

1. Look back at your results for Lab 7.2. Which nutrients do you consume too little of?

_____

_____

List at least three foods you could add to your diet in order to increase your consumption of these nutrients:

Food: _____ Rich in: _____

Food: _____ Rich in: _____

Food: _____ Rich in: _____

(**Hint:** To get ideas for new foods to try, go to the Food Groups section of www.ChooseMyPlate.gov and choose the food groups one by one. You will see a listing of fruits, vegetables, grains, protein-rich foods, and dairy foods.)

2. Do you consume too much sugar, protein, saturated fat, or sodium? If so, what foods high in these substances could you reduce or eliminate from your diet? List at least three:

Food: _____ High in: _____

Food: _____ High in: _____

Food: _____ High in: _____

3. How closely did your diet match up with the USDA recommendations? Fill in the blanks below.

Current dairy intake: _____ cups   Recommended dairy intake: _____ cups

Current intake of protein-rich foods: _____ oz.   Recommended intake of protein-rich foods: _____ oz.

Current vegetables intake: _____ cups   Recommended vegetables intake: _____ cups

Current fruits intake: _____ cups   Recommended fruits intake: _____ cups

Current whole grains intake: _____ oz.   Recommended whole grains intake: _____ oz.

How can you adjust your diet to more closely meet recommended intake levels for each food group?

- I would like to increase/decrease my milk intake by _____cups.
- I would like to increase/decrease my meat and beans intake by _____oz.
- I would like to increase/decrease my vegetables intake by _____oz.
- I would like to increase/decrease my fruits intake by _____cups.
- I would like to increase/decrease my whole grains intake by _____oz.

Section II: Short- and Long-Term Goals

Create short- and long-term goals for your healthy eating plan. Be sure to use SMART (specific, measurable, action-oriented, realistic, time-limited) goal-setting guidelines and the information obtained from section 1 of this lab and all of your Lab 7.2 materials. Choose appropriate target dates and rewards for completing your goals.

1. Short-Term Goal (3 to 6 Months)

    a. Goal: _____

    _____

    b. Target Date: _____

    c. Reward: _____

2. Long-Term Goal (12+ Months)

    a. Goal: _____

    _____

    b. Target Date: _____

    c. Reward: _____

Section III: Barriers to Good Nutrition; Strategies for Overcoming Them

1. What barriers or obstacles might hinder your plan for nutrition changes? Indicate your top three nutritional barriers here:

    a. _____

    b. _____

    c. _____

2. Overcoming these barriers to change will be an important step in reaching your goals. List three strategies for overcoming the obstacles listed:

    a. _____

    b. _____

    c. _____

Section IV: Getting Support

List resources you will use to help you change your nutritional behavior and how each of these resources will support your goals:

Friend/partner/relative: _____

School-based resource: _____

Community-based resource: _____

Other: _____

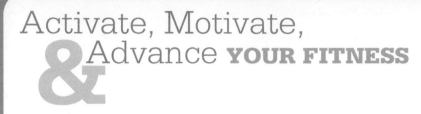

Activate, Motivate, & Advance YOUR FITNESS

ACTIVATE!

Fruits and vegetables are low in calories and important components of a nutritious diet; eating them is helpful for managing your weight. This program can help you successfully increase your vegetable and fruit consumption and variety!

What Do I Need to Do to Eat More Fruits?

KNOW WHAT COUNTS: All fresh, frozen, canned, and dried fruits and 100 percent fruit juices count as fruit.

MORE ABOUT JUICE: Fruit juice can be part of a healthy diet, but even 100 percent fruit juice lacks dietary fiber and it can add extra calories. Most of the fruit you eat should come from whole fruits rather than juice. When choosing juice or canned fruit, look for a notation on the package saying "100% juice" or "fruit canned in 100% fruit juice." Fruit drinks that have little juice are considered sugar-sweetened beverages.

CHOOSE OLD FAVORITES AND NEW: Create a list of fruits you like or want to try for the first time. Remember that fruit may come in different forms (peaches, for example, can be fresh, canned, or frozen).

What Do I Need to Do to Eat More Vegetables?

KNOW WHAT COUNTS: All fresh, frozen, canned, and dried vegetables and 100 percent vegetable juices count.

VARIETY IS KEY: Eat a variety of vegetables, especially dark-green and red and orange vegetables and beans and peas.

CHOOSE OLD FAVORITES AND NEW: Create a list of vegetables you like, types that are available to you, and ones you'd like to try for the first time. Remember that vegetables come in different forms (such as spinach, which you may enjoy fresh, frozen, or canned). A list can help you plan ahead to eat more helpings each day.

Tips to Eating More Fruits and Vegetables

KEEP PRODUCE HANDY: Keep a bowl of whole fruit on the table, on the counter, or in the refrigerator. You can also keep a piece of fruit in your bag for an easy snack. Individual containers of fruits like peaches or applesauce are also easy and convenient. Keep washed and cut vegetables on hand ready for snacking. Carrots, broccoli, cauliflower, bell peppers, and baby tomatoes are all great alone or with dips like hummus, low-fat ranch, or cottage cheese.

CHOOSE MEALS WISELY: Aim for meals that are half fruits and vegetables. Think of building your meal around produce instead of adding produce to a meal based around protein, breads, or rice. Try a salad as a main dish for lunch (go light on the dressing). Include a green salad with your dinner every night. Add beans and peas to salads or get creative and try topping them with dried fruit, oranges, apples, or berries.

When eating out (or in the dining hall) look for options that include the most vegetables, such as a pizza topped with mushrooms and green peppers or a veggie burrito or omelet. Add vegetables such as tomatoes, lettuce, and avocado to your sandwiches and subs. Choose split pea or lentil soups or add beans into other soup choices.

Replace high-calorie foods such as chips or cookies with lower-calorie fruit-based choices such as 100 percent juice smoothies with low-fat yogurt or milk blended with frozen fruit; 100 percent juice frozen fruit bars; yogurt topped with fresh fruit; or even a "baked" apple cooked in the microwave with cinnamon and raisins.

Choose fresh fruits in season because they will likely taste best and cost less.

Always top your cereal (hot or cold), pancakes, and waffles with fruit. Some ideas include sliced bananas, dried fruit, frozen or fresh berries, and chopped apples or peaches. Note that dried fruit such as raisins and cranberries are high in sugars.

COOKING AND SHOPPING: Review the discussion on fresh, canned, and frozen fruits and veggies on page 258. Keep in mind that all three packing options offer good nutrition and that canned and frozen may offer more bang for your produce buck.

If you are cooking, add shredded carrots or canned pumpkin to muffins and breads and chopped or shredded vegetables to soups, stews, casseroles, stir-fries, and tomato sauces.

Buy baked beans or refried beans in cans to use them for side dishes or snacks, such as adding refried beans to a quesadilla.

Buy vegetables that are easy to prepare, such as bags of baby carrots, bagged salad mixes, or lower-sodium canned vegetables or soup. Frozen vegetables are quick and easy to cook in the microwave.

Buy fruits that are dried, frozen, and canned (in water or 100 percent juice) as well as fresh, so that you always have a supply on hand. Choose packaged fruits that do not have added sugars.

Keep vegetables and fruits visible when storing them.

Four-Week Program to Boost Fruit and Vegetable Intake

Very few adults in the United States eat the recommended 5 to 9 cups of fruits or vegetables per day, so this is a program from which most everyone can benefit. Adjust the program to suit your personal meal schedule.

What Counts as a Cup?

In general, what counts as a cup is: 1 cup of fruit, 1 cup of raw or cooked vegetables, 1 cup of 100 percent fruit or vegetable juice, 2 cups of raw leafy greens, or 1/4 cup of dried fruit. Visit www.ChooseMyPlate.gov for more information on portion sizes.

EATING MORE FRUITS AND VEGETABLES PROGRAM

GOAL: To increase your nutrient levels, especially fiber, vitamins, and antioxidants, increase fruit and vegetable intake to 5 cups of fruits and vegetables per day by progressively including them in meals and snacks over four weeks.

	Mon	Tue	Wed	Thurs	Fri	Sat	Sun
Week 1	2 cups of fruits and vegetables	2 cups of fruits and vegetables	2 cups of fruits and vegetables	2 cups of fruits and vegetables	2 cups of fruits and vegetables	2 cups of fruits and vegetables	2 cups of fruits and vegetables
Week 2	3 cups of fruits and vegetables	3 cups of fruits and vegetables	3 cups of fruits and vegetables	3 cups of fruits and vegetables	3 cups of fruits and vegetables	3 cups of fruits and vegetables	3 cups of fruits and vegetables
Week 3	4 cups of fruits and vegetables	4 cups of fruits and vegetables	4 cups of fruits and vegetables	4 cups of fruits and vegetables	4 cups of fruits and vegetables	4 cups of fruits and vegetables	4 cups of fruits and vegetables
Week 4	5 cups of fruits and vegetables	5 cups of fruits and vegetables	5 cups of fruits and vegetables	5 cups of fruits and vegetables	5 cups of fruits and vegetables	5 cups of fruits and vegetables	5 cups of fruits and vegetables

Note: This program assumes you are already eating 1-2 cups of fruits and vegetables per day. If you are eating <1-2 cups of fruits and vegetables per day, increase your intake before beginning the program to 2 cups per day. If you are already eating >2 cups of fruits and vegetables per day, start by adding one more cup of fruit and vegetables each week until you reach 5 cups per day.

MOTIVATE!

Track your fruit and vegetable intake on your personal planner or on an online food planner site (such as www.supertracker.usda.gov). Make note of the meal or snack, types of produce, and amounts. Here are some tips for boosting the nutrition of your choices:

FRUIT: For the benefits of dietary fiber, choose whole or cut-up fruit rather than fruit juice.

Select fruits with more potassium more often; these include bananas, prunes and prune juice, dried peaches and apricots, and orange juice. Try to eat different colors of fruits to make consuming a good variety easier.

VEGETABLES: More often select vegetables that contain higher levels of potassium, such as sweet potatoes, white potatoes, white beans, tomato products (paste, sauce, and juice), beet greens, soybeans, lima beans, spinach, lentils, and kidney beans.

Keep in mind that sauces and seasonings can add calories, saturated fat, and sodium to vegetables. Use the Nutrition Facts label to compare the calories and % Daily Value for saturated fat and sodium in plain and seasoned vegetables.

Prepare foods from fresh ingredients to lower sodium intake. Most of the sodium we eat comes from packaged or processed foods. Buy canned vegetables labeled "reduced sodium," "low sodium," or "no salt added."

ADVANCE!

Now that you have boosted your fruit and vegetable intake, challenge yourself to explore and consume even more produce, or try cooking an old favorite in a new way. Below is a program to help you increase your variety of produce. Choose new varieties from the lists following the program. On days without a new fruit or vegetable in your program, continue incorporating the new varieties from the previous day(s).

INCREASING YOUR FRUIT AND VEGETABLE VARIETY PROGRAM

GOAL: To eat a variety of fruits and vegetables, especially including vegetables from the following sub-groups: dark-green vegetables, red and orange vegetables, and beans and peas, progressively over a four-week period.

	Mon	Tue	Wed	Thurs	Fri	Sat	Sun
Week 1	Try 1 new fruit or vegetable		Try 1 new fruit or vegetable				
Week 2	Try 1 new fruit and 1 new vegetable		Try 1 new fruit and 1 new vegetable				
Week 3	Try 1 new fruit and 1 new vegetable		Try 1 new fruit and 1 new vegetable		Try 1 new fruit and 1 new vegetable		
Week 4	Try 2 new fruits and 2 new vegetables		Try 1 new fruit and 1 new vegetable		Try 2 new fruits and 2 new vegetables		

Common Fruit Choices to Add for Variety

Apples
Apricots
Bananas
Blueberries
Cantaloupe
Cherries
Grapefruit
Grapes
Honeydew

Kiwi fruit
Lemons
Limes
Mangoes
Nectarines
Oranges
Peaches
Pears
Papaya

Pineapple
Plums
Prunes
Raisins
Raspberries
Strawberries
Tangerines
Watermelon

Common Vegetable Choices to Add for Variety

Dark Green
Bok choy
Broccoli
Collard greens
Dark green leafy lettuce
Kale
Mesclun
Mustard greens
Romaine lettuce
Spinach
Turnip greens
Watercress

Red and Orange
Acorn, butternut, or
   hubbard squash
Carrots
Pumpkin
Red peppers
Sweet potatoes
Tomatoes or tomato juice

Beans and Peas
Black beans

Black-eyed peas
Garbanzo beans (chickpeas)
Kidney beans
Lentils
Navy beans
Pinto beans
Soy beans
Split peas
White beans

Starchy
Cassava
Corn
Green peas
Green lima beans
Plantains
Potatoes
Taro
Water chestnuts

Other
Artichokes
Asparagus
Avocado

Bean sprouts
Beets
Brussels sprouts
Cabbage
Cauliflower
Celery
Cucumbers
Eggplant
Green beans
Green peppers
Iceberg (head) lettuce
Mushrooms
Okra
Onions
Turnips
Wax beans
Zucchini

8 Managing Your Weight

LEARNINGoutcomes

LO 8.1 Explain why obesity is both a worldwide trend and a serious concern in America.

LO 8.2 Discuss four effects of body weight and composition on wellness.

LO 8.3 List reasons why some diets work but most fail.

LO 8.4 Describe three major eating disorders.

LO 8.5 Define metabolic rate, set point, and energy balance and relate them to body weight, composition, and weight maintenance.

LO 8.6 Choose a realistic target based on your metabolic rate, activity level, eating habits, and environment and create a behavior change plan for long-term weight management.

MasteringHealth™

Go online for chapter quizzes, interactive assessments, videos, and more!

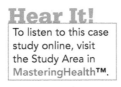

TALIA

"I'm Talia, from Indiana. I'm a freshman at our biggest state college and planning to study social work. My grades are pretty high and I've made lots of friends. It can get crazy, though, with my part-time job on top of studying. A bunch of us have an Econ study group that meets a couple times a week in somebody's room about 9 or 10 at night. We usually get a pizza, some ice cream, or Mexican food—the cafeteria dinner is inedible, except for the desserts! So we're starving by the time our group meets. My only real issue is weight. You've heard of the Freshman 15? Well I have gained at least half that much and my clothes are getting too tight. I wasn't thin to start with, either! I'd like to lose some weight but I've heard that diets don't work—you gain everything back. Should I just buy new clothes?"

Hear It!
To listen to this case study online, visit the Study Area in MasteringHealth™.

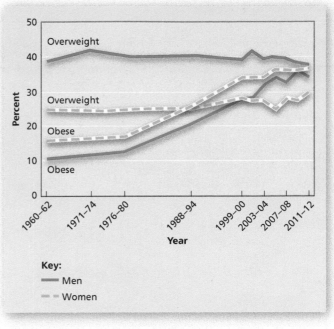

FIGURE **8.1** For the past half century, 25 percent of American women and 40 percent of American men have been overweight despite massive government campaigns and personal efforts at weight reduction. Since 1960, the percentage of obese adults has more than doubled. About two-thirds of Americans are now overweight or obese and risk weight-related illnesses.

Source: NCHS E-Stat, "Prevalence of Overweight, Obesity and Extreme Obesity among Adults: United States, Trends 1960–1962 through 2011–2012," National Health and Nutrition Examination Survey.

E xcess weight is a serious issue in America that can harm individual health and that taxes our national resources. More than two-thirds of Americans over age 20 are at an unhealthy weight.[1] About half of adults (33.3 percent of the total adult population) are **overweight** (see **Figure 8.1**), meaning that their body weight is more than 10 percent over the recommended range and their body mass index (BMI) is between 25 and 29.9.[2] The other half (34.9 percent of the total adult population) are **obese**, with a BMI of 30 or above.[3] Less than 5 percent of Americans older than age 20 are **underweight**, with a BMI below 18.5 or a weight 10 percent below the recommended range.[4]

Even more alarming is the trend toward childhood obesity: In the past 25 years, obesity rates for young children more than doubled; for kids aged 6 to 11, the rates nearly tripled; and for adolescents, they more than tripled (**Figure 8.2**, page 280).[5] Overall, 16.9 percent of American children are obese and another 14.9 percent

are overweight.[6] In the past few years, rates have started improving for children under 5 and have plateaued for older kids.[7]

College students have historically been in better shape than other adult populations. However, college students have been gaining weight and body fat, too. A recent study of nearly 3,000 college students indicated that one-quarter to one-half of them are overweight or obese,[8] and with obesity comes increased risk for stroke, heart disease, and diabetes.

As you assess your own diet, exercise, and **weight management** strategies, keep these points in mind:

- Changing your body weight and composition

overweight In an adult, a BMI of 25 to 29 or a body weight more than 10 percent above recommended levels

obese In an adult, a BMI of 30 or more or a body weight more than 20 percent above recommended levels

underweight In an adult, a BMI below 18.5 or a body weight more than 10 percent below recommended levels

weight management A lifelong balancing of calories consumed and calories expended through exercise and activity to control body fat and weight

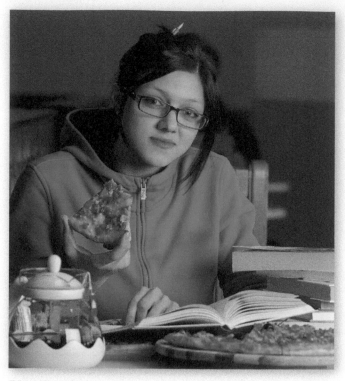

FIGURE **8.2** Calorie intake can soar from mindless snacking on junk food packed with fats and sweeteners.

requires new long-term diet and exercise habits, not short-term fixes.

- Your overall percentage of body fat is more important than your weight or the amount of weight you lose.

- Fast weight loss usually involves a temporary decrease in tissue fluids and often a loss in lean muscle mass, as well. Healthy weight loss means the slow, sustained loss of fat, coupled with increases in muscle mass and the preservation and maintenance of lean body mass.

- Choose the types of calories you consume wisely and learn to equalize your calorie intake and expenditure in an **energy balance** that can help you manage your weight.

This chapter presents the tools and techniques you need to determine a healthy target weight and create a sound plan for reaching and maintaining it. Incorporating weight management into your ongoing wellness program will allow you to realize the significant benefits—physiological, social, and emotional—of sustaining your body mass and body composition within recommended ranges throughout life.

energy balance The relationship between the amount of calories consumed in food and the amount of calories expended through metabolism and physical activity

LO 8.1 Why Is Obesity on the Rise?

In 2015, the World Health Organization (WHO) estimated that 52 percent of the world's adults (more than 1.9 billion people over age 18) were overweight or obese and that the number could increase substantially in the coming decade.[9] Obese adults represent 13 percent of the world's adult population and number more than 600 million worldwide.[10] The WHO coined the term *globesity* to describe this trend. Obesity is a problem in high-income industrialized nations as well as in low- and middle-income developing countries.[11] Diets high in processed fats, meats, sugars, and refined starches provide excess calories, while labor-saving devices and sedentary lifestyles reduce energy expenditure. In developing countries, entire cultures are moving away from traditional diets and manual labor toward mechanization and Western-style junk food.[12] As a result, they are experiencing the same gain in body fat and weight that Americans did three decades ago. Only the poorest countries of sub-Saharan Africa lie outside this worldwide trend.[13]

Several Factors Contribute to Overweight and Obesity in America

In the United States over the last quarter century, the number of obese adults has more than doubled.[14] The map in **Figure 8.3** reveals that obesity rates are distributed unevenly: The southern and Midwestern states show the highest rates. Several factors contribute to the rapid increase.

Overconsumption and Eating Calorie-Dense Foods Americans consume an average of 240 calories more per day now than they did in 1971, according to the Centers for Disease Control and Prevention.[15]

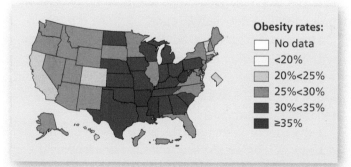

Obesity rates:
No data
<20%
20%<25%
25%<30%
30%<35%
≥35%

FIGURE **8.3** Obesity rates are high nationwide but highest in the Midwest and South.

Source: Centers for Disease Control, "Prevalence of Self-Reported Obesity among US Adults by State and Territory, BRFSS, 2014," 2014, www.cdc.gov

Q&A Exercising for Weight Control: How Well Does It Work?

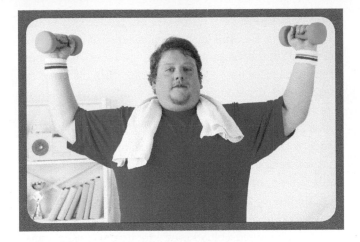

Many people want to lower their BMI but dread counting calories and feeling hungry. They'd like to downsize themselves through exercise alone so they can continue eating the same amount of their usual foods. But will that work? Here's the skinny.

As Chapter 6 explained, exercising can help you lose fat, gain muscle, and drop clothing sizes but it will often leave your weight unchanged or even raise it. So what about exercise and actual weight loss? Researchers know that being sedentary can promote obesity and health risks. They also know that people who break up long periods of sitting with a few minutes of everyday activity—climbing stairs, raking leaves, walking around the block—tend to store less fat and have lower risks for heart disease, diabetes, and related conditions.[1]

As you sit, especially after a meal, blood sugar levels spike, insulin goes up, and fat storage increases in fat (adipose) tissue, allowing weight gain. When you interrupt this process through activity, you stop the fat storage cycle on that occasion.[2]

It seems logical, then, that full-out aerobic exercise and strength training should not just interrupt fat storage but reverse it. Studies show, however, that without calorie restriction (dieting), 30 minutes of vigorous exercise most days for 8 to 16 months will result in minimal weight loss.[3] A full hour each day of vigorous exercise for those same months allowed a typical 150-pound person to drop just 7 or 8 pounds (5 percent of body weight). Few people are willing to make such a determined effort.[4]

What's more, hour-long bouts of heavy exercise tend to precipitate rebound resting and eating a few hours later.[5] If ravenous exercisers aren't careful to interrupt the sitting bouts and avoid filling up with calorie-dense foods, they can erase most or all of the benefits.[6] Researchers conclude that we have similar evolutionary mechanisms to preserve body mass whether dieting or exercising. Thus, we can anticipate only modest weight loss from either approach alone.[7]

However, researchers have another, more hopeful message: People who eat less AND exercise more lose more weight, tend to lose mostly fat rather than lean muscle tissue, and have an easier time keeping weight off.[8] The dual approach also tends to resculpt the body, cutting unhealthy fat from the abdomen and around internal organs.[9]

The answer? Diet + exercise = more weight loss, more fat loss, less muscle loss, and better long-term weight maintenance.

APPLY IT! How much time do you spend sitting each day as you study, attend class, drive your car, and so on? How much time do you spend doing vigorous exercise?

TRY IT! **Today**, keep a log of your "lifestyle exercise." As you move throughout your day, accurately jot down the number of minutes you spend walking, doing chores, and the number of minutes you spend stretching, strength training, or aerobically exercising. **This week**, make a list of new ways to increase both levels of activity and add at least one to any category. Do the same each day for a few days. **In two weeks**, retrack your overall activity to see how many additional minutes you have added to non-exercise and exercise activity.

Sources:
1. P. D. Loprinzi et al., "Association between Biologic Outcomes and Objectively Measured Physical Activity Accumulated in ≥10-Minute Bouts and <10 Minute Bouts," *American Journal of Health Promotion* 27, no. 3 (2013): 143, doi: 10.4278 /ajhp.110916-QUAN-348
2. J. Levine, "Killer Chairs," *Scientific American* 311, no. 5 (November 2014).
3. J. W. Rankin, "Effective Diet and Exercise Interventions to Improve Body Composition in Obese Individuals," *American Journal of Lifestyle Medicine* 9, no. 1 (January/February 2015): 48–62.
4. Ibid.
5. E. Ravussin and C. M. Peterson, "Physical Activity and the Missing Calories," *Exercise and Sport Sciences Reviews* 43, no. 3 (July 2015): 107–8.
6. E. C. Wuorinen, "The Psychophysical Connection between Exercise, Hunger, and Energy Intake," *American Journal of Lifestyle Medicine* 8, no. 3 (May/June 2014): 159–63.
7. D. L. Swift et al., "The Role of Exercise and Physical Activity in Weight Loss and Maintenance," *Progress in Cardiovascular Diseases* 56, no. 4 (January/February 2014): 441–47.
8. Ibid.
9. Rankin, "Effective Diet and Exercise Interventions," 2015.

Without additional exercise, extra calories usually lead to weight gain. Eating certain calorie-dense foods also contributes to weight gain: A 20-year study of more than 120,000 Americans revealed that weight gain was closely associated with consuming refined carbohydrates and fatty foods such as potato chips, potatoes, sugary beverages, and red and processed meats.[16] Recent studies suggest that such foods also trigger fat storage and weight gain by altering the normal balance of intestinal microbes.[17]

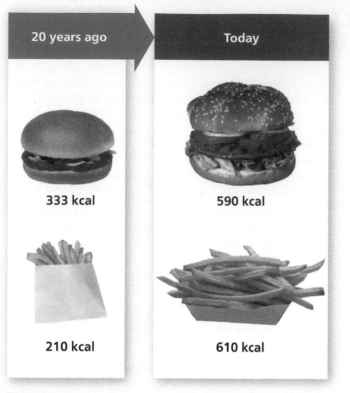

20 years ago	Today
333 kcal	590 kcal
210 kcal	610 kcal

FIGURE **8.4** Today's serving portions are significantly larger than those of past decades. A 25-ounce prime-rib dinner served at one local steak chain contains nearly 3,000 calories and 150 grams of fat. That's twice as many calories and more than three times the fat than many adults need in a whole day, and it's just the meat part of the meal!

Source: Data are from National Heart, Lung, and Blood Institute, "Portion Distortion," April 2015, www.nhlbi.nih.gov/health/educational/wecan/eat-right/portion-distortion.htm

Food portions in restaurants and supermarkets have grown steadily over the past half-century (**Figure 8.4**). Researchers have also found that people don't read their own "fullness signals," or feelings of *satiety,* very well. So, the bigger the portions, the more they will eat overall.[18]

See It!
Watch "Experiment Shows Portion Control is Key to Healthy Eating" at MasteringHealth™.

Easy access to unhealthy food also encourages overeating.[19] Most drugstores, gas stations, schools, and public buildings offer brightly packaged, high-calorie snacks that encourage junk-food sales and consumption.[20] Fast-food franchises offer relatively inexpensive foods loaded with saturated fat, salt, and refined carbohydrates. On average, Americans aged 20 to 39 eat 15 percent of their daily calories from fast food.[21]

Advertising promotes overeating of nutritionally poor

non-exercise activity Routine daily activities such as standing up and walking around that use energy but are not part of deliberate exercise

sweets, sodas and fruit drinks, alcoholic beverages, and salty snacks. Amazingly, one-third of our daily calories come from just a few categories of these highly advertised junk foods.[22]

Too Little Exercise The ease of our modern life is an improvement over the hard physical labor of past generations. Yet the exertion we are spared amounts to hundreds of calories per day that we *don't* burn off as we sit at our desks, drive our vehicles, or change channels with a remote control.[23] Even the layout of modern towns and cities reduces energy expenditure. Walkable neighborhoods with open space for recreation and grocery stores that sell fresh produce have child obesity rates *half* as high as neighborhoods without these amenities.[24] And in neighborhoods with fewer exercise opportunities and poorer food choices, adults are more likely to weigh more and have high blood pressure, heart disease, cancer, diabetes, and other diseases.[25] The bottom line: Being sedentary contributes to illness and early mortality.[26] The Q&A box Exercising for Weight Control: How Well Does It Work? explores the impact of exercise on weight management.

Hereditary and Developmental Factors With all these overconsumption factors in play, why isn't *everyone* overweight? Part of the answer lies in heredity. If most of your relatives are overweight or obese, you are more likely to gain weight during adulthood. If most of your relatives are thin, you are more likely to be thin as well. Researchers have learned that dozens—perhaps hundreds—of genes help determine your weight by controlling metabolic rate, "thriftiness"—the tendency to conserve energy and store fat—and other factors.[27] Food consumption patterns in parents appear to turn some of these weight genes on and off in developing embryos.[28] A mother's consumption of mint, sugar, garlic, alcohol, and other flavors, for example, can generate taste preferences in her infant.[29] And mother mice fed junk-food diets produce pups with addiction-like brain circuitry.[30]

Non-Exercise Activity Uses Energy In recent years, researchers have studied the human "fidget factor": the tendency of some people to use energy by fidgeting, jiggling their head, hands, and feet, and getting up to walk around every few minutes. Studies show that lean people burn 279 to 477 more calories per day than obese people through this type of **non-exercise activity**.[31]

Demographic and Lifestyle Factors A mix of demographic factors both biological and non-biological—

DIVERSITY
Race/Ethnicity, Gender, Life Stage, and Weight

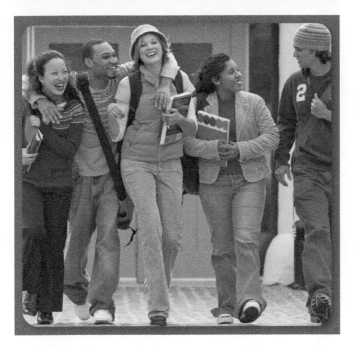

Body weight varies by racial/ethnic group to some degree, based on genes as well as on cultural preferences for food and exercise. Combining the data for males and females, the percentages of overweight and obese adults in the United States are: Pacific Islanders (76.1 percent); Native Americans (72 percent); African Americans (70.7 percent); Hispanic Americans (69.9 percent); whites (62.8 percent); and Asian Americans (38.5 percent).[1] In each group, men have higher rates of overweight and obesity than women with one exception: Rates of both in African American females are 1.5 times higher than in males.[2]

Some ethnic groups appear to have "thrifty genes" that helped their ancestors survive during extended periods

of famine by slowing down metabolism to conserve food energy. In a modern environment of plentiful food, widespread mechanization, and diminished activity, however, "thrifty genes" promote weight gain. Pima Indians are a dramatic example: 90 percent of the adults are overweight and 75 percent are obese.

Weight also varies with life stage. About 8 percent of American infants and toddlers have a high percentile weight for their height.[3] This doubles to 16.9 percent among 2- to 19-year-olds, and then doubles again to more than 30 percent among adults 20 and older. Pregnancy starts the upward-climbing scales for many women. And for both sexes, "middle-age spread" is real: between ages 20 and 44, 57 percent of adults are overweight or obese. Between 44 and 65, that escalates to 70.5 percent and remains high. The percentage drops once again in those over 75 to 56.6 as many of those with the highest BMIs die from chronic diseases.[4]

Women have a tendency to burn fewer calories than men due to their higher level of essential body fat and lower ratio of lean body mass to fat mass. Because muscle cells burn more energy, and because men usually have more muscle tissue than women, men burn 10 to 20 percent more calories than women do, even at rest. Monthly hormonal cycles and pregnancy also increase the likelihood of weight fluctuation and gain. Even so, adult men remain more likely to be overweight than adult women.

Sources:
1. D. L. Blackwell, J. W. Lucas, and T. C. Clarke, "Summary Health Statistics for US Adults: National Health Interview Survey, 2012," National Center for Health Statistics, *Vital and Health Statistics* 10, no. 260 (2014): 83–84.
2. Centers for Disease Control and Prevention, "Health of Black or African American Non-Hispanic Population," updated April 2015, www.cdc.gov/nchs/fastats/black-health.htm
3. C. L. Ogden et al., "Prevalence of Childhood and Adult Obesity in the United States, 2011–2012," *Journal of the American Medical Association* 311, no. 8 (February 26, 2014): 806–14.
4. Blackwell, "Summary Health Statistics," 2014.

including sex, race/ethnicity, culture, education, and economic level—all influence weight. The Diversity box Race/Ethnicity, Gender, Life Stage, and Weight explains the impact of such factors on your body weight and likelihood of overweight or obesity.

Biological and cultural factors interact, of course: Our family and ethnic group influence what, when, and how much we eat, as well as how much we exercise and participate in other activities. A taste for high-fat, high-calorie foods, for instance, may start before birth but is reinforced through family upbringing. The same is true for leisure time activity: 25 percent of

Americans engage in *no* exercise, sports, or other physical activity *at all* during their leisure time.[32] Education and income influence these choices; the higher their education level and earnings, the more physically active people are likely to be.[33]

Additional lifestyle choices also influence body weight. Drinking alcohol is associated with weight gain over time, as are watching television, smoking and then quitting, and sleeping less than six hours or more than eight hours per night.[34]

See It!
Watch "Fast-Paced Movies, TV Shows May Lead to More Snacking" at MasteringHealth™.

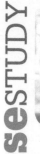

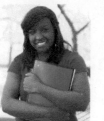

TALIA

"We never worried much about weight in my family. Here, though, a lot of the students talk about weight, go on diets, and even post mean stuff online about people who are heavy. I decided to try to lose that 'Freshman 8' of mine. So I'm using a few of my friends' ideas. I'm drinking two energy drinks every day—Kristen said they cut your appetite and speed up your metabolism. I'm skipping breakfast and catching the last bus to work so I get there faster than walking. And I'm eating more meat to get a high protein diet. That's supposed to be the best one. I don't know if I've lost any weight so far—maybe a little."

APPLY IT! What factors can you list that might contribute to Talia's weight gain? How well do you think her approach is going to work and why? The end-of-chapter labs can help you answer this question.

TRY IT! Write down your BMI using the chart in Figure 6.2 on page 213 or a BMI calculator like the one at www.caloriecontrol.org. Does it represent underweight, healthy weight, overweight, or obesity? Have you gained weight, lost weight, or stayed the same since entering college? What are the main contributors to your own current body composition? Lab 8.1 can help you calculate this.

Hear It!
To listen to this case study online, visit the Study Area in MasteringHealth™.

LO 8.2 How Do My Weight and Body Composition Affect My Wellness?

A leading nutritionist has written that body weight sits at the center of an intricate web of health and disease.[35] Indeed, research shows you are more likely to remain healthy throughout life if (1) your BMI is between 21 and 23 if you are a woman and 22 and 24 if you are a man; (2) you maintain approximately the same BMI and waist size throughout your adult life; and (3) your body's fat deposits occur around your hips and thighs rather than your abdomen. High BMIs and abdominal fat (indicated by a large waist size) are associated with higher risk for several chronic diseases.[36]

Being underweight is an important but far less common problem. Fewer than 5 percent of Americans have a BMI under 18.5.[37] Underweight carries its own significant health risks and can result from an unusually fast metabolism, excessive dieting, extreme exercise, eating disorders, smoking, or illness.

Body Weight Can Promote or Diminish Your Fitness

A stable, healthy-range BMI goes hand in hand with regular exercise and physical activity. Maintaining weight and BMI within recommended ranges increases energy and reduces likelihood of injury during fitness activities.

Overweight and underweight can contribute to poor fitness. Overweight can lead to a downward fitness spiral: An over-accumulation of body fat can strain bones, joints, and muscles and make exercising harder and injury more likely. Resulting stiffness and pain, in turn, make exercising even more difficult. They also make it harder to work and carry out daily activities such as walking up stairs, carrying books or grocery bags, shoveling snow, and getting in and out of vehicles.

Underweight can lead to muscle wasting as the body breaks down muscle tissue for energy when fat stores are low. Muscle wasting, in turn, can lead to weakness and declining ability to exercise and accomplish daily tasks. These inevitably reduce both fitness and wellness.

Body Weight Can Have Social Consequences

Being overweight can subject a person to significant discrimination in education, employment, health care, and social interactions, starting in childhood.[38] "Weight stigma," or prejudice against overweight and obese people, is widespread in society and often starts with parents and teachers of overweight youngsters. Researchers have discovered, for example, that parents spend less money sending their overweight children to college than they do their thinner children.

Adult attitudes rub off on children. Preschoolers are more likely to describe overweight kids their own age as "mean, ugly, or stupid."[39] In addition, obesity contributes to breast development and other signs of early puberty in a sizeable fraction of girls by age 7—which leads to taunting and self-consciousness.[40]

Weight stigma is also quite common among employers. Overweight job applicants suffer discrimination, get hired less often, and get fired more often than thinner individuals with similar qualifications.[41] Weight stigma is even pronounced among health professionals, including specialists who treat the obese![42]

As Talia discovered, the online cyberbullying practice called "fat shaming" is increasingly common and can be hurtful, depressing, and even destructive.[43] Negative self-images and beliefs can lead to discouragement, shame, hopelessness, and in many, to eating "comfort foods" that temporarily boost mood but cause more fat storage and weight gain.[44] Researchers consider anti-fat bias to be a serious societal issue in need of more study and creative solutions. Awareness that weight management can boost energy, positive self-esteem, and physical wellness is a good starting place.

Body Weight Can Influence Your Risk for Chronic Disease

People with excess body fat have higher levels of several serious chronic diseases, including heart disease, stroke, type 2 diabetes, sleep apnea, arthritis, and cancer (**Figure 8.5**).[45] Specific cancers linked to high BMI include cancers of the prostate, colon, rectum, esophagus, pancreas, kidney, gallbladder, ovary, cervix, liver, breast, uterus, and stomach.[46]

Accumulation of fat around the waist (a 40-inch waistline or higher for a man, or a 35-inch waistline or higher for a woman) increases the risk for developing metabolic syndrome. This serious medical condition is a combination of abdominal fat deposits, high blood cholesterol, high blood pressure, and insulin resistance or full-fledged type 2 diabetes.[47] Ominously, American waistlines jumped an extra inch in just the past decade to an overall mean of 38.7 inches (98.5 cm).[48] Fortunately, though, losing even a few pounds can bring measurable health benefits.[49] For example, test subjects with early signs of diabetes dropped their risk of developing the full-blown disease by 10 percent for every kilogram (2.2 pounds) of weight they lost.[50]

Body Weight Can Affect Your Life Expectancy

You can expect to live longer if your body weight and BMI are within recommended ranges. As **Figure 8.6** on page 286 shows, being fit significantly reduces mortality risk, especially when combined with healthy weight. Being obese (a BMI of 30 or above) cuts an average of six to seven years from the life of a non-smoker and 13 to

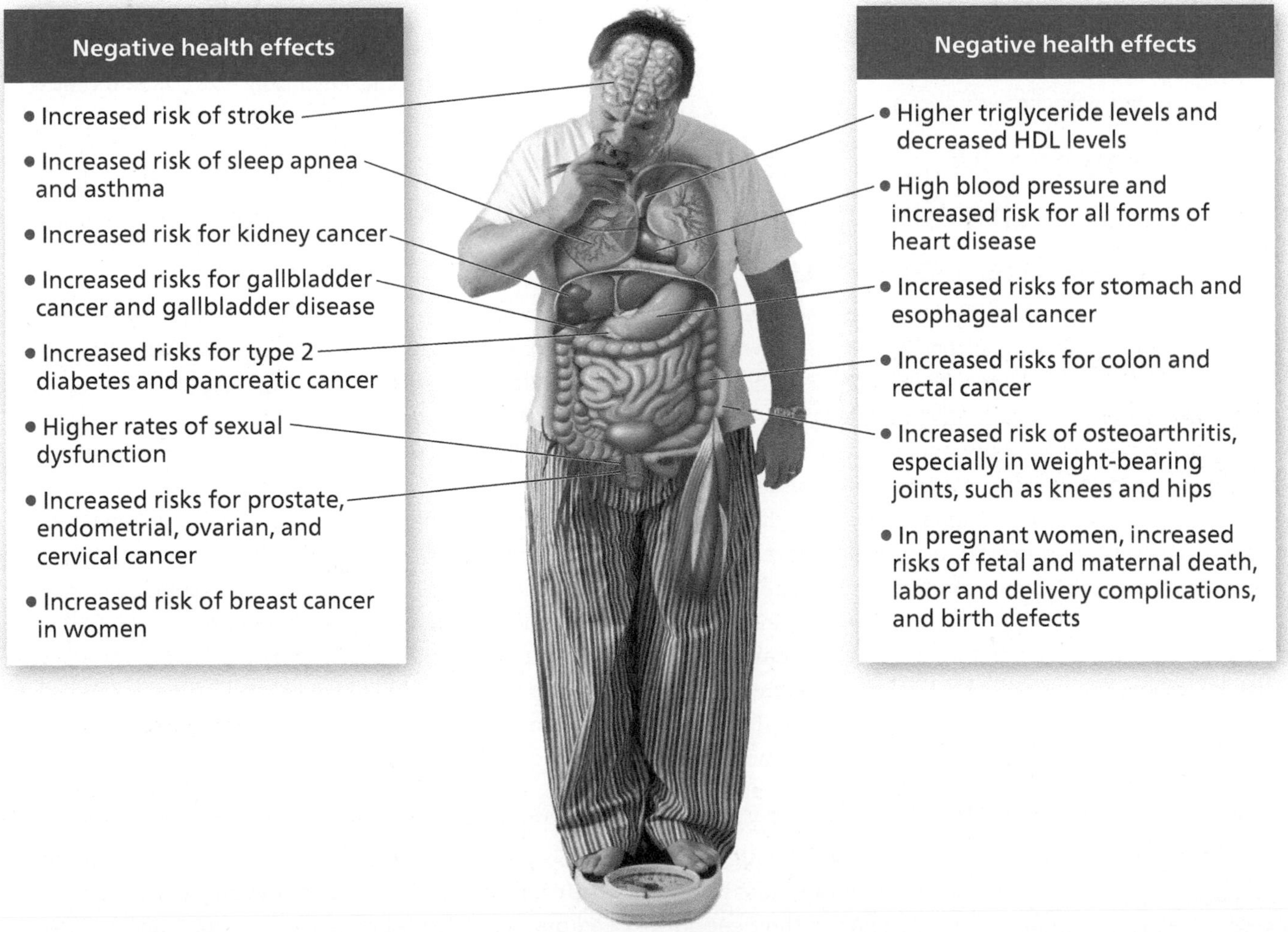

Negative health effects

- Increased risk of stroke
- Increased risk of sleep apnea and asthma
- Increased risk for kidney cancer
- Increased risks for gallbladder cancer and gallbladder disease
- Increased risks for type 2 diabetes and pancreatic cancer
- Higher rates of sexual dysfunction
- Increased risks for prostate, endometrial, ovarian, and cervical cancer
- Increased risk of breast cancer in women

Negative health effects

- Higher triglyceride levels and decreased HDL levels
- High blood pressure and increased risk for all forms of heart disease
- Increased risks for stomach and esophageal cancer
- Increased risks for colon and rectal cancer
- Increased risk of osteoarthritis, especially in weight-bearing joints, such as knees and hips
- In pregnant women, increased risks of fetal and maternal death, labor and delivery complications, and birth defects

FIGURE **8.5** Body weight can influence the risks for chronic disease.

14 years from a smoker.[51] Americans' average life expectancy could actually begin to decline because obesity is so prevalent and can shorten life so dramatically.[52]

Underweight people have a shorter life expectancy than normal-weight or overweight people.[53] The statistics reflect the fact that a low BMI is characteristic of patients with illnesses such as cancer, uncontrolled diabetes, and disordered eating. Some researchers argue that people who are underweight but *not* ill and who are careful to get complete daily nutrition may actually realize greater longevity.[54] Underweight associated with poor nutrition, however, can lead to life-shortening conditions such as anemia, susceptibility to disease and infection, slower recovery from illness, muscle wasting and weakness, and osteoporosis and bone fractures.

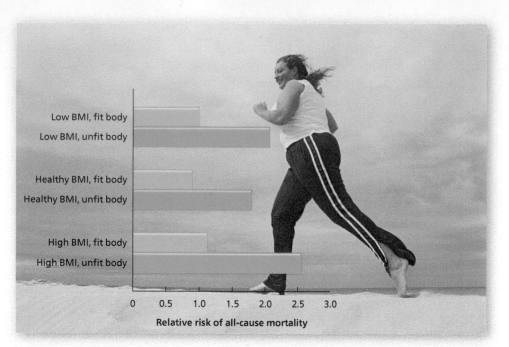

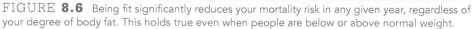

FIGURE **8.6** Being fit significantly reduces your mortality risk in any given year, regardless of your degree of body fat. This holds true even when people are below or above normal weight.

Source: C. D. Lee et al., "Cardiorespiratory Fitness, Body Composition, and All-Cause and Cardiovascular Disease Mortality in Men," *American Journal of Clinical Nutrition* 69, no. 3 (1999): 373–80. Used by permission of the American Society for Nutrition. Also reference 76, Lin et al. (2015).

LO 8.3 Why Do Most Diets Succeed in the Short Term but Fail in the Long Run?

Overweight or obese Americans face a discouraging cultural phenomenon. Most media images show slim people or buffed-up athletes. This leads to high levels of body dissatisfaction and, in turn, fuels a $30 billion per year diet industry. Many people are convinced that they will successfully lose weight if they can simply find the right diet. They bounce from one highly publicized diet to another: low-fat, high carbohydrate; low carbohydrate, high protein; and so on. Experts agree that any calorie-cutting diet can produce weight loss in the short term. They also acknowledge that most people's attempts at weight loss will fail in the long run unless they change their eating habits permanently

weight cycling The pattern of repeatedly losing and gaining weight, from illness or dieting

yo-yo dieting A series of diets followed by eventual weight gain

rigid diets Weight-loss regimens that specify strict rules on calorie consumption, types of foods, and eating patterns

and make sustained exercise and activity part of their daily lives. Let's look more closely at diets and dieting.

Diets Often Lead to Weight Cycling

Do you know someone who is dieting? A survey by the American College Health Association indicated that almost 40 percent of college students dieted to lose weight within the previous month.[55] Dismayingly, three-quarters of dieters will regain their weight within two years (or sooner) after a major diet. Most will wind up in a process called **weight cycling**—a pattern of repeatedly losing and regaining weight.

Weight experts refer to this pattern as **yo-yo dieting**. Yo-yo dieting may have significant health consequences such as high blood pressure, diabetes, and other chronic diseases. It's not clear why weight cycling is associated with physical health problems, but when researchers controlled for all other effects, they found that gaining and losing the same 5 pounds over and over appears to create risk in and of itself.[56] For this reason, they emphasize the importance of maintaining weight loss once achieved.

Some diet plans and foods promise quick weight loss with no hunger and very little effort. These diets usually backfire. One major reason is that they are rigid. **Rigid diets** specify rules like "eat only cabbage soup and grapefruit," or "eliminate all fats and oils" or "never eat sugar." Because rigid diets are unpleasant and restrictive, cravings build up and people "fall off the wagon." Once they do, they have a tendency to binge. Psychologists call this the "what the hell effect."[57] The result is more anxiety, depression, and a higher percentage of body fat than people on more flexible plans.[58]

Live It!
Complete Worksheet 21 All-or-Nothing Thinking at MasteringHealth™.

In contrast, **flexible diets** are based on energy balancing of calories eaten and burned. They focus on portion size and make allowances for variations in daily routine, appetite, and food availability. For example, if you go to a party and overeat, a flexible diet allows you to cut extra calories the next day and increase your exercise to compensate. As a result, people tend to stay on flexible diets longer and, in the process, learn better long-term eating habits.

Everyone who restricts calorie intake will experience some degree of lowered metabolism as the body "defends" its fat stores. That's why even in a sensible diet, weight loss tends to slow down after an initial quick drop and why the long-held rule that you must cut 3,500 calories to lose a pound of fat is not strictly correct.[59] The same energy conservation appears to be true for calorie expenditure through exercise. It also explains why people tend to gain back some or all of the weight they lose, and ultimately, why we must change our eating and exercise habits permanently to successfully maintain a lower weight and BMI.

Our Built-In Appetite Controls Make Diets Less Effective

Our bodies have a complicated set of internal chemical signals and control mechanisms that tell us when to eat, how much to eat, how much fat our bodies should store, and how we should respond when those fat stores start to shrink.[60] For example, we produce powerful appetite stimulants such as leptin and ghrelin. Rising and falling levels of these hormones stimulate appetite and, along with it, food seeking and eating behaviors.

Our numerous gut microbes play a surprising role in controlling appetite and fat storage, especially in response to sweeteners, both caloric and non-caloric.[61] Bacterial cells in the intestines thrive on sweeteners and release compounds that can cause glucose intolerance (a forerunner of diabetes) and promote fat storage (that can lead to overweight or obesity). On average, Americans consume more than 100 pounds of sugars and artificial sweeteners per person per year.

And our sleep cycles and other circadian rhythms are linked to body weight: Sleeping less than six hours per night can increase ghrelin levels, and in turn appetite and weight gain.[62] Late-night snacking can have a

magnified effect based on those same circadian factors. The infographic Weight Loss Myth-busters on page 296 reveals the importance of *what* and *when* you eat (rather than simply how much you eat).

The body's own fat cells also play a role. In adults, widely distributed white fat cells store energy and help control blood levels of fats and sugars. The body's white fat stokes the appetite, leading to thicker and thicker fat layers and higher risks of obesity, diabetes, and heart disease.[63] Small groups of localized brown fat cells primarily burn energy to help heat the body in response to cold or starvation. And recently discovered beige fat cells—embedded throughout the widespread white fat tissue—can ramp up and burn extra calories, especially after exercise or when chilled.[64] Many researchers now believe that manipulating fat cells with various proteins, hormones, and even immune factors could provide new ways to control weight and fight obesity.[65] In the meantime, do-it-yourself measures to ramp up fat-burning include regular aerobic exercise, avoiding sweeteners and other foods that promote fat storage, and keeping your environment chilly rather than overheated.[66]

Commercial and Medical Interventions Range from Bogus to Beneficial

Most over-the-counter products—"fat burners," "starch blockers," muscle stimulators, supplements, and other diet aids—are ineffective or even dangerous. Prescription drugs and bariatric (weight-loss) surgery do help some people. Both have serious side effects, however, and are viable options for only a minority of overweight and obese people (see the Q&A box Do Diet Drugs and Surgery Work?).

Brand-name diet plans and programs span a wide range of approaches and have a widely varied track record. Some dictate high protein and low carbs, others the reverse; others emphasize cutting out most dietary fat or eating mainly foods with a low glycemic index. **Table 8.1** compares several brand-name diets, typical outcomes, and expert recommendations based on a major recent study.[67]

See It!
Watch "Low-Carb Diet Trumps Low Fat in Study" at MasteringHealth™.

The bottom line: Most diets will work to some degree if you cut calories and increase exercise. However, nearly all dieters gain back their weight over time *unless they permanently adopt new habits*. A weight-loss

flexible diets Weight-loss regimens that focus on portion size and make allowances for variations in daily routine, appetite, and food availability

TABLE 8.1 Name-Brand Diets Compared

Diet	Type of Diet Based on Nutrients	Notable Pluses	Notable Minuses
Atkins	• Low carbohydrate • High protein (55 percent or more) • High fat	Short term: • Maximum weight loss • More fat loss, less loss of lean muscle tissue • Drop in blood fats, sugars	Long term: • Elevated blood fats • Increased inflammation • Increased risk of chronic diseases (cardiovascular, diabetes, cancer, Alzheimer's)
DASH USDA My Pyramid Weight Watchers Jenny Craig	• High carbohydrate (50 to 60 percent) • Moderate protein (15 to 20 percent) • Moderate fat (20 to 30 percent)	• Moderate weight loss • Behavioral support from peers, leaders • Can promote long-term behavioral change	• Diets allow some refined sugars • Can promote elevated blood fats, sugars, inflammation, disease risk over long term
Dr. Dean Ornish American Heart Association Volumetrics	• High carbohydrate • Low protein • Low fat	• Moderate to good weight loss • Less back sliding at one year • Encourage fiber, low-glycemic, low-density foods	• Tendency to lose more lean tissue/less fat tissue than high-protein diets • Adherence challenging; very low fat leads to unpalatable foods
Zone Biggest Loser	• Moderate carbohydrate (40 to 50 percent) • High protein (~30 percent) • Moderate fat (25 to 30 percent)	• Promises more fat loss, less lean loss with adherence • Encourages exercise and permanent lifestyle change	• Weight loss slower, less dramatic than on high-protein diets • Low-calorie counts, careful balancing of nutrients make adherence challenging

Advice from the experts: Any diet will promote weight loss in the short term. Some work more quickly in the short term. Some have less back sliding than others at one year. Some promote health risks in the long term. Consumers should pick a diet they can best adhere to, add exercise, and concentrate on permanent lifestyle changes.

Sources:
1. B. C. Johnston et al., "Comparison of Weight Loss among Named Diet Programs in Overweight and Obese Adults: A Meta-Analysis," *Journal of the American Medical Association* 312, no. 9 (2014): 923–33.
2. L. Van Horn, "A Diet by Any Other Name Is Still about Energy," *Journal of the American Medical Association* 312, no. 9 (2014): 900–1.

diet, in other words, is not a time-limited event; it's a prolonged life path that can lead to weight management and wellness. Behavioral support can be very helpful in this and campus health centers can usually recommend local support groups or programs to attend, as Talia does in this chapter's case study.

Enlisting the personal encouragement of friends, roommates, and family members can also be important. If people undermine your efforts to eat or exercise, tell them firmly that you need support—or space. We consider more tools for effective weight loss and management later in this chapter.

disordered eating Atypical, abnormal food consumption that diminishes wellness but is usually neither long-lived nor disruptive to everyday life

eating disorders Disturbed patterns of eating, dieting, and perceptions of body image that have psychological, environmental, and possibly genetic underpinnings and that lead to consequent medical issues

LO 8.4 What Are Eating Disorders?

Skipping meals, downing diet supplements, and binging on junk food are all forms of disordered eating: atypical, abnormal food consumption. **Disordered eating** diminishes your wellness but can be short-lived. One recent study suggests that 25 to 40 percent of female college students report body image, weight management, and out-of-control eating problems that amount to disordered eating.[68] Actual **eating disorders** are long-lasting, disturbed patterns of eating, dieting, and body perceptions with psychological, environmental, and possibly genetic underpinnings. Eating disorders disrupt relationships, emotions, and concentration, and can lead to physical injury, hospitalization, and even death. They require diagnosis and treatment from a psychiatrist or other physician.

Recognizing an eating disorder in yourself or a loved one can lead to treatment that improves or stops the behavior. The statements in **Figure 8.7** on page 290 can

Q&A Do Diet Drugs and Surgery Work?

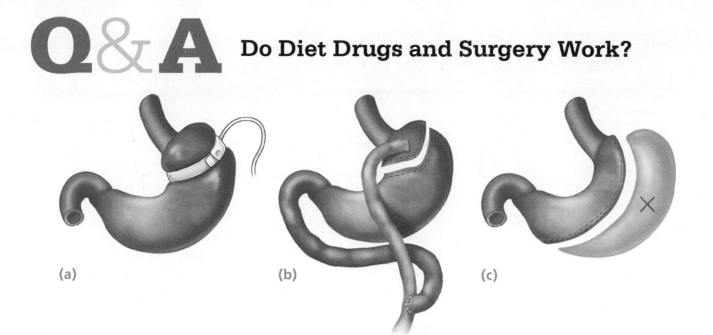

(a)　　　(b)　　　(c)

Millions of people think, "I hate diets and exercise but I need to lose a lot. Maybe the answer is prescription diet drugs or even surgery." Are these good solutions? Are they even realistic? Consider these facts.

- Nearly all physicians want proof that a patient has tried but not succeeded at well-organized diet and exercise regimens before considering drugs or surgery.[1]

- Weight loss drugs are serious compounds with significant side effects and typically modest success. Several types block cravings or appetite while others block fat absorption. Virtually all are short-term (three-month to one-year) adjuncts to long-term diets and exercise. A few "off-label" drugs—intended for seizures, depression, diabetes, and other conditions—trigger some weight loss as a side effect.[2] When the drugs work well, weight loss ranges from 3 to 10 percent of body weight; patients usually regain some of this once they stop taking the medications.[3] Side effects can include anxiety, irritability, insomnia, headache, nausea, fatigue, flatulence, urgent elimination, and fecal spotting.[4]

- Approved patients tend to have BMIs of 30 or greater or BMIs of 27 or higher *plus* serious chronic diseases that could be improved through weight loss (for example, heart disease or type 2 diabetes. Some are also smokers and have other risk factors like high blood pressure, blood sugar, or cholesterol.[5]

- Over-the-counter drugs and supplements have a bad reputation for costing a lot and doing little, with negative or harmful effects. The list includes ephedrine (now banned), laxatives, cold and sinus pills, *Hoodia gordonii*, St. John's wort, bitter orange, ginseng, ginkgo, and BMPEA from the *Acacia rigidula* shrub.[6]

- Researchers are developing new drugs and devices including pills that create fullness by expanding once swallowed, implanted electronic devices that block hunger circuits, and others that chemically manipulate a patient's own hormones or gut microbes.[7]

- Surgeons perform more than 100,000 weight-loss surgeries (so-called bariatric procedures) each year for patients with high BMIs who are unable to lose 5 percent or more of their body weight through lifestyle changes. This surgery can be temporary or permanent and is often a last-ditch remedy for obese people with chronic diseases or a high risk of developing them. The various types of bariatric surgery average about $25,000 per operation, and tend to greatly reduce the stomach's capacity to hold and digest food. The drawings compare three bariatric procedures. In (a), an adjustable gastric band greatly restricts stomach size. In (b), surgery creates an egg-sized stomach pouch and bypasses the rest of the stomach. In (c), surgical removal of most stomach tissue leaves a narrow "gastric sleeve."[8] Most patients do lose significant amounts of weight but most regain some or all of it within a few years even with just a tiny stomach pouch remaining. Medical complications are common.

APPLY IT! Do you, a friend, or a loved one qualify for weight loss drugs or surgery? If yes, list their particular criteria. What are their alternatives to these serious medical treatments?

Sources:
1. J. Jin, "Medications for Weight Loss: Indications and Usage," *Journal of the American Medical Association* 313, no. 21 (2015): 2196.
2. D. Schumacher, "Pharmacological Management of the Obese Patient," *American Journal of Lifestyle Medicine* 9 (March/April 2015): 137–56.
3. S. Z. Yanovski and J. A. Yanovski, "Long-Term Drug Treatment for Obesity: A Systematic and Clinical Review," *Journal of the American Medical Association* 311, no. 1 (2014): 74–86; Schumacher, "Pharmacological Management," 2015.
4. Yanovski, "Long-Term Drug Treatment," 2014.
5. Schumacher, "Pharmacological Management," 2015.
6. A. O'Connor, "Study Warns of Diet Supplement Dangers Kept Quiet by FDA," *New York Times Alternative Medicine Now*, April 7, 2015, A-1.
7. A. Pollack, "Early Results Arrive on Weight-Loss Pills That Expand in the Stomach," *New York Times*, June 23, 2014, 2; T. Hampton, *Journal of the American Medical Association* 313, no. 8 (2015): 785.
8. P. R. Schauer et al., "Bariatric Surgery versus Intensive Medical Therapy for Diabetes—3-Year Outcomes," *New England Journal of Medicine* 370 (May 22, 2014): 2002–13; L. Sjostrom et al., "Association of Bariatric Surgery with Long-Term Remission of Type 2 Diabetes and with Microvascular and Macrovascular Complications," *Journal of the American Medical Association* 311, no. 22 (2014): 2297–304.

Eating disorder	Disordered eating	Food preoccupied/obsessed	Concerned well	Food is not an issue
• I regularly stuff myself and then exercise, vomit, use diet pills or laxatives to get rid of the food or calories. • My friends/family tell me I am too thin. • I am terrified of eating fat. • When I let myself eat, I have a hard time controlling the amount of food I eat. • I am afraid to eat in front of others.	• I have tried diet pills, laxatives, vomiting, or extra time exercising in order to lose or maintain my weight. • I have fasted or avoided eating for long periods of time in order to lose or maintain my weight. • I feel strong when I can restrict how much I eat. • Eating more than I wanted to makes me feel out of control.	• I think about food a lot. • I feel I don't eat well most of the time. • It's hard for me to enjoy eating with others. • I feel ashamed when I eat more than others or more than what I feel I should be eating. • I am afraid of getting fat. • I wish I could change how much I want to eat and what I am hungry for.	• I pay attention to what I eat in order to maintain a healthy body. • I may weigh more than what I like, but I enjoy eating and balance my pleasure with eating with my concern for a healthy body. • I am moderate and flexible in goals for eating well. • I try to follow Dietary Guidelines for healthy eating.	• I am not concerned about what others think regarding what and how much I eat. • When I am upset or depressed I eat whatever I am hungry for without any guilt or shame. • Food is an important part of my life but only occupies a small part of my time.

Body dysmorphic disorder	Distorted body image	Body preoccupied/obsessed	Body acceptance	Body ownership
• I often feel separated and distant from my body—as if it belongs to someone else. • I don't see anything positive or even neutral about my body shape and size. • I don't believe others when they tell me I look OK. • I hate the way I look in the mirror and often isolate myself from others.	• I spend a significant amount of time exercising and dieting to change my body. • My body shape and size keeps me from dating or finding someone who will treat me the way I want to be treated. • I have considered changing or have changed my body shape and size through surgical means so I can accept myself.	• I spend a significant time viewing my body in the mirror. • I spend a significant time comparing my body to others. • I have days when I feel fat. • I am preoccupied with my body. • I accept society's ideal body shape and size as the best body shape and size.	• I base my body image equally on social norms and my own self-concept. • I pay attention to my body and my appearance because it is important to me, but it only occupies a small part of my day. • I nourish my body so it has the strength and energy to achieve my physical goals.	• My body is beautiful to me. • My feelings about my body are not influenced by society's concept of an ideal body shape. • I know that the significant others in my life will always find me attractive.

FIGURE **8.7** Thought patterns associated with healthy and disordered eating habits exist on a continuum, as do thought patterns associated with positive and negative body image.

Adapted from Smiley/King/Avery: Campus Health Service. Original continuum, C. Schislak, *Preventive Medicine and Public Health.* Copyright 1996 Arizona Board of Regents. Used with permission.

help you recognize eating disorders. People with a related syndrome called **body dysmorphic disorder** (BDD) have unrealistic and negative self-perceptions such as believing they look fat even when they are rail thin or feeling underdeveloped when their muscle size is average.

They can become obsessed with this supposed physical "defect" and take ill-advised actions, such as consuming energy drinks to "speed up metabolism" or taking "strength" supplements to enlarge muscles.[69] BDD is

also common in young people with diabetes, cancer, skeletal conditions, and other chronic conditions.[70]

The three most common types of eating disorders are anorexia nervosa, bulimia nervosa, and binge eating disorder. About 20 million American women and 10 million American men meet the criteria for one of these disorders during their lifetimes.[71]

Eating Disorders Have Distinctive Symptoms

Anorexia nervosa is a persistent, chronic eating disorder characterized by deliberate food restriction and severe, life-threatening weight loss (**Figure 8.8** on page 291). People with anorexia first restrict their intake

body dysmorphic disorder A psychological syndrome characterized by unrealistic and negative self-perception focusing on a perceived physical defect

anorexia nervosa A persistent, chronic eating disorder characterized by deliberate food restriction and severe, life-threatening weight loss

Live It!
Complete Worksheet 25 Out of Control or Overcontrol? at MasteringHealth™.

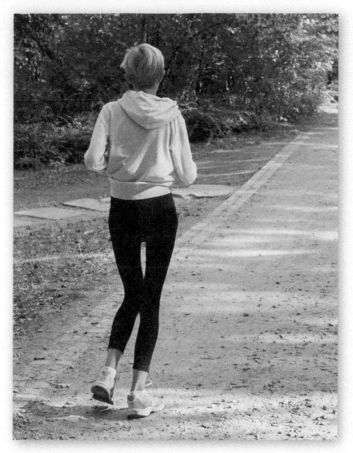

FIGURE **8.8** Anorexia nervosa is characterized by severe, life-threatening weight loss.

Binge eating disorder (BED), a variation of bulimia, involves binge eating but usually no purging, laxatives, exercise, or fasting. Individuals with BED often wind up significantly overweight or obese but tend to binge much more often than does the typical obese person.

See It!
Watch "EDNOS: Most Dangerous, Unheard of Eating Disorder" at MasteringHealth™.

Eating Disorders Can Be Treated

Because eating disorders have complex physical, psychological, and social causes that unfold over many years, there are no quick or simple solutions. Still, eating disorders *are* treatable, and the primary goal is to stop the potentially life-threatening behaviors and the physical damage they can cause to the bones, teeth, throat, esophagus, stomach, intestines, heart, and other organs. Once medically stabilized, the patient can begin long-term therapy. Often, the patient comes from a family that overemphasizes achievement, body weight, and appearance. Genetic susceptibility can also play a role.[73] Therapy focuses on the psychological, social, environmental, and physiological factors that have contributed. In therapy—and often with the help of eating disorder support groups—patients develop new eating behaviors, build self-confidence, deal with depression, and find constructive ways to handle life's problems.

LO 8.5 What Concepts Must I Understand to Achieve My Weight Goals?

How can you frame a personal plan for tracking and modifying calorie intake and expenditure? Key concepts include understanding the role of metabolic rates, recognizing your body's set point, and understanding the energy balance equation. Taking lessons from successful weight maintainers can also help you set and achieve realistic weight goals.

Recognize the Role of Your Metabolic Rate

Your body consumes as much as 60 to 70 percent of your daily calorie intake—typically between 900 and 1800 calories per day—to sustain

of high-calorie foods, then of almost all foods, and then purge what they do eat through vomiting or using laxatives. They sometimes fast or exercise compulsively as well. Symptoms include refusal to maintain a BMI of 18.5 or more; intense fear of gaining weight; disturbed body perception; and in teenage girls and women, amenorrhea (cessation of menstruation) for three months or more. Five to 20 percent of anorexics eventually die from medical conditions brought on by vitamin or mineral deficiencies or physiological results of starvation. This gives anorexia the highest death rate of any psychological illness.[72]

Bulimia nervosa is characterized by frequent bouts of binge eating followed by purging (self-induced vomiting), laxative abuse, or excessive exercise. Bulimics tend to consume much more food than most people would during a given time period and feel a loss of control over it. They often binge and purge in secret. A physician may diagnose bulimia in a patient who binges and purges at least twice a week for three months. People with bulimia also have BDD: They are obsessed with their bodies, weight gain, and their appearance to others. Unlike those with anorexia, however, people with bulimia are often normal weight. Treatment appears to be more effective for bulimia than for anorexia.

bulimia nervosa An eating disorder characterized by frequent bouts of binge eating followed by purging (self-induced vomiting), laxative abuse, or excessive exercise

binge eating disorder (BED) A variation of bulimia that involves binge eating but usually no purging, laxatives, exercise, or fasting

functions such as heartbeat, breathing, and maintenance of body temperature.[74] The rate at which your body consumes food energy to sustain these basic functions is your **basal metabolic rate (BMR)**. Your **resting metabolic rate (RMR)** is slightly higher because it includes the energy you expend to digest food.

BMR can be influenced by your activity level and your body composition. The more lean tissue you have, the greater your BMR; the more fat tissue you have, the lower your BMR. The higher your fitness level, the greater your ratio of lean tissue to fat mass is likely to be, and the more energy you will burn while exercising and at rest. Cardiovascular and strength-building exercises contribute most directly to speeding up BMR.

Recognize Your Body's Set Point

Perhaps you've noticed that your body is programmed around a certain weight or **set point** that it returns to fairly easily when you gain or lose a few pounds. Many dieters reach a plateau after a certain amount of weight loss and can't seem to trim off more pounds. This plateau is due, in part, to a downshifted metabolism balancing out lower calorie intake: The person's energy balance is now at a weight-maintenance, not a weight-loss, level. To "outsmart" and reset the set point, a dieter must lose weight slowly and increase exercise.

basal metabolic rate (BMR) Your baseline rate of energy use, dictated by your body's collective metabolic activities

resting metabolic rate (RMR) Basal metabolic rate plus the energy expended in digesting food

set point A preprogrammed weight that your body returns to easily when you gain or lose a few pounds

negative caloric balance A state in which the amount of calories consumed in food falls short of the amount of calories expended through metabolism and physical activity

positive caloric balance A state in which the amount of calories consumed in food exceeds the amount of calories expended through metabolism and physical activity

isocaloric balance A state in which the amount of calories consumed in food is approximately the same as the amount of calories expended through metabolism and physical activity

Balance Your Energy Equation

Long-term weight management relies on a theoretical balancing of your energy equation—that is, equalizing the calories you eat and those you burn through metabolism and exercise. As explained earlier, the physiology of appetite and weight is more

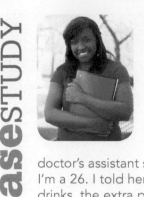

complex and involves what and when you eat, how much you eat, the intensity of your exercise, and other factors. Still, to lose or gain weight, you must deliberately "unbalance" that equation for a while. Expending more calories than you consume should cut fat and weight due to a **negative caloric balance** (**Figure 8.9** on page 293). Consuming more calories than you burn should add fat and weight due to a **positive caloric balance**. Once you reach a desirable BMI, you should be able to maintain your weight through **isocaloric balance**—consuming and expending roughly the same number of calories on a given day.

Accurate tracking is important! Dieters often underestimate how many calories they consume and overestimate how many they burn off with exercise.[75] **Lab 8.1** can help you calculate your current energy balance and set goals for a better balance. Alternatively, you can log on to www.ChooseMyPlate.gov to get a target number for calorie consumption based on your age, sex, and level of daily moderate or vigorous activity. The Super-Tracker feature provides calorie counts for specific foods and portions so you can keep track of how many calories you consume each day. See the end-of-chapter online resources for additional trackers. A few commercial

Do It!

Access these labs at the end of the chapter or online at MasteringHealth™.

programs such as Weight Watchers also help most people track their dieting, even though long-term losses tend to be modest.

LO 8.6 How Can I Create a Successful Plan for Weight Management?

Let's look at the steps you can take to manage your weight.

Assess Your Current Weight and Choose a Realistic Goal

Review Figure 6.2 on page 213 to find healthy weight and BMI ranges based on height. If your body fat percentage is low and your muscle development is high, your healthy weight and your BMI will be on the higher end of the range. The same is also true if your frame size is large. If your body fat percentage is high and your muscle development is low, your healthy weight will be in the middle-to-low end of the range. This is also true if your frame size is medium or small. Knowing these factors will help you determine a realistic weight and body composition goal.

Contemplate Weight Management

If you are satisfied with your current weight, you can simply pursue and refine your application of good nutritional principles and regular exercise. If you are in the dissatisfied majority, use the assessment of your current weight and BMI to choose a realistic weight goal based on no more than a 10 percent initial loss or gain. Even if you don't need weight change now, you can use the specifics in this section to stabilize your current weight and maintain it for the next few decades. Readiness requires motivation, commitment, goals, and a positive attitude.

Prepare for Better Weight Management

- **Think about your beliefs and attitudes.** Do you see yourself as a hopeless victim of "bad genes," overwork, or low budget? Think you are too young to worry about your weight? Or do you believe that you can take effective control of your body composition and weight through eating intelligently, limiting your calorie intake,

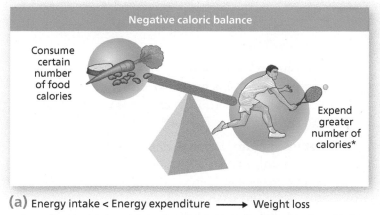

(a) Energy intake < Energy expenditure ⟶ Weight loss

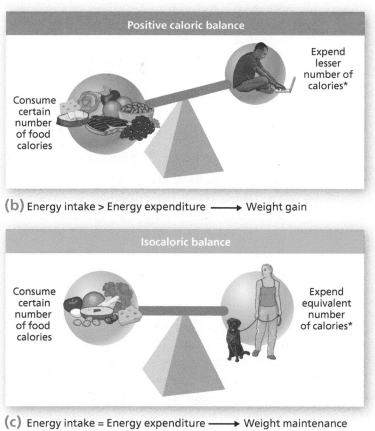

(b) Energy intake > Energy expenditure ⟶ Weight gain

(c) Energy intake = Energy expenditure ⟶ Weight maintenance

FIGURE **8.9** On any given day, each of us has a personal energy equation with either a negative caloric balance, a positive caloric balance, or an isocaloric balance. Over time, this equation helps determine our body weight.

*You expend calories through metabolism, activity, and exercise.

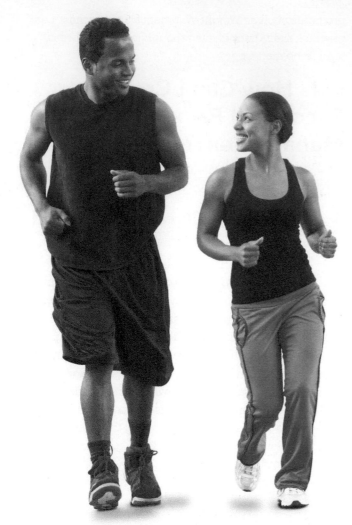

Lab 8.3 will help you get started by identifying and eliminating junk food from your diet.

- **Visualize new behaviors.** What specific new behaviors will you adopt to improve your BMI and body composition? Here are some good choices: Choose only nutritious low-glycemic foods. Avoid junk food. Track the numbers of servings you eat from each food group. Exercise most days of the week. Keep a log of your daily and weekly exercise. Ask friends to support you.

Take Action

- **Commit to your goals.** Behavior change requires commitment. Thinking and talking about your commitment with friends is helpful; so is writing it down and showing it to someone.

- **Set up support.** Solicit the help of people you can trust to support your efforts. Let's say it is 9:30 p.m., you've finished studying and you're hungry, but you've already eaten the 1800 calories on your day's food plan. A supportive friend might say, "Let's fill up on some veggies and take a walk. You'll be glad you stuck with your program!"

The GetFitGraphic Weight Loss Mythbusters on page 296 examines a common weight loss myth—all calories are created equal—and why food choices and timing count.

Establish a Regular Exercise Program

Physical activity is central to changing weight (loss or gain) and maintaining it in order to reduce fat but sustain and build lean tissue.[76] In addition to following a healthy diet, you may need to add 30 to 60 minutes per day of extra activity. The good news is that activity is cumulative: Add 7 minutes of stair-climbing here, plus 11 minutes of brisk walking across campus there, plus 20 minutes of stationary biking, and so on. Aerobic exercise is the best way to burn calories and lose stored fat and body weight.[77]

The greater the frequency, intensity, and time spent on an activity, the more energy you use and the more calories you burn. There are other considerations for choosing types of fitness exercise as well. The larger the muscle groups you use, the more you boost your metabolism and, in turn, your calorie expenditure. Kickboxing and vigorous biking, for example, use the thigh, calf, and gluteus muscles as well as those that move and support your torso. By contrast, lifting small hand weights works

and establishing a program of regular exercise? Talk with others or write in your journal to clarify your attitudes.

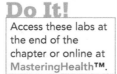
Live It!
Complete Worksheet 23 Why Do You Eat? at MasteringHealth™.

- **Consider your goals.** Motivating goals are usually personal and extended, such as looking good, feeling fit and capable, and staying well over a period of years. Avoid one-shot goals like looking good for a beach trip or a sports match; these can lead to weight cycling. Concentrate on additional long-term goals such as increasing self-esteem, feeling more energetic, and relieving stress. Write out your specific goals in Lab 8.2.

- **Identify barriers to change.** What keeps you from changing or maintaining your weight? A lack of information about good weight management techniques? Consuming too much fat and sugar and too many refined carbohydrates? Snacking late at night? Eating triggers that encourage overconsumption? Lack of social or emotional support? Lack of exercise? Identify your barriers and brainstorm solutions to them.

TABLE 8.2 Calories Burned through Activity

Activity, Sport, or Exercise	Calories You Expend per Minute If You Weigh...		
	110 lb	150 lb	190 lb
Aerobics, 10" step	7.0	9.5	12.0
Basketball, pick-up	7.0	9.5	12.0
Biking, slow	5.3	7.1	9.0
Dancing, moderate pace	4.2	5.7	9.0
Downhill skiing, moderate pace	5.5	7.5	9.5
Frisbee, casual	2.6	3.6	4.5
Golf, walking and pulling clubs	4.4	6.0	7.5
Jogging, moderate pace	5.3	7.1	9.0
Kickboxing	8.8	12.0	14.7
Ping-pong	3.5	4.8	6.0
Soccer, non-competitive	6.1	8.3	10.5
Softball	4.4	6.0	7.5
Stair climbing, 40 stairs/minute	6.1	8.3	10.2
Swimming	8	10	13
Walking	3.1	4.2	6.6
Watching TV	1.0	1.4	1.8

Source: These figures are adapted from a classic and very complete source: F. I. Katch, V. L. Katch, and W. D. McArdle, *Calorie Expenditure Charts*, (Ann Arbor, MI: Fitness Technologies Press, 1996). Similar calorie counts are available in the activity tracker at www.ChooseMyPlate.gov and on exercise apps.

mainly the smaller muscles of the hand, wrist, and lower arms. **Table 8.2** lists caloric expenditures for several popular activities, sports, and exercises for adults of different weight levels.

Achieve Weight Maintenance

Weight maintenance is similar in principle to weight change. The tools are the same, but with weight maintenance, your daily calorie goal for weight management will be isocaloric. It's essential to choose healthy foods, then track the calories you consume. A weekly weigh-in is also crucial. Many people plateau at a particular body weight and need to maintain that level for a few months before losing more weight. The skills you employ during an interim phase of weight maintenance will be excellent practice for the rest of your life! Once sustaining and tracking good nutrition and performing daily

exercise and activity become your normal routine, it should become easier for you to change and maintain your body weight.

Take Lessons from Successful Weight Maintainers

Most people who sustain a normal, healthy weight over decades engage in a physically active lifestyle, averaging a combined hour per day of moderate to vigorous physical activity.[78] They don't skip meals; they eat breakfast every day. They eat a nutritious diet that is low in refined carbohydrates, high-glycemic foods, and saturated fats; high in fruits, vegetables, whole grains, nuts and beans; has moderate levels of lean protein; and has a high volume but a low calorie density. And they avoid sodas and juice drinks sweetened with sugar, corn syrup, or artificial sweeteners.

caseSTUDY

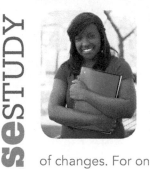

TALIA

"My weight group is really helping. I've lost 5 pounds and my clothes definitely fit better now. The surprising thing is I don't feel like I'm on a diet—I'm not starving all the time. I've made a lot of changes. For one thing, I found some decent things to eat in the cafeteria that I hadn't noticed before. The fruit and the salads are helping me feel full much longer. I don't eat late in the evening any more—I got a few of my Econ study friends to meet in my room *before* dinner and to share better snacks—nuts and plain popcorn instead of junk food. I'm eating breakfast now. And I still make it to work on time because I bought a used bike and I ride it every day. If this is a "diet," I think I can stay on it for a long time!"

APPLY IT! Which of Talia's changes may be helping her lose weight without feeling hungry all the time? What similar changes could you make to your own food routines, whether or not you want to lose weight? What about changes you could make in your activity and exercise? And what about snack timing?

TRY IT! Make one food change per week and one exercise change. Stop after you add three of each and jot down how well they are working for you. Lab 8.2 shows some other ways to set up and track a food plan.

Hear It!

To listen to this case study online, visit the Study Area in MasteringHealth™.

WEIGHT LOSS MYTHBUSTERS

ALL CALORIES ARE EQUAL:
It doesn't matter *what* you eat as long as you limit calories.

FALSE!

During a one-year trial, dieters consuming a **low-carb** diet lost more fat and weight and developed better levels of blood fats than did dieters on a low fat, high-carb diet.[1]

Researchers found that *over time*, a low-carb diet can increase your cholesterol levels (a measure of risk for heart disease). Therefore, a **low-glycemic** diet proved to be the best for weight maintenance.[2]

Evidence is waning for the calorie imbalance hypothesis and building for the hormone hypothesis: Quickly digested carbohydrates cause spikes in insulin that tell fat cells to store fat.[3]

ALL CALORIES ARE EQUAL:
It doesn't matter *when* you eat as long as you limit calories.

FALSE!

Lean mice allowed to eat all types of foods 24 hours per day became obese...

...while those who ate only within a 9- to 12-hour window and *fasted* during the other 12 to 15 hours remained lean.

6 p.m. to 6 a.m.: Fasting

6 a.m. to 6 p.m.: Access to food

Restricting food consumption to 12 or fewer consecutive hours promotes weight loss and maintenance. A beneficial pattern is eating meals no earlier than 6 a.m. and no later than 6 p.m. and then avoiding any consumption during the rest of the evening and night.[4]

Erratic sleep-wake cycles such as those in jet-lagged travelers and shift workers disturb gut bacteria and lead to obesity and glucose intolerance (high blood sugar). If you pull frequent all-nighters, beware![5]

CHANGE

Tips for Weight Management

Try these ideas for reframing weight loss in your mind, rather than jumping right in to a diet regimen:

Live It!
Complete Worksheet 22 It Doesn't Last If You Fast at MasteringHealth™.

- Snacks are a simple place to start. Most people add snacks between their regular meals and wind up with a daily total that's too high. If you do snack, try eating smaller meals. And reach for high-fiber, low-glycemic foods such as fresh fruit, unbuttered popcorn, nuts, or vegetable sticks and low-fat yogurt dip instead of chips, fries, sweets, or cheese-covered anything.

- Consider yourself successful if you lose ½ to 1 pound per week. Faster weight loss stimulates too much hunger, slows down metabolism, and loses lean tissue.

- Avoid feeling famished by choosing high-volume, nutrient-dense foods such as lean protein, veggie-packed clear soups, salads with light dressing, whole grains, fruits, vegetables, and beans. These will fill you more quickly and control hunger longer.

- Eat mindfully rather than mindlessly. Set out a portion or portions of food on a plate, then sit and savor each bite. Avoid munching while you drive, ride, watch TV, or study.

- Watch out for late-night eating. Try fasting for 12 hours between dinner and breakfast to see if it makes a difference. If you get up early, you may need to finish dinner earlier the night before to reach a full 12-hour period.

- Avoid added sugars and artificial sweeteners, particularly in drinks. Drinks sweetened with sugar, corn syrup, and even no-cal sweeteners like aspartame and sucralose affect your gut bacteria and can lead to extra fat storage. Alcoholic drinks also pack a lot of calories and stimulate the appetite.

- Sleep well. Get seven hours of sleep each night or more. Sleep deprivation triggers greater levels of hunger and eating.

- Increase everyday non-exercise activity like taking the stairs instead of the elevator. Break up long stretches of sitting by getting up to walk around every hour or so.

- Increase organized physical activity to meet daily exercise goals of 30 to 60 minutes of moderate to vigorous activity. Pick something fun so you look forward to it!

- If you are dieting, consider joining a support group. Support groups help most people lose at least a small amount of weight and keep it off. Programs like Weight Watchers aim for daily tracking, slow loss, and permanent changes to eating and exercise habits.

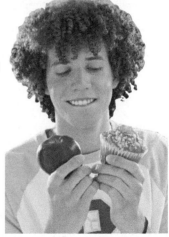

- Use an online or smartphone application to track calories, weight and BMI, keep food diaries, calculate body fat, calculate caloric expenditures through exercise, and so on. You'll still need your own motivation and adherence, but these high-tech tools can make tracking your information and getting support easier and more fun!

Successful weight maintainers are realistic—of body image and goals for weight and BMI. They stay conscious of situations that trigger overeating and apply strategies to avoid them. They are self-motivated. They stay informed. They keep track and consciously balance their food intake and energy expenditure. That way, they know when they've "fallen off the wagon" and can quickly rebalance eating and exercise when their weight starts to creep up.[79]

People who are successful at maintaining a healthy weight typically have tools for coping with problems and handling life stresses. They assume responsibility for their lifestyle behaviors, know where to seek help and access community resources, and have a supportive network of friends and family.[80]

Maintaining recommended weight and BMI confers so many benefits that once you master the needed skill set, you'll rarely miss the junk food you used to eat. Nor will you mind the few minutes it will take each day to track energy consumed and expended. The rewards in lifelong wellness are easily worth the trade-offs!

Study Plan

chapter summary

LO 8.1 Why Is Obesity on the Rise?

- Eating too much and doing too little has created a global obesity crisis. Huge portions and too much fat, sugar, salt—especially in processed foods—contribute too many daily calories. Most people exercise too little due to labor-saving devices, neighborhood layout, sedentary lifestyles, and other factors.

LO 8.2 How Do My Weight and Body Composition Affect My Wellness?

- Being over- or underweight contributes to low self-esteem and to poor fitness, making exercise more difficult, injury more likely, and leading to less and less activity.

- People with high BMI are at increased risk for many types of acute and chronic diseases.

LO 8.3 Why Do Most Diets Succeed in the Short Term but Fail in the Long Run?

- Most Americans diet but gain back all the weight they lose. This cycling is discouraging and creates health risks. The body has complex mechanisms to preserve fat stores through increased appetite. Maintaining weight loss is difficult and requires permanent changes to eating and exercise habits.

- Most over-the-counter diet products are ineffective, and prescription diet drugs and surgery are medically unavailable to most people.

LO 8.4 What Are Eating Disorders?

- Eating disorders are long-lasting, disturbed patterns of eating, dieting, and body perceptions that can disrupt lives, lead to physical harm, and even cause death.

- Eating disorders include anorexia nervosa, bulimia nervosa, and binge eating disorder (BED). All require medical and psychological intervention and long-term support.

LO 8.5 What Concepts Must I Understand to Achieve My Weight Goals?

- Daily calorie expenditure includes basal and resting metabolic rates plus calories expended through activity.

- Set point is a metabolic plateau based on your body's tendency to defend fat stores. Long-term management of weight and body composition requires lifestyle changes to reset this to a lower level.

- To stabilize your weight, you must balance your energy: Calories consumed must equal calories expended through exercise.

LO 8.6 How Can I Create a Successful Plan for Weight Management?

- Assess your current weight, choose a realistic goal, apply behavioral change steps, and create a specific plan for improved diet and exercise.

review questions

LO 8.1 1. The World Health Organization coined the term *globesity* to promote an understanding of
a. global hunger.
b. rising obesity rates in underdeveloped countries.
c. rising obesity rates in developed countries.
d. the epidemic of obesity in the global population.

LO 8.1 2. If more than 20 percent above the recommended weight range, a person who is 5'8" tall is considered
a. overweight.
b. obese.
c. at ideal weight.
d. at his or her set point.

LO 8.2 3. Indicate the body system least likely to be affected negatively by excess body weight.
a. Cardiovascular system (heart and lungs)
b. Digestive system (gallbladder, kidneys, colon)
c. Musculoskeletal system (bones and joints)
d. Integumentary system (skin and hair)

LO 8.3 4. Getting up, walking around, and jiggling your feet when seated are all examples of
a. positive caloric balance.
b. set point.
c. resting metabolism.
d. non-exercise activity.

review questions CONTINUED

LO 8.3 **5.** Weight cycling is
a. a pattern of repeatedly losing and regaining weight.
b. characterized by rigid diets.
c. characterized by flexible diets.
d. uncommon.

LO 8.4 **6.** Anorexia nervosa is characterized by
a. frequent bouts of binge eating followed by self-induced vomiting.
b. deliberate food restriction and severe, life-threatening weight loss.
c. going on diet after diet.
d. obesity.

LO 8.5 **7.** To lose weight, you must
a. lower your basal metabolic rate.
b. achieve a new isocaloric balance.
c. raise your resting metabolic rate.
d. unbalance caloric intake and expenditure.

LO 8.5 **8.** The rate at which your body consumes food energy to sustain basic functions is your
a. basal metabolic rate.
b. resting metabolic rate.
c. BMI.
d. set point.

LO 8.6 **9.** A BMI of 16 in a woman indicates
a. overweight.
b. underweight.
c. normal weight.
d. obesity.

LO 8.6 **10.** Successful weight maintainers are most likely to do which of the following?
a. Eat two or three nutritious snacks between regular-sized meals to curb hunger
b. Consume beverages with non-nutritive sweeteners to avoid refined carbohydrates
c. Choose a diet that is very low in fat and protein
d. Eat high volume foods with low calorie density

critical thinking questions

LO 8.1 **1.** What do you see as the greatest contributor to "globesity"? Defend your answer.

LO 8.2, LO 8.6 **2.** How do height, physical build, and musculature affect recommended weight and BMI?

LO 8.3 **3.** List at least three reasons why most dieters regain most or all of their lost weight.

LO 8.7 **4.** List several effective tools for successful weight management. Is one more important than the others? If so, discuss.

check out these eResources

- **Calorie Control Council** The Healthy Weight Tool Kit provides tabs for you to count food calories, calculate the calories you burn through specific activities, determine your BMI, keep a food diary, and assess your nutrients. **www.caloriecontrol.org**
- **Centers for Disease Control and Prevention** Learn more about the health risks related to overweight and obesity. **www.cdc.gov/healthyweight/**
- **The Center for Eating Disorders at Sheppard Pratt** Go to the Eating Disorders Information section of this website to find an online self-assessment to learn if you or a friend has signs of an eating disorder. **http://eatingdisorder.org**

- **National Institutes of Health** You can use the online calculator to find your current BMI. **www.nhlbi.nih.gov/health/educational/lose_wt/**
- **US Department of Agriculture** The USDA ChooseMyPlate Supertracker provides tools for:
  o looking up nutritional information on foods.
  o tracking and recording daily calories consumed.
  o tracking and recording calories expended through physical activity.
  o managing your weight.
  www.supertracker.usda.gov

LEARN A SKILL

CALCULATING ENERGY BALANCE AND SETTING ENERGY BALANCE GOALS

MasteringHealth™

Name: _____ Date: _____

Instructor: _____ Section: _____

Materials: Calculator, access to Internet (optional)

Purpose: To learn how to calculate energy balance and set realistic goals for calorie intake and energy expenditure.

Directions: Complete the following sections.

Section I: Calculating BMR and Energy Expenditure

Your basal metabolic rate (BMR) is the rate at which you burn calories to sustain life functions at rest at a normal room temperature. Your activities, fitness level, stress level, and many other things will affect your BMR.

1. Calculate your BMR (the method shown here uses the Harris-Benedict formula):

Men

   1. BMR = 66 + (6.3 × weight in pounds) + (12.9 × height in inches) − (6.8 × age in years)

   2. BMR = 66 + (   ) + (   ) − (   )

   3. BMR = _____ calories

Women

   1. BMR = 655 + (4.3 × weight in pounds) + (4.7 × height in inches) − (4.7 × age in years)

   2. BMR = 655 + (   ) + (   ) − (   )

   3. BMR = _____ calories

2. Estimate your total energy expenditure (EE):
Total energy expenditure takes into account your amount of activity within a 24-hour period. You can calculate your energy expenditure by keeping an activity log and adding up the calories expended during any non-sleep time. To do this, use the physical activity tracking tool on the ChooseMyPlate website (www.ChooseMyPlate.gov). Another way to estimate total energy expenditure is to use the following calculations. Choose your level of activity on *average* and use that formula to calculate your energy expenditure (EE).

    Multiply your BMR by the appropriate activity factor, completing ONE equation that follows:

- If you are *sedentary* (little or no exercise):

  EE = _____ (BMR) × 1.2 = _____ calories

- If you are *lightly active* (light exercise/sports 1–3 days/week):

  EE = _____ (BMR) × 1.375 = _____ calories

- If you are *moderately active* (moderate exercise/sports 3–5 days/week):

  EE = _____ (BMR) × 1.55 = _____ calories

- If you are *very active* (hard exercise/sports 6–7 days/week):

  EE = _____ (BMR) × 1.725 = _____ calories

- If you are *extra active* (very hard daily exercise/sports & physical job or 23-day training):

  EE = _____ (BMR) × 1.9 = _____ calories

Section II: Calculating Energy Balance

1. Estimated calorie INTAKE (consult your answer to Lab 7.2, Question 4)

_____ calories

2. Estimated calorie EXPENDITURE (EE from Section I)

_____ calories

3. Subtract your EXPENDITURE (#2) from your INTAKE (#1) to get:

Out-of-balance calories = _____ calories

Section III: Tools for Your Weight Management Plan

1. What was your caloric intake from your dietary analysis? _____ What was your energy expenditure? _____ What was your overall energy balance? _____

- Energy balance (200 calories): You are supplying your body with its energy needs and maintaining current weight.
- Negative energy balance (−201 calories): You are expending more energy than you are eating and should be losing weight.
- Positive energy balance (+201 calories): You are eating more energy than you are expending and should be gaining weight.

2. Do you want or need to lose body fat? YES or NO

3. What is your **goal** for your body fat percentage? _____

4. Complete the following calculations to figure out how many pounds of fat you need to lose in order to reach this goal:

- Find your **current fat weight**:

_____ (current weight, lb) × _____ (current % body fat, expressed as a decimal) = _____ current fat weight (lb)

- Find your **lean body mass (LBM)**:

_____ (weight, lb) − _____ (fat weight, lb) = _____ LBM (lb)

- Find your **target body weight**:

_____ (LBM) ÷ (1 − goal % body fat expressed as a decimal) = _____ target body weight (lb)

- Find the lb of fat loss needed to reach your body fat percentage goal:

_____ (current weight, lb) − _____ (target weight, lb) = _____ fat loss needed (lb)

5. If you lose 1 pound of fat per week (500 calorie deficits per day), how many weeks will you take to lose your desired fat weight? _____

6. Brainstorm ways that you can get to a −500 calorie deficit per day through diet and exercise/activity changes.

DIET CHANGE (lower by 250 calories)

_____

_____

_____

_____

_____

ACTIVITY CHANGE (increase by 250 calories)

_____

_____

_____

_____

_____

DO IT!

LAB
8.2

PLAN FOR CHANGE

YOUR WEIGHT
MANAGEMENT PLAN

MasteringHealth™

Name: _____ **Date:** _____

Instructor: _____ **Section:** _____

Materials: None

Purpose: To create an appropriate weight management goal, you must apply behavior change tools and make a plan to implement your goals.

Directions: Complete the following sections.

Section I: Short- and Long-Term Goals

1. Short-Term Goals

- My three-month *or* six-month (circle one) % body fat goal is _____ %.

- My three-month *or* six-month (circle one) weight goal is _____ lb.

- My three-month *or* six-month (circle one) BMI goal is _____ kg/m².

2. Long-Term Goals

a. Based on my current weight, BMI, and % body fat:

- My one-year % body fat goal is _____ %.

- My one-year weight goal is _____ lb.

- My one-year BMI goal is _____ kg/m².

b. I plan to reach that goal by consuming about _____ calories per day and adding _____ activity calories per day.

Section II: Diet Obstacles and Strategies

1. Negative Food and Eating Triggers

Eating and food preferences can be triggered by emotions, social situations, and the sights and smells around you.

a. Fill out the following table exploring your negative food and eating triggers. For example, a situational trigger for you eating sugary foods may be "attending holiday parties."

Diet Behavior	Emotional Triggers	Social Triggers	Situational Triggers
Eating More Food			
Eating Late at Night			
Eating More Often			
Eating Sugary Foods			
Eating Fatty Foods			
Eating Fast Foods			
Eating Out			
Others:			

   b.   List three strategies to overcome or manage your food and eating triggers:

     (1) _____

     (2) _____

     (3) _____

2. Changing Food Patterns

   a.   I will eat LESS of the following foods and beverages:

     _____

     _____

   b.   For good nutrition and weight management goals, I will replace the above foods and beverages with the following:

     _____

     _____

Section III: Exercise and Activity Obstacles and Strategies

1. Reducing Sedentary Behaviors

   a.   Evaluate your sedentary activities in the space below. List your top three sedentary activities (not including time spent in class), the number of days per week you do them, and how many minutes per day.

	Sedentary Activity	Days/Wk	Min/Day
1			
2			
3			

   b.   Which sedentary activity could you replace with physical activity or even supplement with physical activity (such as exercising while you watch TV, or stretching while on your cell phone)? Write down three ideas for replacing sedentary activities with more active ones.

     (1) _____

     (2) _____

     (3) _____

2. Listing Activity Obstacles

List a few of the obstacles to replacing sedentary activity with more energy-intensive physical activity, along with strategies for overcoming these obstacles.

Activity Obstacle	Strategy to Overcome
(1) _____	_____
(2) _____	_____
(3) _____	_____

Section IV: Getting Support

1. I feel supported in my weight goals by these people:

_____

Here's what they do that assists me:

_____

2. I need additional support from these people:

_____

Here's what I need to ask for:

_____

3. **If I need group or medical support**, here are a few places to seek it: student health service, family physician, local hospital, local Weight Watchers chapter, online groups. If needed, I would be inclined to use _____ for support.

Section V: Rewards

1. When I make the **short-term** behavior change described earlier, my reward will be:

_____

Target date _____

2. When I make the **long-term** behavior change described earlier, my reward will be:

_____

Target date _____

DO IT!
LAB
8.3

ASSESS YOURSELF
JUNK FOOD DETECTIVE

MasteringHealth™

Name: _____ **Date:** _____

Instructor: _____ **Section:** _____

Materials: Paper, pen, access to Internet

Purpose: To investigate your typical snack and fast foods and find better substitutes.

Directions: Complete the following list of instructions.

Section I: Favorite Snack and Fast Foods

1. Make a list of six snack or fast foods that you like to eat.

a. _____

b. _____

c. _____

d. _____

e. _____

f. _____

Section II: Investigate Your Favorites

1. Using nutrition labels or Internet information (e.g., nutritional sites on the websites of fast-food franchises), analyze *your typical serving* of each food and record in the blanks provided.

Note: On ingredient lists, added sugars may be called *sucrose, evaporated cane juice, concentrated grape juice, fructose, high fructose corn syrup, corn syrup, mannitol, sorbitol, xylitol, hydrogenated starch hydrosylates.*

Refined grains may be called *enriched wheat flour, white flour, bleached wheat flour, durum wheat semolina, de-germed cornmeal, enriched rice (white rice).* (If the label doesn't list 100 percent whole wheat, rice, oats, and so on, it's probably refined grain.)

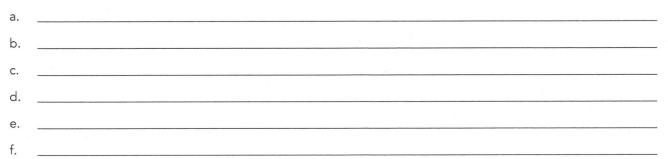

Snack/ Fast Food	Total Calories	Saturated Fat (calories)	*Trans* Fat (grams)	Sodium (milligrams)	Cholesterol (grams)	Refined Grain Carbohydrates (grams)	Added Sugars (grams)

Section III: Rate Your Junk Food

The USDA www.ChooseMyPlate.gov website recommends these criteria for the nutrients you just analyzed:

Calories from saturated fat: Less than 10 percent of total calories (plug in your daily calorie allowance based on Lab 8.1)

***Trans* fat:** Avoid

Sodium: For certain adults (everyone over 51, African Americans, everyone with high blood pressure, diabetes, or kidney disease) less than 1500 milligrams of sodium per day; for all other adults, less than 2300 milligrams per day

Cholesterol: Less than 300 milligrams per day

Grains: Half of daily total should be whole grains, half or less refined grains

Added sugars: Minimize

1. Using these criteria, analyze your typical serving of your six favorite snacks or fast foods against these recommendations. Rate your list in order from 1 to 6, with 1 having the fewest negatives and the least impact on your daily quotients, 2 the next least, and so on, up to 6, the junk food with the most negatives and the highest impact on your nutritional quotients.

Snack/Junk Food	Rating (1–6)
a. _____	_____
b. _____	_____
c. _____	_____
d. _____	_____
e. _____	_____
f. _____	_____

Section IV: Find New Favorites

1. Take the three foods on your list with the highest scores (4, 5, and 6), and for each, name a lower-calorie, more nutritious substitute.

Snack/Junk Food		Nutritious Substitute
a. _____	→	_____
b. _____	→	_____
c. _____	→	_____

Have fun trying these new foods! (If you are on a weight loss or maintenance diet, don't forget portion control.)

Section V: Reflection

1. Changes to your diet begin with motivation. Name three personal reasons why you would be better off by permanently reducing the amount of junk food in your diet.

a. _____

b. _____

c. _____

2. Rewards are another important part of behavior change. Name three non-caloric rewards you could give yourself for avoiding junk foods on three occasions.

a. _____

b. _____

c. _____

Activate, Motivate, & Advance YOUR FITNESS

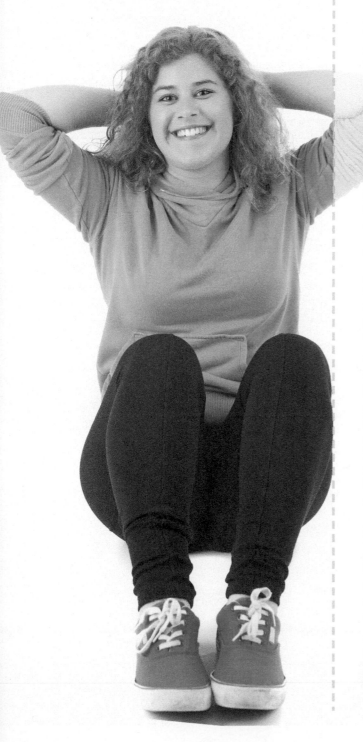

ACTIVATE!

With weight management, progression is the key. Start slowly and go at your own pace, building up stamina and strength. Eventually, you will increase the time and the intensity of your workouts and the sessions become easier. Follow these programs to gradually increase the number of minutes you train each week, the intensity of each session, and the calories you burn with each workout.

What Do I Need?

SHOES AND CLOTHING: The right shoes and clothes can go a long way toward keeping you comfortable and injury free. Refer to the Chapter 3 cardiorespiratory programs for tips on choosing exercise clothing and shoes.

Where Do I Start?

AT HOME: Start with walking! Whether indoors or outdoors, walking is the easiest way to add more activity to your day. Walk on flat surfaces that give like a track or treadmill. As you progress, add inclines and harder surfaces and/or increase your pace or your overall minutes each week.

Walking is a great way to get started, but incorporating *resistance training* will increase your muscular fitness, change your body composition, and boost your overall weekly calorie expenditure. Start by using your own body weight against gravity to increase muscular endurance and strength. Using a sturdy chair, a towel or a mat, and maybe a few household items (e.g., books in your backpack) will help you balance, and add comfort and additional resistance. As you progress, you can add equipment like a band, tubing, stability ball, or medicine ball to provide more resistance.

AT THE GYM: Walking on a treadmill is a great option and offers less impact than cement and asphalt. An elliptical machine is another good option that reduces the stress placed on hips, knees, ankles, and feet. If your gym has a pool, use it. Water walking (shallow or deep) is a great way to move your body without stressing your joints. Water also adds resistance to your workout and, of course, the pool can help you stay cool!

A gym provides access to a wide variety of equipment for resistance training. You will be able to incorporate the use of barbells (long bars with weights attached or slots to add weight plates), dumbbells (smaller, handheld weights), benches (flat, incline, decline), plus cable stations and the latest the industry has to offer.

TECHNIQUE: Safe and effective training really depends on proper technique. Be sure to read through each of the previous chapters for detailed exercise descriptions and learn proper technique and form. If you are unable to maintain good form, simply decrease the weight, the speed of the movement, the number of repetitions, or the length of your workout session.

Warm-Up and Cool-Down

A good warm-up and cool-down consists of simply doing your activity of choice at a slower pace and easing into and out of your training session. Once you have cooled down, include a few more dynamic moves or try a bit of foam rolling. Then perform your static stretches for improved flexibility. (Review Chapter 5 programs for more ideas and descriptions of stretches.)

Four-Week Weight Management Programs

Whether you choose the beginner or intermediate level, increase your overall calorie expenditure gradually so you can prevent injury. Adjust intensity, volume, and training days to suit your personal fitness level and schedule.

BEGINNER WEIGHT MANAGEMENT PROGRAM

Start here if you have a BMI of 30 or greater, or if you have been sedentary for more than three months.

GOAL: Increase cardiorespiratory exercise frequency to three days a week and time to 15 minutes continuously per session, 100+ minutes/week; also incorporate resistance training two days a week.

	Mon	Tue	Wed	Thurs	Fri	Sat	Sun
Week 1	Cardio, 10 min × 3	Resistance, 1 circuit	Cardio, 10 min × 3	Resistance, 1 circuit	Cardio, 10 min × 3		
	Cardio workout: Walk 10 minutes continuously 3× (morning, afternoon, evening) *Resistance circuit workout: Do each exercise for 60 seconds with 15-second rests between exercises.*						
Week 2	Cardio, 10 min × 3	Resistance, 2 circuits	Cardio, 10 min × 3	Resistance, 2 circuits	Cardio, 10 min × 3	Cardio, 10 min × 3	
	Cardio workout: Walk 10 minutes continuously, 3× (morning, afternoon, evening) *Resistance circuit workout: Do each exercise for 60 seconds with 15-second rests between exercises, 60-second rests between circuits.*						
Week 3	Cardio, 15 min × 3	Resistance, 2 circuits	Cardio, 15 min × 3	Resistance, 2 circuits	Cardio, 15 min × 3		
	Cardio workout: Walk 15 minutes continuously, 3× (morning, afternoon, evening) *Resistance circuit workout: Do each exercise for 60 seconds with no rest between exercises, 60-second rests between circuits.*						
Week 4	Cardio, 15 min × 3	Resistance, 3 circuits	Cardio, 15 min × 3	Resistance, 3 circuits	Cardio, 15 min × 3	Cardio, 15 min × 3	
	Cardio workout: Walk 15 minutes continuously, 3× (morning, afternoon, evening) *Resistance circuit workout: Do each exercise for 45 seconds with 10-second rests between exercises, 60-second rests between circuits.*						

Order of Resistance Circuit Exercises for Home Workout

Squat
Push-Up or Modified Push-Up
Lunge
Plank or Modified Plank
Row with Resistance Band or Dumbbell
Lat Pull-Down with Resistance Band
Side Bridge (each side)
Back Extension

Order of Resistance Circuit Exercises for Facility Workout

Chest Press
Squat or Leg Press Machine
Upright Row
Leg Extension
Rows
Overhead Press
Lat Pull-Down
Biceps Curl
Triceps Extension
Plank

MOTIVATE!

Track your weight management exercise program—make note of days, actual exercises, sets, reps, load amounts, and rest intervals. Here are a few additional tips to keep you moving:

MOTIVATING MEASUREMENTS: A weekly weigh-in is the most accurate measure of progress and can be a source of encouragement. This check-in will also help you get back on track if you lose motivation.

BAN THE NEGATIVE BODY-TALK: Stop your negative self-talk and start anew! Surround yourself with positive comments, upbeat training partners, and true supporters of your new healthy behaviors and lifestyle. Stay focused. Remember your goals. Be patient with yourself and acknowledge how much you have already accomplished!

TAKE A LITTLE "YOU" TIME: Make fitness and nutrition a priority. Take time for you—schedule your favorite fitness activity (a stroll, your yoga DVD, pool time) and keep the appointment as you would for any other priority.

KEEP A DIGITAL PHOTO LOG: Take a "before" picture, and take a new picture each week. It may sound like the last thing you want to do. However, it can remind you of just how far you've come and keep you motivated to continue. This also works for your meals (especially when you eat out). Take pictures of your meals and gain a different perspective on what you are eating, how much, and when.

ADVANCE!

Ready for more?

INTERMEDIATE WEIGHT MANAGEMENT PROGRAM

Start here if you have a BMI of 25 to 29, or if you already exercise at least two days a week, or if you simply want to take your weight management program to the next level.

GOAL: Increase cardiorespiratory exercise frequency to five days a week and time to 30 minutes continuously per session, 300+ minutes/week; also incorporate resistance training three days a week.

	Mon	Tue	Wed	Thurs	Fri	Sat	Sun
Week 1	Walk/jog 15 min continuously, ×3 (morning, afternoon, evening)	Resistance, 2 circuits	Walk/jog 15 min continuously, ×3 (morning, afternoon, evening)	Resistance, 2 circuits	Walk/jog 15 min continuously, ×3 (morning, afternoon, evening)	Walk/jog 20 min continuously, ×2 (morning, evening)	
	Resistance circuit workout: Do each exercise for 60 seconds with 10-second rests between exercises, 60-second rests between circuits.						
Week 2	Walk/jog 20 min continuously, ×3 (morning, afternoon, evening)	Walk/jog 15 min + Resistance, 2 circuits	Walk/jog 20 min continuously, ×3 (morning, afternoon, evening)	Walk/jog 15 min + Resistance, 2 circuits	Walk/jog 20 min continuously, ×3 (morning, afternoon, evening)	Walk/jog 25 min continuously, ×2 (morning, evening)	
	Resistance circuit workout: Do each exercise for 60 seconds with 10-second rests between exercises, 60-second rests between circuits.						
Week 3	Walk/jog 25 min continuously, ×3 (morning, afternoon, evening)	Walk/jog 15 min + Resistance, 3 circuits	Walk/jog 25 min continuously, ×3 (morning, afternoon, evening)	Walk/jog 15 min + Resistance, 3 circuits	Walk/jog 25 min continuously, ×3 (morning, afternoon, evening)	Walk/jog 30 min continuously, ×2 (morning, evening)	
	Resistance circuit workout: Do each exercise for 60 seconds with 10-second rests between exercises, 60-second rests between circuits.						
Week 4	Walk/jog 30 min continuously, ×3 (morning, afternoon, evening)	Walk/jog 15 min + Resistance, 3 circuits	Walk/jog 30 min continuously, ×3 (morning, afternoon, evening)	Walk/jog 15 min + Resistance, 3 circuits	Walk/jog 30 min continuously, ×3 (morning, afternoon, evening)	Walk/jog 15 min + Resistance, 3 circuits	
	Resistance circuit workout: Do each exercise for 60 seconds with 10-second rests between exercises, 60-second rests between circuits.						

Order of Resistance Circuit Exercises for Home Workout

Squat + Overhead Press with Resistance Band or Dumbbells
Push-Up or Modified Push-Up
Lunge + Biceps Curl with Resistance Band or Dumbbells
Row with Resistance Band or Dumbbells
Lat Pull-Down with Resistance Band
Triceps Extension with Resistance Band or Dumbbells
Oblique Curl
Plank or Modified Plank
Back Extension

Order of Resistance Circuit Exercises for Facility Workout

Squats or Leg Press Machine
Chest Press
Leg Extension
Overhead Press
Leg Curl
Upright Row
Lunge + Biceps Curl with Resistance Band or Dumbbells
Rows
Lat Pull-Down
Pullover
Plank
Abdominal Curl
Back Extension

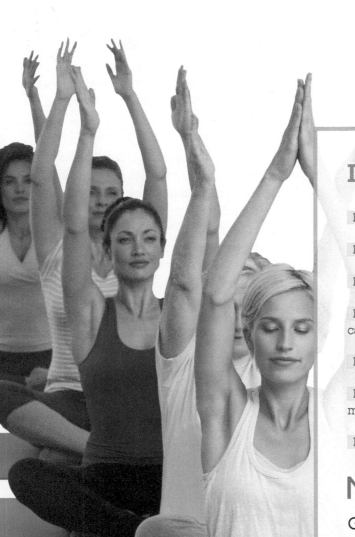

Managing Stress

9

LEARNINGoutcomes

LO 9.1 Define stress.

LO 9.2 Describe how your body responds to stress.

LO 9.3 Explain how stress can harm your body.

LO 9.4 List the kinds of harm stress can cause to your cardiovascular, immune, and other body systems.

LO 9.5 Identify the major sources of stress.

LO 9.6 Describe effective tools for stress management.

LO 9.7 Create your own stress management plan.

MasteringHealth™

Go online for chapter quizzes, interactive assessments, videos, and more!

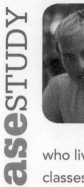

case STUDY

CORY

"Hi, I'm Cory. I'm a junior, majoring in biology. I'm from Denver, Colorado, and just transferred schools to be closer to my dad, who lives alone and has diabetes. I take five classes, I work part time as a lab assistant, and I'm up late every night studying so that I can keep up my grades for applying to medical school. I've always been able to work under pressure, but I have to admit, these past few months have been rough. I am constantly worn out, worried about my dad, and I can barely stay awake in class sometimes. I know that medical school will be even harder, so maybe I should just get used to living like this! But I am so tired of feeling dragged out."

Hear It!

To listen to this case study online, visit the Study Area in MasteringHealth™.

---

stress A disturbance in physical and/or emotional state due to a real or perceived threat, aggravation, or excitement that disturbs the body's "normal" physiological state and to which the body must try to adapt

stressor A physical, social, or psychological event or circumstance to which the body tries to adapt; stressors are often threatening, unfamiliar, disturbing, or exciting

stress response A set of physiological changes initiated by your body in response to a stressor

eustress Stress based on positive circumstances or events; can present an opportunity for personal growth

distress Stress based on negative circumstances or events, or those perceived as negative; can diminish wellness

Everyone feels stress at least some of the time, be it from traffic, competition to enroll in the courses you need, job hunting, fast-changing technology, or a hectic pace that seems to accelerate yearly. Over time, stress can diminish the enjoyment of life and wreak havoc on our health and well-being. Money and health care top the list of Americans' worries.[1] Learning to deal with specific issues and learning

general stress-management techniques are all important to any complete wellness program.

This chapter explains the stress response, details the ways accumulated stress can affect your health, and proposes several helpful strategies you can use to counteract stress. Using the stress-management tools in this chapter, you can better face the pressures of college life and beyond.

LO 9.1 What Is Stress?

In a recent national survey, college students reported stress as the biggest impediment to their academic success, with a greater impact on achievement than colds, flu, sleep difficulty, relationship issues, and all other concerns.[2] But what, exactly, is stress?

The term **stress** is commonly used in many different ways. In this book, we'll define stress as a disturbance in an individual's physical and/or emotional state due to a real or perceived threat, aggravation, or excitement that disturbs the person's "normal" physiological state and to which the body must try to adapt. Any event that disrupts your body's "normal" state is a **stressor**. A stressor can be physical, such as an uncomfortably heavy backpack. It can also be emotional, like the anxiety you feel before a major exam. The term for the physical effect of a stressor is the **stress response**: the set of physiological changes initiated by your body's nervous and hormonal signals. The stress response prepares the brain, heart, muscles, and other organs to respond to a perceived threat or demand.

A more traditional view of stress includes the concepts of both positive stress and negative stress. Positive stress, or **eustress**, presents an opportunity for personal growth, satisfaction, and enhanced well-being. Eustress can invigorate us and motivate us to work harder and achieve more. Entering college, starting a job, and developing a new relationship are all challenges that can produce eustress. Negative stress, or **distress**, can result from negative stressors such as academic pressures, relationship discord, or money problems. It can even result from an overload of positive stressors such as graduating from college, getting married, moving to a new state, and starting a new job all in the same week. Distress can reduce wellness by promoting cardiovascular disease, impairing immunity, or causing mental and emotional dysfunction. With the right mindset and effective management skills, you can divert the pressures of college life toward better coping skills.[3]

LO 9.2 How Does My Body Respond to Stress?

As you sit down in the lecture hall to take your hardest midterm exam, you realize your heart is pounding, your breathing has quickened, your hands are sweating, you have "butterflies" in your stomach, and you feel a sense of dread. You are experiencing a stress response.

The Stress Response

Here's what happens during the seconds that your body initiates a stress response and in the minutes and hours as the response continues (**Figure 9.1**):

1. Your senses perceive and your brain interprets something as a threat; in the preceding example, an exam that will determine half your grade.

2. The threat triggers a region of your brain called the *hypothalamus* to release a hormone that in turn triggers your pituitary gland to secrete **adrenocorticotropic hormone (ACTH)** into your blood.

> **adrenocorticotropic hormone (ACTH)** A hormone secreted by the pituitary gland that causes adrenal glands to secrete cortisol
>
> **cortisol** The body's main stress hormone, secreted by the cortex or outer layer of the adrenal glands located on top of the kidneys; stimulates the sympathetic nervous system; can also damage or destroy neurons

3. ACTH travels through the bloodstream and reaches the outer zone of each adrenal gland (located on top of each kidney). ACTH causes the adrenal glands to secrete **cortisol**, your body's main stress hormone.

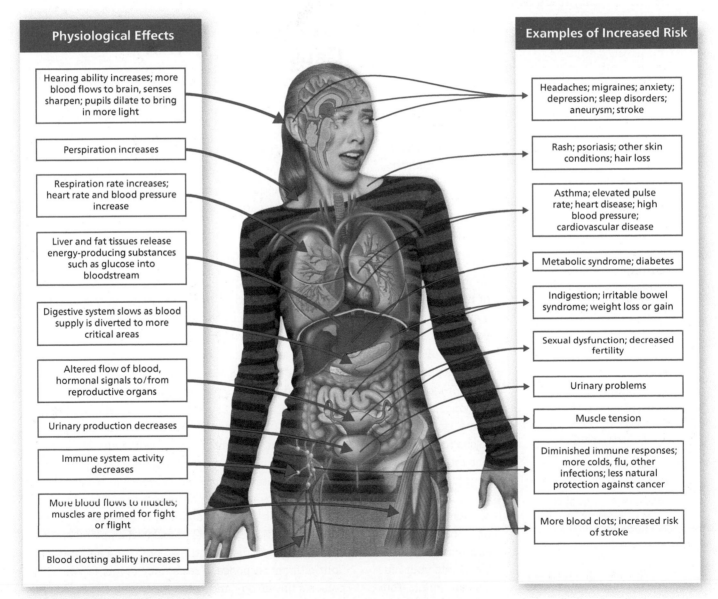

Physiological Effects

- Hearing ability increases; more blood flows to brain, senses sharpen; pupils dilate to bring in more light
- Perspiration increases
- Respiration rate increases; heart rate and blood pressure increase
- Liver and fat tissues release energy-producing substances such as glucose into bloodstream
- Digestive system slows as blood supply is diverted to more critical areas
- Altered flow of blood, hormonal signals to/from reproductive organs
- Urinary production decreases
- Immune system activity decreases
- More blood flows to muscles; muscles are primed for fight or flight
- Blood clotting ability increases

Examples of Increased Risk

- Headaches; migraines; anxiety; depression; sleep disorders; aneurysm; stroke
- Rash; psoriasis; other skin conditions; hair loss
- Asthma; elevated pulse rate; heart disease; high blood pressure; cardiovascular disease
- Metabolic syndrome; diabetes
- Indigestion; irritable bowel syndrome; weight loss or gain
- Sexual dysfunction; decreased fertility
- Urinary problems
- Muscle tension
- Diminished immune responses; more colds, flu, other infections; less natural protection against cancer
- More blood clots; increased risk of stroke

FIGURE **9.1** The stress response.

At the same time, nerve signals from your brain and spinal cord reach and stimulate the central zone of each adrenal gland. Both adrenals respond by releasing two additional stress hormones that ready the body for quick action: **epinephrine** (also called adrenaline) and **norepinephrine** (or noradrenaline).

4. Traveling inside the bloodstream, cortisol reaches specific *target cells* within the body fat and within several organs, including the liver and intestines. Cortisol quickly triggers target cells to convert stored fat, protein, and carbohydrate molecules into glucose. Soon, more glucose is circulating in the blood, supplying the whole body—especially the brain and skeletal muscles—with the extra energy needed to respond to the stressor.

5. The epinephrine and norepinephrine released into the blood rapidly reach target cells in the heart, lungs, stomach, intestines, sense organs, and muscles. Along with signals from sympathetic nerves, these additional stress hormones ready the vital organs for responses that promote survival: fleeing from or confronting the threat. This physiological reaction is called the **fight-or-flight response**.

If you have ever jammed on your car or bicycle brakes to avoid an accident, you have probably felt a jolt of epinephrine. As part of the fight-or-flight response, your pupils dilate, enabling you to see more clearly. The air passages in your lungs also dilate, allowing more oxygen to enter. Your heart beats faster and pumps more blood into your muscles and brain. Your sweat glands release more sweat, and blood is directed away from your hands and feet toward your large muscles and body core; this can make your hands feel cold and clammy. Your digestive action slows down or stops, and your bladder function slows down, since neither process is crucial to short-term survival. Primed in all these ways, your body is ready to handle the stressor, at least in the short term.

After the short-term stressor subsides, your nervous system returns the body to its "normal" state with slower heartbeats, normal breathing rate, normal digestion, and so on. The stress-reduction techniques you will learn later deliberately encourage the body's return to this more relaxed state.

However, if stress continues over long periods, the body's heightened responses can begin to damage various organs and organ systems, as we see shortly (see Figure 9.1).

LO 9.3 Why Does Stress Cause Harm?

Why is chronic stress harmful? After all, if a truck is speeding toward you, your fight-or-flight response could save your life. However, if you are faced with financial hardship or excessive work pressures for years on end, your extended stress response can become chronic and start to harm your health. Two insightful models help explain how *sustained* stress can cause damage over time.

Historic Model: The General Adaptation Syndrome

In the 1930s, biologist Hans Selye studied the response of laboratory rats to painful physical or emotional stressors. He discovered that a wide variety of stressors—such as extreme heat, extreme cold, forced exercise, or surgery—all provoked the same general set of changes in the rats' bodies. Selye proposed a model he called the **general adaptation syndrome (GAS)**, based on these reactions (**Figure 9.2**, page 315).[4] Central to Selye's GAS model is the idea that stress disrupts the body's stable internal environment or *steady state*. Physiological mechanisms work to keep internal conditions (e.g., body temperature, blood-oxygen content, blood pH, and blood sugar levels) within certain "normal" ranges. Scientists use the term **homeostasis** to describe the body's steady state. Selye's model postulated an *alarm stage* in which a stressor disrupts the steady state and triggers a fight-or-flight response; a *resistance stage*, in which a person's physiology and behavior adjust, and build resistance to the stressor; and an *exhaustion stage* during

---

epinephrine (adrenaline) One of two stress hormones released by adrenal glands that readies your body for quick action by stimulating sympathetic nerves

norepinephrine (noradrenaline) One of two stress hormones secreted by adrenal glands that readies your body for quick action by increasing arousal

fight-or-flight response A physiological reaction induced by nervous and hormonal signals that readies the heart, lungs, brain, muscles, and other vital organs and systems in ways that promote survival: fleeing from or confronting a threat

general adaptation syndrome (GAS) A historical model proposed by Hans Selye; it attempts to explain the body's stress response with three stages called alarm, resistance, and exhaustion

homeostasis A state of physiological equilibrium wherein various physiological mechanisms maintain internal conditions (e.g., pH, salt concentration, and temperature) within certain viable ranges

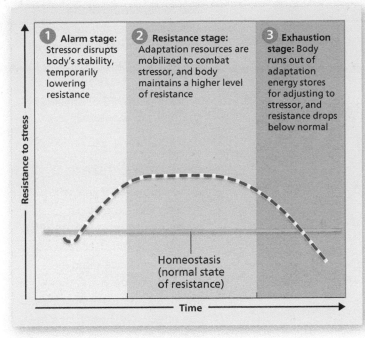

1 **Alarm stage:** Stressor disrupts body's stability, temporarily lowering resistance

2 **Resistance stage:** Adaptation resources are mobilized to combat stressor, and body maintains a higher level of resistance

3 **Exhaustion stage:** Body runs out of adaptation energy stores for adjusting to stressor, and resistance drops below normal

Resistance to stress

Homeostasis (normal state of resistance)

Time

FIGURE **9.2** The general adaptation syndrome model

which the body runs out of resources to successfully adapt to the stressor, resulting in physical or mental illness.

Live It!
Complete Worksheet 8 Stress Reaction at MasteringHealth™.

The general adaptation syndrome recognized that sustained stress can take a toll on wellness. However, scientists have since revisited some of Selye's work and the concept of an "exhaustion stage"—the idea that illness results from running out of resources to adapt to a stressor.[5] They now believe that over time, the stress response *itself* can damage the body and increase the risk of illness, as we will see in the next section.

Allostatic Load

Today's stress researchers use the term **allostasis** to describe the many simultaneous changes that occur in the body to maintain homeostasis, and they use the term **allostatic load** to refer to the long-term wear and tear on the body caused by prolonged allostasis.[6]

If your body's ability to shut off the stress response becomes impaired—even after the stressor has disappeared—allostatic load can result. This cumulative failure to adapt allows high levels of stress hormones to remain in the bloodstream (**Figure 9.3**).[7] Your body can also fail to adapt by releasing too *few* stress hormones, thus it cannot mount an adequate stress response. Allostatic load and failed adaptation can result from a string of stressful events over a long period of time—a classic result of allostatic load is the development of

stress-induced high blood pressure (hypertension).

A person's behavior and choices can also result in allostatic load. For example, some people perceive stress as a positive challenge and respond to it by exercising more, meditating, getting extra sleep, and avoiding drugs and alcohol—all behaviors that can minimize allostatic load and help prevent the damage of chronic stress. Others perceive stress as inevitably negative and respond to it by exercising less, staying up late, drinking more, or starting to smoke or take drugs. Such counterproductive measures actually heighten allostatic load and increase one's susceptibility to developing illness.

allostasis The many simultaneous changes that occur in the body to maintain homeostasis

allostatic load The long-term wear-and-tear on the body that is caused by prolonged allostasis

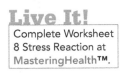

case STUDY

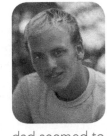

CORY

"I knew this year was going to be a challenge—transferring to a new school and taking upper-level classes. The first month actually went okay. I liked my classes, my dad seemed to be doing better, and I got used to getting by on five hours of sleep each night. Then sometime in September I caught a cold that didn't go away for four weeks! I was coughing all night, could barely pay attention in class, and did badly on one of my midterms. Now I have to work even harder to make up for the low grade."

APPLY IT! List Cory's main sources of stress. Which would you classify as *eustress* and which would you classify as *distress*? How might the allostatic load model explain what is happening with Cory?

TRY IT! Make a list of your own major sources of stress, organizing them into eustress and distress. Labs 9.1 and 9.3 can help you with this list. How does stress affect your body and mind? What do you do when you feel stressed out? If you typically choose unhealthy responses to stress, list some alternative healthy responses you'd like to try.

Hear It!
To listen to this case study online, visit the Study Area in MasteringHealth™.

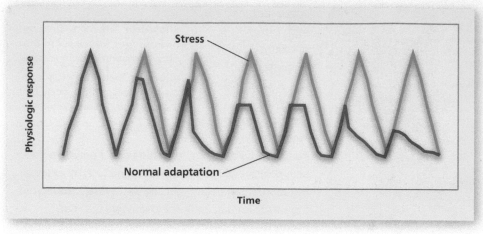

FIGURE **9.3** Allostatic Load: The Current Model. The blue line shows a typical stress response to repeated "hits" from chronic stressors. The response line will rise and then fall as allostatic mechanisms return the body to its normal steady state. The red line shows that in some people, repeated "hits" can lead to a wearing down of stress responses over time; this allows physiological damage to accumulate.

Adapted from B. S. McEwen, "Protective and Damaging Effects of Stress Mediators," *New England Journal of Medicine* 338 (January 15, 1998): 171–79, doi: 10.1056/NEJM199801153380307

LO 9.4 What Kinds of Harm Can Stress Cause?

Studies indicate that 40 percent of deaths and 70 percent of disease in the United States are related, in whole or in part, to stress.[8] Ailments related to chronic stress include heart disease, diabetes, cancer, asthma, headaches, ulcers, low back pain, depression, sleep disorders, and the common cold.[9]

See It!
Watch "Stress Can Damage Women's Health" at MasteringHealth™.

Stress and Cardiovascular Disease

Perhaps the most studied and documented health consequence of unresolved stress is cardiovascular disease (CVD). Research on this topic has demonstrated the impact of chronic stress on heart rate, blood pressure, heart attack, and stroke.[10] Historically, the increased risk of CVD from chronic stress has been linked to increased plaque buildup due to elevated cholesterol, hardening of the arteries, alterations in heart rhythm, and increased and fluctuating blood pressure. Research also points to metabolic abnormalities, insulin resistance, and inflammation in blood vessels as major contributors to heart disease.[11] Recent studies show that when stress increases anger, anxiety, depression, and other negative emotions, the body produces more inflammation-inducing chemicals (cytokines) that can

psychoneuroimmunology (PNI) Science of the interaction between the mind and the immune system

lead to hardening of the arteries.[12] Researchers have identified direct links between the incidence and progression of CVD and stressors such as job strain, caregiving, bereavement, and natural disasters.[13]

Stress and the Immune System

A growing area of scientific investigation known as **psychoneuroimmunology (PNI)** explores the intricate relationship between the mind's response to stress and the immune system's ability to function effectively. Research suggests that too much stress over a long period can negatively impact various aspects of the cellular immune response.[14] Whereas a short-term fight-or-flight response is usually protective, prolonged stress depresses the ability of certain white blood cells, known as killer T cells, to protect the body from infections and from cancer cells that arise in a patient's own body.[15] Stress also activates genes in human immune cells that lead to more inflammation—an important cause of heart disease, diabetes, and other illnesses.[16]

Stress and Other Physical Effects

Prolonged stress can have other physical effects, as well:

- **Weight gain.** Stress hormones can increase food consumption—particularly high-fat and high sugar foods—as well as the tendency to store belly fat. Eating sugar actually decreases the production of cortisol, which explains why many stressed-out people crave sugary treats and why stress can lead to weight gain.[17] Fat tissue itself can even send chemical signals to the brain that help dampen the stress response or keep it rolling. Stress is thus one cog in the complicated metabolic machinery underlying obesity.[18]

- **Hair and skin problems.** Stress can worsen psoriasis and trigger hair loss, either temporarily or permanently.[19]

- **Diabetes.** People under stress often eat poorly, drink alcohol to excess, take drugs, eat junk food, or get too little sleep. All of these can alter blood sugar levels and aggravate pre-existing cases of type 2 diabetes or promote their development. In addition, the stress response itself increases both inflammation-causing cytokines and the levels of glucose circulating in the blood, and both contribute directly to type 2 diabetes.[20]

- **Digestive problems.** People under stress can experience nausea, vomiting, stomach pain, intestinal pain, or diarrhea. Stress hormones can cause existing digestive problems to flare. A classic example is irritable bowel syndrome.[21] Researchers can actually calm anxious behavior in lab mice that they stress out in mazes by altering their gut microbes.[22] This suggests that normalizing your gut ecology through healthy food habits could alleviate both the outward signs of stress and its underlying physiology.

- **Loss of libido.** Even in young people, stress can alter normal levels of sex hormones, possibly leading to erectile dysfunction, emotional swings, and loss of sex drive.[23]

If you experience any of these problems, a trip to the student health center may help you discover links to stress and solutions to the problems.

Stress, the Mind, and the Emotions

Stress may be one of the single greatest contributors to mental impairment and disability and to emotional dysfunction in industrialized nations. One of the most common impairments is disrupted short-term memory, including the memory required for spatial tasks and word recall.[24] Animal studies show that stress hormones can actually shrink the brain's memory center (the *hippocampus*) and negatively impact verbal and other memory functions.[25] Stress causes a flood of natural brain enzymes that disrupt neural connections in the hippocampus, impairing thought and memory.[26] One experimental drug that blocks part of the normal stress response also improves memory and perhaps someday will lead to effective memory drugs.[27]

Stress can lead to mental disorders, as well. Environmental stressors, including money and work pressures, family responsibilities, relationship conflict, and health issues, can heighten your emotional responses and trigger depression, anxiety, addiction, and other disorders. (See the Q & A box Can Stress Affect Your Emotional Wellness? on page 319.)[28]

When stress is severe, an individual's responses may develop into **post-traumatic stress disorder (PTSD)**. Traumas that can trigger PTSD include wartime experiences, rape, near-death experiences in accidents, witnessing a murder or death, being caught in a natural disaster, or a terrorist attack.

LO 9.5 What Are the Major Sources of Stress?

The American Psychological Association reports that young adults (ages 18 to 33) experience the highest stress levels of any adult group, and are most bothered by issues related to work, money, and health.[29] More than half of those surveyed report lying awake during the past month due to stress.[30] A large annual survey of college students found that more than half blamed stress for lowering their grades and other aspects of academic performance to some degree.[31]

Young adults in college can experience a flood of new stressors. Around 30 percent of freshmen report feeling frequently overwhelmed by their work loads, and only half feel that their mental health is above average or higher.[32] Female students report dieting and weight gain as stressful, while male students worry more about being underweight, having relationship issues, and using drugs and alcohol.[33]

Sources of Stress Can Be Internal or External

We must all readjust constantly to those around us, to our separate expectations, and to our overall social and environmental circumstances. Examining the demands you face, your interactions, and details of your history and environment can help you identify your sources of stress and learn new ways to cope (**Figure 9.4**, page 318).

Live It!
Complete Worksheet 9 Stress Tolerance Test at MasteringHealth™.

Change Any time change—whether good or bad—occurs in your normal routine, you experience stress—the more changes and adjustments you must make, the more likely stress will impact your health. For example, leaving home to start college, adjusting to a new schedule, and learning to live with strangers in unfamiliar housing can all cause sleeplessness and anxiety and keep your body in a continual fight-or-flight mode.

Performance Demands We experience stress when we must meet higher standards or unfamiliar demands. In college, competition for grades, athletic positions, club memberships, internships, graduate school acceptance, and job interviews can exert considerable pressure. We can lessen the impact of such demands by setting priorities and realistic deadlines.

post-traumatic stress disorder (PTSD) An acute stress disorder caused by experiencing an extremely traumatic event

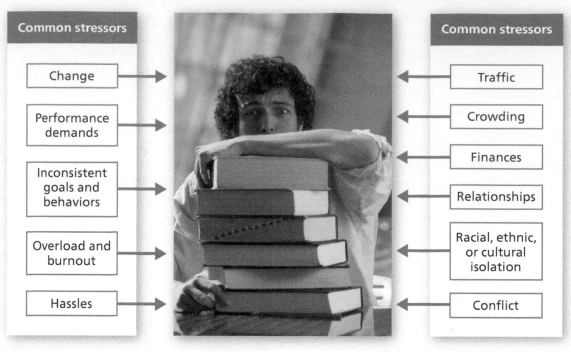

Change

Performance demands

Inconsistent goals and behaviors

Overload and burnout

Hassles

Traffic

Crowding

Finances

Relationships

Racial, ethnic, or cultural isolation

Conflict

FIGURE **9.4** Which of these stressors impact you?

Inconsistent Goals and Behaviors The negative effects of stress can be magnified when we fail to match our goals with our actions. For instance, you may want good grades. But if you party and procrastinate throughout the term, your goals and behaviors are inconsistent. Behaviors that are consistent with your goals—for example, studying harder and partying less to achieve good grades—help alleviate stress.

Overload and Burnout Time pressure, responsibilities, course work, tuition, and high expectations for yourself and those around you—coupled with a lack of support—can lead to *overload:* a state of feeling overburdened, unable to keep up, and longing for escape. Overload pushes some students toward depression, overeating, too much video-gaming, or substance abuse; others respond by using stress-management tools to alleviate tension before it piles up. Unrelieved overload can lead to *burnout,* a state of stress-induced physical and mental exhaustion. Graduate students and postdoctoral candidates often report stress levels high enough to diminish motivation, creativity, and productivity.[34]

Hassles Petty annoyances and frustrations may seem unimportant if taken one by one: getting stuck in a long line at the bookstore, for example, or finding out that a school administrator has miscalculated your transferrable credit hours. However, minor hassles can build to a major meltdown if you perceive those aggravations negatively and let the feelings mount. Appraising difficult situations positively—seeing them as temporary challenges rather than calamities—is the key to resilience, the capacity for mental and emotional stability.[35]

Traffic and Crowding Environmental stress results from events occurring in the physical environment. People living in crowded urban environments, especially lower socioeconomic neighborhoods, experience more stress from traffic, crowding, and related problems such as noise, crime, pollution, and a high cost of living. They have a greater risk of stress-related disorders such as anxiety and depression.[36] Rural people tend to experience different stressors such as limited employment opportunities and decreased services.

Finances The majority of students worry about paying college expenses and most have to take out loans. The GetFitGraphic Dealing with Stress over Debt in College on page 321 shows how many students have learned to cope with that significant source of stress.

Relationships Relationships with friends, partners, family members, and co-workers can be important sources of strength and support, but they can also be stressful. Staying connected can improve our mental, emotional, and physical health. Problematic relationships, however, can diminish our self-esteem and overall wellness. Stress can even be "contagious" and raise cortisol levels in people as they watch friends or even strangers coping with stressful situations.[37]

Q&A Can Stress Affect Your Emotional Wellness?

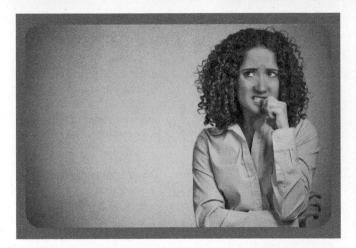

A large national survey of college student's health reveals significant levels of emotional distress: Most respondents report feeling overwhelmed and/or exhausted, very sad, anxious, or lonely within the past year.[1] A sizeable minority reported hopelessness, anger, and/or depression.[2] More than one-sixth of the students polled had received a diagnosis or treatment for anxiety in the past 12 months, and many singled out problems with sleep, finances, school work, and relationships.[3]

Stress and heightened emotions have complicated but very real interconnections: Many students experience high stress levels when they arrive at college based on their previous school and home life, including pressure to stay safe, get good grades, excel at sports, stay out of trouble, join activities, have a big social circle, and get accepted into a desirable school.[4] The new social and academic challenges of college can add to these and push people over an emotional dam. Financial worries and overusing electronic devices can turn up the pressure.[5] What's more, some people are "prewired" to experience stress based on heritable, developmental, and early environmental factors, and are all the more vulnerable to heightened feelings of sadness, worry, anger, and depression.[6]

Because stress and emotions have intertwined physiological roots, applying the stress-management techniques outlined in this chapter can help you manage feelings. Physical activity is a potent alleviator. So are yoga, meditation, and other relaxation methods. The tools outlined on pages 320–329 can help build self-esteem, self-confidence, and skills for handling life stressors.

If negative emotions become severe enough to interfere with studying or daily routines, seek help from your student health service, campus counseling center, or a community-based mental health professional. If depression threatens to derail you, call a local depression or suicide hotline. Even when feelings seem overwhelming, it is possible to take charge and improve emotional wellness, step by step.

Sources:
1. American College Health Association, *American College Health Association-National College Health Assessment II: Towson University Executive Summary, Spring, 2015* (Hanover, MD: American College Health Association, 2015).
2. Ibid.
3. Ibid.
4. J. Hoffman, "Anxiety Tests Colleges," *New York Times*, June 2, 2015, D1.
5. Ibid.
6. A. S. Fox et al., "Intergenerational Neural Mediators of Early-Life Anxious Temperament," *Proceedings of the National Academy of Sciences* (2015): 201508593, doi: 10.1073/pnas.1508593112; H. Zaidan et al., "Prereproductive Stress to Female Rats Alters Corticotropin Releasing Factor Type 1 Expression in Offspring," *Biological Psychiatry* 74, no. 9: 680–87; A. C. Maartje et al., "Maternal Prenatal Stress Is Associated with the Infant Intestinal Microbiota," *Psychoneuroendocrinology* (2015), doi: 10.1016/j.psyneuen.2015.01.006

Racial, Ethnic, or Cultural Isolation Students who act, speak, or dress differently from the norm sometimes face additional pressures. Whether due to race, ethnicity, religious affiliation, age, physical handicap, or sexual orientation, these students may become victims of subtle and not-so-subtle forms of bigotry, insensitivity, harassment, or hostility. For example, more than 886,000 international students attended American colleges and universities in 2014.[38] These students often experience homesickness, language barriers, and cultural differences and suffer significantly more stress-related emotional and physical illnesses than do their American counterparts.[39] Befriending and communicating with foreign students can help them succeed.

Conflict Conflict occurs when we have to choose between competing motives, behaviors, or impulses, or when we face incompatible demands, opportunities, needs, or goals. For example, what if your best friend wanted you to help her cheat on an exam, but you didn't feel right about it? College students often experience stress because their own developing set of beliefs conflicts with the values they learned from their parents.

What stresses do you face, and how are they affecting you? **Lab 9.1** charts many common sources of stress for college students and others. Completing this lab will help you measure your current stress level. Reading

Do It!
Access these labs at the end of the chapter or online at MasteringHealth™.

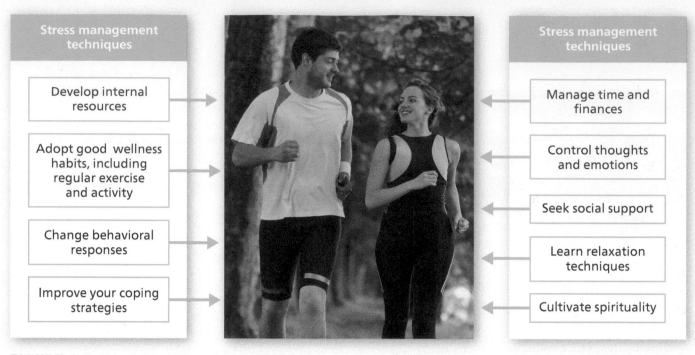

Stress management techniques		Stress management techniques
Develop internal resources		Manage time and finances
Adopt good wellness habits, including regular exercise and activity		Control thoughts and emotions
Change behavioral responses		Seek social support
Improve your coping strategies		Learn relaxation techniques
		Cultivate spirituality

FIGURE **9.5** There are many effective techniques for helping you manage stress.

through the next section will then supply a series of helpful stress-reduction strategies and tools for using them.

LO 9.6 How Can I Manage Stress?

Most young adults (62 percent) do try to reduce their stress levels, but studies show their techniques are often ineffective and sometimes add to rather than resolve their problems.[40] **Figure 9.5** on this page summarizes a low-key, multipronged approach to stress management.

Develop Internal Resources for Coping with Stress

When you perceive that your personal resources are sufficient to meet life's demands, you experience little or no stress. By contrast, when you perceive that life's demands exceed your coping resources, you are likely to feel strain and distress.

appraisal The interpretation and evaluation of information provided to the brain by the senses

psychological hardiness Personal characteristics of control, commitment, and an embrace of challenge that help individuals cope with stress

Self-Esteem and Self-Efficacy

Several coping resources influence whether you assess the stress in your life with a positive **appraisal** or a negative one. Two of the most important

coping resources are *self-esteem* and *self-efficacy*. Self-esteem is a sense of positive self-regard, or how you feel about yourself. Self-efficacy is a belief or confidence in personal skills and performance abilities. Researchers consider self-efficacy one of the most important personality traits that influence psychological and physiological stress responses.[41] Low self-esteem or low self-efficacy can heighten your self-perception of stress, increase your feelings of helplessness in coping with stress, and contribute to depression.[42] Conversely, boosting your own self-esteem and self-efficacy can diminish your stress response and in some cases, improve cognitive performance.[43]

Hardiness Psychologists often characterize people with so-called Type A personalities as hard-driving, competitive, and time-driven. They define people with Type B personalities, in contrast, as relaxed, non-competitive, and tolerant. Researchers once believed that Type A characteristics put people at greater risk of heart attacks than Type B traits.[44] Now they see personality as more complex, with most people expressing a mix of personality traits and influences.

Psychological hardiness, for example, may negate stress associated with hard-driving Type A behavior. Psychologically hardy people tend to express control, commitment, and a willingness to embrace challenge.[45] People with a sense of control can accept responsibility for their behaviors and change self-defeating ones. People with a sense of commitment have good self-esteem

DEALING WITH STRESS OVER DEBT IN COLLEGE

GETFITGRAPHIC

Figuring out how to manage one's money can be tough for college students and owing money on credit cards and loans can be a major strain in college and beyond. A recent survey of 15,000 college students found that 60 percent worried often or very often about meeting regular expenses, and over half also worry frequently about paying for school.[1]

A recent survey of 18,795 American college students found that

STRESS OVER FINANCES

OVER 70%
FEEL **STRESS** OVER THEIR **FINANCES** IN GENERAL.[1]

ABOUT 35%
REPORT THEIR WORRY WAS **TRAUMATIC** OR VERY DIFFICULT TO HANDLE.[2]

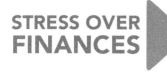

64% of students take loans for college costs

35.5% use loans as their main funding source

24.8% have **$10,000** or more in loan debt

WORRY OVER STUDENT LOANS
20% of students expect to have **$50,000** or more in loan debt by graduation[3]

WORRY OVER CREDIT CARDS

31.9% of students have 1 credit card

24.6% of students have 2 or more credit cards[4]

$499 The average annual balance on student credit cards in a recent year[5]

Avoid mounting debt now.

▶ **BUY ONLY** items you truly need—and pay cash when you can.

▶ **PAY BILLS** on time to protect your financial reputation for future borrowing.

▶ **CONSIDER DEBT** as a last resort, not a first choice.

▶ **KEEP A MINIMUM** of credit cards and try to pay the total balance each month.

and a strong sense of their life's purpose. People who embrace challenge see change as an opportunity for personal growth. Psychologists have studied hardiness extensively, and many believe this personality trait underlies an individual's ability to cope with stress. Resilience extends this by enabling such individuals to find and use resources for their own wellness.[46]

Adopt Good Wellness Habits

Good exercise, eating, and sleep habits make a big different in your body's ability to handle day-to-day stressors. The same is true for avoiding substance abuse. These habits not only improve your wellness, they also diminish the negative effects of stress and reduce allosteric load.

Exercise, Fun, and Recreational Activity One of the most helpful things you can do to combat stress is to improve your overall level of fitness. Exercise helps prevent both physical and mental disorders with stress as an underlying mind/body link. The stress that increases along with mental and emotional disturbances also triggers metabolic changes that thicken belly fat, elevate blood pressure and cholesterol, and contribute to cardiovascular disease.[47] The more you sit in front of a computer, a television, or an electronic game, the higher your risk of stress, anxiety, and sleep problems.[48]

Exercise can literally reprogram the way stressed, anxious, or depressed test subjects perceive environmental stimuli: It can remove some of the threat and negativity they formerly saw and help to alleviate mental and emotional symptoms.[49] Something as simple as a short walk in a park or other green setting can decrease brooding over problems.[50] Deliberately replacing a slump-shouldered "depressive walk" with a bouncing "happy walk" can actually improve your mood.[51] And meeting the American College of Sports Medicine standards for weekly *vigorous* exercise (see Chapter 2) objectively reduces feelings of stress, anxiety, and depression and improves sleep.[52]

Eat Well Eating nutrient-dense foods rather than fast foods and junk foods gives you more mental and physical energy, improves your immune responses, and helps you stay at a healthy weight. Undereating, overeating, or eating nutrient-poor foods can contribute to your stress levels and potential for depression. Many vendors claim that vitamins and supplements reduce stress, but most of these claims are unsupported. Vitamin and mineral supplementation beyond your daily requirements may only add to your stress—financial stress, that is!

Get Enough Sleep Sleep is central to wellness. As explained in the box How Does Sleep Affect My Performance and Mood? on page 323, sleep loss hinders learning, memory, academic work, and body performance. It can also depress mood and prompt feelings of stress, anger, and sadness. *Sound* sleep is important, too. Some people find that inexpensive earplugs or eye masks block sleep-disturbing sound and light. Others require a quieter, darker room or more considerate roommates to solve their sleep problems.

Live It!
Complete Worksheet 4 Sleep Inventory at MasteringHealth™.

Avoid Alcohol and Tobacco Both drinking and smoking can disrupt sleep patterns during the night. Alcohol can disrupt the length of time it takes you to fall asleep as well as the sequence and duration of your sleep states.[53] In particular, alcohol decreases REM sleep and dreaming, and can negatively affect memory, motor skills, and concentration.[54] The nicotine in tobacco is both highly addictive and acts as a mild stimulant that can increase anxiety and decrease sleep.

Change Your Behavioral Responses

What should be your first step toward making positive changes? Recognize that stress is harming your fitness, wellness, relationships, or productivity. Start by assessing all aspects of a stressor, examining your typical response, determining ways to change it, and learning to cope. Often, you cannot change the stressors you face: the death of a loved one, the stringent requirements of your major, stacked-up course assignments, and so on. You can, however, manage your reactions to them.

Assess the Stressor List and evaluate the stressors in your life. Can you change the stressor itself? If not, you can still change your behavior and reactions to reduce the levels of stress you experience. For example, if you have a heavy academic workload, such as five term papers due for five different courses during the same semester, make a plan to start the papers early and space your work evenly so you can avoid panic over deadlines and all-night sessions to finish them on time.

Change Your Response If something causes you distress—a habitually messy roommate, for example—you can (1) express your anger by yelling; (2) pick up the mess yourself but then leave a nasty note; (3) use humor to get your point across; or (4) initiate an even-tempered, matter-of-fact conversation about the problem. Before you respond, think through the most effective choice. Humor and laughter are surprisingly good ways to de-escalate tense situations and benefit your wellness generally. Laughter can boost your immune response, not to mention lightening your mood and even bringing extra oxygen into your lungs![55] A calm, rational conversation can work well, too.

Q&A How Does Sleep Affect My Performance and Mood?

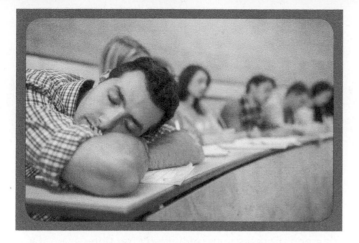

Sleep experts suggest that adults aged 18 to 64 need about seven to nine hours of sleep per night (depending on individual physiology).[1] However, college students average fewer hours than this and 94 percent of students feel tired two to seven mornings per week.[2] In addition, the typical student sleeps less at the end of a semester than at the beginning due to the accumulation of assignments and exams.

Losing an hour or two of sleep actually does matter, even to young, active, healthy college students. And researchers can detect the impact after a single night of poor or limited sleep. Numerous sleep studies confirm the following:

- Sleep loss degrades learning and memory; students who stay up later at night and get less sleep tend to have lower grade point averages than earlier, longer sleepers.[2]

- Longer sleep benefits physical performance. A study of Stanford University men's basketball players showed that extending sleep by an hour or two for several weeks improved their shooting accuracy, reaction time, and sprinting speed.[3] Sleep deprivation diminished the strength and heart rate of martial arts performers, whereas normal sleep enhanced it.[4] Conversely, physical activity benefits sleep; those who exercise regularly get better sleep and feel less sleepy during the day.[5]

- Sleep loss degrades health and appearance. A single sleepless night turns on genes in fat and muscle tissue that can impair glucose tolerance, a precursor to obesity and diabetes.[6] Sleeping less than 5.5 hours per night is also linked to increased snacking, weight gain, and subjective judgments of a less healthy, less attractive, more tired appearance.[7]

- Sleep affects the immune system. Getting too little sleep leaves you less-protected from colds, and can lead to a longer, more dragged-out recovery.[8] Sleep deprivation causes the activity of white blood cells to decline, and they have a harder time fending off infections.[9]

- Sleep affects mood. Sleep deprivation can increase feelings of stress, anger, anxiety, and sadness.[10] These emotional states can, in turn, make sleeping even harder. Feeling extremely stressed out and having a negative emotional response to that stress is, in fact, the best predictor that a student will have sleep problems.[11]

Poor sleep is defined as getting fewer-than-recommended hours of sleep, having irregular bedtimes and rising times, and experiencing interrupted sleep. To improve your sleep:

- go to bed and wake up at as regular a time as possible;

- sleep in a room that is quiet, dark, cool (not cold), and ventilated (but not too drafty);

- get regular exercise, but avoid a heavy cardio workout within an hour or two of bedtime (light stretching and mild cardio are usually fine);[12]

- avoid caffeine in the afternoon and evening;

- avoid excess alcohol.

Sources:
1. National Sleep Foundation, "How Much Sleep Do We Really Need?" 2015, www.sleepfoundation.org
2. American College Health Association, *American College Health Association-National College Health Assessment II: Reference Group Executive Summary*, 2015; J. Peszka, D. Mastin, and J. Harsh, "Sleep Hygiene, Chronotype, and Academic Performance during the Transition from High School through Four Years of College" [presented at the 25th annual meeting of the Associated Professional Sleep Societies (SLEEP), Minneapolis, Minnesota, 2011].
3. C. D. Mah et al., "The Effects of Sleep Extension on the Athletic Performance of Collegiate Basketball Players," *Sleep* 34, no. 7 (2011): 943–50.
4. N. Souissi et al., "Effects of Time-of-Day and Partial Sleep Deprivation on Short-Term Maximal Performances of Judo Competitors," *Journal of Strength and Conditioning Research* 27, no. 9 (2013).
5. National Sleep Foundation, "Physical Activity Impacts Overall Quality of Sleep," 2015, www.sleepfoundation.org; P. D. Loprini and B. J. Cardinal, "Association between Objectively Measured Physical Activity and Sleep, NHANES 2005–2006," *Mental Health and Physical Activity* 4, no. 2 (2011): 65–69.
6. J. Cedernaes et al., "Acute Sleep Loss Induces Tissue-Specific Epigenetic and Transcriptional Alterations to Circadian Clock Genes in Men," *Journal of Clinical Endocrinology and Metabolism* (2015): 2015–284.
7. A. V. Nedeltcheva et al., "Sleep Curtailment Is Accompanied by Increased Intake of Calories from Snacks," *American Journal of Clinical Nutrition* 89, no. 1 (2009): 126–33; S. Patel et al., "Sleeping Less Linked to Weight Gain," *American Thoracic Society* (2006).
8. E. J. Olson, "I'm Having Trouble Sleeping Lately. Does This Increase My Chances of Getting Sick?" *Mayo Clinic Patient Care and Health Information*, June 9, 2015, www.mayoclinic.org
9. K. Ackermann et al., "Diurnal Rhythms in Blood Cell Populations and the Effect of Acute Sleep Deprivation in Healthy Young Men," *Sleep* 36, no. 7 (2012): 933 40.
10. B. A. Marcks, "Co-Occurrence of Insomnia and Anxiety Disorder: A Review of the Literature," *American Journal of Lifestyle Medicine* 3, no. 4 (2009): 300–9.
11. L. A. Verlander, J. O. Benedict, and D. P. Hanson, "Stress and Sleep Patterns of College Students," *Perceptual Motor Skills* 88, no. 3 (1999): 893–98.
12. M. Burman and A. King, "Exercise as Treatment to Enhance Sleep," *American Journal of Lifestyle Medicine* 4, no. 6 (2010): 500–14.

Improve Your Coping Strategies

Good coping strategies can help relieve stress; poor ones can actually make it worse. Researchers have found that college students can better tolerate stress when they deliberately relax through such practices as yoga or meditation; exercise in an extracurricular sport or activity; listen to music; and seek support from family, friends, or teachers.[56] Coping strategies that leave stress levels unchanged include taking a trip, reading a book, sitting quietly, surfing the Internet, writing in a journal, singing, or playing an instrument. Coping strategies that actually lead to more stress include cleaning a room or apartment, calling a (presumably unsupportive) friend or relative, spending time on an Internet social network, taking a study break, going shopping, eating, using drugs or alcohol, or watching a movie. A separate study showed that students who could apply many different coping strategies are more likely to have positive outcomes when confronted with traumatic life events.[57]

Prepare Before Stressful Events Thinking things through before a potentially stressful event may help you avoid destructive or ineffective responses and tolerate escalating stress levels. For example, practicing for a speaking event in front of friends may help you find and correct rough spots, and in turn, lower your levels of stress during the actual speech.

Downshift Many people experience stress because they want to "have it all": a college diploma, a successful career, a family, a wide circle of friends, possessions, status in the community, and so on. But some are lowering their stress by **downshifting**—moving to a simpler life. Here are examples of downshifting:

- Step back to a simpler life by, for example, moving from a large urban area to a smaller town.

- Change from a hectic high-pressure career to a low-key profession that you enjoy for itself, not for the salary it commands.

- Remove the clutter of unused things in your home or scale back to fewer, less-expensive possessions.

Manage Your Time and Finances

Many of us create stress for ourselves through ineffective habits for managing time and finances. Habits are learned behaviors, and you can *unlearn*

---

downshifting Forming new values that include stepping back to a simpler life

---

bad habits or replace them with new habits that serve you better. Here is what to aim for.

Manage Your Time Time—or our perceived lack of it—is one of our biggest stressors. If you learn to handle demands in a more streamlined, efficient way, you can leave more time for other things, such as studying and having fun. To get a handle on time management, work through **Lab 9.2**. The following tips can also help:

> **Do It!**
> Access these labs at the end of the chapter or online at MasteringHealth™.

- **Use a calendar**—paper or electronic—to help you keep track of due dates, events, and commitments.

- **Multitask only when it's truly appropriate.** Save multitasking for things that take less concentration, such as doing the laundry and paying bills. Give important tasks your undivided attention—even if it means ignoring texts and phone calls.

- **Break up big tasks.** Divide big tasks like finishing a term paper into smaller segments and allocate a certain amount of time to each piece. If you find yourself floundering in a task, move on and come back to it when you are refreshed.

- **Clean your desk.** Periodically weed out unneeded papers and file the useful ones in separate folders. Promptly read, respond to, file, or toss mail into the recycle bin.

- **Accommodate your natural rhythms.** If you are a morning person, study and write papers in the morning, and take breaks when you start to slow down.

- **Avoid overcommitment.** Set your school and personal priorities and don't be afraid to say no to things you cannot or should not take on.

- **Avoid interruptions.** When you have a project that requires total concentration, schedule uninterrupted time and spend it in a quiet library carrel or equivalent spot.

- **Manage your time online.** See the Tools for Change box Solutions for Internet Stress on page 325.

- **Remember that time is precious.** Look for things to value in each day. Moments spent worrying over rather than enjoying life are a tremendous waste!

Manage Your Finances Higher education can impose a huge financial burden on parents, students, and communities. Nearly two-thirds of students report "some" or "major" concerns regarding their ability to pay college tuition and expenses.[58]

TOOLS FOR > CHANGE

Solutions for Internet Stress

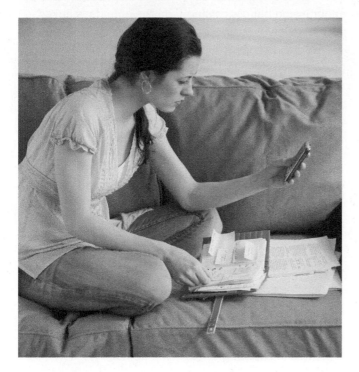

Eight of 10 students find Internet use to be "'close to' or 'as vital' as air, water, food, and shelter."[1] More than 87 percent follow and post to Facebook and 60 percent admitted to checking their smartphones "compulsively."[2] Another two-thirds spend as much or more time with friends online as they do in person.[3] And 81 percent of students play video games—sharpening their spatial skills but, when done in excess, threatening their academic performance.[4]

Even if it seems fun and stimulating, screen time increases stress in surprising ways. Here are a few tips for balancing your time on- and off-line.

- **Check less often for messages.** A study of students, professors, and others monitored stress levels during one week of *unlimited* daily access to email followed by one week of *limited* daily access. Deliberate cutting back turned out to reduce stress as effectively as a meditation session.[5] This relaxation effect, the researchers think, is in large part because limited checking spares a person the mental effort of flipping back-and-forth between tasks. Cutting back to three check-ins per day saved students time and stress.

- **Replace violent video games with funny, uplifting games.** Playing challenging games can lead to a

sense of competency that helps the gamer manage real-world situations and emotions. Playing violent games, however, leads to a more hostile view of the world that makes handling problems more difficult.[6] Try substituting cheerful games, at least some of the time.

- **Try stress-relieving smartphone apps.** Some people prefer to de-stress using an electronic device, and for them there are apps like Personal Zen and Buddhify. Personal Zen trains your brain to focus on positive, non-threatening stimuli while ignoring negative, stress-stoking stimuli. Buddhify guides you through meditation aids for traveling, going to sleep, taking a work break, and so on.[7]

- **Consider counseling.** Students can usually get help for anxiety, sleep issues, screen "addiction," and other stress-related problems from counselors at the student health service. For the non-screen-addicted, there's an online version of therapy: A service called Lantern connects users to licensed therapists by phone and text messages for a small monthly fee.[8]

- **Change what you drink.** Many students consume tea, coffee, coffee drinks, and energy drinks such as Red Bull or Monster, thinking this will boost their mood and make them more alert. High caffeine levels, however, can increase your blood pressure, blood sugar, and feelings of anxiety and jitteriness. At the same time, excess caffeine can disturb your sleep and fray your concentration. Ironically, the more energy drinks a student consumes per week, the lower his or her academic performance is likely to be![9] Monitor—and perhaps cut down—the amount of caffeine you consume. More than 400 milligrams per day is unsafe and you may feel side effects from half that.[10]

1. S. Deatherage et al., "Stress, Coping, and Internet Use of College Students," *Journal of American College Health* 62, no. 1 (January 2014): 40–46.
2. 2014 Cisco Connected World Technology Report, "Cisco Business Insights," accessed August 2015, www.slideshare.net
3. Ibid.
4. S. R. Burgess et al., "Video Game Playing and Academic Performance in College Students," *College Student Journal* 46, no. 2 (June 2012).
5. K. Kushlev and E. Dunn, "Checking Email Less Frequently Reduces Stress," *Computers in Human Behavior* 43, (2015): 220–28.
6. J. A. Bonus, A. Peebles, and K. Riddle, "The Influence of Violent Video Game Enjoyment on Hostile Attributions," *Computers in Human Behavior* 52 (2015): 472.
7. A. Carrns, "A Start-Up Offers Online Therapy for Anxiety and More," *New York Times*, October 25, 2014, B5.
8. Ibid.
9. M. L. Pettit and K. A. DeBarr, "Perceived Stress, Energy Drink Consumption, and Academic Performance among College Students," *Journal of American College Health* 59, no. 5 (2011).
10. Mayo Clinic Staff, "Caffeine: How Much Is Too Much?" April 14, 2014, www.mayoclinic.org

Control Your Thoughts and Emotions

Just as we learn to manage our time and finances, we can learn to manage how we think and react to events and to our emotions.

Manage Your Thinking Our "negative scripts" about ourselves contribute to our stress. When we see ourselves as unable to cope (i.e., when we have low self-efficacy), we tend to handle life's problems and stresses less effectively. You can change negative scripts to more positive ones, however. And in the process, you can diminish stress, boost your self-esteem, and monitor your self-talk to reduce negative and irrational responses. Focus on your current capabilities rather than on past problems.

Here are specific actions you can take to develop better mental skills for stress management:

- **Worry constructively.** Don't waste time and energy worrying about things you can't change or events that may never happen.

- **Perceive life as changeable.** If you accept that change is a natural part of living and growing, the jolt from changes will become less stressful.

- **Consider alternatives.** Remember, there is seldom only one appropriate action. Anticipating options will help you plan for change and adjust more rapidly.

- **Moderate your expectations.** Aim high but be realistic about your circumstances and motivation.

- **Don't rush into action.** Think before you act, especially before taking an action that involves risk. One interesting study showed that women under stress take fewer risks whereas men under stress take more risks.[59] Rather than getting stressed by daily obstacles and negative outcomes, sit back, evaluate the situation, choose a reasoned response, and plan ways to avoid future negative occurrences.

- **Take things less seriously.** Try to keep the real importance of things in perspective. Ask yourself: How much will a situation or event matter in two weeks? Six months?

Manage Negative Emotions and Anger Stress management involves learning to identify emotional reactions that are based on irrational beliefs and negative self-talk. Identifying those can allow you to deal with the belief or emotion in a healthy and appropriate way.

> **Live It!**
> Complete Worksheet 11 Anger Log at MasteringHealth™.

Anger management is particularly important. Anger can be constructive if it mobilizes us to stand up for ourselves or accomplish something others think we are incapable of. However, a habit of responding angrily when our wants or desires are thwarted can be destructive. The inverse is also true: A habit of boiling with anger inside but concealing it on the outside is linked with high levels of anxiety.[60]

Hotheaded, short-fused people are at risk for health problems. Numerous studies show that anger can significantly increase the risk of heart disease. Stress hormones released during anger may constrict blood vessels in the heart or actually promote clot formation, which can trigger a heart attack.[61] Strategies for controlling and redirecting anger include:

- Practice problem-solving techniques instead of complaining

- Seek objective opinions and constructive advice from friends

- Anticipate situations that trigger your anger and brainstorm solutions in advance

- Learn to express your feelings constructively

- Learn how to de-escalate from anger by taking deep breaths or counting to 10

- Keep a journal to observe your own reactions and progress in controlling anger

Seek Social Support

Making, keeping, and spending time with supportive friends helps you deal with adversity.[62] Social interactions are important buffers against the effects of stress: A person who is well integrated socially is only half as likely to die from any cause at any age than is a person with few or no sources of social support.[63] One research team found that friendly in-person hugs could actually help protect recipients from catching the common cold. By comparison, spending most of one's social time connecting to people via cell phones and computers could actually increase the likelihood of catching a cold.[64] Clearly, social connectedness is important to wellness. And supportiveness is key; reaching out to friends or relatives who knock you down emotionally becomes a stressor in itself.

The flip side of social connectedness is social isolation, and it, too, has important health implications. Compared to students with a network of friends, isolated students experience more stress, poorer moods, and lower quality sleep.[65] Studies have found damaging changes to the cardiovascular, immune, and nervous systems of chronically lonely people and these changes may explain why isolated individuals have a higher risk of heart disease, infection, and depression.[66] This research also suggests that a person's actual number of social contacts is less important than the subjective experience of feeling unpopular or lonely.[67]

While friends can be important stress reducers, people sometimes need the help of a counselor or support group. Most schools offer counseling services at no cost for short-term crises. Clergy, instructors, and dorm supervisors also may be helpful resources. If university services are unavailable or if you are concerned about confidentiality, most communities offer low-cost counseling through mental health clinics. You may be able to find a stress-reduction program or support group through one of these professional resources. Many individual counselors and classes teach stress-reduction techniques.

Learn Relaxation Techniques

Deliberate relaxation techniques can be beneficial tools for preventing and reducing stress, and interest in these techniques has doubled in the past 15 years. More than 20 million American adults now practice yoga and 18 million have used some form of mindfulness meditation.[68] These techniques tend to focus the mind and breathing. Here are some of the most popular examples.

Relaxation Breathing When we're tense, we often breathe shallowly in the upper chest or even hold our breath, but this kind of breathing can increase anxiety.[69] **Relaxation breathing**—inhaling deeply and rhythmically and involving the abdominal muscles—can help relieve tension and increase oxygen levels in the blood. This, in turn, can boost energy and sharpen thinking. Relaxation breathing, also called *diaphragmatic breathing,* is easy and can be done sitting or lying down, alone or in a small group, and for a few minutes or longer. The object is to expand the lungs fully by drawing downward with the diaphragm and outward with the abdomen, then releasing fully.

Progressive Muscle Relaxation **Progressive muscle relaxation (PMR)** releases tension in the muscles, muscle group by muscle group. To do PMR, lie down in a quiet, comfortable place and devote 10 or 20 minutes to gradually letting go of accumulated stiffness and tension in the affected muscles. You can do this alone or in a group as a way to relax and refresh yourself fully. Some people also use it as a means of falling asleep.

Mindfulness Meditation There are dozens of forms of meditation. Most involve sitting quietly for 15 to 30 minutes and focusing on breathing, body sensations, and detaching from stray thoughts and worries. Researchers have confirmed that meditating reduces the stress response and can show significant reduction after just three days of 25-minute sessions.[70] Meditation also cuts symptoms of inflammation, boosts the immune response, and improves mental functioning.[71] Additionally, meditation shifts brain activity from the right prefrontal lobe—associated with unhappiness, anger, and distress—toward the left prefrontal lobe, which is associated with happiness and

See It!

Watch "Meditation Becoming More Popular Among Teens" at MasteringHealth™.

relaxation breathing Inhaling deeply and rhythmically, expanding and then relaxing the abdomen; this breathing technique can help relieve tension and increase oxygen intake

progressive muscle relaxation (PMR) A stress-management technique that identifies tension stored in the muscles and releases it, one muscle group at a time

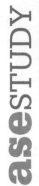
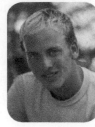

CORY

"This semester was getting out of control. I was exhausted but would have trouble falling asleep, so that was a vicious cycle. I stopped working out—which I used to do twice a week but just didn't have the time for anymore. And I caught another cold at the end of October. My dad started joking that he was healthier than I was! I had to cut out something so I dropped my only elective, Spanish, even though I liked it. I used the extra time to start going back to the gym, and that actually seemed to give me back some energy. I honestly think just those two things alone helped me to get through the rest of the semester. Now, I just need to ace my MCATs . . ."

APPLY IT! What kinds of stress-related problems was Cory exhibiting? Review the section on stress-management tools. Which strategies did Cory employ?

TRY IT! **Today**, make a list of the stress-management strategies you use. Lab 9.2 can help you with that. Using that same list, put a check by the techniques that seem to be the most effective for you. **This week**, start observing your periods of stress and ways of coping more carefully. Lab 9.3 will start you doing some of these same activities. Keep a simple diary of when you feel more stressed and what to do when this happens. Do you see patterns in the timing of your stress periods and how you respond? **In two weeks**, take one pattern—let's say a recurrent stress associated with commuting to campus—and note three ways you could improve this pattern and your response to it. Over the next few days, try each of your ways for coping with the stressor.

Hear It!

To listen to this case study online, visit the Study Area in MasteringHealth™.

---

biofeedback A stress-management technique that teaches you to alter automatic physiological responses such as body temperature, heart rate, or sweating

hypnosis A medical and psychiatric tool that trains people to focus on one thought, object, or voice and to become unusually responsive to suggestion

enthusiasm. See Program 9.1 at the end of this chapter for guidance on beginning a meditation practice.

Yoga Yoga, a set of stretching, relaxation, and breathing movements based on ancient Indian practices, has both physiological and psychological effects. Researchers have documented physical benefits to flexibility and muscular strength as well reductions in stress, anxiety, and chronic pain, and even increased adherence to other kinds of physical exercise programs.[72] Program 9.2 at the end of this chapter will guide you through several yoga routines.

Biofeedback **Biofeedback** involves monitoring physical stress responses such as brain activity, blood pressure, muscle tension, and heart rate with a special machine and then learning to consciously alter these responses. Biofeedback is effective for several stress-related conditions, including high blood pressure, headaches, irritable bowel syndrome, and asthma.[73]

Hypnosis **Hypnosis** trains a person to focus on one thought, object, or voice and to become unusually responsive to suggestion. A qualified hypnotherapist can implant a suggestion that directs a patient to resist habits such as smoking or overeating or to lessen phobias such as fear of snakes or air travel. The patient then learns to induce a state of self-hypnosis as a way to relax deeply and reinforce the behavioral changes.

People who exercise regularly and practice one or more of the relaxation methods listed above can achieve effective relief from stress symptoms. Many will also see improvement in medical conditions that are worsened by stress.

Cultivate Spirituality

Several medical studies have discovered correlations between spirituality and wellness. Prayer, for example, elicits the same relaxation response attained through other stress-management techniques: lowered blood pressure, heart rate, breathing and metabolism, and a more vigorous immune response.[74] Spirituality is also correlated with a reduced *perception* of stress in one's life.

Developing spirituality can be more than just an internal process. It can also be a social process that enhances your relationships with others. The abilities to give and take, speak and listen, and forgive and move on are integral to any process of spiritual development.

Live It!

Complete Worksheet 7 Developing Your Spirituality at MasteringHealth™.

LO 9.7 How Can I Create My Own Stress Management Plan?

At the end of this chapter, you will find tools to help you reduce your stress levels.

- **Lab 9.1** helps you assess situations that leave you susceptible to chronic stress. Using this information, target one or more behaviors that increase your stress.

- Evaluate the behavior(s) you have chosen. Identify your stress-producing behavior patterns. What can you change now or in the near future? Select one stress-producing behavior pattern that you want to change. For instance, **Lab 9.2** will help you manage your time more effectively.

- Use **Lab 9.3** to devise an action plan and create a behavior change contract. As you learned earlier, your behavior change contract should include your long-term goals for change, your short-term goals, the rewards you will give yourself for reaching these goals, potential

Do It!
Access these labs at the end of the chapter or online at MasteringHealth™.

obstacles along the way, and strategies for overcoming these obstacles.

Chart your progress in your journal. At the end of a week, evaluate how successful you were in following your plan. What helped you to be successful? What obstacles to change did you encounter? What will you do differently next week? After you assess yourself, make a plan and revise it as needed. Are your short-term goals attainable? Are the rewards satisfying? Do you need to enlist the help of your peers or professionals? If you think you need professional support, start by consulting the student health service for advice and direction on finding suitable counselors, therapists, or support groups.

See It!
Watch "'Generation Stress:' Tips for Millenials to Reduce Stress" at MasteringHealth™.

Study Plan

chapter summary

LO 9.1 **What Is Stress?**

- Stress is a disturbance of a person's normal state of equilibrium brought on by environmental or emotional stressors. The physiological stress response prepares the body to respond to the demand or perceived threat in a way that allows a return to normalcy.

LO 9.2 **How Does My Body Respond to Stress?**

- The physiological chain of events in the stress response starts when you perceive a stressor. The brain release of ACTH leads the adrenal glands to secrete cortisol and other stress hormones. These activate organs in various body systems to respond to the perceived threat.

LO 9.3 **Why Does Stress Cause Harm?**

- The general adaptation syndrome holds that stress disrupts the body's steady state, leading to alarm, resistance, and eventually an exhaustion of the resources needed to adapt to the stressor. This exhaustion allows illnesses to take hold.

- The allostatic load model holds that the body undertakes many simultaneous changes (allostasis) in response to a disturbance of homeostasis. Prolonged allostasis in response to chronic stress can cause allostatic load in which the body's own stress hormones cause accumulated wear and tear on organ systems.

LO 9.4 **What Kinds of Harm Can Stress Cause?**

- Stress can increase the heart rate and blood pressure and raise the risk of heart attack and stroke; decrease immunity and increase susceptibility to aberrant or invading cells; cause weight gain; alter blood sugar levels and contribute to pre-diabetes or diabetes; lead to indigestion, irritable bowel syndrome, and other digestive problems; diminish sexual drive and performance; and affect the skin and hair.

LO 9.5 **What Are the Major Sources of Stress?**

- Both internal and external factors can lead to stress, including change, performance demands, inconsistent goals and behaviors, overload, the physical environment, relationships, racial and cultural factors, and interpersonal conflict.

LO 9.6 **How Can I Manage Stress?**

- Build self-esteem and self-efficacy.
- Increase exercise and recreational activity.
- Improve diet and sleep and avoid substance use and abuse.
- Change your behavioral responses to cope and prepare for stressors.
- Manage your time, finances, thinking, and emotions.
- Seek social support.
- Learn relaxation techniques.

LO 9.7 **How Can I Create My Own Stress Management Plan?**

- Assess your stressors and stress responses and create a behavior change contract that puts the various kinds of stress management tools to work in your life.

review questions

LO 9.1 **1.** Graduating from college and moving to a new city can create stress as well as provide an opportunity for growth. This type of stress is called
  a. strain.
  b. distress.
  c. eustress.
  d. adaptive response.

LO 9.2 **2.** The physiological instinct to flee from or confront a threat is called
  a. homeostasis.
  b. the fight-or-flight response.
  c. allostasis.
  d. allostatic load.

LO 9.3 **3.** *Homeostasis* describes
  a. the body's "normal" or "steady state."
  b. long-term wear-and-tear on the body.
  c. sustained stress.
  d. the exhaustion stage of the general adaptation syndrome.

LO 9.3 4. Contemporary researchers have modified one stage of Hans Selye's general adaptation syndrome. Which one is it?
a. The alarm stage
b. The resistance stage
c. The allostasis stage
d. The exhaustion stage

LO 9.3 5. *Allostatic load* refers to
a. changes that occur in the body to maintain homeostasis.
b. long-term wear-and-tear on the body caused by stress.
c. the first stage of the general adaptation syndrome.
d. eustress.

LO 9.4 6. Which of the following statements is true?
a. Stress reduces the risk of cardiovascular disease.
b. Stress improves immune system function.
c. Stress alleviates depression and anxiety.
d. Stress reduces overall health and wellness.

LO 9.5 7. Change, hassles, performance demands, and burnout are all examples of
a. psychosocial sources of stress.
b. environmental sources of stress.
c. internal sources of stress.
d. homeostasis.

LO 9.6 8. Effective stress management includes
a. getting by on little sleep.
b. reducing exercise and physical activity to allow more time for studying.
c. eating fast food and junk food to save money and provide comfort.
d. avoiding alcohol and tobacco.

LO 9.6 9. *Relaxation breathing* refers to
a. inhaling deeply and rhythmically to relieve tension and increase oxygen levels in the blood.
b. progressive muscle relaxation.
c. monitoring physical stress responses and then consciously working to alter those responses.
d. biofeedback.

LO 9.6 10. What stress-fighting technique allows people to become unusually responsive to suggestion?
a. Meditation
b. Massage
c. Biofeedback
d. Hypnosis

LO 9.7 11. Creating a behavior change contract for stress management includes all but
a. rewarding yourself for small successes.
b. identifying short-term goals.
c. keeping a list of each failed attempt.
d. identifying long-term goals.

critical thinking questions

LO 9.1, LO 9.3 1 Compare and contrast distress and eustress. In what ways are both types of stress potentially harmful?

LO 9.2 2. Describe five steps in the body's physiological response to stress.

LO 9.3 3. Compare the general adaptation syndrome and allostatic load.

LO 9.4 4. What are some of your own health issues that arise from chronic stress?

LO 9.5 5. List several important sources of stress for college students, and explain how social support, self-esteem, personality, and coping strategies may make a person more or less susceptible.

LO 9.6 6. Which stress management tools have you tried and which could you add after reading this chapter?

check out these eResources

- **American Foundation for Suicide Prevention** Important tips on suicide prevention, including warning signs and risk factors. **www.afsp.org**
- **American Psychological Association** Information on a wide range of mental health and emotional issues. **www.apa.org/topics**
- **Buddhify** and **Personal Zen** Two sites offering mobile phone apps that can help you de-stress. **buddhify.com** and **www.personalzen.com**

- **Mayo Clinic** and **American College of Sports Medicine** Two sites with information on how exercise can help you reduce stress. **www.mayoclinic.org** and **www.acsm.org**
- **National Center for Complementary and Integrative Health** Resources for using yoga and meditation to manage stress. **https://nccih.nih.gov**

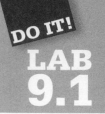

ASSESS YOURSELF
HOW STRESSED
ARE YOU?

MasteringHealth™

Name: _____ Date: _____

Instructor: _____ Section: _____

Purpose: To uncover your major stressors and your stress levels during the past year.

Directions: Learning to "de-stress" starts with an honest examination of your life experiences and your reactions to stressful situations. Respond to each section, assigning points as directed. Total the points from each section, then under Section III: Scoring, add them and compare to the life-stressor scale.

Section I: Recent History

In the last year, how many of the following major life events have you experienced? (Give yourself five points for each event you experienced; if you experienced an event more than once, give yourself 10 points, etc.)

1.	Death of a close family member or friend	_____
2.	Ending a relationship (whether by your own choice or not)	_____
3.	Major financial issue(s) jeopardizing your ability to stay in college	_____
4.	Major move, leaving friends, family, and past activities behind	_____
5.	Serious illness (your own)	_____
6.	Serious illness (of someone close to you)	_____
7.	Marriage or entering a serious relationship	_____
8.	Loss of a beloved pet	_____
9.	Involvement in a legal dispute or issue	_____
10.	Involvement in a hostile, violent, or threatening relationship	_____
Total Points		_____

Section II: Self-Reflection

For each of the following, indicate where you are on the scale of 0 to 5, then add up the points.

		Strongly Disagree				Strongly Agree	
1.	I have a lot of worries at home and at school.	0	1	2	3	4	5
2.	My friends or family members put too much pressure on me.	0	1	2	3	4	5
3.	I am often distracted and have trouble focusing on schoolwork.	0	1	2	3	4	5
4.	I am highly disorganized and do assignments at the last minute.	0	1	2	3	4	5
5.	My life seems to have far too many crisis situations.	0	1	2	3	4	5
6.	I spend a lot of time sitting; I don't have time to exercise.	0	1	2	3	4	5
7.	I don't have enough control in decisions that affect my life.	0	1	2	3	4	5
8.	I wake up most days feeling tired/like I need a lot more sleep.	0	1	2	3	4	5
9.	I often feel that I am alone and don't fit in very well.	0	1	2	3	4	5
10.	I have few friends or people with whom to share thoughts/feelings.	0	1	2	3	4	5
11.	I am uncomfortable in my body and wish I could change my looks.	0	1	2	3	4	5
12.	I'm unsure of whether my major will lead to a job after graduation.	0	1	2	3	4	5

(Continued)

		Strongly Disagree				Strongly Agree	
13.	If I have to wait, I quickly become irritated and upset.	0	1	2	3	4	5
14.	I get upset with myself unless I'm the best in activities and classes.	0	1	2	3	4	5
15.	World events upset me and I'm angry about people's behavior.	0	1	2	3	4	5
16.	I'm overloaded and there are never enough hours in the day.	0	1	2	3	4	5
17.	I feel uneasy when I'm caught up, relaxing, or doing nothing.	0	1	2	3	4	5
18.	I often check emails/tweets/text messages during the night.	0	1	2	3	4	5
19.	I seldom get enough alone time each day.	0	1	2	3	4	5
20.	I worry about whether or not others like me.	0	1	2	3	4	5
21.	I am struggling in my classes and worry about failing.	0	1	2	3	4	5
22.	My relationship with my family is distant and unsupportive.	0	1	2	3	4	5
23.	I tend to be critical and think negatively about the people I observe.	0	1	2	3	4	5
24.	Most people are selfish and distrustful and I'm careful around them.	0	1	2	3	4	5
25.	Life is basically unfair and most of the time, I can't change things.	0	1	2	3	4	5
26.	I give more than I get in relationships with people.	0	1	2	3	4	5
27.	What I do is often not good enough and I should do better.	0	1	2	3	4	5
28.	My friends would describe me as highly stressed and quick to react to people and events with anger and/or frustration.	0	1	2	3	4	5
29.	My friends are always telling me I "need a vacation to relax."	0	1	2	3	4	5
30.	Overall, the quality of my life right now isn't all that great.	0	1	2	3	4	5
Total Points							

Section III: Scoring

Total your points from Sections I and II: _____

The following scores are not meant to be diagnostic, but they do serve as an indicator of potential problem areas. If your scores are:

0–50, your stress levels are low. It is still worth examining areas where you did score points and taking action to reduce your stress levels further.

51–100, your stress levels are moderate, and you may need to reduce certain stresses in your life. Long-term stress and pressure can be counterproductive. Consider what you can do to change your perceptions, your behaviors, or your environment.

101–150, your stress levels are high, and you are probably quite stressed. Examine your major stressors and begin making a plan right now to reduce your stress levels. Delaying this action could lead to significant stress-related problems that affect your wellness, your grades, your social life, and your future!

151–200, you are carrying very high stress and without some significant changes, you could be heading for some serious difficulties. Locate a campus counselor with whom you can share the major issues you just identified as causing stress. Aim to get more sleep and exercise and find time to relax. Surround yourself with people who are supportive and make you feel safe and competent.

Section IV: Reflection

Were you surprised by your total stress score? Go back over the list of stressors and find two that you could eliminate with simple actions. Write them here along with the action for each.

Stressor _____ Action _____

Stressor _____ Action _____

DO IT!

LAB
9.2

LEARN A SKILL

MANAGING YOUR TIME

MasteringHealth™

Name: _____   **Date:** _____

Instructor: _____   **Section:** _____

Purpose: Learn a concrete way to manage your time so you can accomplish the things you want to.

Section I: Analyzing Your Time

Every evening for a week fill out the following table, listing how much time you spent doing each activity that day.

Activity	Monday	Tuesday	Wednesday	Thursday	Friday	Saturday	Sunday	Total Hours
Getting ready								
On the road								
In class								
Working for pay								
Exercising								
Eating								
Studying								
Watching TV or movies								
Using computer (school)								
Using computer (recreational)								
Spending time with friends								
Leisure activities								
Sleeping								
Other (specify)								

At the end of the week, total the hours for each activity. Are there any activities that you would like to do more or less frequently? You can use the rest of this lab to clarify your goals and set up your calendar so that you accomplish the things that you want to accomplish.

Section II: Clarify Your Goals and Create Your Task List

1. On a piece of paper, or in a journal, list your goals down the left side. Goals can be anything from "go to nursing school" to "learn to play racquetball." Make the goals specific. Instead of "be more musical," come up with a concrete goal such as "learn to play guitar."

2. On the right side of the paper, break each of your goals down into specific tasks. For example, as part of the nursing school goal, you might add "make a list of possible schools" to the task list.

3. Next, prioritize the tasks by numbering them in order of importance.

Section III: Enter Your Tasks Onto Your Calendar

In your calendar, write the commitments you already have—classes, job, exercise, rehearsals, and so on. Be sure to look at the schedule you filled out in Section I. Now is your chance to think about what activities you want to continue and which you would like to curb.

When you have all of your commitments written in, you'll be able to see windows of free time in your schedule. Now review your task list from Section II and choose the most important tasks to put in your free time. Make sure these tasks are things that are really important to you to accomplish.

Section IV: Make it Happen

Go over your schedule at the start of each day. This gives you a chance to prepare for the day and remember things that you need to take with you. At the end of the day, cross off tasks you were able to accomplish and rearrange (or delete) tasks that you didn't do.

Section V: Reflection and Evaluation

1. Describe any times you found yourself procrastinating. What do you think caused that? Were you bored? Were you overwhelmed? What specific thing could you do next time to get back on track quicker? For example, if you were overwhelmed, is there an advisor you could talk to who could help you prioritize?

_____

_____

_____

2. Did you check your schedule each morning, write in tasks, check them off, and do weekly planning? If not, what got in the way? What could you do differently next time?

_____

_____

_____

3. Did you find other people encroaching on your time? What happened? How could you handle that differently next time?

_____

_____

_____

4. Review your goals and tasks for the next week, adjust the list to reflect tasks you've accomplished or any other changes, and then block off time on your calendar for the most important items. Remember that time management is an ongoing exercise. Spend at least 20 minutes at the start of your week planning for the upcoming week, then stay focused on the goals you want to accomplish!

DO IT!

**LAB
9.3**

PLAN FOR CHANGE

YOUR PERSONAL STRESS-
MANAGEMENT PLAN

MasteringHealth™

Name: _____ Date: _____

Instructor: _____ Section: _____

Purpose: To develop a stress-management plan that targets the key sources of stress in your life.

Section I: Examine Your Behavior and Attitudes

1. Enter your results from the Scoring section of Lab 9.1 here:

Score: _____ Stress level: _____

Suggested actions: _____

2. Do you feel that stress is a problem in your life right now?   ☐ Yes   ☐ No

If your score indicated high levels of stress in Lab 9.1, and yet you don't see stress as an issue to address, consider your readiness for change.

Section II: Identify Major Sources of Stress

After reviewing your entries in the stress survey in Lab 9.1, describe your main sources of stress, grouping them into the following categories:

College

_____

_____

Family

_____

_____

Fitness/Wellness Issues

_____

_____

Social Issues

_____

_____

Money Matters

_____

_____

Time-Management Issues

_____

_____

Section III: Set Realistic Goals

Use this chart to rank your top five stressors from Section II, in order of urgency. Note ways to modify or eliminate each stressor. Note stress-reduction techniques that you can apply when the stressor arises.

	Stressors	Can I Modify or Eliminate the Stressor? Y/N	Can I Reduce Stress Symptoms? Y/N
Most urgent	1.		
⇓	2.		
⇓	3.		
⇓	4.		
Least urgent	5.		

Section IV: Devise a Strategy and an Action Plan

Use this section to target the most urgent source of stress in your life first, and then address additional stressors as you feel ready to work on them.

1. Stressor: _____

2. Is it possible that I will need help from others? ☐ Y ☐ N

If yes, ask yourself the following:

What professional resources are available where I live, work, or go to school? _____

_____

_____

How can I get my friends or family involved? _____

_____

3. List general strategies for modifying or eliminating environmental stressors that apply to more than one of your most urgent examples: _____

_____

4. What stress-management techniques can I use to relieve my own ongoing or recurrent symptoms of stress? (Consider relaxation breathing, progressive muscle relaxation, visual imagery, meditation, yoga, improved fitness, improved diet, better time-management skills, and enhanced spiritual connectedness.)

_____

_____

5. How can I plan ahead to avoid this stressor in the future?

_____

_____

6. How will I reward myself for sticking to my plan? _____

_____

Section V: Create a Behavior Change Contract

Use the information from Section IV to develop a behavior change contract that targets the stressor(s) you selected. A basic behavior change contract is included at the front of this book.

Section VI: Reflection

How will you be better off by reducing the top stressors in your life?

_____

_____

Activate, Motivate, & Advance YOUR WELL-BEING

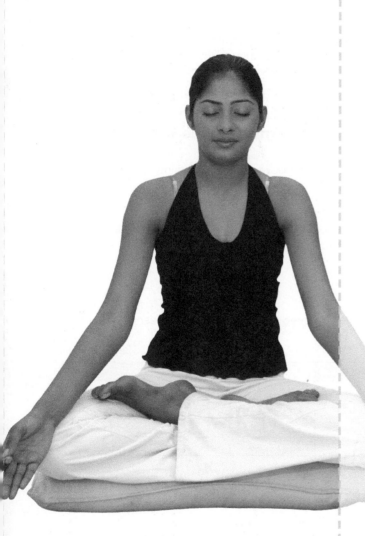

ACTIVATE!

Mindfulness meditation is a popular relaxation activity. We all experience tension from worrying about or anticipating our problems. Meditation can help us relax and compose ourselves. It instills a sense of well-being that improves many aspects of life. People who meditate regularly often enjoy a realistic sense of optimism, enhanced intimacy, more satisfying social relations, and a stronger ability to pay attention. In short, meditation brings physical, emotional, and intellectual enhancement.

What Do I Need?

LOCATION: You may meditate in your own living space, but be on the lookout for quiet places to meditate on campus, indoors or out.

TIME: If you live with others, plan to sit at a quiet time of the day, perhaps before your roommates get up or after they leave. Turn off your cell phone. Place a timer, such as a watch or digital alarm clock, in your meditation area so that you can set it and not have to be concerned with keeping track of time while you meditate.

POSTURE: Sitting on the floor with crossed legs is the best posture for meditation. Place your hands in your lap or on your thighs, whichever is comfortable for you. Sit on a firm cushion that supports your spine and lifts your buttocks higher than your knees.

The advantage of this posture is stability. The broad base supports you, inviting relaxation at the physical and mental level. The spine is self-supported and this discourages sleepiness and promotes balanced energy. Meditation is very much a physical activity.

If sitting on the floor is too uncomfortable, use a kneeling bench or sit on a firm chair such as a folding chair or a dining room chair. Sit toward the forward edge of the chair—don't lean against the backrest.

CLOTHING: Loose-fitting pants allow the abdomen to relax and the thighs to rotate outward, and bare feet are most comfortable for sitting cross-legged.

How Do I Start?

FOCUS ON YOUR BREATH: Close your eyes and draw your attention to the area of your abdomen that moves while breathing. Mindfully observe the movement of your abdomen as you inhale (outward abdomen movement) and exhale (inward abdomen movement). Make soft mental notes, "out" and "in."

Noticing the breath is the primary activity of meditation. It helps to sharpen and strengthen your attention.

- Don't exaggerate your breathing, let it be natural. Don't use your imagination to create an image of the breath, just attend to the sensations that are actually occurring.

- If your mind wanders, gently reapply your attention to your breath. You cannot control your mind with your will power. Relax! Make a mental note, "wandering, wandering," and focus on your breath again. Already you are learning about stress and how to let go.

- To avoid boredom, sleepiness, and wandering thoughts, notice the breath from the beginning, through the middle, to the end. By focusing on the sensations—stretching, tightness, swelling; then softness, cascading, and deflation—you will feel stress leave you.

- As you become more skilled, your attention will become sustained and steadier for longer periods of time. Gradually your mind will settle down and your body will relax. This composure of mind and body is energizing, bright, and pleasant.

FOCUS ON ANY FEELINGS OF DISCOMFORT: Physical pain or mental pain can be difficult for the body and mind. In trying to push them away, you may experience tension and stress. Turn toward what you have been avoiding and the rewards will be immediate.

- When physical pain or mental displeasure arises for you, track and scrutinize the sensation. Apply a soft mental label, like "pain" or "disliking," three or so times. Keep track of sensations you perceive as painful, like pressure, hardness, and heat, for example. The fear of pain will lose its grip as you see that pain is just a collection of intense sensations.

- When you are disturbed by thinking about someone you dislike, try saying this mantra: "If I have hurt, harmed, or offended anyone knowingly or unknowingly, may I be forgiven." Repeat that several times and then continue with this: "And anyone who may have hurt, harmed, or offended me knowingly or unknowingly, I freely forgive them."

- When the strength of attention on the discomfort weakens, turn back to your breath to make a fresh start, setting aside the negativity. Your composure will grow as you focus on the breath.

END THE SESSION by moving slowly. Take a little time to stretch and rest, write in your journal, and transition from quiet and stillness into activity.

- Wait 20 minutes or so before making phone calls, texting, or getting into conversations.

Four-Week Beginning Meditation Program

When you first sit down, take a few minutes to record notes. Write down what you observe about your breath. The purpose of this exercise is to enhance your ability to pay attention to the breath as it is, in the same spirit as if you were an artist who kept a sketchbook in which to record things seen during the day.

BEGINNER MEDITATION PROGRAM

Start at this level if you are new to meditation or have been away from your meditation practice for a year or more.

GOAL: Sit for 15 minutes every other day for four weeks.

	Mon	Tue	Wed	Thurs	Fri	Sat	Sun
Week 1	15 min		15 min		15 min		15 min
Week 2		15 min		15 min		15 min	
Week 3	15 min		15 min		15 min		15 min
Week 4		15 min		15 min		15 min	

MOTIVATE!

Keep a meditation journal to track the changing quality of your meditation experiences. Here are some additional meditation motivators:

ACCEPT THE CHALLENGE: Learning to meditate may sound simple, but it is a challenge! To do it, you must meet and overcome doubt, boredom, desire, irritability, and restlessness. Remember that being able to meet life's challenges with a calm mind is a valuable thing—worth working for.

FACE DISTRACTIONS: If you keep wanting to get up and eat something or check for text messages, then observe each mental interruption, acknowledge it, and let it go.

ENJOY THE FREEDOM: To detach from discomfort and taking things personally is a great relief. It is uplifting to relax in the face of annoyances that previously would have provoked resistance and retaliation. Introspection gives rise to insight and inner freedom.

JOIN A GROUP: Beginners can find it motivating to join a meditation class with a teacher. You may be able to find a meditation class through a yoga center, through your fitness instructor, or in a local alternative newspaper. If you sit with a group, you will enjoy the inspiration and support of the group energy and can begin to feel confident about the benefits of daily practice. If you can't find an established group, consider forming your own group of people with similar goals.

ATTEND A RETREAT: In addition to a weekly group, you may want to deepen your learning by going on a silent retreat. Retreats may be for a weekend or for as long as three months! Some retreats are specifically for young people.

ADVANCE!

Meditation is a lifelong affair. When you learn how to meditate, you learn how to be attentive and reflective all the time. You will want to meditate every day. People often find that 45 minutes to an hour daily is enough to see real effects in personality, friendships, and ability to concentrate on work.

INTERMEDIATE MEDITATION PROGRAM

Start at this level if you have been consistently meditating for 15 to 20 minutes three to four days a week for three months or more.

GOAL: Sit for 20 minutes five days a week, working up to sitting daily for a minimum of 20 minutes.

	Mon	Tue	Wed	Thurs	Fri	Sat	Sun
Week 1	20 min	20 min		20 min	20 min		
Week 2	20 min	20 min	20 min	20 min	20 min		
Week 3	20 min	20 min	20 min	20 min	20 min	20 min	
Week 4	20 min	20 min	20 min	20 min	20 min	20 min	20 min

Activate, Motivate, & Advance YOUR WELL-BEING

ACTIVATE!

Yoga is a fun physical and psychological practice that incorporates stretching, relaxation, and breathing movements to bring greater balance to body and mind. Yoga's benefits range from enhancing flexibility and muscular strength to reducing tension and stress. The postures can renew and invigorate the body through stretching and strengthening. Breathing techniques can release tension and stress and bring an overall calmness of mind and spirit. This program will help you get started with basic yoga.

What Do I Need?

MATERIALS: Choose a mat that will provide traction as well as cushioning. You may also want to use blocks and straps. They help support the body for postures that might be challenging, especially in the beginning.

LOCATION: You can practice yoga anywhere big enough to lay down a mat. Choose a space that is calm, quiet, and comfortable in light and temperature.

CLOTHING: Wear comfortable clothing that allows you to move freely.

How Do I Start?

BREATHING: Your breath (referred to as *pranayama* in yoga exercises) is the most important part of yoga. Aim for deep breaths, inhaling and exhaling from the belly. Never force or strain your breathing.

- The most common breath used during yoga is called *ujjayi* (pronounced *ooo-ja-i-aa*). Practice this breath while in a seated position. Once you can sustain your ability to breathe in this manner, begin using it during yoga practice.

- To perform ujjayi breathing, inhale and exhale slowly and deeply through the nose. You will begin to slightly constrict the passage of air. Your breathing will sound like Darth Vader or like you are trying to fog up a pair of glasses.

- During your yoga practice, every time you lift your chest, inhale, and when you drop your chest, exhale. If you are holding a pose, breathe deeply and slowly so you can hear yourself breathe.

TECHNIQUES: Yoga postures focus on aligning the body. Follow these techniques as you practice the different poses:

- Maintain an active back extension using core strength, with a neutral spine and pelvis.

- During forward bending, hinge from the hips, engaging the abdominal muscles, and keep your knees soft to maintain length and strength in the spine. Avoid bending from the lumbar spine. When returning to a neutral spine from a forward bend, soften your knees and use the muscles in your legs to push you back to a neutral position.
- Keep your shoulders relaxed and down away from your ears to avoid tension in your neck and shoulders. Keep your head in line with the spine. You can look up, center, or down, as long as your head remains a natural extension of the spine.
- To avoid unnecessary stress to the low back when coming into and out of forward bending in standing poses, sweep your arms out to the sides instead of bringing your arms out in front of you.
- To prevent joint injuries and muscular imbalances, distribute your weight evenly onto your hands and/or feet when setting the foundation of a pose. Always keep your knees in line with your toes.

Four-Week Yoga Program

Examples of the poses you'll perform are on pages 345–346. Hold each pose for one count of breath as you inhale and one count of breath as you exhale.

- Start each session with corpse pose for one minute, which means you will simply lie down on your back, close your eyes, and scan your body for any tension. Breathe with slow, deep inhales and exhales; if you notice any tension in some area of your body, release it as you exhale.
- For greater relaxation and meditation, end each session with the corpse pose for 5 to 10 minutes.

BEGINNER YOGA PROGRAM

Start here if you're new to yoga or if you've practiced yoga in the past but have taken a break.

GOAL: Practice a basic yoga sequence two to four times a week, building to a total of 120 minutes by week four (30 to 60 minute sessions).

	Mon	Tue	Wed	Thurs	Fri	Sat	Sun
	T	T	T	T	T	T	T
Week 1	20			20			
Week 2	25		25		25		
Week 3	30		30		30		
Week 4	30		30		30		30

T = Total time of session in minutes.

Order of Poses

Corpse Pose
Cat/Cow
Spinal Balance
Downward Facing Dog
Warrior 1 (left foot forward, right foot back, and anchored to the floor)
Triangle
Downward Facing Dog
Warrior 2 Cat/Cow

Extended Angle
Corpse Pose
Downward Facing Dog
Warrior 1 (right foot forward, left foot back, and anchored to the floor)
Triangle
Warrior 2
Extended Angle

MOTIVATE!

The entire yoga practice is about relaxing and listening inwardly to reduce tightness, anxiety, and mind chatter. Keeping a yoga journal of how you feel when doing each pose can help you become aware of your own practice. Here are some other motivators to keep you going when your mind and body want to quit:

NO TIME? NEVER MIND! If you are having difficulty committing to a longer practice, start with some deep breathing, neck circles, and then reach your arms up and stretch long. You're already on your way to feeling the benefits of stretching and breathing!

FIND A FRIEND: Find a friend who will encourage you to stick with your yoga program or even join you. Use the power and motivation of holding each other accountable and committed to the practice.

TRY A NEW STYLE: There are many different styles of yoga. Seek out classes that sound fun at your school, gym, or local yoga studio. *Bikram* yoga is done in a very hot room, *Iyengar* emphasizes alignment and perfecting poses, and *vinyasa* is a flowing series that warms and energizes the body in an aerobic practice.

ADVANCE!

Now it's time to become even more present with your breath and dedicate yourself to building a healthier body and a calmer mind. Start each session with corpse pose (one minute) and end each session by sustaining corpse pose for 5–10 minutes.

INTERMEDIATE YOGA PROGRAM

Start here if you have been practicing yoga consistently two to three times a week for two months or more.

GOAL: Practice a basic yoga sequence three to five times a week, building to 250 minutes of yoga per week and six counts of breath per pose by week four.

	Mon		Tue		Wed		Thurs		Fri		Sat		Sun	
	T	B	T	B	T	B	T	B	T	B	T	B	T	B
Week 1	40	1I 1E			40	1I 1E			40	1I 1E				
Week 2	40	1I 1H 2E			40	1I 1H 2E			40	1I 1H 2E			40	1I 1H 2E
Week 3	40	2I 1H 2E			40	2I 1H 2E	40	2I 1H 2E	40	2I 1H 2E			40	2I 1H 2E
Week 4	50	2I 2H 2E			50	2I 2H 2E	50	2I 2H 2E	50	2I 2H 2E			30	2I 2H 2E

T = Total time of session in minutes.
B = Counts per breath (or for holding the breath) for each pose. For example,
1I = inhale for 1 count; 1H = hold the breath for 1 count; 1E = exhale for 1 count.

Order of Poses

Repeat this sequence the more your body adjusts to the added time.

Cat/Cow
Spinal Balance
Downward Facing Dog
Warrior 1 (left foot forward, right foot back and anchored to the floor)
Warrior 2
Triangle
Extended Angle
Triangle
Warrior 2
Warrior 1
Extended Angle
Downward Facing Dog
Cat/Cow

Downward Facing Dog
Warrior 1 (right foot forward, left foot back and anchored to the floor)
Warrior 2
Triangle
Extended Angle
Triangle
Warrior 2
Warrior 1
Extended Angle
Downward Facing Dog
Cat/Cow
Corpse Pose

BASIC YOGA POSES

Cat/Cow

Strengthens: Core stabilizers, neck, and shoulders

Stretches: Core stabilizers

Getting into the pose: From all fours, with your wrists on the floor directly under your shoulders and your knees directly under

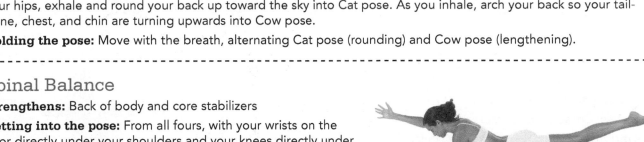

your hips, exhale and round your back up toward the sky into Cat pose. As you inhale, arch your back so your tailbone, chest, and chin are turning upwards into Cow pose.

Holding the pose: Move with the breath, alternating Cat pose (rounding) and Cow pose (lengthening).

Spinal Balance

Strengthens: Back of body and core stabilizers

Getting into the pose: From all fours, with your wrists on the floor directly under your shoulders and your knees directly under your hips, extend one arm forward and lift the opposite leg backward, so your arm, torso, and leg form one straight line.

Holding the pose: Keep your core stabilizer muscles active to support your midsection. Look toward the ground and focus on lengthening, instead of lifting higher. Avoid collapsing into the supporting shoulder. After holding one side for the recommended time, alternate sides.

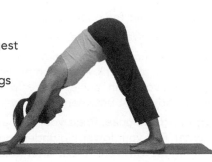

Downward Facing Dog

Strengthens: Upper body

Stretches: Shoulders, hamstrings, calves, and latissimus dorsi (or "lats," your largest back muscles)

Getting into the pose: Start in Child's pose on the floor, face down, with your legs tucked under you (so you are sitting on your heels) and your arms extended outwards. From Child's pose, with your palms flat on the floor, shoulder width apart, come up onto all fours, tucking your toes under and pressing your hips high and back away from your hands. Straighten your legs (if appropriate), and lift your knee caps upward while pressing your heels down.

Holding the pose: Lift your tailbone while pushing your palms forward and your heels back and down. Let your chest, shoulders, head, and neck sink toward the floor, and breathe into your back. Make sure your weight is equally distributed across your hands and into your thumbs and fingers.

Warrior 1

Strengthens: Quads and glutes

Stretches: Latissimus dorsi and hip flexors

Getting into the pose: From a lunge, with heel-to-heel alignment, point your front toes straight ahead, with your back foot turned outward so your heel is the furthest point away from you. Lift your arms up, bending the front knee to 90 degrees, keeping it over the ankle. Bring your chest and naval forward without lifting your back heel.

Holding the pose: Let your lower body sink and lift your upper body. Move away from your navel, stretching the mat out in both directions. Avoid moving your front knee past your front ankle. Bring your arms behind your ears and draw your chin back gently. After holding one side for the recommended time, alternate sides.

Warrior 2

Strengthens: Quads and glutes

Stretches: Chest and adductors

Getting into the pose: From a wide stance, float your arms out at shoulder height. Point your front toes straight ahead, keeping your back heels flat and pushed out so they are the furthest point away from you. Bend your front knee to 90 degrees and keep it over your front ankle. Keep your hips level and point your navel toward the side.

Holding the pose: The focal point is your front fingertips. Continue stretching away from the center of your body so your lower body drops and your upper body lifts. Maintain your front knee to ankle alignment. Relax your shoulders and collarbones down. After holding one side for the recommended time, alternate sides.

Triangle

Strengthens: Torso and legs

Stretches: Waist and hamstrings

Getting into the pose: From Warrior 2, straighten your forward leg, reaching forward with your hand and back with the hips. Hinging over towards your front leg, rest your front hand on your shin, ankle, or the floor. Revolve your chest toward the sky, imagining your body is flat between two panes of glass and in line with the heels.

Holding the pose: Press your feet away from one another, and expand away from the center. Roll your lower hip under and avoid letting your torso, neck, and head fall out of alignment with your heels. After holding one side for the recommended time, alternate sides.

Extended Angle

Strengthens: Quads and glutes

Stretches: Groin, adductors, waist

Getting into the pose: From a wide stance (such as a lunge), turn your front toes straight ahead with your back toes turned in slightly. Bend your front knee, and bring down your front arm until your hand is inside the front foot, lining your arm up with your lower leg. Extend your top arm to the sky, and if comfortable, look up.

Holding the pose: Your chest revolves upwards as your shoulder presses into your knee. Drop your hips down and press them forward, keeping them in alignment with your heels. There should be a straight line from your back heel to your fingertips. After holding one side for the recommended time, alternate sides.

Reducing Your Risk of Cardiovascular Disease

10

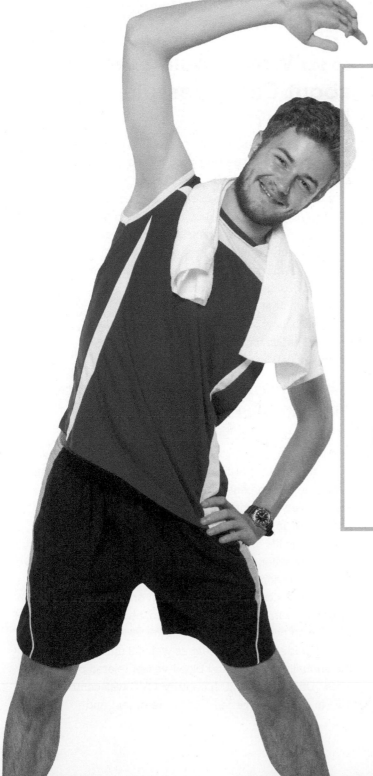

LEARNINGoutcomes

LO 10.1 Define cardiovascular disease (CVD), explain why a college student should be concerned about CVD, and list the human and economic impacts of CVD.

LO 10.2 Explain how CVD affects the heart and blood vessels and list some symptoms CVD can cause.

LO 10.3 Describe various forms of CVD, including hypertension, atherosclerosis, stroke, heart disease, and others.

LO 10.4 Outline the main risk factors for CVD, including those you can and cannot control.

LO 10.5 Create a plan and apply behavior-change skills to lower your own risk of CVD.

MasteringHealth™

Go online for chapter quizzes, interactive assessments, videos, and more!

DARYL

"Hi, I'm Daryl. I'm a junior, majoring in education. I'm also a jazz pianist and I play at clubs around town about three times a week. I love jazz, and the gigs help me pay my college tuition.

"I think I'm pretty healthy—I've never been hospitalized for anything—but I do have a family history of heart disease. Both of my grandfathers died from heart attacks when they were in their 40s. My dad died of a stroke when I was 10, and my mom is currently taking pills for high blood pressure and high cholesterol. I know I'm still young, but with my family history, I'm worried. Is it too early for me to start doing something to protect myself? What should I do? And how can I help my mom?"

Hear It!
To listen to this case study online, visit the Study Area in MasteringHealth™.

TABLE **10.1 Six Leading Causes of Death in the United States**	
Cause	Number of deaths
Heart disease	611,105
Cancer	584,881
Chronic lower respiratory diseases	149,209
Accidents (unintentional injuries)	130,557
Stroke	128,978
Alzheimer's disease	84,767

Data from Centers for Disease Control and Prevention and National Center for Health Statistics, "Leading Causes of Death," October 2015, www.cdc.gov

LO 10.1 Why Should I Worry about Cardiovascular Disease?

As a college student, your most pressing concerns are probably things like getting good grades, paying tuition, and landing a job. CVD could be the furthest thing from your mind. However, it is not too early to start learning about CVD. For many people, the earliest manifestations of heart and blood vessel diseases take root during childhood and early adulthood, especially if they are overweight or obese.[6] While family history plays an important role, lifestyle choices that you make now—such as whether to smoke, how often to exercise, how you manage stress, and your habits day to day—can also greatly influence your risk.

Live It!
Complete Worksheet 39 Healthy Heart IQ at MasteringHealth™.

Cardiovascular Disease Is America's Biggest Killer

CVD and stroke account for about 29 percent of all deaths in the United States each year—more than any other single cause of death in America.[7] In fact, CVD has been the leading cause of death in the United States almost every year since 1900. If we completely eliminated CVD in the United States, experts estimate that our average life expectancy would rise by almost seven years.[8] Together, heart disease and strokes kill more Americans each year—both men *and* women and people of various races—than cancer or any other cause (see the Diversity box Men, Women, and Cardiovascular Disease on page 349).

CVD is a global problem as well; 18 million people die annually of heart- and blood-vessel-related problems.[9] Until the mid-20th century, CVD was common only in affluent societies. Today, treatment and

---

Cardiovascular disease (CVD) describes diseases of the heart and blood vessels brought on by a buildup of fatty accumulations that restrict or block blood flow. CVD can have devastating consequences such as a heart attack or stroke, which are the number one and number six leading causes of death in America (**Table 10.1**).[1]

You may think that cardiovascular problems strike only old people. In fact, about 40 percent of women and men between the ages of 20 and 49 have some indicators of CVD including elevated blood pressure and blood levels of cholesterol.[2] Of those under 40, 9 to 15 percent have actual CVD.[3] The rates of high blood pressure, high cholesterol, and CVD nearly double during middle age.[4] Overall, one-third of adult Americans have CVD; by retirement age and older, the number reaches three-quarters.[5]

cardiovascular disease (CVD) A disease of the heart and/or blood vessels

DIVERSITY
Men, Women, and Cardiovascular Disease

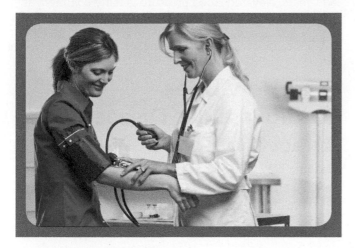

Many people know that heart attacks and other outcomes of cardiovascular disease are the leading causes of death in American men. Fewer realize, however, that cardiovascular disease is the leading cause of death in American women as well. The most recent American Heart Association statistics show that all forms of CVD claimed 398,086 female victims and 402,851 male.[1] This figure for women is higher than the number of female lives lost to all forms of cancer, diabetes, and lung diseases *combined*.

Many students also don't realize that cardiovascular disease affects young people, too. The American Heart Association considers seven measures (non-smoking, BMI, diet, exercise, blood pressure, blood cholesterol, and blood glucose) in its assessment of ideal cardiovascular health. Only 8 percent of American adults between ages 20 and 39, including both men and women, have even five out of seven ideal measures.[2] Although all the numbers are below 28 percent for both sexes, women are more likely than men to have four, five, or six of the ideal measures and men are more likely than women to have just one, two, or three of the measures.

When less-than-ideal prevention leads to outright cardiovascular disease, men and women show different patterns and symptoms. For example:

- Men tend to develop coronary heart disease 10 to 15 years earlier than women, and throughout the world, this fact accounts for men's shorter life expectancies.[3] Women rarely have heart attacks before menopause (early 50s), but they catch up to men by their 80s.[4]

- Men and women experience different heart attack symptoms. Men tend to experience the classic "squeezing" sensation in the chest, pain in the chest or arm, and/or shortness of breath. Women, however, are less likely to feel these symptoms. Instead, they are more likely to experience shortness of breath, weakness or fatigue, a cold sweat, or dizziness. If they feel any localized pressure, it tends to be between the shoulder blades rather than in the chest or arm. Women are also more likely than men to have early warning symptoms up to one month before a heart attack, including unusual fatigue, sleep disturbances, shortness of breath, indigestion, and anxiety.[5] However, because they often don't recognize these symptoms as a heart attack, women are more likely than men to delay treatment and die from the initial attack.

- Looking at cardiovascular disease as a whole, men are more likely to have heart attacks, while women with CVD are more likely to have strokes. This is perhaps based on the smaller diameter of women's blood vessels and the greater tendency for men under stress to display high blood pressure and women under stress to form blood clots.[6]

APPLY IT! For both sexes, most risk factors remain the same as do the steps you can take to prevent CVD. The American Heart Association calls these Life's Simple Seven:

1. Don't smoke
2. Eat better
3. Get active
4. Manage your blood pressure
5. Stay at a healthy weight
6. Manage your blood sugar
7. Manage your blood cholesterol.[7]

Sources:
1. American Heart Association, "Statistical Fact Sheet 2015 Update: Women and Cardiovascular Disease," 2015, www.heart.org; D. Mozaffarian et al., "Heart Disease and Stroke Statistics—2016 Update," *Circulation* 133, no. 4 (2015), doi: 10.1161/CIR.0000000000000350; D. Mozaffarian et al., "Executive Summary: Heart Disease and Stroke Statistics—2016 Update," *Circulation* 133 (2016): 447–54, doi: 10.1161/CIR. 0000000000000366
2. Mozaffarian et al., "Heart Disease and Stroke Statistics," 2015.
3. H. Beltran-Sanchez, C. E. Finch, and E. M. Crimmins, "Twentieth Century Surge of Excess Male Mortality," *Proceedings of the National Academy of Sciences* 112, no. 29 (2015), doi: 10.1073/pnas.142194112
4. Ibid.
5. Mozaffarian et al., "Heart Disease and Stroke Statistics," 2015.
6. Z. Samad et al., "Sex Differences in Platelet Reactivity and Cardiovascular and Psychological Response to Mental Stress in Patients with Stable Ischemic Heart Disease," *Journal of the American College of Cardiology* 64, no. 16 (2014): 1669–78, doi: 10.1016/j.jacc.2014.04.087
7. American Heart Association, "My Life Check—Life's Simple Seven," updated August 10, 2015, www.heart.org

prevention have markedly improved death rates in high-income countries while low- and middle-income countries are shouldering 80 percent of the global burden of CVD in terms of health costs, premature deaths, and lost productivity.[10] The GetFitGraphic on page 351 illustrates the prevalence of CVD around the world as well as simple preventive measures—the so-called "simple seven"—that could eliminate much of this burden.[11]

Cardiovascular Disease Can Greatly Decrease Your Quality of Life

Even when CVD is not fatal, it can seriously impact daily life. Heart attack and stroke survivors may lose their ability to walk, talk, read, exercise, or carry out other daily activities. CVD can cause chest pain, shortness of breath, and damage to internal organs. It can also require expensive drugs, which have their own negative side effects.

Cardiovascular Disease Can Begin Early in Life

Childhood and early adolescence are often when people first start experiencing the risk factors for CVD—poor diet, lack of exercise, BMI above 25, and smoking.[12] Obese children already show many physical markers for CVD, including type 2 diabetes, high blood pressure, high LDL ("bad") cholesterol levels, and high blood sugar levels.[13] One research team even looked at very early indicators of CVD risk in 1- to 5-year-old children. They found that kids with the lowest levels of vitamin D through diet and sunlight had the highest levels of the cholesterol associated with CVD risk in adults.[14]

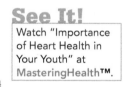

See It!
Watch "Importance of Heart Health in Your Youth" at MasteringHealth™.

A now-classic study of blood vessel tissue from 3,000 young people between the ages of 15 and 34 who had died of accidents, homicides, or suicides discovered glistening streaks of fat and fatty buildup inside some of their blood vessels—deposits that marked the unmistakable beginnings of CVD. The researchers found early signs of CVD in 2 percent of males aged 15 to 19. They also observed advanced markers of CVD in 20 percent of males and 8 percent of females in the 30- to 34-year-old age group. The young people who died with blood vessel deposits already starting to accumulate had, during their short lives, displayed poorer diet, less exercise, higher BMI, and/or more smoking than the young people who died lacking those deposits.[15]

plaques A pinpoint area of fatty, waxy debris that accumulates at a site along the inner wall of an artery or arteriole

One result of such vessel buildup is elevated blood pressure. Young teens who watch TV and snack on junk food for a couple of hours a day already show higher blood pressure readings, as do obese teens.[16] By the college years, elevated blood pressure is fairly common, as the Diversity box College Students and Hypertension explains on page 352.

LO 10.2 How Does Cardiovascular Disease Affect the Body?

Learning how CVD affects your body will help you understand why it causes the symptoms it does and what you can do to keep your cardiovascular system healthy.

Cardiovascular Disease Affects the Heart and Blood Vessels

Your body contains trillions of living cells, all needing a continuous supply of oxygen and energy compounds. The cardiovascular system—the heart and blood vessels—does the critical work of delivering that oxygen and energy *to* your cells. It also removes carbon dioxide and other waste products *from* your cells. (To review the anatomy of the cardiovascular system, see Chapter 3.)

Throughout the body, the walls of blood vessels are smooth inside and out. The walls of the arteries, which carry oxygen-rich blood away from the heart, are strong and elastic; the walls of the veins, which carry oxygen-depleted blood back toward the heart, are thinner and more fixed in diameter. In a healthy cardiovascular system, blood can flow freely down the long narrow opening in the middle of each vessel. The heart's ventricles fill smoothly and forcibly push blood out into the arteries. Tight-closing valves help prevent blood from flowing backward. The circulating blood reaches all the distant capillary beds in the brain, limbs, kidneys, skin, and other organs. It then returns quickly to the heart through the veins.

Atherosclerosis Lifestyle and genetic factors can cause deposits of fatty, waxy, yellowish, sludge-like debris called *atheromas* to accumulate inside arteries and smaller arterioles. Other substances such as calcium salts, cholesterol, cellular waste, blood clotting proteins, and white blood cells can accumulate around the atheromas, enlarging and solidifying the yellowish deposits into hardened blockages called **plaques**. These plaques, in turn, can bulge inward and restrict the vessels' inner

WHAT IS THE IMPACT OF CARDIOVASCULAR DISEASE ON SOCIETY?

CVD takes a huge toll on the U.S. and globally: it affects over 80% of Americans at some point during their lives and costs billions of dollars in annual medical expenses. Here are a few figures and facts about the impact of CVD on society.

HOW COMMON IS CVD IN THE U.S.?

The prevalence of CVD increases with age, affecting 4 out of 5 Americans by the age of 80.[1]

Age	Male	Female
20–39 years old	11.9%	10.0%
40–59 years old	40.5%	35.5%
60–79 years old	69.1%	67.9%
80 years & older	84.7%	85.9%

What are the annual MEDICAL COSTS of CVD in the U.S.?

Coronary heart disease	**$215.6**
Hypertension	**$46.4**
Stroke	**$33.6**
Other	**$24.6**
TOTAL	**$320.2**

Estimated costs in billions, 2010[2]

CVD RISKS and contributing FACTORS

- ☑ Age
- ☑ Sex
- ☑ Hereditary factors
- ☑ Smoking
- ☑ High blood pressure
- ☑ High blood cholesterol
- ☑ Physical inactivity
- ☑ Obesity and overweight
- ☑ Diabetes
- ☑ Stress
- ☑ Alcohol or drugs
- ☑ Diet

WHAT CAN I DO TO PREVENT CVD?

Although there are some risk factors that you cannot control (such as heredity, age, gender, and race), taking these steps may lessen your CVD risk:

- ☑ Don't smoke
- ☑ Eat a nutritious diet
- ☑ Exercise regularly
- ☑ Maintain a healthy weight
- ☑ Reduce stress
- ☑ Control diabetes
- ☑ Don't abuse drugs & alcohol

What is the global burden of annual CVD DEATHS?

Estimates rounded to the nearest thousand[4]

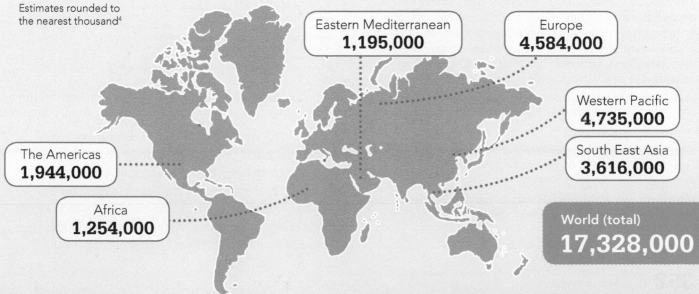

Eastern Mediterranean
1,195,000

Europe
4,584,000

Western Pacific
4,735,000

South East Asia
3,616,000

The Americas
1,944,000

Africa
1,254,000

World (total)
17,328,000

DIVERSITY
College Students and Hypertension

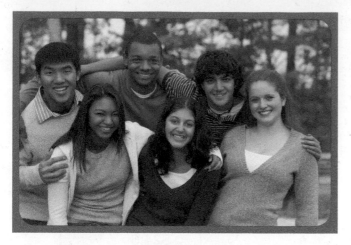

In a large recent survey of American college students, 4.4 percent report being treated for hypertension (high blood pressure) within the past year.[1] Does this mean students don't have to worry about blood pressure problems and related cardiovascular diseases?

Unfortunately, no. As rates of overweight and obesity rise among teens and young adults, indicators of present and future CVD rise as well. The same major survey found that 36.6 percent of American college students have a BMI indicating overweight (BMI 25 to 29.9) or obesity (BMI 30 to 40).[2]

A recent study of more than 700,000 adolescents found that as BMI increases, so do one or both blood pressure readings.[3] And experts are beginning to focus on prehypertension (blood pressure between 120/80 mm Hg and 139/89 mm Hg) as a good indicator of current and future cardiovascular problems.[4]

As hypertension began to appear in young people in the 1980s and 1990s, scientists began looking for the very earliest indicators and re-categorized prehypertension as a problem to watch in kids, teens, and young adults.[5] They found that about 30 percent of high school students have at least one reading in the prehypertension or hypertension range.[6] Elevated readings in one's teens or 20s—even if only in the prehypertension range—are associated with increased risk of atherosclerosis and other forms of CVD in middle age.[7]

A recent analysis of graduate students' heart health provides an instructive view for all students: Researchers collected data for three years during the students' graduate work and found that most of the students exercised at least three days per week, had BMIs under 25, and had healthy levels of blood glucose and fats. However, more than 25 percent had either hypertension or prehypertension; 30 percent got too little exercise, and a large majority (80.6 percent) ate few fruits and vegetables. In addition, over the three years, their exercise levels for both aerobic and strength training dropped, as did their sleep duration.[8] What this suggests is that even among highly educated young people, the effort of staying well begins to taper off as professional demands rise. With this decline come the seeds of future cardiovascular disease.

APPLY IT! The time to form good health habits is not in middle age when chronic diseases start to manifest themselves, but rather in your teens and 20s when body weight, blood pressure, and blood fats and sugars begin to climb. Hypertension can have devastating long-term effects on nearly every organ of the body. But here's the good news: Long-term studies show that young people with healthy blood pressure and few or no risk factors for CVD are much less likely to miss work or suffer disabilities of any kind later in life.[9]

Sources:
1. American College Health Association, *American College Health Association: National College Health Assessment II, Towson University Executive Summary, Spring 2015* (Hanover, MD: American College Health Association, 2015).
2. Ibid.
3. Y. Arbel et al., "Trends in Adolescents Obesity and the Association between BMI and Blood Pressure: A Cross Sectional Study in 714,922 Teenagers," *American Journal of Hypertension* (March 2015), doi: 10.1093/ajh/hpv007
4. N. B. Allen et al., "Blood Pressure Trajectories in Early Adulthood and Subclinical Atherosclerosis in Middle Age," *Journal of the American Medical Association* 311, no. 5 (2014): 490–97; S. Kishi et al., "Cumulative Blood Pressure in Early Adulthood and Cardiac Dysfunction in Middle Age: The CARDIA Study," *Journal of the American College of Cardiology* 65, no. 25 (2015): 2679–87, doi:10.1016/j.jacc.2015.04.042
5. K. M. Redwine and B. Falkner, "Progression of Prehypertension to Hypertension in Adolescents," *Current Hypertension Reports* 14, no. 6 (December 2012): 619–25.
6. A. A. Acosta et al., "Prevalence of Persistent Prehypertension in Adolescents," *Journal of Pediatrics* 160, no. 5 (May 2012): 757–61.
7. American Heart Association News, "Young Heart Health Linked to Better Overall Health in Later Years," November 16, 2014, http://newsroom.heart.org/news/sunday-news-tips-27755332?preview=83a9
8. Allen et al., "Blood Pressure Trajectories," 2014.
9. S. B. Racette, "Exercise and Cardiometabolic Risk Factors in Graduate Students: A Longitudinal, Observational Study," *Journal of American College Health* 62, no. 1 (January 2014): 47–56.

arterial stenosis A narrowing of the inner channel of arteries and smaller arterioles due to the buildup of a sludge-like layer of fatty, waxy debris

atherosclerosis Hardening or stiffening of the arteries as plaque accumulates, often at injury sites, in the inner linings of arteries

channels. This narrowing is called **arterial stenosis**. Plaques and blood clots can eventually grow large enough to block blood flow through the vessel (see **Figure 10.1**) or even cause the vessel to rupture.

The process of accumulation and restriction in blood vessels is known as **atherosclerosis** (from the Greek words *athero*, meaning "gruel," and *sclerosis*, meaning

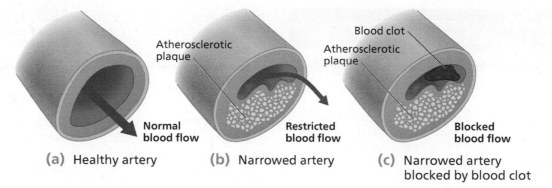

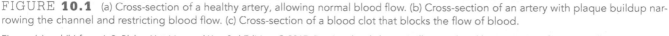

FIGURE 10.1 (a) Cross-section of a healthy artery, allowing normal blood flow. (b) Cross-section of an artery with plaque buildup narrowing the channel and restricting blood flow. (c) Cross-section of a blood clot that blocks the flow of blood.

Figures (a) and (b) from J. S. Blake, *Nutrition and You*, 3rd Edition, © 2015. Reprinted and electronically reproduced by permission of Pearson Education, Inc., Upper Saddle River, New Jersey.

"hardness"). Atherosclerosis is a major factor in many forms of CVD. The buildup process can take decades, but atherosclerosis can start in childhood, especially in the overweight and obese.[17]

Arteries with plaques on their walls transport less blood and are stiffer and less flexible. Just as the pressure builds up in a hose if you block normal water flow with your thumb, plaque buildup and channel narrowing can increase pressure within the blood vessels. The buildup can occur in the arteries that supply the heart, brain, kidneys, or other organs, or in peripheral arteries (often in the legs). Plaque in these areas can cause heart attacks, strokes, pain, and poor wound healing. Unhealthy habits, including smoking, chronic stress, inactivity, high alcohol consumption, high blood sugar, high blood pressure, obesity, and unfavorable levels of certain fats and cholesterol in the blood can all increase the speed and severity of atherosclerosis and, in turn, contribute to CVD.[18] Atherosclerotic CVD is America's leading cause of death and disability.[19]

In recent years, medical researchers have studied the role of *inflammation* in atherosclerosis. Inflammation is an immune response that causes redness and swelling in response to injury. Researchers think that the immune system recognizes plaque as abnormal and tries to wall off the deposits. Ironically, this low-grade inflammation inside blood vessels contributes to further plaque buildup. Eventually, inflammation can cause a bulging plaque deposit to rupture, leading to a blood clot, which, in turn, can cause a heart attack or stroke by blocking a vessel entirely.[20]

Several factors can injure the inner walls of blood vessels and promote inflammation at the injury site.[21] These include high blood levels of LDL (low-density lipoprotein) cholesterol, smoking, hypertension, diabetes mellitus, poor diet, alcohol consumption, and

disease-causing bacteria and viruses. The latter include *Chlamydia pneumoniae* (a common cause of respiratory infections), *Helicobacter pylori* (which can cause ulcers), herpes simplex virus (to which most Americans are exposed by age 5), and cytomegalovirus (another herpes virus transmitted through body fluids and infecting most Americans before age 40).

Several natural substances within the body serve as links between unhealthy lifestyle habits, inflammation in blood vessel walls, and CVD. Stored fat and associated immune cells in a person's fat tissue spew out proteins called *C-reactive proteins* (CRPs)—the more stored fat, the more CRPs. Alcohol consumption and diets low in whole grain, fruits, and green leafy vegetables can lead to higher levels of an amino acid called *homocysteine*.[22] Doctors use both CRPs and homocysteine as markers to predict and diagnose atherosclerosis. Researchers are discovering other blood fats and proteins, that can indicate risk for early stages of the disease.[23]

Lifestyle changes such as regular exercise, weight management, smoking cessation, moderation of alcohol intake, eating less sugar and refined carbohydrates, and consuming more whole grains and fruits and vegetables appear to reduce inflammation and its markers in the blood. Drugs called statins also reduce the inflammation associated with atherosclerosis.[24] CVD experts now believe that millions of Americans with elevated risk of heart attack or stroke should begin taking statin drugs, even if they don't show signs of CVD.[25]

LO 10.3 Cardiovascular Disease Takes Many Forms

Let's look at common forms of CVD and their prevalence in American adults (**Table 10.2**).

TABLE 10.2 Major Types of Cardiovascular Disease and Prevalence of Each

Type of Cardiovascular Disorder or Disease	Prevalence in the United States
Hypertension	80 million
Coronary heart disease (including heart attack)	15.5 million; 660,000 new and 305,000 recurrent heart attacks per year
Angina pectoris	8.2 million
Arrhythmia	2.7 million to 6.1 million
Congestive heart failure	5.7 million
Congenital cardiovascular defects	Eight defects per 1,000 live births
Stroke	6.6 million; 795,000 new or recurrent cases of stroke each year

Data from D. Mozaffarian et al., "Heart Disease and Stroke Statistics—2016 Update: A Report from the American Heart Association," *Circulation* 133, no. 4 (2015), doi: 10.1161/CIR.0000000000000350; D. Mozaffarian et al., "Executive Summary: Heart Disease and Stroke Statistics—2016 Update," *Circulation* 133 (2016): 447–54, doi: 10.1161/CIR. 0000000000000366

Hypertension **Hypertension**, or sustained high blood pressure, is the most common form of CVD. It is also considered a risk factor for other forms of CVD. About 30 percent of all Americans—more than 78 million people—have hypertension.[26] Because it has no initial symptoms, many are unaware that they have the condition.[27] In fact, some experts call hypertension the "silent killer."[28]

Hypertension damages blood vessels and promotes plaque development.[29] As mentioned earlier, plaque deposits and vessel-channel narrowing can in turn increase resistance to blood flow throughout the circulatory system and can cause blood pressure to rise further, creating a damaging cycle. In

hypertension Sustained blood pressure over 139/89 mm Hg

systolic pressure The pressure applied to the walls of the arteries when the heart contracts

diastolic pressure The pressure applied to the walls of the arteries during the heart's relaxation phase

addition to leading to other forms of CVD, hypertension can slow your thinking or make you more susceptible to dementia later in life.[30]

You may think of high blood pressure as an old person's disease. In fact, the earliest signs of it can start in childhood or adolescence and are common by college age. Hypertension can result from consuming too much salt and sugar (see the Q&A box Do Salt and Sugar Increase My Risk of Cardiovascular Disease? on page 355) Other causes of hypertension include kidney or heart abnormalities, aging, inherited tendencies, obesity, sleep apnea, stress, or certain kinds of tumors.

A blood pressure device can help diagnose hypertension. Such devices measure your blood pressure in two parts, expressed as a fraction—for example, 120/80. Both values are measured in millimeters of mercury (mm Hg). The first number refers to **systolic pressure**, the pressure being applied to the walls of the arteries when the heart contracts, pumping blood to the rest of the body. The second value is **diastolic pressure**, the pressure applied to the walls of the arteries during the heart's relaxation phase. During this phase, blood is reentering the heart's chambers, preparing for the next heartbeat.

Blood pressure varies, depending on an individual's weight, age, physical condition, gender, and ethnic background. Systolic blood pressure tends to increase with age, while diastolic blood pressure tends to increase until age 55, and then decline. Generally, men have a greater risk for high blood pressure than women until age 60; at that point, the risks begin to equalize. After age 80, women are more likely to have high blood pressure than men.[31]

For a healthy adult, normal systolic blood pressure is *less than* 120 mm Hg, and normal diastolic blood pressure is *less than* 80 mm Hg.[32] A physician may diagnose *prehypertension* or the potential beginnings of hypertension when blood pressure is above normal, but not yet in the hypertensive range (see **Table 10.3** on this page). Hypertension is usually diagnosed when systolic pressure is 140 or above. When only systolic pressure is high,

TABLE 10.3 Blood Pressure Readings

Classification	Systolic Reading (mm Hg)	Diastolic Reading (mm Hg)
Normal	Less than 120	Less than 80
Prehypertension	120–139	80–89
Hypertension		
Stage 1	140–159	90–99
Stage 2	160 or higher	100 or higher

Note: If systolic and diastolic readings fall into different categories, treatment is determined by the highest category. Readings are based on the average of two or more properly measured, seated readings on each of two or more health care provider visits.

Source: National Heart, Lung, and Blood Institute, "Description of High Blood Pressure," September 2015, www.nhlbi.nih.gov/health

Q&A Do Salt and Sugar Increase My Risk of Cardiovascular Disease?

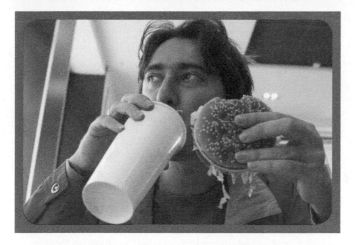

The average American adult consumes 3,592 mg of sodium per day in salt (NaCl)— about 1½ tsp. daily. This is one and a half times more than the recommended 2,300 mg per day for most adults and almost two and a half times more than the USDA-recommended level of 1,500 mg for those over 50, African Americans, and those who have high blood pressure.[1] Government health organizations advocate limiting salt because excess sodium promotes fluid retention. This, in turn, elevates blood pressure and contributes to hypertension and CVD. To get below 2,300 mg, most adults would have to cut overall salt consumption by about half a teaspoon or more.

Most of the salt in our national diet comes from processed foods, not overusing your salt shaker. A single serving of the following foods can equal nearly half of a day's recommended sodium: turkey lunch meat, chicken fingers, canned soup, frozen entrees, cheeseburger, pasta sauce, or barbecued pork. These can supply one third of a day's sodium or more: One slice of pizza, a corn dog, a tablespoon of soy sauce. And these foods are also high in sodium: bread, cheese, chips, cookies.[3]

A population-wide average drop in dietary salt by 1,200 mg/day could cut thousands of new cases of cardiovascular disease, and prevent thousands of strokes, heart attacks, and deaths each year. It would also save $18 billion in annual health care costs.[4] Researchers are currently debating what the ideal consumption levels should be. One Canadian study suggests that 2,300 mg/day is low enough while an American study projects that intake levels above 2,000 mg/day are killing 1.65 million people globally each year.[5] Regardless of the exact figures, it's clear that the typical college diet is loaded with salt and it's a good idea to cut back.

What about sugar? Surprisingly, researchers predict that added sugars and other sweeteners may have an even greater impact on CVD than salt.[6] The average American consumes 15 percent of daily calories as added sugars (sucrose, corn syrup, brown sugar, honey, agave syrup, concentrated fruit juice, and so on). That's 300 to 450 calories in a 2,000 to 3,000 calorie per day diet. Most of this extra sugar comes from sweetened sodas, sports drinks, energy drinks, coffee drinks, and tea drinks. Pastries, desserts, candy, ice cream, cookies, energy bars, and other sweets contribute significant amounts as well.

Like salt, sugar takes a toll on our cardiovascular health by increasing weight gain and by raising both glucose and triglyceride levels in the blood. Consuming an extra 2.6 ounces per day of corn syrup (the amount in two or three sweetened drinks) doubles a person's risk for high systolic blood pressure.[7] And public health statistics show a clear danger: Those who consume the highest levels of added sugars (25 percent of daily calories or more) double their risk of dying from CVD.[8] Eating rapidly digested carbohydrates such as sugars, white bread, white rice, or French fries promotes the inflammation that leads to weight gain, CVD, diabetes, and other conditions. Eating slowly digested carbohydrates such as whole grains, beans, and fruits and vegetables fights inflammation and lowers risk.[9]

As with other CVD risks, learning to reduce salt and sugar is best accomplished early. Healthy ingrained eating habits can begin to protect you as a young adult.

Sources:
1. Centers for Disease Control and Prevention, "Sodium Intake among US Adults—26 States, the District of Columbia, and Puerto Rico, 2013," *Morbidity and Mortality Weekly Report* 64, no. 25 (July 3, 2015): 695–98.
2. Centers for Disease Control and Prevention, "Get the Facts: Sources of Sodium in Your Diet," accessed August 2015, www.cdc.gov
3. Ibid.
4. K. Bibbins-Domingo et al., "Projected Effect of Dietary Salt Reductions on Future Cardiovascular Disease," *New England Journal of Medicine* 362, no. 7 (2010): 590–99.
5. D. Mozaffarian et al., "Global Sodium Consumption and Death from Cardiovascular Causes," *New England Journal of Medicine* 371 (2014): 623–34.
6. J. J. DiNicolantonino and S. C. Lucan, "The Wrong White Crystals: Not Salt but Sugar as Aetiological in Hypertension and Cardiometabolic Disease," *Open Heart* 1, no. 1 (2014): e000167, doi: 10.1136/openhrt-2014-000167
7. D. I. Jalal et al., "Increased Fructose Associates with Elevated Blood Pressure," *Journal of the American Society of Nephrology* 21, no. 9 (2010): 1543–49.
8. N. V. Dhurandhar and D. Thomas, "The Link between Dietary Sugar Intake and Cardiovascular Disease Mortality: An Unresolved Question," *Journal of the American Medical Association* 313, no. 9 (2015): 959–60.
9. Harvard Health Publications, "Foods That Fight Inflammation," *Harvard Women's Health Watch*, July 1, 2014, www.health.harvard.edu/staying-healthy/foods-that-fight-inflammation

the condition is *isolated systolic hypertension*, the most common form of high blood pressure in older Americans.

If you are diagnosed with prehypertension or hypertension in college, you can—and should—do something about it. Prehypertension in early adulthood usually precedes hypertension and heart disease in middle age.[33] Successful lifestyle modifications include maintaining a healthy weight, exercising regularly, managing stress, reducing dietary salt and sugar, and eating a healthy diet.[34] You may also need to work with your physician to lower your blood pressure through prescription drugs.

Coronary Heart Disease Atherosclerosis in the heart's main blood vessels causes **coronary heart disease (CHD)** or **coronary artery disease (CAD)**. More than 15 million Americans have coronary heart disease. Of all the types of CVD, CHD is the greatest killer. Each year, an estimated 1.09 million Americans suffer a new or recurrent heart attack.[35] The American Heart Association calculates that approximately every 34 seconds, someone has a heart attack in the United States and every 84 seconds, someone dies.[36]

A heart attack, also called a **myocardial infarction (MI)**, occurs when an area of the heart suffers permanent damage after plaque or a blood clot blocks the heart muscle's normal blood supply. Even flat, nonblocking plaques increase your risk of heart attack.[37] But when the plaques bulge or a clot forms, they can dramatically slow or stop blood flow and deprive the surrounding tissue of oxygen. If the blockage is extremely minor, an otherwise healthy heart will adapt over time as small blood vessels reroute needed blood through other areas.

When heart blockage is more severe, however, a person can experience the symptoms of a heart attack and will require life-saving support. The Tools for Change box *In the Event of a Heart Attack, Stroke, or Cardiac Arrest* (on page 357) describes how you should respond if you or someone near you experiences such symptoms. Surprisingly, recent research indicates that nearly half of the time, heart attacks are "silent"—they lack dramatic symptoms such as chest pain or shortness of breath.[38] This makes CVD prevention and management all the more important.

Angina Pectoris Atherosclerosis and other circulatory impairments may reduce the heart's blood and oxygen supply and cause a condition called **ischemia**. People with ischemia often suffer from varying degrees of chest pain, also called **angina pectoris**. The American Heart Association estimates that 8.2 million Americans suffer from angina.[39] Many people experience short episodes of angina whenever they exert themselves. Symptoms range from slight indigestion to a feeling that the heart is being crushed. Generally, the more severe the oxygen deprivation, the more severe the chest pain. Treatments range from rest to nitroglycerin tablets, which relax vessels and lessen the heart's workload; *beta-blockers*, which slow heart beat and lower blood pressure; and calcium channel blockers, which lessen painful spasms of the coronary arteries.

Arrhythmias An **arrhythmia**, or irregular heartbeat, is relatively common: Many millions of Americans experience one of the various forms each year.[40] The disturbed heartbeat rhythm can take several forms: racing heart in the absence of exercise or anxiety (*tachycardia*); an abnormally slow heartbeat (*bradycardia*); or a sporadic, quivering pattern called *fibrillation*. **Fibrillation** renders the heart extremely inefficient at pumping blood through the vessels. If a fibrillation event or a series of fibrillations go untreated, the condition can be fatal.

Even without CVD, you may feel heart arrhythmias from drinking too much caffeine or from the nicotine in tobacco. Mild cases like this are seldom life-threatening. If you develop a severe case due to disease, you may require drug therapy or a pacemaker.

Congestive Heart Failure More than 5.7 million Americans suffer from **congestive heart failure (CHF)** each year.[41] In CHF, the heart muscle is damaged or overworked, the pumping chambers are taxed to the

---

coronary artery disease (CAD) or coronary heart disease (CHD) Atherosclerosis (the buildup of plaque deposits) in the main arteries that supply oxygen and other materials to the heart muscle

myocardial infarction (MI) Medical term for a heart attack; involves permanent damage to an area of the heart muscle brought on by a cessation of normal blood supply

ischemia A damaging reduction in the blood (and therefore the oxygen supply) to a region of the heart, brain, or other organ

angina pectoris Chest pain due to ischemia, or reduction in blood flow to the heart muscle and surrounding tissues

arrhythmia Irregular heartbeat; can involve abnormally fast or slow heartbeat or the disorganized, sporadic beat of fibrillation

fibrillation A sporadic, quivering heartbeat pattern that results in inefficient pumping of blood

congestive heart failure (CHF) A cardiovascular disease in which the heart muscle is damaged or overworked, and the heart lacks the strength to keep blood circulating normally through the body

TOOLS FOR CHANGE

In the Event of a Heart Attack, Stroke, or Cardiac Arrest

APPLY IT! Knowing what to do in a cardiovascular emergency could save a friend's life—or your own.

Warning Signs of a Heart Attack

- Uncomfortable pressure, fullness, squeezing, or pain in the center of the chest (more likely in men) or between the shoulder blades (more likely in women), lasting two minutes or longer
- Jaw pain and/or shortness of breath
- Pain spreading to the shoulders, neck, or arms
- Dizziness, fatigue, fainting, sweating, and/or nausea

Not all of these warning signs occur in every heart attack. For instance, a woman's heart attack may show up as shortness of breath, fatigue, and jaw or shoulder blade pain or pressure, stretched out over hours rather than minutes. If any of these symptoms appear, don't wait. Get help immediately!

Warning Signs of a Stroke

- Sudden numbness or weakness, especially on one side of the body, affecting face, arm, and/or leg
- Sudden mental confusion, especially trouble speaking or understanding words
- Sudden vision problems in one or both eyes
- Sudden dizziness, loss of balance, lack of coordination, or trouble walking
- Sudden severe headache without apparent cause

Warning Signs of a Cardiac Arrest

- Sudden loss of responsiveness (won't respond if tapped on either shoulder)
- Normal breathing stops (tilt head up; check for breathing for five seconds)

Know What to Do before an Emergency Strikes

- Find out which hospitals in your area have 24-hour emergency cardiac care.
- Determine (in advance) the hospital or medical facility that is nearest your home, school, and office, and tell your family and friends to call this facility in an emergency.
- Keep a list of emergency rescue service numbers next to your telephone and in your pocket, wallet, or purse. Remember 911 if you don't have time to call emergency rescue numbers.

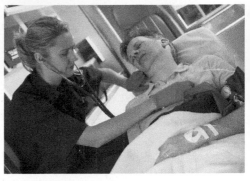

- If you have chest or jaw discomfort that lasts more than two minutes, call the emergency rescue service or 911. Do not drive yourself to the hospital unless there is no other alternative.

TRY IT! Be a Lifesaver during a Crisis

- If you are with someone who is showing signs of a heart attack or stroke and the warning signs last for two minutes or longer, act immediately.
- Expect a denial. It is normal for a person with chest discomfort to deny the possibility of anything as serious as a heart attack. Don't take no for an answer. Insist on taking prompt action.
- Call 911 or an emergency rescue service, or get to the nearest hospital emergency room that offers 24-hour emergency cardiac care.
- If you are with someone in cardiac arrest and if you are properly trained, give chest compressions and mouth-to-mouth breathing. Continual chest compressions appear to be more important for adult heart attack victims; combined compressions and breathing (CPR or cardiopulmonary resuscitation) seem to be more important for children having a heart, stroke, or breathing-related emergency. Get instructions on which to use from a 911 operator, emergency medical technician, or other rescue personnel if possible.
- An automated external defibrillator (AED) may save a person during cardiac arrest. These devices are increasingly common in public places—workplaces, restaurants, health clubs, sports stadiums, schools, shopping centers, airports, hotels, and so on. Cultivate the habit of noticing their location in case of emergency.

Source: Adapted from American Heart Association, "Warning Signs of Heart Attack, Stroke, and Cardiac Arrest," accessed August 28, 2015, www.americanheart.org

limit, and the heart becomes too weak to keep blood circulating normally through the body. The weakened heart pumps out less blood through the arteries. As a result, less blood flows back through the veins to the heart. As the blood begins to back up, body tissues become congested: Pooling blood enlarges the heart, making it even less efficient, and fluid accumulates in the legs, ankles, or lungs, where it can cause swelling or difficult breathing. Many factors can cause CHF including heart defects, infection, heart attack, hypertension, or even cancer treatments.

CHF can be fatal if undiagnosed and untreated, but most cases respond well to drug treatment. Doctors often prescribe diuretics ("water pills") to increase urination and reduce fluid accumulation. Drugs such as digitalis increase the heart's pumping action, and vasodilators expand blood vessels so blood can flow through more easily and reduce the heart's workload.

Congenital Heart Disease **Congenital heart disease**, meaning heart disease present at birth, affects about 8 of every 1,000 live births in the United States.[42] A baby may be born with a slight *heart murmur,* an audible sound due to an irregular heart valve that allows turbulent blood flow through the heart. Some children outgrow such heart murmurs and have no further problems. Others, however, can have more serious congenital irregularities in their heart anatomy or function that require surgical repair. Causes may include hereditary factors, a mother's case of rubella (German measles) or certain other infections during pregnancy, or the mother's use of alcohol or drugs during fetal development. Advances in treatment continually improve the prospects for people with congenital heart defects.

Stroke The American Heart Association estimates that 6.6 million Americans alive today have suffered a stroke at some point in their lives. Each year more than 795,000 people experience a new or recurrent stroke, and 129,000 of them die, making stroke the fifth leading cause of death.[43]

Just as a heart attack can occur when a blocked vessel starves part of the heart of needed oxygen, a

congenital heart disease Heart disease present at birth

stroke A sudden loss of function in a region of the brain caused by blockage in or rupture of a blood vessel, leading to oxygen deprivation, cell damage, or death

stroke is a sudden loss of function in part of the brain caused by blockage or rupture of a blood vessel. The resulting oxygen deprivation can damage or kill brain cells. *Ischemic*

strokes are due to a plaque-blocked vessel or a floating blood clot that lodges in a vessel and cuts off blood supply to a brain region. *Hemorrhagic* strokes occur when a blood vessel bursts, spilling blood rather than transporting it and damaging that unsupplied area through oxygen deprivation.

Factors that can contribute to stroke include family history, advancing age, atherosclerosis, heart disease, CHF, hypertension, smoking, diabetes, sedentary lifestyle, obesity, heavy drinking, and stimulant drugs.[44] Genetics can play a role, as well: African Americans are more than twice as likely to suffer a stroke than those of other races.[45]

Some strokes are mild and cause only temporary dizziness, slight weakness, or numbness. If a stroke affects a large or crucial region of the brain, it may cause speech impairments, memory problems, loss of motor control, or death. About 10 percent of major strokes are preceded—days, weeks, or months earlier—by *transient ischemic attacks (TIAs)*, brief interruptions of the blood supply to the brain that cause only temporary dizziness, weakness, paralysis, numbness, or other symptoms.[46] In recent years, stroke deaths have dropped by more than 20 percent thanks to better diagnosis, better surgical options, new clot-busting drugs that can be injected immediately after a stroke has occurred, better aftercare for stroke patients, and campaigns to teach awareness and avoidance of risk factors.

LO 10.4 What Are the Main Risk Factors for Cardiovascular Disease?

CVD is an unfortunate reality. However, you can modify many individual risk factors. By identifying your risks and understanding which risks you can control (see **Lab 10.1**), you can lower your chances of developing CVD.

Do It!
Access these labs at the end of the chapter or online at MasteringHealth™.

Risks You Can Control

Experts have identified at least 10 significant risk factors for CVD: tobacco use, hypertension, high blood fats, overweight/obesity, physical inactivity, type 2 diabetes, metabolic syndrome, uncontrolled stress, poor nutrition, and heavy alcohol consumption. The more risk factors you have, the greater your chances of heart attack, stroke, angina, atherosclerosis, and other forms of CVD.[47] However, since lifestyle choices underlie many of these risk factors, changes to daily habits can often help. Let's look at these risk factors more closely.

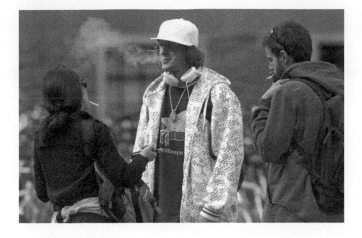

Tobacco Use In 1964, the Surgeon General of the United States asserted that smoking was the greatest risk factor for heart disease. Today, more than 46,000 annual deaths from CVD are directly related to smoking.[48] Cigarette smokers are two to four times more likely to develop coronary heart disease than nonsmokers.[49] Evidence also indicates that chronic exposure to second-hand smoke in the environment increases a *non-smoker's* risk of CVD by 25 to 30 percent and that CVD, in turn, kills an estimated 42,000 nonsmokers each year.[50]

How does tobacco use damage the heart? There are two plausible explanations. One is that nicotine increases heart beat rate, heart output, blood pressure, and oxygen use by heart muscles. The heart is forced to work harder to obtain sufficient oxygen. The other explanation is that chemicals in smoke damage and inflame the lining of the coronary arteries, allowing cholesterol and plaque to accumulate, increasing blood pressure, and forcing the heart to work harder. In addition, chemicals in smoke increase blood clotting and the chance of heart attack.

With the advent of e-cigarettes, smoking rates are rising among teens, college students, and other young adults. Like traditional tobacco products, e-cigarettes deliver nicotine and many kinds of cancer-producing and lung-damaging vaporized chemicals. Early evidence suggests that over time, e-cigarettes will also contribute to CVDs.[51] Chapter 13 covers e-cigarette use in more detail.

Hypertension We have seen that hypertension can damage artery walls and lead to atherosclerosis. Hypertension damages the body in many other ways too. It can:

- Weaken artery walls and lead to an *aneurysm,* an abnormal, blood-filled bulge in a blood vessel that has the potential to rupture.

- Damage coronary arteries, enlarge the heart, or weaken the heart muscle.
- Affect blood vessels in the brain, causing strokes and TIAs, promoting dementia, and impairing cognitive function.
- Injure delicate blood vessels in the kidneys and eyes, leading to kidney damage or failure and impaired vision or vision loss.

In addition, hypertension can reduce sexual function, disrupt sleep, and magnify the bone loss of osteoporosis.[52]

Thousands of young adults have undiagnosed hypertension, and this is significant because early blood pressure changes tend to lead to heart disease in middle age.[53] Reducing dietary sugar, sodium, and saturated fats can help lower blood pressure, as can managing stress and taking certain prescription drugs. Maintaining a healthy weight is especially important: Among some female students, a gain of just 1.5 pounds raised blood pressure by three to five points. Luckily, weight *loss* can *lower* blood pressure.[54]

High Levels of Fats in Your Blood *Hyperlipidemia*— or high levels of cholesterol, triglycerides, and other fats (lipids) in the blood—is correlated with increased risk of several CVDs. According to one report, more than 50 percent of American men aged 65 and older and 40 percent of American women aged 65 or older are on some type of anti-hyperlipidemia medication, such as "statins" (e.g., Lipitor) and other drugs designed to reduce blood fats.[55] Unfortunately, many of these medications carry significant risks of their own. In addition, many people use these medications as "crutches" and continue to eat high-fat foods, assuming that the medications will keep them safe from CVD.

Diets high in saturated fats and/or *trans* fats can raise blood cholesterol levels and contribute to atherosclerosis. They can also switch on the body's blood-clotting system, making the blood thicker and stickier. All of these blood changes increase the risk of heart attack or stroke. **Table 10.4** on page 360 shows recommended levels for blood cholesterol. People with several risk factors for CVD should follow the most stringent range of the guidelines for blood cholesterol.

Total cholesterol levels are just one measure of CVD risks. Another is the ratio of "bad" to "good" cholesterol. Low-density lipoprotein (LDL), often referred to as "bad" cholesterol, contributes to plaque buildup on artery walls. High-density lipoprotein (HDL), or "good" cholesterol, removes plaque from artery walls, thus serving as a protector. In theory, if LDL levels get too high relative to

TABLE 10.4 LDL, Total, and HDL Cholesterol and Triglycerides (mg/dL) Levels for Adults

LDL Cholesterol	
Less than 100	Desirable
100–129	Near desirable to above desirable
130–159	Borderline high
160 or higher	High
Total Cholesterol	
Less than 200	Desirable
200–239	Borderline high
240 or higher	High
HDL Cholesterol	
Less than 40	Low; major risk factor for heart disease
60 or higher	Desirable; lower your risk for heart disease
Triglycerides	
Below 150	Normal and desirable

Source: National Heart, Lung, and Blood Institute, "What Is Cholesterol?" August 2015, www.nhlbi.nih.gov/health

HDL levels, plaque will accumulate inside arteries and lead to cardiovascular problems. The LDL/HDL ratio can increase because of too much saturated fat in the diet, lack of exercise, high stress levels, or genetic predisposition.

Another type of blood fat, the *triglycerides*, also promote atherosclerosis. As people get older, heavier, or both, their triglyceride and cholesterol levels tend to rise. No one has yet proved that high triglyceride levels cause atherosclerosis and thus underlie CVD. However, these blood fats may contribute to faster plaque development. People who eat the most sugar have higher blood triglycerides (as well as higher weight) and their risk of dying from CVD is two to three times higher.[56]

You can learn your LDL, HDL, total cholesterol, and triglyceride levels with a fasting blood test (no eating or drinking for 12 hours before the test). Compare your numbers to Table 10.4 and discuss their significance with your health provider.

Overweight and Obesity
Being overweight or obese can strain the heart, forcing it to push blood through "extra" miles of capillaries that supply each pound of fat. A heart that must continuously move blood through an overabundance of vessels has to work harder and may become weakened

metabolic syndrome A group of metabolic conditions occurring together that increase a person's risk of heart disease, stroke, and diabetes

or damaged. The same high-fat, high-sugar, high-calorie diets that lead to overweight and obesity can also contribute to plaque formation.

Overweight people are more likely to develop heart disease and stroke even if they have no other CVD risk factors.[57] This is especially true for people who tend to store fat around the upper body and waist (an "apple" shape) as opposed to those who tend to store fat around the hips and thighs (a "pear" shape). Losing as little as 5 to 10 percent of your body weight can significantly lower blood cholesterol.[58] Cardiovascular experts are urging doctors to consider and treat obesity as a disease, not just a lifestyle problem.[59]

See It! Watch "Mediterranean Diet Could Help Reduce Heart Disease" at MasteringHealth™.

Physical Inactivity
A sedentary lifestyle is one of the most significant risk factors for CVD. Elevating your heart rate and blood flow through moderate to vigorous activity benefits the heart muscle and helps prevent plaque deposits on artery walls. Conversely, inactivity makes the heart muscle less efficient and allows plaque to build up. Even modest levels of low-intensity physical activity—walking, gardening, housework, dancing—are beneficial if done regularly and over the long term.

Despite the clear benefits of regular exercise, about 30 percent get none at all and only about half of Americans over age 18 meet widely accepted guidelines for 150 minutes per week of moderate activity or 75 minutes of vigorous activity.[60] Teens who watch two hours or more of TV per day and college students with the highest levels of smartphone use are also the most sedentary.[61]

Diabetes Mellitus
Chronic diseases are interrelated: People who have one tend to have others. This connection is especially clear when it comes to diabetes and CVD. Diabetes significantly increases the risk for CVD even if blood sugar levels are well controlled. When they're uncontrolled, the risks are even higher. People with diabetes have death rates from CVD that are almost twice as high as those of people without diabetes.[62] The risk is so great, in fact, that many physicians consider someone with pre-diabetes or the early stages of diabetes to have the same risks as someone who has already had his or her first heart attack. Diabetics also tend to have increased blood fat levels and atherosclerosis, and their small blood vessels tend to deteriorate, particularly in the eyes and extremities.

Metabolic Syndrome
Metabolic syndrome refers to a cluster of obesity-related risk factors associated with

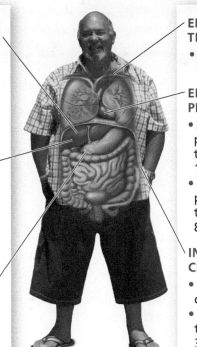

HIGH LEVELS OF C-REACTIVE PROTEIN
- Liver produces C-reactive protein
- Levels above 10 mg/L indicate inflammation in the body

REDUCED BLOOD HDL CHOLESTEROL
- *Men:* Less than 40 mg/dL
- *Women:* Less than 50 mg/dL

ELEVATED FASTING BLOOD GLUCOSE
- Greater than or equal to 100 mg/dL

ELEVATED BLOOD TRIGLYCERIDES
- Greater than or equal to 150 mg/dL

ELEVATED BLOOD PRESSURE
- *Systolic* blood pressure greater than or equal to 130 mm Hg
- *Diastolic* blood pressure greater than or equal to 89 mm Hg

INCREASED WAIST CIRCUMFERENCE
- *Men:* Greater than or equal to 40 inches
- *Women:* Greater than or equal to 34.6 inches

FIGURE **10.2** Risk factors associated with metabolic syndrome.

CVD and type 2 diabetes.[63] People with metabolic syndrome have several characteristics in common (see **Figure 10.2**):

- Abdominal obesity, meaning a large waistline (40 inches in men or 34.6 inches in women, or larger)

- Elevated levels of triglycerides in the blood (150 mg/dL or higher)

- Low levels of "good cholesterol" (HDLs below 40 mg/dL in men or 50 mg/dL in women)

- High blood pressure (130/89 mm Hg or higher)

- High levels of the sugar glucose in the blood (100 mg/dL or higher after fasting)

- High levels of C-reactive protein (more than 10 mg/L), indicating inflammation

The American Heart Association estimates that one-quarter to one-third of the American population over age 20 has metabolic syndrome.[64] By definition, they have multiple risk factors for CVD, and thus their overall risk of developing cardiovascular illness is high.

The prevalence of metabolic syndrome in adolescents and young adults is causing concern among many health professionals.[65] According to another study, 43 percent of college students had at least one of the indicators.[66] Poor nutrition (specifically low intake of fruits and vegetables and high intake of sweetened

beverages), poor fitness levels, and being overweight all increase the risk of metabolic syndrome.[67] The message is clear: Being young does not make you immune to metabolic syndrome and its multiple risk factors for CVD.

Other Controllable Factors Stress can be a risk factor for CVD. Your body's stress response can raise blood pressure and trigger blood-clotting and heart rhythm abnormalities.[68] Stress can also foster habits that promote CVD, such as overeating, smoking, or poor sleep. Disrupted sleep, insomnia, sleep apnea, snoring, traffic noise, and a lack of social support have all been linked to higher CVD risk.[69]

Poor nutrition also increases CVD risk. Too much saturated fat, salt, and refined carbohydrates and too little fiber and too few fruits and vegetables all heighten risk, while improved nutrition lowers it. Updated guidelines by the American Heart Association and American College of Cardiologists urge people to stop worrying about specific foods and the *occasional* treat of ice cream or cake and to strive for an overall healthy eating pattern.[70]

Although some studies suggest that *moderate* amounts of alcohol may help lower the risk of CVD, excessive alcohol consumption can raise blood triglycerides, trigger arrhythmias, raise blood pressure, promote obesity, and contribute to heart failure and strokes. (Chapter 13 discusses normal and excessive drinking levels.) Stimulant drugs, such as amphetamines or cocaine, can also trigger strokes—even in young people.[71]

Risks You Cannot Control

Unfortunately, there are risk factors for CVD that you cannot control, but knowing about them can help you plan for the right kinds of action. The list includes heredity, age, gender, and race. Doctors now have formulas that enable them to calculate a person's 10-year risk and lifetime risk of dying from CVD and can use this information in treating patients and helping them to prevent CVD.[72]

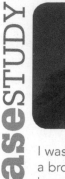

DARYL

"I took my mom in for a check-up the other day. The good news is that the things she's doing—diet, exercise, pills—have brought her blood pressure and cholesterol down since the last check-up. While I was sitting in the waiting room, though, I read a brochure about risk factors for heart disease. I knew genetics was a factor, but I was surprised at how many other risk factors I had: not being very active (unless you count playing the piano!), breathing in other people's smoke at jazz clubs, too much fast food, and stress."

APPLY IT! What else could Daryl do to assess his risk for cardiovascular disease? What risk factors for cardiovascular disease do you have?

TRY IT! **Today**, sort your risk factors by "controllable" and "non-controllable" and place them in order of greatest risk. Lab 10.1 can help you accomplish this. **This week**, list ways you could change your lifestyle to reduce your vulnerability for the top three controllable risk factors. **In two weeks**, list ways to work on each listed item. These will overlap, so boil your lifestyle ideas down to one set and begin!

Hear It!
To listen to this case study online, visit the Study Area in MasteringHealth™.

Heredity A family history of CVD—that is, CVD in several generations of an extended family—appears to increase risk significantly. The inherited trait of blood type predicts risk, too: With type O blood as a standard, those with type A are 5 percent more likely to develop CVD, those with type B are 11 percent more likely, and those with type AB are 23 percent more likely.[73] Several other inherited factors have surprising, even bizarre connections to CVD risk: Baldness, hairy ears, short adult height, and a diagonal crease on your earlobes can each increase—even double—your risk![74] Researchers are working on explanations. In the meantime, be aware that your genes, your fetal and home environment, and your learned patterns of diet, exercise, and stress all contribute to risk and can alert you to work toward prevention.

Age Seventy-five percent of all heart attacks occur in people over age 65. The risk for CVD increases with age for both sexes.[75] As we've seen, though, atherosclerosis can begin in kids and teens. Many people under age 65—even a significant number of college students—take a baby aspirin every day to prevent heart attack and stroke. Recent federal guidelines, however, discourage that practice in those younger than 50 or older than 69.[76] The risk of stomach bleeding and allergic reactions to aspirin tend to outweigh the CVD benefits in those groups; people between 50 and 69 should consult a physician before beginning daily aspirin.[77]

Gender Men are at greater risk for CVD until about age 60, when risk begins to equalize between the sexes.[78] A man's risk is magnified if his ancestors came from Northern Europe.[79] A woman's risk is greater the earlier menstruation starts (menarche) and stops (menopause); her risk is lower the longer she breastfeeds.[80] Women under age 35 have a fairly low risk of CVD unless they have high blood pressure, kidney problems, or diabetes. The risks rise in all women over 35, especially those who smoke and also take oral contraceptives.[81]

Race Members of certain racial/ethnic groups may face increased CVD risk (see **Figure 10.3**).[82] African

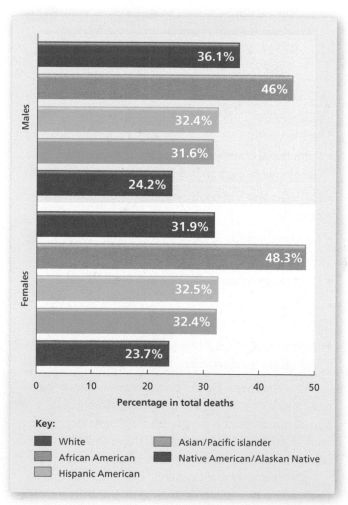

FIGURE 10.3 Ethnicity and Cardiovascular Deaths. Cardiovascular disease claims a disproportionate number of African Americans.

Source: D. Mozaffarian et al., "Heart Disease and Stroke Statistics—2015 Update," *Circulation* 131, no. 4 (2014): e29–e322.

Americans have the highest rates of CVD, followed by Caucasian Americans and Mexican Americans. Rates for Asian Americans are below 25 percent.[83] A recent study revealed that black males have higher levels of aldosterone, a hormone produced by the adrenal glands on the kidneys and involved in the body's water and salt retention and excretion. Naturally higher levels of aldosterone increase sodium and water retention, raise blood pressure, and cause changes to the heart, even in black males aged 15 to 19.[84]

LO 10.5 How Can I Avoid Cardiovascular Disease?

People often wait until they get a scary medical diagnosis before changing their habits. If you have risk factors for CVD, the earlier you confront them, the better your chances of avoiding CVD later. This includes prehypertension or blood pressure above 120/80 mm Hg in young adulthood.

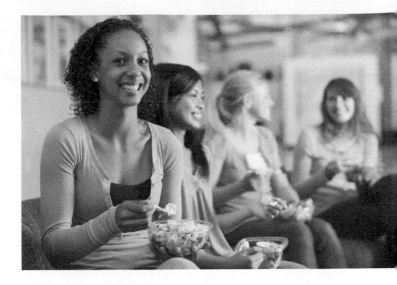

Live It!

Complete Worksheet 38 Cardiovascular Risk Assessment at MasteringHealth™.

Lower Your Controllable Risks

Here are specific behavioral tips for reducing the risk factors you can control.

Don't Use Tobacco According to the American Heart Association, smoking is the greatest preventable cause of disease and death. Even light smoking—just two cigarettes per day—increases your CVD risk. When people stop smoking, regardless of how long or how much they have smoked, their risk of heart disease declines. Women appear to recover lung function more fully than men.[85] Since secondhand smoke is a potent risk factor, avoid smoky places when possible. Avoid all forms of tobacco, since nicotine increases blood pressure, heart rate, blood clotting, and plaque buildup.

Eat Well There are numerous ways you can promote cardiovascular health through better nutrition. The American Heart Association recommends the following:[86]

- Use at least as many calories as you consume.

- In your diet, emphasize fruits and vegetables, whole grains, low-fat dairy products, skinless poultry and fish, nuts and legumes, and healthy vegetable oils.

- Limit saturated fat, trans fat, sodium, red meat, and sweeteners.[87]

- Drink alcohol in moderation.

- Be aware of portion sizes, especially while dining out.

Individual studies on foods reveal important details about risk and protection. Apples, raisins, citrus fruit, hot peppers, blueberries, and strawberries contain specific compounds that cut LDL levels, lower blood pressure, open blood vessels, or lower cardiovascular risks in other ways.[88] The fiber in unrefined whole-grain foods can help lower cholesterol and help you feel full. The omega-3 fatty acids in fish such as salmon and trout may lower the risk of death from coronary artery disease. Nuts and vegetable oils also contain omega-3 and omega-6 fatty acids. Vegetable oils high in monounsaturated fats, such as canola oil, can actually help reduce the metabolically active belly fat that increases your risk of CVD.[89]

Eating red meat is linked to higher risks of CVD and cancer.[90] Low-carbohydrate, high-protein diets that concentrate on animal proteins can significantly increase CVD risk.[91] Eating three or more egg yolks per week can accelerate plaque formation in blood vessels.[92]

The DASH (Dietary Approaches to Stop Hypertension) diet, based on National Institutes of Health research, emphasizes a list very similar to the American Heart Association's recommendations. The Tools for Change box The DASH Diet on page 364 provides details.

Exercise Regularly Regular cardiovascular exercise strengthens heart muscle and helps keep the blood vessels resilient. Performing 30 to 60 minutes or more of moderate to vigorous activity most days of the week will help prevent CVD. Strength training and flexibility are also important components of your exercise plan for cardiovascular wellness, helping you to maintain muscle mass, speed up metabolism, control weight, and prevent injury.

The DASH Diet

APPLY IT! Originated by researchers for the National Institutes of Health, the DASH diet (Dietary Approaches to Stop Hypertension) is a set of nutritional guidelines that can help you reduce blood pressure.

TRY IT! Below are some of the highlights. Within the serving ranges, go for the lower numbers if you eat 2,000 calories or fewer per day:

- Consume four to six servings of fruits and four to six servings of vegetables each day.
- Consume two to four servings of fat-free or low-fat dairy products.
- Eat at least three whole-grain foods each day as well as high-fiber foods such as beans to get enough dietary fiber.
- Choose protein-rich food containing heart-healthy fats. Examples are nuts and seeds (three to five servings per week) and fatty fish such as salmon. Consume no more than 1.5 to 2.5 servings of fish, skinless poultry, or the leanest meats (check labels) per day.
- Be careful to get recommended levels of sodium, potassium, magnesium, and calcium.
- Reduce your intake of red meat, high-fat dairy products, and other sources of saturated fat.
- Cut back on empty calories by limiting food containing white flour, added sugars, white rice, and other quickly digested foods that spike blood sugar.

You can find the entire DASH eating plan online at http://dash-diet.org/what_is_the_dash_diet.asp

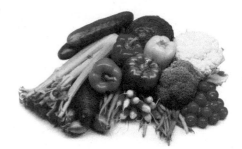

Manage Your Stress The physiological stress response raises blood pressure, speeds the heart rate, and floods the bloodstream with glucose. All of these, in turn, can promote CVD by damaging the blood vessels and contributing to atherosclerosis. See Chapter 9 for important stress-reduction tools that can lower your risk of CVD.

Control Diabetes Because elevated sugar levels in the blood greatly increase the risk for heart disease, stroke, and artery disease, people with diabetes are at tremendous risk. The very factors that contribute to the development of type 2 diabetes (obesity, hypertension, elevated blood cholesterol and triglycerides, inactivity) are additional risks for CVD. As Chapter 11 explains in detail, careful diet, increased exercise, and medication help most diabetics control their condition and lower their CVD risk.

Avoid Alcohol and Drug Abuse If you drink, keep your consumption below one drink per day if you are a woman and two per day if you are a man. Greater consumption raises blood sugar and triglyceride levels. Avoid recreational drugs, especially stimulants, since they increase heart rate and blood pressure.[93]

Study Plan

chapter summary

LO 10.1 Why Should I Worry about Cardiovascular Disease?

- Cardiovascular disease, America's biggest killer, accounts for 29 percent of all deaths.
- CVD kills 18 million people per year worldwide, mostly in low- and medium-income countries.
- CVD can greatly diminish your quality of life.
- CVD starts in childhood or adolescence and elevates blood pressure in a significant percentage of college students.

LO 10.2 How Does Cardiovascular Disease Affect the Body?

- CVD causes atherosclerosis throughout the body. Plaque build-up leads to vessel narrowing and hypertension.
- The human immune system sees plaque as foreign and tries to wall it off. This low-grade inflammation inside of blood vessels can lead to more plaque and to ruptures that can cause heart attacks or strokes.

LO 10.3 Cardiovascular Disease Takes Many Forms

- Hypertension is the most common form of CVD.
- In **coronary heart disease (CHD)** or **coronary artery disease (CAD)**, atherosclerosis occurs in the heart's main blood vessels. This can reduce heart function and can trigger heart attacks.

- Ischemia reduces the heart's blood and oxygen supply, often leading to chest pain.
- Heart arrhythmias include racing heart (tachycardia), slow heart (bradycardia), or the irregular pattern called fibrillation.
- In congestive heart failure, a weakened heart muscle pumps less blood and oxygen and leads to fluid accumulation in the extremities.
- About 8 babies per 1,000 are born with a congenital heart defect such as a heart murmur due to a valve defect.
- Stroke is the fifth leading cause of death in America.

LO 10.4 What Are the Main Risk Factors for Cardiovascular Disease?

- CVD risks you can control include tobacco use; hypertension; high levels of cholesterol, triglycerides, and other fats in the blood; overweight and obesity; physical inactivity; diabetes mellitus; metabolic syndrome; stress; disrupted sleep; and poor nutrition.
- CVD risks you cannot control include inherited tendencies, advancing age, gender, and race/ethnicity.

LO 10.5 How Can I Avoid Cardiovascular Disease?

- Lower your controllable risks by avoiding tobacco use and exposure to second-hand smoke; eating a heart-healthy diet; exercising regularly; managing your stress; controlling diabetes; and avoiding alcohol and drug abuse.

review questions

LO 10.1 1. Cardiovascular disease and stroke are responsible for about _____ of deaths in the United States each year.
a. one-half
b. one-tenth
c. one-sixth
d. one-third

LO 10.2 2. Each of the following explains CVD damage to the blood vessels except
a. atherosclerotic hardening.
b. arrhythmia.
c. plaque formation.
d. inflammation.

LO 10.2 3. Which of the following is characteristic of cardiovascular disease?
a. Joint pain
b. Feeling energized
c. Having no symptoms at all
d. Dry skin

LO 10.3 4. Which of the following is an example of cardiovascular disease (CVD)?
a. Diabetes
b. Diastolic pressure
c. Coronary heart disease
d. Systolic pressure

LO 10.3 **5.** Which of the following accurately describes *hypertension*?
a. Sustained high blood pressure
b. A thickening or hardening of the arteries
c. Heart blockage
d. Irregular heartbeat

6. When atherosclerosis occurs in the heart's main blood vessels, it is called
a. peripheral artery disease.
b. coronary artery disease.
c. inflammation.
d. homocysteine.

LO 10.4 **7.** Which of the following is a significant risk factor for CVD?
a. Regular exercise
b. Stress management
c. Underweight
d. Tobacco use

LO 10.4 **8.** A person with metabolic syndrome is likely to have which one of the following?
a. Abdominal obesity or a large waistline
b. Depressed levels of triglycerides in the blood
c. High levels of "good" cholesterol (HDLs)
d. Hypoglycemia or low blood sugar

LO 10.4 **9.** Low-density lipoprotein (LDL) is often referred to as
a. "good" cholesterol.
b. "bad" cholesterol.
c. diabetes mellitus.
d. metabolic syndrome.

LO 10.5 **10.** Each of these can help you avoid CVD except
a. switching from tobacco to e-cigarettes.
b. following the DASH diet.
c. observing the Simple 7.
d. getting moderate exercise most days of the week.

critical thinking questions

LO 10.1, LO 10.2, LO 10.3 **1.** Discuss the evidence that people in your age group are at risk for developing CVD.

LO 10.2 **2.** Describe the atherosclerosis process and explain the medical term *atherosclerotic cardiovascular disease*.

LO 10.2, LO 10.5 **3.** Discuss specific ways that exercise and dietary changes can help prevent CVD.

LO 10.3, LO 10.4, LO 10.5 **4.** List six different forms of CVD. Compare and contrast their risk factors, symptoms, and prevention.

check out these eResources

- **American College of Sports Medicine** The fastest way to find a good discussion of the weekly sessions you need to protect your heart and blood vessels is to simply enter "ACSM Cardio Guidelines—Guidelines for Cardiorespiratory Fitness Training" on your device's search engine. **www.acsm.org**
- **American Heart Association** Learn more about the roles of high blood pressure and diabetes in cardiovascular disease. **www.heart.org**
- **Heart Insight** This online magazine has helpful articles including tips on mobile devices, apps, and wearable sensors. **http://heartinsight.heart.org/**

- **National Heart, Lung, and Blood Institute** Learn more about the medical history of America's war on heart and vascular diseases, and recommendations for diet, exercise, and lifestyle. **www.nhlbi.nih.gov**
- **World Heart Federation** Global perspective on cardiovascular disease. The "Heart Facts" tab on the home page takes you to fact sheets on diseases and risks, as well as to books, videos, and other resources. **www.world-heart-federation.org**

ASSESS YOURSELF

UNDERSTAND YOUR
OVERALL CVD RISK

MasteringHealth™

Name: _____ Date: _____

Instructor: _____ Section: _____

Purpose: To engage you in thinking critically about your own risk factors for CVD.

Directions: Complete each of the following questions about CVD risk and total your points in each section—the higher the score, the greater your risk. If you answered "don't know" for any question, talk to your parents or other family members as soon as possible to find out whether you have any unknown risks.

Section I: Assess Risk Factors You Cannot Control: Your Family History of CVD

	Yes	No	Don't Know
1. Do any of your primary relatives (mother, father, grandparents, siblings) have a history of heart disease or stroke?	1	0	
2. Do any of your primary relatives (mother, father, grandparents, siblings) have diabetes?	1	0	
3. Do any of your primary relatives (mother, father, grandparents, siblings) have high blood pressure?	1	0	
4. Do any of your primary relatives (mother, father, grandparents, siblings) have a history of high cholesterol?	1	0	
5. During the time you lived at home, did your family consume red meat and high-fat dairy products several times per week?	1	0	
Total for Section I = _____			

Section II: Assess Risk Factors You Can Control: Your Lifestyle Choices

	Yes	No	Don't Know
1. Do you have high blood pressure?	1	0	
2. Is your total cholesterol level higher than recommended? (See Table 10.4)	1	0	
3. Have you been diagnosed as pre-diabetic or diabetic?	1	0	
4. Do you smoke three or more cigarettes per day?	1	0	
5. Would you describe your life as being highly stressful?	1	0	
Total for Section II = _____			

Section III: Assess Additional Risks You Can Control: Other Factors and Choices

1. How would you best describe your current BMI?	
<18.5 (1 point)	25–29.9 (1 point)
18.5–24.9 (0 point)	≥30 (2 points)

2. How would you describe your level of exercise?	
Moderate activity for 30 to 60 minutes on fewer than three days per week, plus fewer than three cardio workouts per week and fewer than two strength-training workouts per week	1 point
Moderate activity for 30 to 60 minutes most days of the week, plus three cardio workouts and two strength-training workouts per week	0 points
Moderate activity for 60 minutes or more most days of the week, plus more than three cardio workouts and two strength-training workouts per week	0 points

3. How would you describe your dietary behaviors?	
I eat more than the recommended number of calories each day.	1 point
I eat about the recommended number of calories/day for my age, BMI, and activity level.	0 points
I eat fewer than the recommended number of calories each day.	0 points

4. Which of the following best describes your typical dietary behavior?	
I eat several servings of red meat per week and consume saturated fat from other meats and high-fat dairy products most days.	1 point
I eat from the major food groups, trying hard to get the recommended fruits and vegetables.	0 points
Whenever possible, I try to substitute olive oil or canola oil for other forms of dietary fat.	0 points

Total for Section III = _____

Scoring: Look at each section. If your total score for that section is 0, your CVD risk is minimal. Keep up the good work! If your score is between 1 and 3, your risk is moderate and you should initiate some change to lower it. If you score a 4 or 5, you should make substantial changes in those factors that you can control. Your behavior change plan for the chapter will help, and you can get additional advice from your instructor.

Section IV: Reflection

1. What are your risk factors for CVD? Identify any behaviors that put you at risk for CVD. What can you change right now? What can you change in the future to reduce your risk?

_____

_____

_____

_____

2. Which risk factors for CVD are outside your control? What can you do to reduce your risk of CVD, even though you have some uncontrollable risk factors?

_____

_____

_____

_____

Activate, Motivate, & Advance YOUR FITNESS

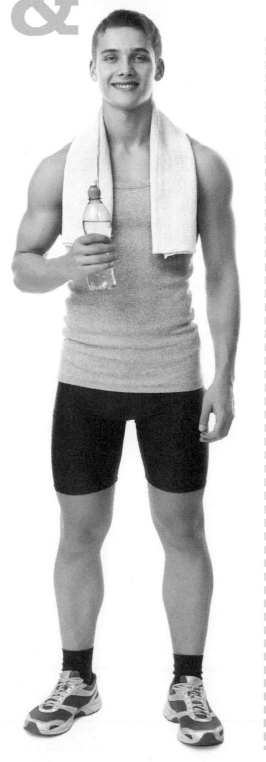

Pull all your fitness programs together to create a comprehensive personal program—one that meets your own long-term goals. First, identify which exercises work for you and which ones you'd like to modify (refer to Figure 4.10 on page 137–150, Figure 5.7 on pages 185–190, and Figure 5.8 on pages 191–192). Then, look at the following sample programs. Start at your current level and modify for your own preferences and rate of improvement.

ACTIVATE!
Warm-Up & Cool-Down

Warming-up prior to exercise is crucial! Start with gentle cardio-respiratory exercises for 5 to 10 minutes. After breaking a light sweat, add dynamic movements that increase your range of motion.

After your exercise session, cool down by moving at a slower pace until your heart rate and temperature fall to comfortable levels. Finish your cool-down with a few stretches.

Total Fitness Programs

Adjust intensity, volume, and training days to suit your personal fitness level and schedule.

Start here if you are new to exercise or if you have not exercised for more than three months.

GOAL: Establish a consistent pattern of activity and exercise, gradually increasing time, intensity, and variety over four weeks. Follow warm-up and cool-down guidelines above for each exercise session.

WEEK 1	Activities*	Time/Distance OR Sets/Reps	Intensity/Wt**
Sunday	**Cardio:** Walk	5 min	L
Monday	**Cardio:** Walk	5 min	L
	Muscle: Push-Up	10 reps, 1 set	BW
	Muscle: Abdominal Curl	15 reps, 1 set	BW
Tuesday	**Cardio:** Walk	8 min	M
Wednesday	**Cardio:** Walk	8 min	M
	Muscle: Push-Up	10 reps, 1 set	BW
	Muscle: Abdominal Curl	15 reps, 1 set	BW
Thursday	Rest Day		
Friday	**Cardio:** Walk	10 min	M
Saturday	Rest Day		
WEEK 2	Activities	Time/Distance OR Sets/Reps	Intensity/Wt
Sunday	**Cardio:** Walk	10 min	L
	Stretch: Hip Flexor Stretch	1 rep, 15 seconds	
	Stretch: Calf Stretches	1 rep, 15 seconds	
Monday	**Cardio:** Walk	10 min	M
	Muscle: Push-Up	8 reps, 2 sets	BW
	Muscle: Abdominal Curl	10 reps, 2 sets	BW
Tuesday	**Cardio:** Walk	10 min	M
Wednesday	**Cardio:** Walk	10 min	M
	Muscle: Push-Up	12 reps, 1 set	BW
	Muscle: Abdominal Curl	18 reps, 1 set	BW
Thursday	Rest Day		
Friday	**Cardio:** Walk	15 min	M
	Stretch: Hip Flexor Stretch	1 rep, 15 seconds	
	Stretch: Calf Stretches	1 rep, 15 seconds	
Saturday	Rest Day		
WEEK 3	Activities	Time/Distance OR Sets/Reps	Intensity/Wt
Sunday	**Cardio:** Walk	15 min	L
	Stretch: Hip Flexor Stretch	1 rep, 15 seconds	
	Stretch: Calf Stretches	1 rep, 15 seconds	
	Stretch: Shin Stretch	1 rep, 15 seconds	
Monday	**Cardio:** Walk	10 min	M
	Muscle: Push-Up	8 reps, 2 sets	BW
	Muscle: Abdominal Curl	10 reps, 2 sets	BW
	Muscle: Lunge	10 reps, 1 set	BW
Tuesday	**Cardio:** Walk	15 min	M
Wednesday	**Cardio:** Walk	10 min	M
	Muscle: Push-Up	15 reps, 1 set	BW
	Muscle: Abdominal Curl	20 reps, 1 set	BW
	Muscle: Lunge	12 reps, 1 set	BW
Thursday	Rest Day		
Friday	**Cardio:** Walk	20 min	M
	Stretch: Hip Flexor Stretch	1 rep, 15 seconds	
	Stretch: Calf Stretches	1 rep, 15 seconds	
	Stretch: Shin Stretch	1 rep, 15 seconds	
Saturday	Rest Day		

(Continued)

WEEK 4	Activities	Time/Distance OR Sets/Reps	Intensity/Wt
Sunday	**Cardio:** Walk **Stretch:** Hip Flexor Stretch **Stretch:** Calf Stretches **Stretch:** Shin Stretch **Stretch:** Hamstrings Stretch	20 min 2 reps, 10 seconds 2 reps, 10 seconds 2 reps, 10 seconds 2 reps, 10 seconds	L
Monday	**Cardio:** Walk **Muscle:** Push-Up **Muscle:** Abdominal Curl **Muscle:** Lunge **Back Health:** Arm/Leg Extensions **Stretch:** Pectoral and Biceps Stretch **Stretch:** Shoulder Stretch	15 min 10 reps, 2 sets 12 reps, 2 sets 10 reps, 2 sets 10 reps, 1 set 1 rep, 15 seconds 1 rep, 15 seconds	M BW BW BW BW
Tuesday	**Cardio:** Walk	20 min	M
Wednesday	**Cardio:** Walk **Muscle:** Push-Up **Muscle:** Abdominal Curl **Muscle:** Lunge **Back Health:** Arm/Leg Extensions **Stretch:** Pectoral and Biceps Stretch **Stretch:** Shoulder Stretch	15 min 20 reps, 1 set 25 reps, 1 set 15 reps, 1 set 10 reps, 1 set 2 reps, 10 seconds 2 rep, 10 seconds	M BW BW BW BW
Thursday	Rest Day		
Friday	**Cardio:** Walk **Stretch:** Hip Flexor Stretch **Stretch:** Calf Stretches **Stretch:** Shin Stretch **Stretch:** Hamstrings Stretch	20 min 2 reps, 10 seconds 2 reps, 10 seconds 2 reps, 10 seconds 2 reps, 10 seconds	M
Saturday	Rest Day		

*Cardiorespiratory (Cardio)** activities can vary from walking, running, cycling, hiking, elliptical/treadmill training, stationary cycling, fitness classes, and/or swimming. Choose your activities based on equipment/facility availability and your personal preference.
Intensity is listed as Light/Lifestyle (L), Moderate (M), or Vigorous (V) (see Figure 2.1, page 31). **Weight (Wt)** listed as Body Weight (BW).
Resistance Training (Muscle) Exercises: See Figure 4.10 (pages 137–150) for exercise descriptions and photos.
Stretching Exercises: See Figure 5.7 (pages 185–190) for exercise descriptions and photos.
Back Health Exercises: See Figure 5.8 (pages 191–192) for exercise descriptions and photos.

INTERMEDIATE PERSONAL FITNESS PROGRAM

Start here if you already exercise two days a week.

GOAL: Meet the minimum FITT guidelines for cardiorespiratory, muscle, and flexibility fitness by the end of four weeks. Follow warm-up and cool-down guidelines for each exercise session.

WEEK 1	Activities*	Time/Distance OR Sets/Reps	Intensity/Wt**
Sunday	Rest Day		
Monday	**Cardio:** Walk/Run **Muscle:** Exercises 1-3 below **Stretch:** Exercises 1-3 below	20 min 8 reps, 1 set 1 rep, 15 seconds	L BW or 65%
Tuesday	Rest Day		
Wednesday	**Cardio:** Walk/Run **Muscle:** Exercises 1-3 below **Stretch:** Exercises 1-3 below	20 min 10 reps, 1 set 1 rep, 15 seconds	L BW or 65%
Thursday	Rest Day		
Friday	**Cardio:** Walk/Run	20 min	M
Saturday	Rest Day		

(Continued)

WEEK 2	Activities	Time/Distance OR Sets/Reps	Intensity/Wt
Sunday	Rest Day		
Monday	**Cardio:** Walk/Run **Muscle:** Exercises 1-5 below **Stretch:** Exercises 1-4 below	25 min 12 reps, 1 set 1 rep, 20 seconds	M BW or 65%
Tuesday	Rest Day		
Wednesday	**Cardio:** Walk/Run **Muscle:** Exercises 1-5 below **Stretch:** Exercises 1-4 below	30 min 12 reps, 1 set 1 rep, 20 seconds	L BW or 70%
Thursday	Rest Day		
Friday	**Cardio:** Walk/Run **Stretch:** Exercises 1-4 below	30 min 1 rep, 20 seconds	M
Saturday	Rest Day		
WEEK 3	Activities	Time/Distance OR Sets/Reps	Intensity/Wt
Sunday	Rest Day		
Monday	**Cardio:** Walk/Run **Muscle:** Exercises 1-6 below **Back Health:** Exercises 1-2 below **Stretch:** Exercises 1-4 below	30 min 8 reps, 2 sets 10 reps, 1 set 2 reps, 15 seconds	M BW or 75%
Tuesday	Rest Day		
Wednesday	**Cardio:** Walk/Run **Muscle:** Exercises 1-6 below **Stretch:** Exercises 1-5 below	35 min 10 reps, 2 sets 2 reps, 15 seconds	M BW or 75%
Thursday	Rest Day		
Friday	**Cardio:** Walk/Run **Stretch:** Exercises 1-5 below	30 min 2 reps, 15 seconds	M
Saturday	**Cardio:** Walk/Run	35 min	M
WEEK 4	Activities	Time/Distance OR Sets/Reps	Intensity/Wt
Sunday	Rest Day		
Monday	**Cardio:** Walk/Run **Muscle:** Exercises 1-8 below **Back Health:** Exercises 1-3 below **Stretch:** Exercises 1-5 below	35 min 12 reps, 2 sets 10 reps, 1 set 2 reps, 20 seconds	M BW or 70%
Tuesday	Rest Day		
Wednesday	**Cardio:** Walk/Run **Muscle:** Exercises 1-8 below **Back Health:** Exercises 1-3 below **Stretch:** Exercises 1-5 below	40 min 15 reps, 2 sets 12 reps, 1 set 2 reps, 20 seconds	M BW or 70%
Thursday	Rest Day		
Friday	**Cardio:** Walk/Run **Cardio:** Intervals (30 sec on: 1 min recover) **Stretch:** Exercises 1-6 below	30 min Repeat 4 times 2 reps, 20 seconds	M V
Saturday	**Cardio:** Walk/Run **Stretch:** Exercises 1-6 below	45 min 2 reps, 20 seconds	M

*Cardiorespiratory (Cardio) activities can vary from walking, running, cycling, hiking, elliptical/treadmill training, stationary cycling, fitness classes, and/or swimming. Choose your activities based on equipment/facility availability and your personal preference.
Intensity is listed as Light/Lifestyle (L), Moderate (M), or Vigorous (V) (see Figure 2.1, page 31). **Weight (Wt) listed as Body Weight (BW) or percent of 1RM.
Resistance Training (Muscle) Exercises: See Figure 4.10 (pages 137–150) for exercise descriptions and photos.
1) Push-Up, 2) Abdominal Curl, 3) Squat or Lunge, 4) Row, 5) Plank (hold 20 to 40 sec), 6) Heel Raise, 7) Overhead Press, 8) Lat Pull-Down.

(Continued)

Stretching Exercises: See Figure 5.7 (pages 185–190) for exercise descriptions and photos.
1) Hip Flexor Stretch, 2) Pectoral and Biceps Stretch, 3) Calf Stretches, 4) Hamstrings Stretch, 5) Shoulder Stretch, 6) Neck Stretches.
Back Health Exercises: See Figure 5.8 (pages 191–192) for exercise descriptions and photos.
1) Arm/Leg Extensions, 2) Cat Stretch, 3) Back Bridge.

MOTIVATE!

Keep a log of your active days, actual exercises, time spent, and repetitions/sets. Is your motivation lagging? Find a workout partner, view a new exercise video online, add exercise to your commute, get out to nature areas, or download a new app with ready-made fitness sessions! The bottom line: *keep moving.* Make a commitment to yourself to be active for a long, healthy life!

ADVANCE!

Once you've established your exercise program, try out this more advanced program.

ADVANCED PERSONAL FITNESS PROGRAM

Start here if you already exercise three to four days a week.

GOAL: Consistently meet FITT guidelines for cardiorespiratory, muscle, and flexibility fitness and increase intensity levels over four weeks. Follow warm-up and cool-down guidelines for each exercise session.

WEEK 1	Activities*	Time/Distance OR Sets/Reps	Intensity/Wt**
Sunday	Rest Day		
Monday	**Cardio:** Walk/Run **Muscle:** Exercises 1-6 below **Back Health:** Exercises 1-2 below **Stretch:** Exercises 1-5 below	30 min 10 reps, 2 sets 10 reps, 1 set 2 reps, 15 seconds	M BW or 70%
Tuesday	Rest Day		
Wednesday	**Cardio:** Walk/Run **Muscle:** Exercises 1-6 below **Stretch:** Exercises 1-5 below	35 min 10 reps, 2 sets 2 reps, 15 seconds	M BW or 75%
Thursday	Rest Day		
Friday	**Cardio:** Walk/Run **Stretch:** Exercises 1-6 below	35 min 2 reps, 15 seconds	M
Saturday	**Cardio:** Walk/Run	40 min	M
WEEK 2	**Activities**	**Time/Distance OR Sets/Reps**	**Intensity/Wt**
Sunday	Rest Day		
Monday	**Cardio:** Walk/Run **Muscle:** Exercises 1-8 below **Back Health:** Exercises 1-3 below **Stretch:** Exercises 1-7 below	35 min 12 reps, 2 sets 12 reps, 1 set 2 reps, 20 seconds	M BW or 75%
Tuesday	Rest Day		
Wednesday	**Cardio:** Walk/Run **Muscle:** Exercises 1-8 below **Back Health:** Exercises 1-3 below **Stretch:** Exercises 1-7 below	40 min 15 reps, 2 sets 15 reps, 1 set 2 reps, 20 seconds	M BW or 70%
Thursday	Rest Day		
Friday	**Cardio:** Walk/Run **Cardio:** Intervals (30 sec on: 1 min recover) **Stretch:** Exercises 1-6 below	35 min Repeat 4 times 2 reps, 20 seconds	M V
Saturday	**Cardio:** Walk/Run **Stretch:** Exercises 1-8 below	45 min 2 reps, 20 seconds	M

(Continued)

WEEK 3	Activities	Time/Distance OR Sets/Reps	Intensity/Wt
Sunday	Rest Day		
Monday	**Cardio:** Walk/Run **Muscle:** Exercises 1-10 below **Back Health:** Exercises 1-3 below **Stretch:** Exercises 1-8 below	40 min 6 reps, 2 sets 20 reps, 1 set 2 reps, 20 seconds	M BW or 85%
Tuesday	**Cardio:** Walk/Run **Cardio:** Intervals (30 sec on: 1 min recover) **Stretch:** Exercises 1-4 below	30 min Repeat 4 times 1 rep, 20 seconds	M V
Wednesday	**Cardio:** Walk/Run **Muscle:** Exercises 1-10 below **Back Health:** Exercises 1-3 below **Stretch:** Exercises 1-8 below	40 min 8 reps, 2 sets 25 reps, 1 set 2 reps, 20 seconds	M BW or 85%
Thursday	Rest Day		
Friday	**Cardio:** Walk/Run **Cardio:** Intervals (30 sec on: 1 min recover) **Stretch:** Exercises 1-7 below	45 min Repeat 5 times 2 reps, 20 seconds	M V
Saturday	**Cardio:** Walk/Run **Stretch:** Exercises 1-9 below	50 min 2 reps, 25 seconds	M
WEEK 4	Activities	Time/Distance OR Sets/Reps	Intensity/Wt
Sunday	**Stretch:** Exercises 1-9 below	2 reps, 25 seconds	
Monday	**Cardio:** Walk/Run **Muscle:** Exercises 1-10 below **Back Health:** Exercises 1-3 below **Stretch:** Exercises 1-8 below	45 min 10 reps, 2 sets 15 reps, 2 sets 2 reps, 20 seconds	M BW or 80%
Tuesday	**Cardio:** Walk/Run **Cardio:** Intervals (45 sec on: 1 min recover) **Stretch:** Exercises 1-4 below	35 min Repeat 5 times 2 reps, 15 seconds	M V
Wednesday	**Cardio:** Walk/Run **Muscle:** Exercises 1-10 below **Back Health:** Exercises 1-3 below **Stretch:** Exercises 1-8 below	50 min 12 reps, 2 sets 20 reps, 2 sets 2 reps, 20 seconds	M BW or 80%
Thursday	Rest Day		
Friday	**Cardio:** Walk/Run **Cardio:** Intervals (45 sec on: 45 sec recover) **Stretch:** Exercises 1-7 below	55 min Repeat 6 times 2 reps, 25 seconds	M V
Saturday	**Cardio:** Walk/Run **Stretch:** Exercises 1-9 below	60 min 2 reps, 30 seconds	M

***Cardiorespiratory (Cardio)** activities can vary from walking, running, cycling, hiking, elliptical/treadmill training, stationary cycling, fitness classes, and/or swimming. Choose your activities based on equipment/facility availability and your personal preference.

****Intensity** is listed as Light/Lifestyle (L), Moderate (M), or Vigorous (V) (see Figure 2.1, page 31). **Weight (Wt)** listed as Body Weight (BW) or percent of 1RM.

Resistance Training (Muscle) Exercises: See Figure 4.10 (pages 137–150) for exercise descriptions and photos.
1) Push-Up, 2) Abdominal Curl, 3) Squat or Lunge, 4) Row, 5) Plank (hold 30 to 60 sec), 6) Heel Raise, 7) Overhead Press, 8) Lat Pull-Down, 9) Oblique Curl, 10) Triceps Extension.

Stretching Exercises: See Figure 5.7 (pages 185–190) for exercise descriptions and photos.
1) Hip Flexor Stretch, 2) Pectoral and Biceps Stretch, 3) Calf Stretches, 4) Hamstrings Stretch, 5) Shoulder Stretch, 6) Neck Stretches, 7) Quadriceps Stretch, 8) Gluteal Stretch, 9) Upper Back Stretch.

Back Health Exercises: See Figure 5.8 (pages 191–192) for exercise descriptions and photos.
1) Arm/Leg Extensions, 2) Cat Stretch, 3) Back Bridge.

Appendix

Answers to End-of-Chapter Review Questions

Chapter 1
1. b; 2. a; 3. b; 4. b; 5. d; 6. b; 7. b; 8. a; 9. a

Chapter 2
1. b; 2. c; 3. d; 4. a; 5. a; 6. b; 7. d; 8. d; 9. b; 10. d

Chapter 3
1. a; 2. d; 3. c; 4. a; 5. a; 6. c; 7. a; 8. d; 9. c; 10. d

Chapter 4
1. d; 2. a; 3. d; 4. a; 5. b; 6. a; 7. c; 8. b; 9. a; 10. c

Chapter 5
1. d; 2. a; 3. c; 4. b; 5. b; 6. d; 7. d; 8. b; 9. d; 10. a

Chapter 6
1. c; 2. d; 3. a; 4. c; 5. b; 6. b; 7. a; 8. c; 9. a; 10. d

Chapter 7
1. c; 2. d; 3. d; 4. c; 5. d; 6. d; 7. d; 8. a; 9. a; 10. d; 11. c; 12. c

Chapter 8
1. d; 2. b; 3. d; 4. d; 5. a; 6. b; 7. d; 8. a; 9. b; 10. d

Chapter 9
1. c; 2. b; 3. a; 4. d; 5. b; 6. d; 7. a; 8. d; 9. a; 10. d; 11. c

Chapter 10
1. d; 2. b; 3. c; 4. c; 5. a; 6. b; 7. d; 8. a; 9. b; 10. a

References

Chapter 1

1. American College Health Association, *American College Health Association—National College Health Assessment II: Reference Group Executive Summary, Fall 2015* (Hanover, MD: American College Health Association, 2016).

2. Ibid.

3. National Wellness Institute, "The Six Dimensions of Wellness," 2015, http://www.nationalwellness.org/?page=Six_Dimensions&hhSearchTerms=%22Definition+and+Wellness%22

4. Ibid.

5. K. Berkman and I. Karvachi, "A Historical Framework for Social Epidemiology: Social Determinants of Population Health," in *Social Epidemiology*, eds. K. Berman and I. Karvachi (New York: Oxford University Press, 2014).

6. Ibid.; University of California, Davis, Student Health and Counseling Services, "Intellectual Wellness," accessed May 2016; National Wellness Institute, "The Six Dimensions of Wellness," 2015.

7. G. Gignanc, A. Karlamglou, and S. Wee, "Emotional Intelligence as a Unique Predictor of Individual Differences in Humor Styles and Humor Appraisal," *Personality and Individual Differences* 56 (2014): 34–39.

8. R. Wilson, "Special Report: Epidemic of Anguish," *Chronicle of Higher Education* (August 31, 2015): 2–26, http://images.results.chronicle.com/Web/TheChronicleofHigherEducation/%7B5d9743b6-cfdc-4ac2-a629-1e59acdaf08b%7D_AD-CHE-MentalHealth.pdf

9. National Alliance on Mental Illness, "Mental Health by the Numbers: Mental Health Facts—Children and Teens Infographic," 2015, http://www.nami.org/Learn-More/Mental-Health-By-the-Numbers

10. Ibid.; National Alliance on Mental Illness, "College Survey: 50 Percent of College Students with Mental Health Problems Who Withdraw from School Because of Mental Health Issues Never Access College Mental Health Services," accessed May 2016.

11. Conference Board Annual Report, August 2015, www.prnewswire.com/news-releases/us-job-satisfaction-at-lowest-level-in-two-decades-80699752.html

12. T. C. Premuzic, "Does Money Really Affect Motivation? A Review of Research," *Harvard Business Review*, April 10, 2013, https://hbr.org/2013/04/does-money-really-affect-motiv#

13. Centers for Disease Control and Prevention, "Physical Activity and Health: The Benefits of Physical Activity," June 4, 2015, https://www.cdc.gov/physicalactivity/basics/pa-health/; D. Aune et al., "Physical Activity and Risk of Type 2 Diabetes: A Systematic Review and Dose Response Meta-Analysis," *European Journal of Epidemiology* 30, no. 7 (2015): 529–42; C. Lang et al., "The Relationship between Physical Activity and Sleep from Mid-Adolescence to Early Adulthood: A Systematic Review of Methodological Approaches and Meta-Analyses, " *Sleep Medicine Reviews* 28 (August 2015), doi: 10.1016/j.smrv.2015.07.004. Epub 2015 Aug 5.

14. Centers for Disease Control and Prevention, National Center for Health Statistics, "How Healthy Are We?" Table 7, February 2016, http://www.cdc.gov/nchs/fastats/life-expectancy.htm; World Bank, "Life Expectancy at Birth, Total (Years), http://data.worldbank.org/indicator/SP.DYN.LE00.IN?page=4HO; World Health Organization, "Global Health Observatory Data: Infant Mortality," 2016, http://www.cdc.gov/nchs/fastats/life-expectancy.htm; World Bank, "Life Expectancy at Birth, Total (Years), http://data.worldbank.org/indicator/SP.DYN.LE00.IN?page=4HO; World Health Organization, "Global Health Observatory Data: Infant Mortality," 2016, http://www.who.int/gho/child_health/mortality/neonatal_infant_text/en/

15. C. Murray et al., "Global, Regional, and National Disability-Adjusted Life Years (DALYs) for 306 Diseases and Injuries and Healthy Life Expectancy (HALE) for 188 Countries, 1990–2013: Quantifying the Epidemiological Transition," *Lancet* 386, no. 10009 (2015), http://www.thelancet.com/journals/lancet/article/PIIS0140-6736(15)61340-X/fulltext; World Health Organization, "Global Observation Repository, Life Expectancy Data by Country," 2013.

16. Centers for Disease Control and Prevention, National Vital Statistics System–National Center for Health Statistics, WISQUARS, "Ten Leading Causes of Death by Age, United States, 2013," 2015, http://www.cdc.gov/injury/wisqars/pdf/leading_causes_of_death_by_age_group_2013-a.pdf

17. R. Shah et al., "Association of Fitness in Young Adulthood with Survival and Cardiovascular Risk: The Coronary Artery Risk Development in Young Adults (CARDIA) Study," *JAMA Intern Medicine* 176, no. 1 (November 30, 2015), doi: 10.1001/jamainternmed.2015.6309; B. Spring et al., "Healthy Lifestyle Change and Subclinical Atherosclerosis in Young Adults: Coronary Risk Development in Young Adults (CARDIA) Study," *Circulation* (2014), http://circ.ahajournals.org/content/early/2014/04/28/CIRCULATIONAHA.113.005445.full.pdf+html

18. D. Hupin et al., "Even a Low Dose of Moderate-to-Vigorous Physical Activity Reduces Mortality by 22% in Adults Aged ≥ 60 Years: A Systematic Review and Meta-Analysis," *British Journal of Sports Medicine* (2015), doi: 10.1136/bjsports-2014-094306; P. I. Janssen et al., "Years of Life Gained Due to Leisure-Time Physical Activity in the US," *American Journal of Preventative Medicine* 44, no. 1 (2013): 23–29.

19. C. E. Garner et al., "American College of Sports Medicine Position Stand: Quantity and Quality of Exercise for Developing and Maintaining Cardiorespiratory, Musculoskeletal, and Neuromotor Fitness in Apparently Healthy Adults: Guidance for Prescribing Exercise," *Medicine and Science in Sports and Exercise* 43, no. 7 (2011): 1334–59.

20. Centers for Disease Control and Prevention, National Center for Chronic Disease Prevention and Health Promotion–Division of Nutrition, Physical Activity, and Obesity, "State Indicator Report on Physical Activity, 2014," 2015, http://www.cdc.gov/physicalactivity/downloads/pa_state_indicator_report_2014.pdf?s_cid=bb-DNPAO-SIRPA2014-002&utm_source=external&utm_medium=banner&utm_content=DNPAO-SIRPA2014-002&utm_campaign=

21. Ibid.

22. C. L. Ogden et al., "Prevalence of Childhood and Adult Obesity in the United States, 2011–2012," *JAMA* 2014. 311, no. 8: 806–14, doi: 10.1001/jama.2014.732

23. World Health Organization, "Global Status Report on Noncommunicable Diseases, 2014," Chapter 7, 2014, http://apps.who.int/iris/bitstream/10665/148114/1/9789241564854_eng.pdf

24. Healthy People 2020, "Framework: The Vision, Mission, and Goals of *Healthy People 2020*," https://www.healthypeople.gov/

25. USGovernmentSpending.com, "US Health Care Spending," 2016, http://www.usgovernmentspending.com/spend.php?title=US_Health_Care_Spending&expand=10&meta=health, "US Health Care Spending," 2016, http://www.usgovernmentspending.com/spend.php?title=US_Health_Care_Spending&expand=10&meta=health

26. L. Lorenzoni, A. Belloni, and F. Sassi, "Health Care Expenditures and Health Policy in the USA versus Other High Spending OECD Countries," *Lancet* 384, no. 9937 (2014): 83–92, doi: http://www.thelancet.com/journals/lancet/article/PIIS0140-6736(14)60571-7/fulltext

27. US Department of Health and Human Services, "Affordable Care Act: About the Law," October 2015.

28. S. Collins, P. Rasmussen, and M. Doty, "Gaining Ground: America's Health Insurance Coverage and Access to Care after the Affordable Care Act's First Open Enrollment Period," 2014, http://www.commonwealthfund.org/publications/issue-briefs/2014/jul/health-coverage-access-aca

29. Ibid.

30. J. Prochaska, C. DiClemente, and J. Norcross, "In Search of How People Change: Application to Addictive Behaviors," *American Psychologist* 47, no. 9 (1983): 1102–14.

31. Centers for Disease Control and Prevention, "FastStats: Exercise or Physical Activity," 2015, http://www.cdc.gov/nchs/fastats/exercise.htm

32. A. Rogers and Members of the 2015 Dietary Guidelines Advisory Group, "Scientific Report of the 2015 Dietary Guidelines Advisory Committee: Advisory Report to the Secretary of Health and Human Services and the Secretary of Agriculture," February 2015, https://health.gov/

dietaryguidelines/2015-scientific-report/PDFs/Scientific-Report-of-the-2015-Dietary-Guidelines-Advisory-Committee.pdf

33. Ibid.

34. American College Health Association, *ACHA-NCHA II: Undergraduate Students Reference Group Data Report, Spring 2015* (Hanover, MD: American College Health Association, 2015); K. M. Leung et al., "Predictors of Physical Activities in Non-Traditional College Students" (abstract of paper presented at American Alliance for Health, Physical Education, Recreation, and Dance Annual Convention, Charlotte, North Carolina, April 2013).

35. R. Rhodes and C. Yao, "Models Accounting for Intention-Behavior Discordance in the Physical Activity Domain: A User's Guide, Content Overview, and Review of Current Evidence," *International Journal of Behavioral Nutrition and Physical Activity* 12, no. 9 (2015), doi: 10.1186/s12966-015-0168-6; M. Koring et al., "Synergistic Effects of Planning and Self-Efficacy on Physical Activity," *Health Education and Behavior* 39, no. 2 (2012): 152–58.

36. K. Bell et al., "Does the Hand That Controls the Cigarette Packet Rule the Smoker? Findings from Ethnographic Interviews with Smokers in Canada, Australia, the United Kingdom, and the USA," *Social Science and Medicine* 142 (2015): 136–44.

37. G. M. Hochbaum, *Public Participation in Medical Screening Programs: A Socio-Psychological Study*, Department of Health Education and Welfare, PHS Publication no. 572 (Washington, DC: US Government Printing Office, 1958); I. M. Rosenstock, V. J. Strecher, and M. H. Becker, "Social Learning Theory and the Health Belief Model," *Health Education & Behavior* 15, no. 2 (1988): 175–83, doi: 10.1177/109019818801500203

38. G. T. Doran, "There's a S.M.A.R.T. Way to Write Management's Goals and Objectives," *Management Review* 70, no. 11 (1981): 35–36

GETFITGRAPHICS References

1. D. Belsky et al., "Cardiorespiratory Fitness and Cognitive Function in Midlife: Neuroprotection or Neuroselection," *Journal of Neurology* 77, no. 4 (2015): 607–17.

2. L. Brinke et al., "Aerobic Exercise Increases Hippocampal Volume in Older Women with Probable Mild Cognitive Impairment: A 6-Month Randomised Controlled Trial," *British Journal of Sports Medicine* 49 (2015): 248–54, doi: 10.1136bjsports-2013-093184

3. T. Tarumi and R. Zhang, "The Role of Exercise-Induced Cardiovascular Adaptation in Brain Health," *American College of Sports Medicine* 43, no. 4 (2015): 181–89.

4. C. Lees and J. Hopkins, "Effect of Aerobic Activity on Cognition, Academic Achievement, and Psychosocial Function in Children: A Systematic Review of Randomized Controlled Trials," *Preventing Chronic Disease* (2013).

5. A. Singh et al., "Physical Activity and Performance at School: A Systematic Review of the Literature Including a Methodological Quality Assessment," *Archives of Pediatrics and Adolescent Medicine* 166, no. 1 (2012): 49–55.

6. T. Archer and D. Garcia, "Physical Exercise Influences Academic Performance and Well-Being in Children and Adolescents," *International Journal of School and Cognitive Psychology* 1 (2014): e102, doi: 10.4172/ijscp.1000e102

7. J. Nyberg et al., "Cardiovascular and Cognitive Fitness at Age 18 and Risk of Early-Onset Dementia," *Brain, A Journal of Neurology* (2014), doi: http://dx.doi.org/10.1093/brain/awu041

8. C. Boyle et al., "Physical Activity, Body Mass Index, and Brain Atrophy in Alzheimer's Disease," *Neurobiology of Aging* 36, no. 1 (2015): S194–S202.

Chapter 2

1. R. Vigen et al., "Association of Cardiorespiratory Fitness with Total, Cardiovascular, and Non-Cardiovascular Mortality across 3 Decades of Follow Up in Men and Women," *Circulation, Cardiovascular Quality and Outcomes* 5, no. 3 (2012): 358–64.

2. N. Zhu et al., "Cardiorespiratory Fitness and Brain Volume and White Matter Integrity: The CARDIA Study," *Neurology* 84, no. 23 (2015): 2347–53.

3. H. Suominen, "Muscle Training for Bone Strength," *Aging Clinical and Experimental Research* 18, no. 2 (2006): 85–93.

4. K. Small, L. McNaughton, and M. Matthews, "A Systematic Review into the Efficacy of Static Stretching as Part of a Warm-Up for the Prevention

of Exercise-Related Injury," *Research in Sports Medicine* 16, no. 3 (2008): 213–31.

5. L. O. Mikkelsson et al., "Adolescent Flexibility, Endurance Strength, and Physical Activity as Predictors of Adult Tension Neck, Low Back Pain, and Knee Injury: A 25-Year Follow-Up Study," *British Journal of Sports Medicine* 40, no. 2 (2006): 107–13; M. J. Spink et al., "Foot and Ankle Strength, Range of Motion, Posture, and Deformity Are Associated with Balance and Functional Ability in Older Adults," *Archives of Physical Medicine and Rehabilitation* 92, no. 1 (2011): 68–75.

6. T. D. Brutsaert and E. J. Parra, "What Makes a Champion? Explaining Variation in Human Athletic Performance," *Respiratory Physiology and Neurobiology* 151, no. 2–3 (2006): 109–23.

7. I. Mujika and S. Padilla, "Detraining: Loss of Training-Induced Physiological and Performance Adaptations—Part I: Short-Term Insufficient Training Stimulus," *Sports Medicine* 30, no. 2 (2000): 79–87.

8. I. Mujika and S. Padilla, "Detraining: Loss of Training-Induced Physiological and Performance Adaptations—Part II: Long-Term Insufficient Training Stimulus," *Sports Medicine* 30, no. 3 (2000): 145–54.

9. I. Mujika and S. Padilla, "Cardiorespiratory and Metabolic Characteristics of Detraining in Humans," *Medicine and Science in Sports and Exercise* 33, no. 3 (2001): 413–21; I. Mujika and S. Padilla, "Muscular Characteristics of Detraining in Humans," *Medicine and Science in Sports and Exercise* 33, no. 8 (2001): 1297–303; J. T. Lemmer et al., "Age and Gender Responses to Strength Training and Detraining," *Medicine and Science in Sports and Exercise* 32, no. 8 (2000): 1505–12; M. S. Lo et al., "Training and Detraining Effects of the Resistance vs. Endurance Program on Body Composition, Body Size, and Physical Performance in Young Men," *Journal of Strength and Conditioning Research* 25, no. 8 (2011): 2246–54.

10. Mujika and Padilla, "Detraining: Loss of Training-Induced Physiological and Performance Adaptations—Part II," 2000.

11. E. S. George, R. R. Rosenkranz, and G. S. Kolt, "Chronic Disease and Sitting Time in Middle-Aged Australian Males: Findings from the 45 and Up Study," *International Journal of Behavioral Nutrition and Physical Activity* 10, no. 20 (2013), www.ijbnpa.org

12. Office of Disease Prevention and Health Promotion, US Department of Health and Human Services, *2008 Physical Activity Guidelines for Americans: Be Active, Healthy, and Happy!* ODPHP Publication no. U0036 (Washington, DC: US Department of Health and Human Services, 2008).

13. World Health Organization, "Global Recommendations on Physical Activity for Health," Global Strategy on Diet, Physical Activity, and Health, www.who.int; C. E. Garner et al., "American College of Sports Medicine Position Stand: Quantity and Quality of Exercise for Developing and Maintaining Cardiorespiratory, Musculoskeletal, and Neuromotor Fitness in Apparently Healthy Adults: Guidance for Prescribing Exercise," *Medicine and Science in Sports and Exercise* 43, no. 7 (2011): 1334–59.

14. B. W. Ward et al., "Early Release of Selected Estimates Based on Data from the 2014 National Health Interview Survey," National Center for Health Statistics, June 2015, www.cdc.gov

15. Office of Disease Prevention and Health Promotion, US Department of Health and Human Services, Healthy People 2020, "2020 Objectives and Goals: Physical Activity," http://healthypeople.gov

16. J. M. Conn, J. L. Annest, and J. Gilchrist, "Sports and Recreation-Related Injury Episodes in the US Population, 1997–99," *Injury Prevention* 9, no. 2 (2003): 117–23.

17. M. N. Sawka et al., "American College of Sports Medicine Position Stand: Exercise and Fluid Replacement," *Medicine and Science in Sports and Exercise* 39, no. 2 (2007): 377–90.

18. H. H. Fink, A. E. Mikesky, and L. A. Burgoon, *Practical Applications in Sports Nutrition*, 4th ed. (Sudbury, MA: Jones and Bartlett Publishers, 2013).

19. American College of Sports Medicine, *ACSM's Guidelines for Exercise Testing and Prescription*, 9th ed. (Baltimore: Lippincott Williams & Wilkins, 2014).

20. Ibid.

21. K. Melzer et al., "Physical Activity and Pregnancy: Cardiovascular Adaptations, Recommendations, and Pregnancy Outcomes," *Sports Medicine* 40, no. 6 (2010): 493–507.

22. A. N. Blaize, K. J. Pearson, and S. Newcomer, "Impact of Maternal Exercise during Pregnancy on Offspring Chronic Disease Susceptibility," *Exercise and Sport Science Reviews* 43, no. 4 (July 15, 2015);

M. Carolan-Olah, M. Duarte-Gardea, and J. Lechuga, "A Critical Review: Early Life Nutrition and Prenatal Programming for Adult Disease," *Journal of Clinical Nursing* 24, no. 23–24 (August 9, 2015).

23. American College of Obstetricians and Gynecologists, "ACOG Committee Opinion No. 267: Exercise during Pregnancy and the Postpartum Period," *Obstetrics & Gynecology* 99, no. 1 (2002): 171–73.

24. R. Myrna-Bekas et al., "Mood Changes in Individuals Who Regularly Participate in Various Forms of Physical Activity," *Human Movement* 13, no. 2 (2012): 170–77.

25. B. Kwan and A. Bryan, "Affective Response to Exercise as a Component of Exercise Motivation: Attitudes, Norms, Self-Efficacy, and Temporal Stability of Intentions," *Psychology of Sport and Exercise* 11, no. 1 (2010): 71–79.

26. J. F. Sallis and K. Glanz, "The Role of Built Environments in Physical Activity, Eating, and Obesity in Childhood," *The Future of Children* 16, no. 1 (2006): 89–108; H. M. Grow et al., "Where Are Youth Active? Roles of Proximity, Active Transport, and Built Environment," *Medicine and Science in Sports and Exercise* 40, no. 12 (2008): 2071–79.

27. R. Ewing et al., "Relationship between Urban Sprawl and Physical Activity, Obesity, and Morbidity," *American Journal of Health Promotion* 18, no. 1 (2003): 47–57.

28. M. J. Koohsari et al., "Neighborhood Environmental Attributes and Adults' Sedentary Behaviors: Review and Research Agenda," *Preventative Medicine* 77 (2015): 141–49.

29. L. Carrasco, C. Villaverde, and C. M. Oltras, "Endorphin Responses to Stress Induced by Competitive Swimming Event," *Journal of Sports Medicine and Physical Fitness* 47, no. 2 (2007): 239–45.

30. J. Brunet and C. Sabiston, "Exploring Motivation for Physical Activity across the Adult Lifespan," *Psychology of Sport and Exercise* 12, no. 2 (2011): 99–105.

GETFITGRAPHICS References

1. C. E. Matthews et al., "Amount of Time Spent in Sedentary Behaviors and Cause-Specific Mortality in US Adults," *American Journal of Clinical Nutrition* 495, no. 2 (2012): 437–45.

2. E. G. Wilmot et al., "Sedentary Time in Adults and the Association with Diabetes, Cardiovascular Disease, and Death: Systematic Review and Meta-Analysis," *Diabetologia* 55, no. 11 (2012): 2895–905.

3. A. V. Patel et al., "Leisure-Time Spent Sitting and Site-Specific Cancer Incidence in a Large US Cohort," *Cancer Epidemiology, Biomarkers, and Prevention* (June 30, 2015), doi: 10.1158/1055-9965.EPI-15-0237

4. J. G. Z. van Uffelen et al., "Sitting-Time, Physical Activity, and Depressive Symptoms in Mid-Aged Women," *American Journal of Preventive Medicine* 45, no. 3 (2013): 276–81.

5. L. L. Craft et al., "Evidence That Women Meeting Physical Activity Guidelines Do Not Sit Less: An Observational Inclinometry Study," *The International Journal of Behavioral Nutrition and Physical Activity* 4, no. 9 (2012): 122.

6. K. Shuval, "Sedentary Behavior, Cardiorespiratory Fitness, Physical Activity, and Cardiometabolic Risk in Men: The Cooper Center Longitudinal Study," *Mayo Clinic Proceedings* 89, no. 8 (2014): 1052–62.

7. J. P. Buckley et al., "Standing-Based Office Work Shows Encouraging Signs of Attenuating Post-Prandial Glycemic Excursion," *Occupational and Environmental Medicine* 71, no. 2 (2014): 109–11.

8. P. T. Katzmarzyk, "Standing and Mortality in a Prospective Cohort of Canadian Adults," *Medicine and Science in Sports and Exercise* 46, no. 5 (2014): 940–46.

9. C. E. Matthews et al., "Mortality Benefits for Replacing Sitting Time with Different Physical Activities," *Medicine and Science in Sports and Exercise* 47, no. 9 (2015): 1833–40.

10. J. Henson et al., "Associations of Objectively Measured Sedentary Behavior and Physical Activity with Markers of Cardiometabolic Health," *Diabetologia* 56, no. 5 (2013): doi: 10.1007/s00125-013-2845-9

Chapter 3

1. S. Kodama et al., "Cardiorespiratory Fitness as a Quantitative Predictor of All-Cause Mortality and Cardiovascular Events in Healthy Men and Women," *Journal of the American Medical Association* 301, no. 19 (2009): 2024–35, doi: 10.1001/jama.2009.681

2. A. Veijalainen et al., "Associations of Cardiorespiratory Fitness, Physical Activity, and Adiposity with Arterial Stiffness in Children," *Scandinavian Journal of Medicine & Science in Sports* (July 29, 2015).

3. K. S. Palve et al., "Association of Physical Activity in Childhood and Early Adulthood with Carotid Artery Elasticity 21 Years Later: The Cardiovascular Risk in Young Finns Study," *Journal of the American Medical Association* 3, no. 2 (2014): e000594; A. T. Cote et al., "Obesity and Arterial Stiffness in Children: Systemic Review and Meta-Analysis," *Arteriosclerosis, Thrombosis, and Vascular Biology* 35, no. 4 (2015): 1038–44.

4. C. P. Earnest et al., "Maximal Estimated Cardiorespiratory Fitness, Cardiometabolic Risk Factors, and Metabolic Syndrome in the Aerobics Center Longitudinal Study," *Mayo Clinic Proceedings* 88, no. 3 (2013): 259–70; O. Ekblom et al., "Cardiorespiratory Fitness, Sedentary Behaviour, and Physical Activity Are Independently Associated with the Metabolic Syndrome, Results from the SCAPIS Pilot Study," *PLOS ONE* (June 29, 2015): e0131586.

5. J. W. Van Dijk et al., "Exercise and 24-h Glycemic Control: Equal Effects for All Type 2 Diabetes Patients?" *Medicine & Science in Sports & Exercise* 45, no. 4 (2013): 628–35, doi: 10.1249 /MSS.0b013e31827ad8b4

6. D. Schmid and M. F. Leitzmann, "Cardiorespiratory Fitness as a Predictor of Cancer Mortality: A Systematic Review and Meta-Analysis," *Annals of Oncology* 26, no. 2 (2015): 272–78.

7. P. Zhang et al., "Association of Changes in Fitness and Body Composition with Cancer Mortality in Men," *Medicine & Science in Sports & Exercise* 46, no. 7 (2014): 1366–74; S. W. Farrell et al., "Cardiorespiratory Fitness, Different Measures of Adiposity, and Total Cancer Mortality in Women," *Obesity* 19, no. 11 (2011): 2261–67.

8. G. R. Hunter et al., "Exercise Training and Energy Expenditure Following Weight Loss," *Medicine & Science in Sports & Exercise* 47, no. 9 (2015): 1950–57.

9. J. R. Trombold et al., "Acute High-Intensity Endurance Exercise Is More Effective Than Moderate Intensity Exercise for Attenuation of Postprandial Triglyceride Elevation," *Journal of Applied Physiology* 114, no. 6 (2013): 792–800, doi: 10.1152/japplphysiol.01028.2012

10. A. M. Knab et al., "A 45-Minute Vigorous Exercise Bout Increases Metabolic Rate for 14 Hours," *Medicine & Science in Sports & Exercise* 43, no. 9 (2011): 1643–48.

11. M. D. Hoffman and D. R. Hoffman, "Exercisers Achieve Greater Acute Exercise-Induced Mood Enhancement Than Non-Exercisers," *Archives of Physical Medicine and Rehabilitation* 89, no. 2 (2008): 358–63.

12. M. E. Hopkins et al., "Differential Effects of Acute and Regular Physical Exercise on Cognition and Affect," *Neuroscience* 215 (2012): 59–68, doi: 10.1016/j.neuroscience.2012.04.056

13. T. M. DiLorenzo et al., "Long-Term Effects of Aerobic Exercise on Psychological Outcomes," *Preventative Medicine* 28, no. 1 (1999): 75–85.

14. G. M. Cooney et al., "Exercise for Depression," *Cochrane Database of Systematic Reviews* 9 (September 12, 2013): CD004366; V. S. Conn, "Depressive Symptom Outcomes of Physical Activity Interventions: Meta-Analysis Findings," *Annals of Behavioral Medicine* 39, no. 2 (2010): 128–38, doi: 10.1007 /s12160-010-9172-x

15. S. M. Park, Y. S. Kwak, and J. G. Ji, "The Effects of Combined Exercise on Health-Related Fitness, Endotoxin, and Immune Function of Postmenopausal Women with Abdominal Obesity," *Journal of Immunology Research* 2015, no. 830567 (May 14, 2015); J. Romeo et al., "Physical Activity, Immunity, and Infection," *Proceedings of the Nutrition Society* 69, no. 3 (2010): 390–99.

16. M. A. Moro-Garcia et al., "Frequent Participation in High-Volume Exercise Throughout Life Is Associated with a More Differentiated Adaptive Immune Response," *Brain, Behavior, and Immunity* 39 (2014): 61–74.

17. J. E. Ahlskog et al., "Physical Exercise as a Preventive or Disease-Modifying Treatment of Dementia and Brain Aging," *Mayo Clinic Proceedings* 86, no. 9 (2011): 876–84, doi: 10.4065/mcp.2011.0252

18. K. I. Erickson et al., "Exercise Training Increases Size of Hippocampus and Improves Memory," *Proceedings of the National Academy of Sciences USA* 108, no. 7 (2011): 3017–22, doi: 10.1073/pnas.1015950108

19. K. M. Erlandson et al., "Relationship of Physical Function and Quality of Life among Persons Aging with HIV Infection," *AIDS* 28, no. 13 (2014): 1939–43; M. Gomes Neto et al., "A Systematic Review of Effects of Concurrent Strength and Endurance Training on the Health-Related Quality of Life and Cardiopulmonary Status in Patients with HIV/AIDS," *BioMed Research International* 2013, no. 319524 (April 3, 2013).

20. S. I. Mishra et al., "Exercise Interventions on the Health-Related Quality of Life for Cancer Survivors," *Cochrane Database of Systematic Reviews* 8, no. CD007566 (August 15, 2012).

21. M. Benetti, C. L. Araujo, and R. Z. Santos, "Cardiorespiratory Fitness and Quality of Life at Different Exercise Intensities after Myocardial Infarction," *Arquivos Brasileiros de Cardiologia* 95, no. 3 (2010): 399–404.

22. S. Marzolini et al., "The Effects of an Aerobic and Resistance Exercise Training Program on Cognition Following Stroke," *Neurorehabilitation & Neural Repair* 27, no. 5 (2013): 392–402, doi: 10.1177/1545968312465192

23. G. Borg, *Borg's Perceived Exertion and Pain Scales* (Champaign, IL: Human Kinetics, 1998), 27–38.

24. R. J. Robertson et al., "Validation of the Adult OMNI Scale of Perceived Exertion for Cycle Ergometer Exercise," *Medicine & Science in Sports & Exercise* 36, no. 1 (2004): 102–8; A. C. Utter et al., "Validation of the Adult OMNI Scale of Perceived Exertion for Walking/Running Exercise," *Medicine & Science in Sports & Exercise* 36, no. 10 (2004): 1776–80.

25. Centers for Disease Control and Prevention, National Center for Environmental Health's Health Studies Branch, "Frequently Asked Questions (FAQs) about Extreme Heat," reviewed September 2015, http://emergency.cdc.gov/disasters/extremeheat/faq.asp

26. M. N. Sawka et al., "American College of Sports Medicine Position Stand: Exercise and Fluid Replacement," *Medicine & Science in Sports & Exercise* 39, no. 2 (2007): 377–90, doi: 10.1249/mss.0b013e31802ca597

GETFITGRAPHICS References

1. M. Miyashita, S. F. Burns, and D. J. Stensel, "An Update on Accumulating Exercise and Postprandial Lipaemia: Translating Theory into Practice," *Journal of Preventive Medicine & Public Health* 46 (2013): S3–S11, doi: 10.3961/jpmph.2013.46.S.S3

2. G. D. Lewis et al., "Metabolic Signatures of Exercise in Human Plasma," *Scientific Translational Medicine* 2, no. 33 (2010): 33–37, doi: 10.1126/scitranslmed.3001006

3. G. McRae et al., "Extremely Low-Volume, Whole-Body Aerobic-Resistance Training Improves Aerobic Fitness and Muscular Endurance in Females," *Applied Physiology Nutrition and Metabolism* 37, no. 6 (2012): 1124–31, doi: 10.1139/h2012-093

Chapter 4

1. Centers for Disease Control and Prevention, "Division of Nutrition, Physical Activity, and Obesity," 2015, http://www.cdc.gov/nccdphp/dnpao/index.html

2. D. R. Claflin et al., "Effects of High- and Low-Velocity Resistance Training on the Contractile Properties of Skeletal Muscle Fibers from Young and Older Humans," *Journal of Applied Physiology* 111, no. 4 (2011): 1021–30, doi: 10.1152/japplphysiol.01119.2010

3. K. A. Volaklis, M. Halle, and C. Meisinger, "Muscular Strength as a Strong Predictor of Mortality: A Narrative Review," *European Journal of Internal Medicine* 26, no. 5 (2015): 303–10, doi: 10.1016/j.ejim.2015.04.013

4. K. Davison et al., "Relationships between Obesity, Cardiorespiratory Fitness, and Cardiovascular Function," *Journal of Obesity* 2010, no. 191253 (2010), doi: 10.1155/2010/191253; M. Fogelholm, "Physical Activity, Fitness, and Fatness: Relations to Mortality, Morbidity, and Disease Risk Factors: A Systematic Review," *Obesity Reviews* 11, no. 3 (2010): 202–21, doi: 10.1111/j.1467-789X.2009.00653.x; J. G. Stegger et al., "Body Composition and Body Fat Distribution in Relation to Later Risk of Acute Myocardial Infarction: A Danish Follow-Up Study," *International Journal of Obesity* 35, no. 11 (2011): 1433–41, doi: 10.1038/ijo.2010.278

5. Z. Wang et al., "Specific Metabolic Rates of Major Organs and Tissues across Adulthood: Evaluation by Mechanistic Model of Resting Energy Expenditure," *American Journal of Clinical Nutrition* 92, no. 6 (2010): 1369–77, doi: 10.3945/ajcn.2010.29885

6. S. M. Fernando et al., "Myocyte Androgen Receptors Increase Metabolic Rate and Improve Body Composition by Reducing Fat Mass," *Endocrinology* 151, no. 7 (2010): 3125–32, doi: 10.1210/en.2010-0018; R. R. Wolfe, "The Underappreciated Role of Muscle in Health and Disease," *American Journal of Clinical Nutrition* 84, no. 3 (2006): 475–82.

7. J. E. Donnelly et al., "American College of Sports Medicine Position Stand: Appropriate Physical Activity Intervention Strategies for Weight Loss and Prevention of Weight Regain for Adults," *Medicine & Science in Sports & Exercise* 41, no. 2 (2009): 459–71, doi: 10.1249/MSS.0b013e3181949333

8. A. Figueroa et al., "Effects of Diet and/or Low-Intensity Resistance Exercise Training on Arterial Stiffness, Adiposity, and Lean Mass in Obese Postmenopausal Women," *American Journal of Hypertension* 26, no. 3 (2013): 416–23, doi: 10.1093/ajh/hps050

9. J. B Moore et al., "Effects of a 12-Week Resistance Exercise Program on Physical Self-Perceptions in College Students," *Research Quarterly for Exercise and Sport* 82, no. 2 (2011): 291–301.

10. V. A. Cornelissen et al., "Impact of Resistance Training on Blood Pressure and Other Cardiovascular Risk Factors: A Meta-Analysis of Randomized, Controlled Trials," *Hypertension* 58, no. 5 (2011): 950–58, doi: 10.1161/HYPERTENSIONAHA.111.177071; N. Gelecek et al., "The Effects of Resistance Training on Cardiovascular Disease Risk Factors in Postmenopausal Women: A Randomized-Controlled Trial," *Health Care for Women International* 33, no. 12 (2012): 1072–85, doi: 10.1080/07399332.2011.645960; D. Sheikholeslami Vatani et al., "Changes in Cardiovascular Risk Factors and Inflammatory Markers of Young, Healthy, Men after Six Weeks of Moderate or High Intensity Resistance Training," *Journal of Sports Medicine and Physical Fitness* 51, no. 4 (2011): 695–700.

11. E. A. Morra et al., "Long-Term Intense Resistance Training in Men Is Associated with Preserved Cardiac Structure/Function, Decreased Aortic Stiffness, and Lower Central Augmentation Pressure," *Journal of Hypertension* 32, no. 2 (2014): 286–93, doi: 10.1097/HJH.0000000000000035

12. D. P. Leong et al., "Prognostic Value of Grip Strength: Findings from the Prospective Urban Rural Epidemiology (PURE) Study," *Lancet* 386, no. 9990 (2015): 266–73, doi: http://dx.doi.org/10.1016/S0140-6736(14)62000-6

13. H. C. Almstedt et al., "Changes in Bone Mineral Density in Response to 24 Weeks of Resistance Training in College-Aged Men and Women," *Journal of Strength and Conditioning Research* 25, no. 4 (2011): 1098–103, doi: 10.1519/JSC.0b013e3181d09e9d

14. E. A. Marques et al., "Effects of Resistance and Aerobic Exercise on Physical Function, Bone Mineral Density, OPG, and RANKL in Older Women," *Experimental Gerontology* 46, no. 7 (2011): 524–32, doi: 10.1016/j.exger.2011.02.005

15. K. Keller and M. Engelhardt, "Strength and Muscle Mass Loss with Aging Process: Age and Strength Loss," *Muscles, Ligaments, and Tendons Journal* 3, no. 4 (2013): 346–50.

16. C. S. Bickel, J. M. Cross, and M. M. Bamman, "Exercise Dosing to Retain Resistance Training Adaptations in Young and Older Adults," *Medicine & Science in Sports & Exercise* 43, no. 7 (2011): 1777–87, doi: 10.1249/MSS.0b013e318207c15d

17. P. Srikanthan and A. S. Karlamangla, "Muscle Mass Index as a Predictor of Longevity in Older Adults," *American Journal of Medicine* 127, no. 6 (2014): 547–53, doi: 10.1016/j.amjmed.2014.02.007

18. J. Holviala et al., "Effects of Prolonged and Maintenance Strength Training on Force Production, Walking, and Balance in Aging Women and Men," *Scandinavian Journal of Medicine and Science in Sport* 24, no. 1 (2012), doi: 10.1111/j.1600-0838.2012.01470.x

19. M. A. Kostek et al., "Subcutaneous Fat Alterations Resulting from an Upper-Body Resistance Training Program," *Medicine & Science in Sports & Exercise* 39, no. 7 (2007): 1177–85.

20. W. R. Thompson, "Worldwide Survey of Fitness Trends for 2015: What's Driving the Market," *ACSM's Health & Fitness Journal* 18, no. 6 (2014): 8–17, doi: 10.1249/FIT.0000000000000073

21. J. A. Falactic et al., "Effects of Kettlebell Training on Aerobic Capacity," *Journal of Strength and Conditioning Research* 29, no. 7 (2015): 1943–47, doi: 10.1519/JSC.0000000000000845

22. K. Jay et al., "Kettlebell Training for Musculoskeletal and Cardiovascular Health: A Randomized Controlled Trial," *Scandinavian Journal of Work, Environment, and Health* 37, no. 3 (2010): 196–203, doi: 10.5271/sjweh.3136

23. W. H. Otto et al., "Effects of Weightlifting vs. Kettlebell Training on Vertical Jump, Strength, and Body Composition," *Journal of Strength and Conditioning Research* 25, no. 5 (2012): 1199–202, doi: 10.1519/JSC.0b013e31824f233e

24. R. Radaelli et al., "Dose-Response of 1, 3, and 5 Sets of Resistance Exercise on Strength, Local Muscular Endurance, and Hypertrophy," *Journal of Strength and Conditioning Research* 29, no. 5 (2015): 1349–58, doi: 10.1519/JSC.0000000000000758

25. R. L. Cunningham et al., "Androgenic Anabolic Steroid Exposure during Adolescence: Ramification for Brain Development and Behavior," *Hormones and Behavior* 64, no. 2 (2013): doi: 10.1016/j.yhbeh.2012.12.009

26. G. Kanayama et al., "Cognitive Deficits in Long-Term Anabolic-Androgenic Steroid Users," *Drug and Alcohol Dependence* 130, no. 1–3 (2013): 208–14, doi: 10.1016/j.drugalcdep.2012.11.008

27. D. G. Candow et al., "Effect of Different Frequencies of Creatine Supplementation on Muscles Size and Strength in Young Adults," *Journal of Strength and Conditioning Research* 25, no. 7 (2011): 1831–38, doi: 10.1519/JSC.0b013e3181e7419a

28. National Institutes of Health, Medline Plus, "DHEA," updated March 2013, www.nlm.nih.gov

29. W. L. Baker, S. Karan, and A. M. Kenny, "Effect of Dehydroepiandrosterone on Muscle Strength and Physical Function in Older Adults: A Systematic Review," *Journal of the American Geriatrics Society* 59, no. 6 (2011): 997–1002, doi: 10.1111/j.1532-5415.2011.03410.x

30. C. E. Brodeur et al., "The Andro Project: Physiological and Hormonal Influences of Androstenedione Supplementation in Men 35 to 65 Years Old Participating in a High-Intensity Resistance Training Program," *Archives of Internal Medicine* 160, no. 20, (2000): 3093–104.

31. S. Basaria, "Androgen Abuse in Athletes: Detection and Consequences," *Journal of Clinical Endocrinology & Metabolism* 95, no. 4 (2010): 1533–43, doi: 10.1210/jc.2009-1579

32. L. Wideman et al., "Growth Hormone Release during Acute and Chronic Aerobic and Resistance Exercise: Recent Findings," *Sports Medicine* 32, no. 15 (2002): 987–1004.

33. A. Weltman et al., "Effects of Continuous versus Intermittent Exercise, Obesity, and Gender on Growth Hormone Secretion," *Journal of Clinical Endocrinology and Metabolism* 93, no. 12 (2008): 4711–920, doi: 10.1210/jc.2008-0998

34. N. M. Cermak et al., "Protein Supplementation Augments the Adaptive Response of Skeletal Muscle to Resistance-Type Exercise Training: A Meta-Analysis," *American Journal of Clinical Nutrition* 96, no. 6 (2012): 1454–64, doi: 10.3945/ajcn.112.037556

35. M. Williams, "Dietary Supplements and Sports Performance: Amino Acids," *Journal of the International Society of Sports Nutrition* 2, no. 2 (2005): 63–67.

36. P. Lagiou et al., "Low Carbohydrate-High Protein Diet and Incidence of Cardiovascular Diseases in Swedish Women: Prospective Cohort Study," *BMJ* 344 (2012): e4026, doi: http://dx.doi.org/10.1136/bmj.e4026

GETFITGRAPHICS References

1. Centers for Disease Control and Prevention/NCHS, "National Health Interview Survey: January–March 2015, Sample Adult Core Component," 2015, www.cdc.gov

2. American College Health Association, *American College Health Association—National College Health Assessment II (ACHA-NCHA II): Undergraduate Reference Group Executive Summary, Fall 2012* (Hanover, MD: American College Health Association, 2013).

3. E. Santos et al., "Influence of Moderately Intense Strength Training on Flexibility in Sedentary Young Women," *Journal of Strength and Conditioning Research* 24, no. 11 (2010): 3144–49.

4. M. P. Mosti et al., "Maximal Strength Training Improves Bone Mineral Density and Neuromuscular Performance in Young Adult Women," *Journal of Strength and Conditioning Research* 28, no. 10 (2014): 2935–45, doi: 10.1519/JSC.0000000000000493

5. K. Keller and M. Engelhardt, "Strength and Muscle Mass Loss with Aging Process: Age and Strength Loss," *Muscles, Ligaments, and Tendons Journal* 3, no. 4 (2013): 346–50.

Chapter 5

1. H. B. Medeiros, D. S. de Araujo, and C. G. de Araujo, "Age-related Mobility Loss Is Joint-Specific: An Analysis from 6,000 Flexitest Results," *Age* 35, no. 6 (2013): 2399–407, doi: 10.1007/s11357-013-9525-z

2. E. A. Courtney-Long et al., "Prevalence of Disability and Disability Type among Adults—United States, 2013,"*MMWR Morbidity Mortality Weekly Report* 64, no. 29 (2015): 777–83.

3. M. J. Spink et al., "Foot and Ankle Strength, Range of Motion, Posture, and Deformity Are Associated with Balance and Functional Ability in Older Adults," *Archives of Physical Medicine and Rehabilitation* 92, no. 1 (2011): 68–75, doi: 10.1016/j.apmr.2010.09.024

4. D. L. Blackwell, J. W. Lucas, and T. C. Clarke, "Summary Health Statistics for US Adults: National Health Interview Survey, 2012," *Vital Health Statistics* 10, no. 260 (2014).

5. M. Fransen et al., "Exercise for Osteoarthritis of the Knee: A Cochrane Systematic Review," *British Journal of Sports Medicine* (September 24, 2015), pii: bjsports-2015-095424, doi: 10.1136/bjsports-2015-095424; T. O'Dwyer, F. O'Shea, and F. Wilson, "Physical Activity in

Spondyloarthritis: A Systematic Review," *Rheumatology International* 34, no. 7 (2014): 887–902, doi: 10.1007/s00296-014-3141-9; J. K. Cooney et al., "Benefits of Exercise in Rheumatoid Arthritis," *Journal of Aging Research* (2011): 681640, doi: 10.4061/2011/681640

6. F. R. Moyano et al., "Effectiveness of Different Exercises and Stretching Physiotherapy on Pain and Movement in Patellofemoral Pain Syndrome: A Randomized Controlled Trial," *Clinical Rehabilitation* 27, no. 5 (2013): 409–17, doi: 10.1177/0269215512459277

7. D. Perich et al., "Low Back Pain in Adolescent Female Rowers: A Multi-Dimensional Intervention Study," *Knee Surgery, Sports Traumatology, Arthroscopy* 19, no. 1 (2011): 20–29, doi: 10.1007/s00167-010-1173-6

8. I. Calvo-Muñoz, A. Gómez-Conesa, and J. Sánchez-Meca, "Physical Therapy Treatments for Low Back Pain in Children and Adolescents: A Meta-Analysis," *BMC Musculoskeletal Disorders* 14 (2013): 55, doi: 10.1186/1471-2474-14-55

9. P. W. Marshall, J. Mannion, and B. A. Murphy, "Extensibility of the Hamstrings Is Best Explained by Mechanical Components of Muscle Contraction, Not Behavioral Measures in Individuals with Chronic Low Back Pain," *PM&R* 1, no. 8 (2009): 709–18, doi: 10.1016/j.pmrj.2009.04.009

10. E. N. Johnson and J. S. Thomas, "Effect of Hamstring Flexibility on Hip and Lumbar Spine Joint Excursions during Forward-Reaching Tasks in Participants with and without Low Back Pain," *Archives of Physical Medicine and Rehabilitation* 91, no. 7 (2010): 1140–42, doi: 10.1016/j.apmr.2010.04.003

11. National Institute of Neurological Disorders and Stroke, "Low Back Pain Fact Sheet," NIH Publication no. 15-5161 (Bethesda, MD: Office of Communications and Public Liaison, National Institutes of Health, 2015), www.ninds.nih.gov

12. R. J. Johns and V. Wright, "Relative Importance of Various Tissues in Joint Stiffness," *Journal of Applied Physiology* 17, no. 5 (1962): 824–28.

13. M. J. Alter, *The Science of Flexibility* (Champaign, IL: Human Kinetics, 2004); J. M. Soucie et al., "Range of Motion Measurements: Reference Values and a Database for Comparison Studies," *Haemophilia* 17, no. 3 (2011): 500–7, doi: 10.1111/j.1365-2516.2010.02399.x

14. J. Hwang and M. C. Jung, "Age and Sex Differences in Ranges of Motion and Motion Patterns," *International Journal of Occupational Safety and Ergonomics* 21, no. 2 (2015): 173–86, doi: 10.1080/10803548.2015.1029301; P. Aronson et al., "Medial Tibiofemoral-Joint Stiffness in Males and Females across the Lifespan," *Journal of Athletic Training* 49, no. 3 (2014): 399–405, doi: 10.4085/1062-6050-49.2.18

15. R. Simão et al., "The Influence of Strength, Flexibility, and Simultaneous Training on Flexibility and Strength Gains," *Journal of Strength and Conditioning Research* 25, no. 5 (2011): 1333–38, doi: 10.1519/JSC.0b013e3181da85bf

16. E. Peck et al., "The Effects of Stretching on Performance," *Current Sports Medicine Reports* 13, no. 3 (2014): 179–85, doi: 10.1249/JSR.0000000000000052

17. J. E. Bushell, S. M. Dawson, and M. M. Webster, "Clinical Relevance of Foam Rolling on Hip Extension Angle in a Functional Lunge Position," *Journal of Strength and Conditioning Research* 29, no. 9 (2015): 2397–403; K. C. Healey et al., "The Effects of Myofascial Release with Foam Rolling on Performance," *Journal of Strength and Conditioning Research* 28, no. 1 (2014): 61–68.

18. M. N. Houston et al., "The Effectiveness of Whole-Body-Vibration Training in Improving Hamstring Flexibility in Physically Active Adults," *Journal of Sport Rehabilitation* 24, no. 1 (2015): 77–82, doi: 10.1123/JSR.2013-0059

19. J. B. Feland et al., "Whole Body Vibration as an Adjunct to Static Stretching," *International Journal of Sports Medicine* 31, no. 8 (2010): 584–89, doi: 10.1055/s-0030-1254084

20. National Center for Health Statistics, *Health, United States, 2014: With Special Feature on Adults Aged 55–64* (Hyattsville, MD: Centers for Disease Control, 2015), www.cdc.gov/nchs/data/hus/hus14.pdf

21. Ibid.

22. B. I. Martin et al., "Expenditures and Health Status among Adults with Back and Neck Problems," *JAMA* 299, no. 6 (2008): 656–64, doi: 10.1001/jama.299.6.656

23. K. K. Hansraj, "Assessment of Stresses in the Cervical Spine Caused by Posture and Position of the Head," *Surgical Technology International* 25 (2014): 277–79.

24. R. Shiri et al., "The Association between Smoking and Low Back Pain: A Meta-Analysis," *American Journal of Medicine* 123, no. 1 (2010): 87.e7–35, doi: 10.1016/j.amjmed.2009.05.028

25. Ibid.

26. National Institute of Neurological Disorders and Stroke, "Low Back Pain Fact Sheet," 2015.

27. A. J. Teichtahl et al., "Physical Inactivity Is Associated with Narrower Lumbar Intervertebral Discs, High Fat Content of Paraspinal Muscles, and Low Back Pain and Disability," *Arthritis Research & Therapy* 17 (2015): 114, doi: 10.1186/s13075-015-0629-y

28. S. J. Bigos et al., "High-Quality Controlled Trials on Preventing Episodes of Back Problems: Systematic Literature Review in Working-Age Adults," *Spine Journal: Official Journal of the North American Spine Society* 9, no. 2 (2009): 147–68, doi: 10.1016/j.spinee.2008.11.001

29. D. M. Urquhart et al., "Increased Fat Mass Is Associated with High Levels of Low Back Pain Intensity and Disability," *Spine* 36, no. 16 (2011): 1320–25, doi: 10.1097/BRS.0b013e3181f9fb66

30. K. Ohtsuki, "The Immediate Changes in Patients with Acute Exacerbation of Chronic Lower-Back Pain Elicited by Direct Stretching of the Tensor Fasciae Latae, the Hamstrings, and the Adductor Magnus," *Journal of Physical Therapy Science* 24 (2012): 707–9.

GETFITGRAPHICS **References**

1. D. L. Blackwell, J. W. Lucas, and T. C. Clarke, "Summary Health Statistics for US Adults: National Health Interview Survey, 2012," *Vital Health Statistics* 10, no. 260 (2014).

2. C. Kennedy et al., "Psychosocial Factors and Low Back Pain among College Students," *Journal of American College Health* 57, no. 2 (2008): 191–95, doi:10.3200/JACH.57.2.191-196

3. Z. Heuscher et al., "The Association of Self-Reported Backpack Use and Backpack Weight with Low Back Pain among College Students," *Journal of Manipulative Physiological Therapy* 33, no. 6 (2011): 432–37, doi: 10.1016/j.jmpt.2010.06.003

4. North American Spine Society, "Back Pack Safety," www.knowyourback.org

5. P. T. Hakala et al., "Frequent Computer-Related Activities Increase the Risk of Neck-Shoulder and Low Back Pain in Adolescents," *European Journal of Public Health* 16, no. 5 (2006): 536–41.

6. J. P. Auvinen et al., "Is Insufficient Quantity and Quality of Sleep a Risk Factor for Neck, Shoulder, and Low Back Pain? A Longitudinal Study among Adolescents," *European Spine Journal* 19, no. 4 (2010): 641–49, doi: 10.1007/s00586-009-1215-2

7. D. P. Gilkey et al., "Risk Factors Associated with Back Pain: A Cross-Sectional Study of 983 College Students," *Journal of Manipulative and Physiological Therapeutics* 33, no. 2 (2010): 88–95, doi: 10.1016/j.jmpt.2009.12.005

8. National Institute of Neurological Disorders and Stroke, "Low Back Pain Fact Sheet," NIH Publication no. 15-5161 (Bethesda, MD: Office of Communications and Public Liaison, National Institutes of Health, 2015), www.ninds.nih.gov

Chapter 6

1. C. D. Fryar, M. D. Carroll, and C. L. Ogden, "Prevalence of Obesity among Children and Adolescents: United States, Trends 1963–1965 through 2011–2012," *National Center for Health Statistics, Health E-Stats* (2014), www.cdc.gov

2. J. J. Reilly and J. Kelly, "Long-term Impact of Overweight and Obesity in Childhood and Adolescence on Morbidity and Premature Mortality in Adulthood: Systematic Review," *International Journal of Obesity* 35, no. 7 (2011): 891–98, doi: 10.1038/ijo.2010.222; D. S. Freeman, C. L. Ogden, and B. K. Kit, "Interrelationships between BMI, Skinfold Thickness, Percent Body Fat, and Cardiovascular Disease Risk Factors among US Children and Adolescents," *BMC Pediatrics* 15 (2015): doi: 10.1186/s12887-015-0493-6

3. R. An, "Prevalence and Trends of Adult Obesity in the US, 1999–2012," *ISRN Obesity* 2014, no. 185132 (2014), doi: http://dx.doi.org/10.1155/2014/185132

4. National Heart, Lung, and Blood Institute—Expert Panel on the Identification, Evaluation, and Treatment of Overweight in Adults, "Clinical Guidelines on the Identification, Evaluation, and Treatment of Overweight and Obesity in Adults: Executive Summary," *American Journal of Clinical Nutrition* 68, no. 4 (1998): 899–917.

5. L. N. Borrell and L. Samuel, "Body Mass Index Categories and Mortality Risk in US Adults: The Effect of Overweight and Obesity on Advancing Death," *American Journal of Public Health* 104, no. 3 (2014): 512–19, doi: 10.2105/AJPH.2013.301597

6. R. Siren, J. G. Eriksson, and H. Vanhanan, "Waist Circumference Is a Good Indicator of Future Risk for Type 2 Diabetes and Cardiovascular Disease," *BMC Public Health* 12 (2012): 631, doi: 10.1186/1471-2458-12-631

7. V. H. Heyward, *Advanced Fitness Assessment and Exercise Prescription,* 7th ed. (Champaign, IL: Human Kinetics, 2014).

8. J. P. Després, "Body Fat Distribution and the Risk of Cardiovascular Disease: An Update," *Circulation* 126 (2012): 1301–13, doi: 10.1161/CIRCULATIONAHA.111.067264

9. C. S. Fox et al., "Abdominal Visceral and Subcutaneous Adipose Tissue Compartments: Association with Metabolic Risk Factors in the Framingham Heart Study," *Circulation* 116, no. 1 (2007): 39–48.

10. G. Fisher et al., "Effect of Diet with and without Exercise Training on Markers of Inflammation and Fat Distribution in Overweight Women," *Obesity (Silver Spring)* 19, no. 6 (2011): 1131–36, doi: 10.1038 / oby.2010.310

11. B. H. Goodpaster et al., "Effects of Diet and Physical Activity Interventions on Weight Loss and Cardiometabolic Risk Factors in Severely Obese Adults: A Randomized Trial," *JAMA* 304, no. 16 (2010): 1795–802, doi: 10.1001/jama.2010.1505

12. Heyward, *Advanced Fitness Assessment and Exercise Prescription*, 2014.

13. A. S. Jackson et al., "Cross-Validation of Generalised Body Composition Equations with Diverse Young Men and Women: The Training Intervention and Genetics of Exercise Response (TIGER) Study," *British Journal of Nutrition* 101, no. 6 (2009): 871–78; A. J. Chambers et al., "A Comparison of Prediction Equations for the Estimation of Body Fat Percentage in Non-Obese and Obese Older Caucasian Adults in the United States," *Journal of Nutrition, Health, and Aging* 18, no. 6 (2014): 586–90, doi: 10.1007/s12603-014-0017-3

14. D. A. Fields, M. I. Goran, and M. A. McCrory, "Body-Composition Assessment via Air-Displacement Plethysmography in Adults and Children: A Review," *American Journal of Clinical Nutrition* 75, no. 3 (2002): 453–67.

15. Heyward, *Advanced Fitness Assessment and Exercise Prescription*, 2014; S. Leahy et al., "A Comparison of Dual Energy X-Ray Absorptiometry and Bioelectrical Impedance Analysis to Measure Total and Segmental Body Composition in Healthy Young Adults," *European Journal of Applied Physiology* 112, no. 2 (2012): 589–95, doi: 10.1007/s00421-011-2010-4

16. E. E. Helander et al., "Are Breaks in Daily Self-Weighing Associated with Weight Gain?" *PLOS ONE* 9, no. 11 (2014): e113164, doi: 10.1371/journal.pone.0113164

GETFITGRAPHICS **References**

1. S. Luebberding, N. Krueger, and N. S. Sadick, "Cellulite: An Evidence-Based Review," *American Journal of Clinical Dermatology* 16, no. 4 (2015): 243–56, doi: 10.1007/s40257-015-0129-5

2. US National Library of Medicine, National Institutes of Health, Medline Plus, "Cellulite," updated December 2015, www.nlm.nih.gov/medlineplus/ency/article/002033.htm

Chapter 7

1. R. H. Nagler, "Adverse Outcomes Associated with Media Exposure to Contradictory Nutrition Messages," *Journal of Health Communication* 19, no. 1 (2014): 24.

2. US Department of Agriculture, Economic Research Service, "Food Availability and Consumption, Loss-Adjusted Food Availability Data," September 2015, www.ers.usda.gov

3. Spoon University, "Grub Hub Data Reveals Strange College Delivery Trends," August 2014, http://spoonuniversity.com

4. US Department of Agriculture, Agricultural Marketing Service, "How to Buy Fresh Vegetables," Home and Garden Bulletin No. 258, 1994.

5. US Department of Health and Human Services and US Department of Agriculture, *Dietary Guidelines for Americans 2015–2020*, 8th ed., December 2015, www.health.gov; J. S. Morrell et al., "Metabolic Syndrome, Obesity, and Related Risk Factors among College Men and Women," *Journal of American College Health* 60, no. 1 (2012): 82–89.

6. D. A. Dingman et al., "Factors Related to the Number of Fast Food Meals Obtained by College Meal Plan Students," *Journal of American College Health* 62, no. 8 (November/December 2014): 562–69.

7. A. Almohanna et al., "Impact of Dietary Acculturation on the Food Habits, Weight, Blood Pressure, and Fasting Blood Glucose Levels of International College Student," *Journal of American College Health* 63, no. 5 (July 2015): 307–14.

8. K. M. Flegal et al., "Trends in Obesity among Adults in the United States, 2005 to 2014," *Journal of the American Medical Association* 315, no. 21 (2016): 2284–91.

9. S. R. Miller and W. A. Knudson, "Nutrition and Cost Comparisons of Select Canned, Frozen, and Fresh Fruits and Vegetables," *American Journal of Lifestyle Medicine* 8, no. 6 (November/December 2014): 430–37.

10. W. D. Hoyt, S. B. Hamilton, and K. M. Rickard, "The Effects of Dietary Fat and Caloric Content on the Body-Size Estimates of Anorexic Profile and Normal College Students," *Journal of Clinical Psychology* 59, no. 1 (2003): 85–91.

11. J. C. Frankel, "Diet Studies Challenge Thinking on Proteins versus Carbs," *Science* 7, no. 343 (March 2014): 1068; G. Taubes, "Which One Will Make You Fat?" *Scientific American* 309, no. 3 (September 2013); C. B. Ebbeling et al., "Effects of Dietary Composition on Energy Expenditure during Weight Loss Maintenance," *Journal of the American Medical Association* 307, no. 24 (June 27, 2012).

12. N. R. Rodriguez, "Introduction to Protein Summit 2.0: Continued Exploration of the Impact of High Quality Protein for Optimal Health," *American Journal of Clinical Nutrition* 101, no. 6 (June 2015): 1317S–19S.

13. Ibid.

14. Ibid.

15. Physicians Committee for Responsible Medicine, "Analysis of Health Problems Associated with High-Protein, High-Fat, Carbohydrate-Restricted Diets Reported via an Online Registry," May 2004, accessed October 2015, www.pcrm.org

16. Rodriguez, "Introduction to Protein Summit 2.0," 2015.

17. Ibid.

18. E. Ota et al., "Antenatal Dietary Advice and Supplementation to Increase Energy and Protein Intake," *Cochrane Database of Systematic Reviews* 9 (September 12, 2012): CD000032.

19. US Department of Agriculture, Economic Research Service, "Food Availability and Consumption," 2015; American Heart Association, "Sugar 101," accessed October 2015, www.heart.org

20. N. Linos and M. T. Bassett, "Added Sugar Intake and Public Health," *Journal of the American Medical Association* 314, no. 2 (2015): 187; Q. Yang et al., "Added Sugar Intake and Cardiovascular Disease Mortality among US Adults," *Journal of the American Medical Association Internal Medicine* 174, no. 4 (2014): 516–24.

21. D. Quagliani and P. Felt-Gunderson, "Closing America's Fiber Intake Gap: Communication Strategies from a Food and Fiber Summit," *American Journal of Lifestyle Medicine* 1559827615588079 (June 2, 2015).

22. Ibid.; US Food and Drug Administration, "How to Understand and Use the Nutrition Facts Label," February 2012, www.fda.gov; Morrell et al., "Metabolic Syndrome, Obesity, and Related Risk Factors," 2012.

23. K. E. Davis, "The Cholesterol-Lowering Potential of Whole Grains," *American Journal of Lifestyle Medicine* 8, no. 4 (July/August 2014): 231–34.

24. J. Hu et al., "Glycemic Index, Glycemic Load, and Cancer Risk," *Annals of Oncology* 24, no. 1 (2013): 245–51; R. H. Eckel, "Role of Glycemic Index in the Context of an Overall Heart-Healthy Diet," *Journal of the American Medical Association* 312, no. 23 (2014): 2531–41.

25. F. M. Sacks et al., "Effects of High versus Low Glycemic Index Dietary Carbohydrate on Cardiovascular Disease Risk Factors and Insulin Sensitivity: The OmniCarb Randomized Clinical Trial," *Journal of the American Medical Association* 312, no. 23 (2014); Eckel, "Role of Glycemic Index," 2014.

26. Eckel, "Role of Glycemic Index," 2014.

27. Harvard T. H. Chan School of Public Health, "Omega-3 Fatty Acids: An Essential Contribution," *The Nutrition Source*, accessed October 2015, www.hsph.harvard.edu

28. A. Grey and M. Bolland, "Clinical Trial Evidence and Use of Fish Oil Supplements," *JAMA Internal Medicine* 174, no. 3 (2014): 460–62; E. Y. Chew et al., "Effect of Omega-3 Fatty Acids, Lutein/Zeaxanthin, or other Nutrient Supplementation on Cognitive Function: The AREDS2 Randomized Clinical Trial," *Journal of the American Medical Association* 314, no. 8 (2015): 791–801.

29. V. Bouvard et al., "Carcinogenicity of Consumption of Red and Processed Meat," *Lancet Oncology* 16, no. 16 (2015), doi: 10.1016/S1470-2045(15)00444-1

30. Y. Rong et al., "Egg Consumption and Risk of Coronary Heart Disease and Stroke: Dose-Response Meta-Analysis of Prospective Cohort Studies," *BMJ* 346 (2013): e8539.

31. J. Thompson and M. Manore, *Nutrition: An Applied Approach,* 4th ed. (San Francisco: Pearson, 2014).

32. R. J. De Souza et al., "Intake of Saturated and Trans Unsaturated Fatty Acids and Risk of All Cause Mortality, Cardiovascular Disease, and Type 2 Diabetes: Systematic Review and Meta-analysis of Observational Studies," *BMJ* 351 (2015): h3978, doi: http://dx.doi.org/10.1136/bmj.h3978

33. American Heart Association, "What Your Cholesterol Levels Mean," updated October 19, 2015, www.heart.org

34. W. Willett, "The Case for Banning Trans Fats," *Scientific American* 310, no. 3 (March 2014): 13.

35. FDA Consumer Updates, "FDA Cuts Trans Fat in Processed Foods," updated June 16, 2015, www.fda.gov

36. R. Estruch et al., "Primary Prevention of Cardiovascular Disease with a Mediterranean Diet," *New England Journal of Medicine* 368 (February 2013).

37. US Food and Drug Administration, "Mercury Levels in Commercial Fish and Shellfish, 1990–2010," January 2013, www.fda.gov

38. J. May, "Ascorbic Acid Transporters in Health and Disease" (paper given at Linus Pauling Diet and Optimum Health Annual Conference, Portland, Oregon, May 2007).

39. Centers for Disease Control and Prevention, "Most Americans Should Consume Less Sodium," September 30, 2015, www.cdc.gov

40. Centers for Disease Control and Prevention, "CDC Vital Signs: Reducing Sodium in Children's Diets," September 2014, www.cdc.gov

41. Centers for Disease Control and Prevention, "Most Americans Should Consume Less Sodium," 2015.

42. McDonald's, "USA Nutrition Facts for Popular Menu Items," October 22, 2015, http://nutrition.mcdonalds.com/getnutrition/nutritionfacts.pdf

43. F. J. He et al., "Salt Intake and Cardiovascular Mortality," *American Journal of Medicine* 120, no. 1 (2007): e5–e7.

44. J. Midgley et al., "Effects of Reduced Dietary Sodium on Blood Pressure: A Meta-Analysis of Randomized Controlled Trials," *Journal of the American Medical Association* 275, no. 20 (1996): 1590–97.

45. D. Mozaffarian et al., "Global Sodium Consumption and Death from Cardiovascular Causes," *New England Journal of Medicine* 371 (2014): 624–34.

46. Harvard T. H. Chan School of Public Health, "Health Risks and Disease," *The Nutrition Source*, accessed October 2015, www.hsph.harvard.edu

47. K. Hoy and J. D. Goldman, "What We Eat in America: Calcium Intake of the US Population, NHANES 2009–2010," Dietary Data Brief no. 13, September 2014, www.ars.usda.gov

48. National Osteoporosis Foundation, "What Is Osteoporosis?" accessed October 2015, www.nof.org

49. Ibid.

50. Ibid.

51. K. Zeratsky, "What Are the Risks of Vitamin D Deficiency?" Mayo Clinic, Healthy Lifestyle: Nutrition and Healthy Eating, June 15, 2015, www.mayoclinic.org; J. W. Miller et al., "Vitamin D Status and Rates of Cognitive Decline in a Multiethnic Cohort of Older Adults," *JAMA Neurology* 72, no. 11 (September 2015), doi: 10.1001/jamaneurol.2015.2115

52. C. N. Camaschella, "Iron Deficiency Anemia," *New England Journal of Medicine* 372 (2015): 1832–43.

53. Ibid.

54. National Center for Environmental Health, "Second National Report on Biochemical Indicators of Diet and Nutrition in the US Population 2012 Executive Survey," March 2012, www.cdc.gov

55. Ibid.

56. National Institutes of Health, "Dietary Supplement Fact Sheet: Iron," February 2013, http://ods.od.nih.gov

57. Ibid.

58. American Red Cross, "Plasma," accessed October 2015, www.redcrossblood.org

59. A. E. Carroll, "The Persistent Health Myth of 8 Glasses of Water a Day," *New York Times*, August 25, 2015.

60. Mayo Clinic Staff, "Dehydration: Risk Factors," February 12, 2014, www.mayoclinic.org; B. M. Popkin et al., "Water, Hydration, and Health," *Nutrition Review* 68, no. 8 (2010): 439–58.

61. D. C. Nieman et al., "Bananas as an Energy Source during Exercise: A Metabolomics Approach," *PLOS ONE* 7, no. 5 (2012).

62. Consumers Union, "A Guide to the Best and Worst Drinks," *Consumer Reports on Health* (July 2006): 8–9.

63. M. Datta et al. "Food Fortifications and Supplement Use: Are There Health Implications?" *Critical Reviews in Food Science and Nutrition* (July 18, 2014).

64. J. L. Pomeranz and K. D. Brownell, "Can Government Regulate Portion Sizes?" *New England Journal of Medicine* 371 (2014): 1956–58.

65. S. Tavernise and S. Strom, "US to Require Calorie Counts, Even at Movies," *New York Times*, November 25, 2014.

66. Centers for Disease Control and Prevention, "Restaurant Customers Do Use Calorie Information on Menus," *Journal of the American Medical Association* 312, no. 9 (2014): 883; J. Block and C. A. Roberto, "Potential Benefits of Calorie Labeling in Restaurants," *Journal of the American Medical Association* 312, no. 9 (2014): 887–88.

67. US Department of Agriculture, Center for Nutrition Policy and Promotion, "A Brief History of USDA Food Guides," June 2011, www.choosemyplate.gov

68. J. F. Hollis et al., "Weight Loss during the Intensive Intervention Phase of the Weight-Loss Maintenance Trial," *American Journal of Preventative Medicine* 35, no. 2 (2008): 118–26.

69. Bouvard et al., "Carcinogenicity of Consumption of Red and Processed Meat," 2015.

70. J. Sarris et al., "Nutritional Medicine as Mainstream in Psychiatry," *Lancet Psychiatry* 2, no. 3 (2015): 271.

71. B. J. Rolls, E. A. Bell, and B. A. Waugh, "Increasing the Volume of a Food by Incorporating Air Affects Satiety in Men," *American Journal of Clinical Nutrition* 72, no. 2 (2000): 361–68.

72. M. P. Mattson, "What Doesn't Kill You…" *Scientific American* 313, no. 1 (July 2015): 40–45; L. Bell, "For Athletes, Antioxidant Pills May Not Help Performance," *Science News* 187, no. 5 (March 7, 2015).

73. M. W. Moyer, "The Myth of Antioxidants," *Scientific American* 308 (February 2013): 64–67.

74. Mattson, "What Doesn't Kill You…" 2015.

75. Ibid.

76. Ibid; M. Greger, "Plant Power: Eat a Variety of Plant Foods to Boost Nutrition and Health," *American Journal of Lifestyle Medicine* 9, no. 4 (July/August 2015): 278–79; V. Ha et al., "Effect of Dietary Pulse Intake on Established Therapeutic Lipid Targets for Cardiovascular Risk Reduction: A Systematic Review and Meta-Analysis of Randomized Controlled Trials," *Canadian Medical Association Journal* 186, no. 8 (May 13, 2014): E252–62; Patient Education, "Oh, Nuts! Enjoy the Tasty Nutrition and Health Benefits of Nuts," *American Journal of Lifestyle Medicine* 8, no. 1 (January/February 2014): 31–32; G. J. Troup et al., "Stable Radical Content and Anti-Radical Activity of Roasted Arabica Coffee: From In-Tact Bean to Coffee Brew," *PLOS ONE* 10, no. 4 (2015); L. K. Kay, "From A to Shiitake: Japanese Mushrooms May Offer Certain Benefits," *Today's Dietician* 12, no. 11(November 2010): 20.

77. Medline Plus, "Folic Acid in Diet," February 18, 2013, ?www.nlm.nih.gov

78. J. L. Buell et al., "National Athletic Trainers' Association Position Statement: Evaluation of Dietary Supplements for Performance Nutrition," *Journal of Athletic Training* 48, no. 1 (January/February 2013): 124–36.

79. M. N. Sawka, "American College of Sports Medicine Position Stand: Exercise and Fluid Replacement," *Medicine and Science in Sports and Exercise* 39, no. 2 (2007): 377–90.

80. L. M. Burke et al., "Carbohydrates and Fat for Training and Recovery," *Journal of Sports Science* 22, no. 1 (2004): 15–30; L. M. Burke et al., "Guidelines for Daily Carbohydrate Intake: Do Athletes Achieve Them?" *Sports Medicine* 31, no. 4 (2001): 267–99.

81. S. M. Phillips, D. R. Moore, and E. J. Tang, "A Critical Examination of Dietary Protein Requirements, Benefits, and Excesses in Athletes," *International Journal of Sports Nutrition and Exercise Metabolism* 17 (2007): S58–S76.

82. J. L. Ivy and L. M. Ferguson-Stegall, "Nutrient Timing: The Means to Improved Exercise Performance, Recovery, and Training Adaptation," *American Journal of Lifestyle Medicine* 8, no. 4 (July/August 2014): 246–59.

83. K. A. Beals and A. Mitchell, "Recent Recommendations and Current Controversies in Sport Nutrition," *American Journal of Lifestyle Medicine* 9, no. 4 (July/August 2015): 288–97.

84. N. Clark, "Recovering from Hard Exercise," *American Fitness* 30, no. 5 (2012): 64–65.

85. J. B. Anderson et al., *Eat Right! Healthy Eating in College and Beyond* (San Francisco: Benjamin Cummings, 2007).

86. Scientific Report of the 2015 Dietary Guidelines Advisory Committee, "Appendix E-3.7: Developing Vegetarian and Mediterranean-Style Food Patterns," updated November 2, 2015, www.health.gov

87. US Department of Health and Human Services and US Department of Agriculture, *Dietary Guidelines for Americans 2015–2020*, 2015.

88. American Dietetic Association, "Position of the American Dietetic Association: Vegetarian Diets," *Journal of the American Dietetic Association* 109, no. 7 (2009): 1266–82.

89. A. Pan et al., "Red Meat Consumption and Mortality," *Archives of Internal Medicine* 172, no. 7 (2012): 555–63.

90. D. White, "Where's the Beef? Dining Makes Moves Toward Meatless Meals," *University of California at Santa Cruz News,* June 2012, http://news.ucsc.edu

91. L. B. Harvey and H. A. Ricciotti, "Nutrition for a Healthy Pregnancy," *American Journal of Lifestyle Medicine* 8, no. 2 (March/April 2014): 80–87.

92. Ibid.

93. Ibid.

94. Rodriguez, "Introduction to Protein Summit 2.0," 2015.

95. US Department of Health and Human Services and US Department of Agriculture, *Dietary Guidelines for Americans 2015–2020*, 2015.

96. American Diabetes Association, "Making Healthy Food Choices," accessed November 2015, www.diabetes.org

97. Centers for Disease Control and Prevention, "CDC Estimates of Foodborne Illness in the United States," updated January 8, 2014, www.cdc.gov

98. The Organic Trade Association, "Eight in Ten US Parents Report They Purchase Organic Products," April 2013, www.ota.com

99. K. Brandt et al., "Agroecosystem Management and Nutritional Quality of Plant Foods: The Case of Organic Fruits and Vegetables," *Critical Reviews in Plant Sciences* 30, no. 1–2 (2011): 177–97; C. Smith-Spangler et al., "Are Organic Foods Safer or Healthier Than Conventional Alternatives? A Systematic Review," *Annals of Internal Medicine* 157, no. 5 (2012): 348–66.

100. US Environmental Protection Agency, "Pesticides and Foods: Health Problems Pesticides May Pose," May 2012, www.epa.gov

101. G. Pinholster, "AAAS Board of Directors: Legally Mandating GM Food Labels Could 'Mislead and Falsely Alarm Consumers,'" *American Association for the Advancement of Science News*, October 2012, www.aaas.org; World Health Organization, "20 Questions on Genetically Modified Foods," accessed March 2014, www.who.int

102. US Food and Drug Administration, "Food Allergies: What You Need to Know," April 2013, www.fda.gov

103. National Institute of Allergy and Infectious Diseases, "Food Allergy," August 2013, www.niaid.nih.gov

104. R. S. Gupta et al., "The Prevalence, Severity, and Distribution of Childhood Food Allergy in the United States," *Journal of Pediatrics* 128, no. 1 (2011): e9–e17.

105. J. N. Keith et al., "The Prevalence of Self-Reported Lactose Intolerance and the Consumption of Dairy Foods among African American Adults Less Than Expected," *Journal of the National Medical Association* 103 (2011): 36–45.

106. J. Kurman, "Self-Enhancement, Self-Regulation, and Self-Improvement Following Failures," *British Journal of Social Psychology* 45, no. 2 (2006): 339–56.

107. P. A. Cohen, "Hazards of Hindsight: Monitoring the Safety of Nutritional Supplements," *New England Journal of Medicine* 370 (2014): 1277–80.

108. M. Mitka, "Emerging Data Continue to Find Lack of Benefit for Vitamin-Mineral Supplement Use," *Journal of the American Medical Association* 311, no. 5 (2014): 454–55; Buell et al., "National Athletic Trainers' Association Position Statement," 2013.

109. P. A. Cohen et al., "Presence of Banned Drugs in Dietary Drugs Following FDA Recalls," *Journal of the American Medical Association* 312, no. 16 (2014): 1691–93.

110. Ibid.

111. Mitka, "Emerging Data Continue to Find Lack of Benefit for Vitamin-Mineral Supplement Use," 2014; National Institutes of Health, "NIH State of the Science Panel Urges More Informed Approach to Multivitamin/Mineral Use for Chronic Disease Prevention," May 2006, www.nih.gov

112. M. Stampfer and W. Willet, "Folate Supplements for Stroke Prevention: Targeted Trial Trumps the Rest," *Journal of the American Medical Association* 313, no. 13 (2015): 1321–22.

113. B. Frei et al., "Enough Is Enough," *Annals of Internal Medicine* 160, no. 11 (2014): 807.

114. Ibid.

115. Buell et al., "National Athletic Trainers' Association Position Statement," 2013.

GETFITGRAPHICS References

1. US Department of Health and Human Services and US Department of Agriculture, *Dietary Guidelines for Americans 2015–2020*, 8th ed., December 2015, www.health.gov

2. J. S. Morrell et al., "Metabolic Syndrome, Obesity, and Related Risk Factors among College Men and Women," *Journal of American College Health* 60, no. 1 (2012): 82–89; J. Tanton et al., "Eating Behaviours of British University Students: A Cluster Analysis on a Neglected Issue," *Advances in Preventive Medicine* 2015, no. 639239 (2015).

3. Centers for Disease Control and Prevention, "Sodium Fact Sheet," February 2016, www.cdc.gov

4. S. S. Gropper et al., "Weight and Body Composition Changes during the First Three Years of College," *Journal of Obesity* 2012, no. 634048 (2012).

5. American College Health Association, *American College Health Association—National College Health Assessment II: Towson University Executive Summary, Spring 2015* (Hanover, MD: American College Health Association, 2015), www.acha-ncha.org

Chapter 8

1. C. L. Ogden et al., "Prevalence of Obesity among Adults: United States, 2011–2012," NCHS Data Brief, no. 131 (Hyattsville, MD: National Center for Health Statistics, 2013).

2. K. M. Flegal et al., "Prevalence of Obesity and Trends in the Distribution of Body Mass Index among US Adults, 1999–2010," *Journal of the American Medical Association* 307, no. 5 (2012): 491–97.

3. Ogden et al., "Prevalence of Obesity," 2013.

4. C. D. Fryar and C. L. Ogden, "Prevalence of Underweight among Adults Aged 20 and Over: United States, 1960–1962 through 2011–2012," Health E-Stat, National Health and Nutrition Examination Survey, updated September 2014, www.cdc.gov

5. C. D. Fryar et al., "Prevalence of Overweight and Obesity among Children and Adolescents: United States, 1963–1965 through 2011–2012," Health E-Stat, National Health and Nutrition Examination Survey, updated September 2014, www.cdc.gov

6. Ibid.

7. S. A. Cunningham et al., "Incidence of Childhood Obesity in the United States," *New England Journal of Medicine* 370 (2014): 403–11.

8. J. S. Morrell et al., "Metabolic Syndrome, Obesity, and Related Risk Factors among College Men and Women," *Journal of American College Health* 60, no. 1 (2012).

9. World Health Organization, "Fact Sheet No. 311: Obesity and Overweight," updated January 2015, www.who.int

10. Ibid.

11. World Health Organization, "Controlling the Global Obesity Epidemic," 2013, www.who.int

12. D. G. McNeil, "Food Habits Becoming Worse around the World," *New York Times*, Section D, Global Health, February 24, 2015, 3.

13. International Union of Nutritional Sciences, "The Global Challenge," IUNS 2012.

14. Ogden et al., "Prevalence of Obesity," 2013.

15. E. S. Ford and W. H. Dietz, "Trends in Energy Intake among Adults in the United States: Findings from NHANES," *American Journal of Clinical Nutrition* 97, no. 4 (2013): 848–53.

16. D. Mozaffarian et al., "Changes in Diet and Lifestyle and Long-Term Weight Gain in Women and Men," *New England Journal of Medicine* 364, (2011): 2392–404, doi: 10.1056/NEJMoa1014296, available at www.nejm.org

17. C. Wallis, "Gut Reactions," *Scientific American* 310, no. 6 (June 2014).

18. B. Wamsink, J. E. Painter, and J. North, "Bottomless Bowls: Why Visual Cues of Portion Size May Influence Intake," *Obesity Research* 13, no. 1 (2005): 93–100.

19. J. C. Spence et al., "Relation between Local Food Environments and Obesity among Adults," *BMC Public Health* 9 (2009): 192; B. Wansink, "Environmental Factors That Increase the Food Intake and Consumption Volume of Unknowing Customers," *Annual Review of Nutrition* 24 (2004): 455–79.

20. B. Wansink, "Environmental Factors That Increase the Food Intake and Consumption Volume of Unknowing Customers," *Annual Review of Nutrition* 24 (2004): 455–79.

21. C. D. Fryar and R. B. Ervin, "Caloric Intake from Fast Food among Adults: United States, 2007–2010," NCHS Data Brief, no. 144 (Hyattsville, MD: National Center for Health Statistics, 2013).

22. G. Block et al., "Foods Contributing to Energy Intake in the US: Data from NHANES III and NHANES 1999–2000," *Journal of Food Chemistry and Analysis* 17, no. 3–4 (2004): 439–47.

23. National Center for Health Statistics, "Prevalence of Sedentary Leisure-Time Behavior among Adults in the United States," Health E-Stat, National Health and Nutrition Examination Survey, updated February 2010, www.cdc.gov

24. L. D. Frank et al., "Objective Assessment of Obesogenic Environments in Youth: Geographic Information System Methods and Spatial Findings from the Neighborhood Impact on Kids Study," *American Journal of Preventive Medicine* 42, no. 5 (2012): e47–55.

25. M. Papas et al., "The Built Environment and Obesity," *Epidemiological Reviews* 29, no. 1 (2007): 129–43; M. Rao et al., "The Built Environment and Health," *Lancet* 370, no. 9593 (2007): 1111–13.

26. A. Biswas et al., "Sedentary Time and Its Association with Risk for Disease Incidence, Mortality, and Hospitalization in Adults: A Systematic Review and Meta-Analysis," *Annals of Internal Medicine* 162, no. 2 (2015): 123–32, doi: 10.7326/M14-1651

27. Centers for Disease Control and Prevention, "Other Factors in Weight Gain: Genetics," updated May 2015, www.cdc.gov

28. S. E. Ozanne, "Epigenetic Signatures of Obesity," *New England Journal of Medicine* 372 (March 5, 2015): 973–74.

29. E. Underwood, "The Taste of Things to Come: Early Postnatal and Even Prenatal Experiences Shape Culinary Tastes," *Science* 345, no. 6198 (August 15, 2014): 750–51.

30. Ibid.

31. J. A. Levine et al., "Inter-individual Variation in Posture Allocation: Possible Role in Human Obesity," *Science* 307, no. 5709 (2005): 584–86.

32. Centers for Disease Control and Prevention, "Highest Rates of Leisure-Time Physical Inactivity in Appalachia and South: CDC Releases New Estimates for All US Counties," February 16, 2011, www.cdc.gov/media/releases/2011/p0216_physicalinactivity.html

33. National Center for Health Statistics, "Prevalence of Sedentary Leisure-time Behavior," 2010.

34. Mozaffarian et al., "Changes in Diet," 2011.

35. W. Willett, *Eat, Drink, and Be Healthy: The Harvard Medical School Guide to Healthy Eating* (New York: Free Press, 2003), 35.

36. D. Canoy et al., "Body Fat Distribution and Risk of Coronary Heart Disease in Men and Women in the European Prospective Investigation into Cancer and Nutrition in Norfolk Cohort: A Population-Based Prospective Study," *Circulation* 116, no. 25 (2007): 2933–43.

37. Fryar and Ogden, "Prevalence of Underweight," 2014.

38. R. Puhl and K. D. Brownell, "Bias, Discrimination, and Obesity," *Obesity Research* 9, no. 12 (2001): 788–805.

39. D. R. Musher-Eizenman et al., "Body Size Stigmatization in Preschool Children: The Role of Control Attributions," *Journal of Pediatric Psychology* 29, no. 8 (2004): 613–20.

40. D. F. Maron, "Why Girls Are Starting Puberty Early," *Scientific American* 312, no. 5 (May 2015).

41. R. Puhl and K. D. Brownell, "Bias, Discrimination, and Obesity," 2001.

42. M. B. Schwartz et al., "Weight Bias among Health Professionals Specializing in Obesity," *Obesity Research* 11, no. 9 (2003): 1033–39.

43. C. Kronengold, "Body-Shaming + Cyberbullying," *National Eating Disorders Association*, July 7, 2015, www.nationaleatingdisorders.org/blog/body-shaming-cyberbullying

44. S. S. Wang et al., "The Influence of the Stigma of Obesity on Overweight Individuals," *International Journal of Obesity* 28, no. 10 (2004): 1333–37.

45. Obesity: halting the epidemic by making health easier at a glance. 2011 http://www.cdc.gov/chronicdisease/resources/publications/aag/obesity.htm

46. E. Calle et al., "Overweight, Obesity, and Mortality from Cancer in a Prospectively Studied Cohort of US Adults," *New England Journal of Medicine* 348, no. 17 (2003): 1625–38.

47. N. Pandey and V. Gupta, "Trends in Diabetes," *Lancet* 369, no. 9569 (2007): 1256–57.

48. E. S. Ford et al., "Trends in Mean Waist Circumference and Abdominal Obesity among US Adults, 1999–2012," *Journal of the American Medical Association* 312, no. 11 (2014): 1151–53.

49. Mayo Clinic Staff, "Metabolic Syndrome," August 2014, www.mayoclinic.com

50. L. M. Delahanty et al., "Effects of Weight Loss, Weight Cycling, and Weight Loss Maintenance on Diabetes Incidence and Change in Cardiometabolic Traits in the Diabetes Prevention Program," *Diabetes Care* 37, no. 10 (October 2014): 2738–45.

51. C. C. Mann, "Provocative Study Says Obesity May Reduce US Life Expectancy," *Science* 307, no. 5716 (2005): 1716–17.

52. S. J. Olshansky et al., "A Potential Decline in Life Expectancy in the United States in the 21st Century," *New England Journal of Medicine* 352, no. 11 (2005): 1138–45.

53. K. Flegal et al., "Excess Deaths Associated with Underweight, Overweight, and Obesity," *Journal of the American Medical Association* 298, no. 17 (2007): 2028–37; K. M. Flegal and B. I. Graubard, "Estimates of Excess Deaths Associated with Body Mass Index and Other Anthropometric Variables," *American Journal of Clinical Nutrition* 89, no. 4 (2009): 1213–19.

54. L. Fontana et al., "Long-Term Calorie Restriction Is Highly Effective in Reducing the Risk for Atherosclerosis in Humans," *Proceedings of the National Academy of Sciences* 101, no. 17 (2004): 6659–63.

55. American College Health Association, *American College Health Association-National College Health Assessment II: Reference Group Executive Summary Fall 2012*, 2013.

56. Delahanty et al., "Effects of Weight Loss," 2014.

57. C. N. Markey, "Don't Diet!" *Scientific American Mind*, September/October 2015.

58. C. F. Smith et al., "Flexible versus Rigid Dieting Strategies: Relationship with Adverse Behavioral Outcomes," *Appetite* 32, no. 3 (1999): 295–305.

59. K. D. Hall et al., "Quantification of the Effect of Energy Imbalance on Bodyweight," *Lancet* 378, no. 9793 (2011): 826–37.

60. S. Stock et al., "Ghrelin, Peptide YY, Glucose-Dependent Insulinotropic Polypeptide, and Hunger Responses to a Mixed Meal in Anorexic, Obese, and Control Female Adolescents," *Journal of Clinical Endocrinology and Metabolism* 90, no. 4 (2005).

61. A. N. Payne et al., "Gut Microbial Adaptation to Dietary Consumption of Fructose, Artificial Sweeteners, and Sugar Alcohols: Implications for Host-Microbe Interactions Contributing to Obesity," *Obesity Reviews* 13 (2012): 799–809; Wallis, "Gut Reactions," 2014; J. Suez et al., "Artificial Sweeteners Induce Glucose Intolerance by Altering the Gut Microbiota," *Nature* 514 (October 9, 2014): 181–86.

62. R. Leproult and E. Van Cauter, "Role of Sleep and Sleep Loss in Hormonal Release and Metabolism," *Endocrine Development* 17 (2010): 11–21; P. S. Hogenkamp et al., "Acute Sleep Deprivation Increases Portion Sizes and Affects Food Choice in Young Men," *Psychoneuroendocrinology* (2013): S0306–4530.

63. D. S. Ludwig and M. L. Friedman, "Increasing Adiposity: Consequence or Cause of Overeating?" *Journal of the American Medical Association* 311, no. 21 (2014): 2167–68.

64. A. Park et al., "Distinction of White, Beige, and Brown Adipocytes Derived from Mesenchymal Stem Cells," *World Journal of Stem Cells* 6, no. 1 (January 26, 2014): 33–42.

65. M. W. Moyer, "Supercharging Brown Fat to Battle Obesity," *Scientific American* 311, no. 2 (July 15, 2014); K. Grens, "Activating Beige Fat," *The Scientist*, June 5, 2014; R. R. Rao et al., "Meteorin-like Is a Hormone That Regulates Immune-Adipose Interactions to Increase Beige Fat Thermiogenesis," *Cell* (2014), doi: 10.1016/j.cell.2014.03.065; M. Harms and P. Seale, "Brown and Beige Fat: Development, Function, and Therapeutic Potential," *Nature Medicine* 19 (2013): 1252–63, doi: 10.1038/nm.3361

66. D. S. Ludwig, "Increasing Adiposity," 2014; M. W. Moyer, "Supercharging Brown Fat," 2014.

67. B. C. Johnston et al., "Comparison of Weight Loss among Named Diet Programs in Overweight and Obese Adults: A Meta-Analysis," *Journal of the American Medical Association* 312, no. 9 (2014): 923–33.

68. A. Schwitzer and L. Choate, "College Women Eating Disorder Diagnostic Profile and DSM-5," *Journal of American College Health* 63, no. 1 (2015): 73–78.

69. A. J. Jeffers et al., "Energy Drinks, Weight Loss, and Disordered Eating Behaviors," *Journal of American College Health* 62, no. 5 (2014): 336–42; V. George and C. Mayo, "Eating Disorder Risk and Body Dissatisfaction Based on Muscularity and Body Fat in Male University Students," *Journal of American College Health* 62, no. 6 (2014): 407–15.

70. V. Quick, "Social Theory Applied to Body Image and Chronic Illness in Youth," *American Journal of Lifestyle Medicine* 8, no. 1 (January/February 2014): 15–20.

71. National Eating Disorder Association, "Get the Facts on Eating Disorders," 2015, www.nationaleatingdisorders.org/get-the-facts

72. American Psychiatric Association, "Eating Disorders," accessed August 2015, www.psychiatry.org/mental-health/eating-disorders

73. T. K. Clarke et al., "The Genetics of Anorexia Nervosa," *Clinical Pharmacology and Therapeutics* 2, no. 91 (2012): 181–88; C. M. Bulik et al., "The Genetics of Anorexia Nervosa," *Annual Review of Nutrition* 27 (2007): 263–75.

74. Mayo Clinic Staff, "Metabolism and Weight Loss: How You Burn Calories," September 2014, www.mayoclinic.com

75. Loyola Medicine, "4 Top Reasons Why Dieters Do Not Lose Weight," January 2013, www.loyolamedicine.com; D. M. Thomas et al., "Why Do Individuals Not Lose More Weight from an Exercise Intervention at Defined Dose? An Energy Balance Analysis," *Obesity Research* 10, no. 13 (2012): 835–47.

76. Lin et al., "Effects of Exercise Training on Cardiorespiratory Fitness and Biomarkers of Cardiometabolic Health: A Systematic Review and Meta-Analysis of Randomized Controlled Trials," *Journal of the American Heart Association* 4 (2015): e002014[0].

77. L. H. Willis et al., "Effects of Aerobic and/or Resistance Training on Body Mass and Fat Mass in Overweight and Obese Adults," *Journal of Applied Physiology* 12, no. 113 (2012): 1831–37.

77. R. R. Wing and S. Phelan, "Long-Term Weight Loss Maintenance," *American Journal of Clinical Nutrition* 82, no. 1 (2005): 222S–25S.

79. K. Elfhag and S. Rossner, "Who Succeeds in Maintaining Weight Loss?" *Obesity Review* 6, no. 1 (2005): 67–85.

80. Ibid; J. Moreno and C. Johnston, "Success Habits of Weight Losers," *American Journal of Lifestyle Medicine* 6, no. 2 (2012): 113–15; Centers for Disease Control and Prevention, "Keeping It Off," 2011, www.cdc.gov/healthyweight/losing_weight/keepingitoff.html; S. Ramage et al., "Healthy Strategies for Successful Weight Loss and Weight Maintenance: A Systematic Review," *Applied Physiology, Nutrition, and Metabolism* 39 (2014): 1–20; S. Simpson et al., "What Is the Most Effective Way to Maintain Weight Loss in Adults?" *BMJ* 343 (2011): d8042.

GETFITGRAPHICS **References**

1. J. C. Frankel, "Diet Studies Challenge Thinking on Proteins versus Carbs," *Science* 7 (March 2014): 343 (6175), 1068.

2. C. Wanjek and Live Science, "When Dieting, Not All Calories Are Created Equal," *Scientific American* (June 27, 2012).

3. G. Taubes, "Which One Will Make You Fat?" *Scientific American* 309, no. 3 (September 2013).

4. C. B. Ebbeling et al., "Effects of Dietary Composition on Energy Expenditure during Weight Loss Maintenance," *Journal of the American Medical Association* 307, no. 24 (June 27, 2012).

5. L. B. Ray, "You Are Not Just What, but When You Eat," *Science* 347, no. 6217 (January 2, 2015): 39.

6. A. Chaix et al., "Time-Restricted Feeding Is a Preventative and Therapeutic Intervention against Diverse Nutritional Challenges," *Cell Metabolism* 20, no. 6 (December 2, 2014): 991–1005.

7. L. D. Chong, "One Clock for You and Your Microbes," *Science* 346, no. 6211 (November 14, 2014): 823.

Chapter 9

1. American Psychological Association, "American Psychological Association Survey Shows Money Stress Weighing on Americans' Health Nationwide," February 4, 2015, http://www.apa.org/news/press/releases/2015/02/money-stress.aspx

2. American College Health Association, *American College Health Association-National College Health Assessment II: Towson University Executive Summary, Spring 2015* (Hanover, MD: American College Health Association, 2015).

3. A. Tugend, "The Contrarians on Stress: It Can Be Good for You," *New York Times,* October 4, 2014, B4.

4. H. Selye, "The General-Adaptation-Syndrome," *Annual Review of Medicine* 2 (1951): 327–42.

5. M. P. Pettigrew and K. Lee, "The 'Father of Stress' Meets 'Big Tobacco': Hans Selye and the Tobacco Industry," *American Journal of Public Health* 101, no. 3 (March 2011): 411–18.

6. B. McEwen and T. Seeman, "Allostatic Load and Allostasis," John D. and Catherine T. MacArthur Research Network on Socioeconomic Status and Health, University of California at San Francisco (revised 2009).

7. T. M. Beckie, "A Systematic Review of Allostatic Load, Health, and Health Disparities," *Biological Research for Nursing* 14, no. 4 (October 2012): 311–46; D. Mauss et al., "Measuring Allostatic Load in the Workforce: A Systematic Review," *Industrial Health* (National Institute of Occupational Safety and Heath) 53, no. 1 (January 2015): 5–20; A. Steptoe and M. Kivimaki, "Stress and Cardiovascular Disease," *Nature Reviews Cardiology* 9, no. 6 (2012): 360–70.

8. A. Mokdal et al., "Actual Causes of Death in the United States 2000," *Journal of the American Medical Association* 291, no. 10 (2004): 1238–45.

9. Mauss et al., "Measuring Allostatic Load," 2015.

10. Ibid.; E. Backe et al., "The Role of Psychosocial Stress at Work for the Development of Cardiovascular Disease: A Systematic Review," *International Archives of Occupational and Environmental Health* 85, no. 1 (2011): 67–79; A. Steptoe, A. Rosengren, and P. Hjemdahl, "Introduction to Cardiovascular Disease, Stress, and Adaptation," in *Stress and Cardiovascular Disease,* eds. A. Steptoe, A. Rosengren, and P. Hjemdahl (New York: Springer, 2012), 1–14.

11. S. Cohen et al., "Chronic Stress, Glucocorticoid Receptor Resistance, Inflammation, and Disease Risk," *Proceedings of the National Academy of Sciences for the United States of America* (2012), doi: 10.1073/pnas.1118355109

12. P. J. Gianaros et al., "An Inflammatory Pathway Links Atherosclerotic Cardiovascular Disease Risk to Neural Activity Evoked by the Cognitive Regulation of Emotion," *Biological Psychiatry* 75, no. 9 (May 1, 2014).

13. Mauss et al., "Measuring Allostatic Load," 2015; M. Kivimaki et al., "Job Strain as a Risk Factor for Coronary Heart Disease: A Collaborative Meta-Analysis of Individual Participants," *Lancet* 380, no. 9852 (2012): 1491–97; E. Mostofsky et al., "Risk of Acute Myocardial Infarction after the Death of a Significant Person on One's Life. The Determinants of Myocardial Infarction Onset Study," *Circulation* 125, no. 3 (2012): 491–96.

14. A. Romanov et al., "A Secretagogin Locus of the Mammalian Hypothalamus Controls Stress Hormone Release," *EMBO Journal* (October 2014), doi: 10.15252/embj.201488977; J. Campisi et al., "Acute Psychosocial Stress Differentially Influences Salivary Endocrine and Immune Measures in Undergraduate Students," *Physiology and Behavior* 107, no. 3 (2012): 317–21; G. Marshall, ed., "Stress and Immune-Based Diseases," *Immunology and Allergy Clinics of North America* 31, no. 1 (2011): 317–21.

15. P. Payne and M. Crane-Godreau, "The Preparatory Set: A Novel Approach to Understanding Stress, Trauma, and the Body Mind Therapies Frontiers in Human Neuroscience," April 1, 2015, http://dx.doi.org/10.3389/fnhum.2015.00178

16. T. Hampton, "Stress Affects Expression of Inflammatory Genes in Immune Cells," *Journal of the American Medical Association* 311, no. 1 (2014): 19.

17. M. Tryon et al., "Excessive Sugar Consumption May Be a Difficult Habit to Break: A View from the Brain and Body," *Journal of Clinical Endocrinology and Metabolism* 100, no. 6 (2015): 2239.

18. A. D. de Kloet et al., "Adipocyte Glucorcorticoid Receptors Mediate Fat-to-Brain Signaling," *Psychoneuroendocrinology* 56 (2015): 110, doi: 10.1016/j.psyneuen.2015.03.008

19. K. Thorslund et al., "The Expression of Serotonin Transporter Protein Correlates with the Severity of Psoriasis and Chronic Stress," *Archives of Dermatological Research* 305, no. 2 (2013): 99–104; D. K. Hall-Flavin, "Can Stress Cause Hair Loss?" MayoClinic.com, January 14, 2014, www.mayoclinic.com

20. P. J. Gianaros, "An Inflammatory Pathway," 2014; T. Morris et al., "Stress and Chronic Illness: The Case of Diabetes," *Journal of Adult Development* 18, no. 2 (2011): 70–80.

21. National Digestive Diseases Information Clearinghouse (NDDIC), "Symptoms and Causes of Irritable Bowel Syndrome," February 23, 2015, www.niddk.nih.gov

22. M. J. Friedrich, "Unraveling the Influence of Gut Microbes on the Mind," *Journal of the American Medical Association* 313, no. 17 (2015): 1699–1701.

23. V. Bitsika, C. Sharpley, and R. Bell, "The Contribution of Anxiety and Depression to Fatigue among a Sample of Australian University Students: Suggestions for University Counselors," *Counseling Psychology Quarterly* 22, no. 2 (2009): 243–53.

24. M. Agnieszka et al., "Chronic Stress Impairs Prefrontal Cortex-Dependent Response Inhibition and Spatial Working Memory," *Behavioral Neuroscience* 126, no. 5 (2012): 605–19; L. Schwabe, T. Wolf, and M. Oitzl, "Memory Formation under Stress: Quantity and Quality," *Neuroscience and Biobehavioral Reviews* 34, no. 4 (2009): 584–91.

25. M. Marin et al., "Chronic Stress, Cognitive Functioning, and Mental Health," *Neurobiology of Learning and Memory* 96, no. 4 (2011): 583–95; E. Dias-Ferreira et al., "Chronic Stress Causes Frontostriatal Reorganization and Affects Decision-Making," *Science* 325, no. 5940 (2009): 621–25.

26. M. A. van der Kooij et al., "Role for MMP-9 in Stress-Induced Downregulation of Nectin-3 in Hippocampal CA1 and Associated Behavioural Alternations," *Nature Communications* 5, no. 4995 (2014), doi: 10.1038/ncomms5995

27. A. G. Hinnebusch, "Blocking Stress for Better Memory?" *Science* 348, no. 6238 (May 29, 2015): 967–68.

28. American Psychological Association, "Missing the Mark on Stress Management," *The Impact of Stress,* 2012, www.apa.org

29. American Psychological Association, "Stress at Any Age Is Still Stress," *Stress by Generation,* 2012, www.apa.org

30. Ibid.

31. American College Health Association, *American College Health Association-National College Health Assessment II: Towson University Executive Summary, Spring 2015,* 2015.

32. J. H. Pryor et al., *The American Freshman: National Norms Fall 2014* (Los Angeles: Higher Education Research Institute, February 2015), available at http://heri.ucla.edu

33. D. Pedersen, "Stress Carry-Over and College Student Health Outcomes," *College Student Journal* 46, no. 3 (2012): 620–27.

34. C. Arnold, "The Stressed-Out Postdoc," *Science* 345, no. 6196 (August 1, 2014): 594.

35. R. Kalisch et al., "A Conceptual Framework for the Neurobiological Study of Resilience," *Behavioral and Brain Sciences* 38 (2015): e92, doi:10.1017/S0140525X1400082X

36. F. Lederbogen et al., "City Living and Urban Upbringing Affect Neural Social Stress Processing in Humans," *Nature* 474, no. 7352 (2011); C. E. Chloe et al., "Neighbourhood Socioeconomic Status and Biological 'Wear and Tear' in a Nationally Representative Sample of US Adults," *Journal of Epidemiology and Community Health* 64, no. 10 (2010): 860–65.

37. V. Engert et al., "Cortisol Increase in Empathic Stress Is Modulated by Social Closeness and Observation Modality," *Psychoneuroendocrinology* (2014), doi: 10.1016/j.psyneuen.2014.04.005

38. D. Haynle, "Number of International College Students Continues to Climb," *US News and World Report Education,* November 17, 2014, www.usnews.com/education/best-colleges/articles/2014/11/17/number-of-international-college-students-continues-to-climb

39. C. A. Thurber and E. A. Walton, "Homesickness and Adjustment in University Students," *Journal of American College Health* 60, no. 5 (2012): 415–19.

40. American Psychological Association, "Stress by Generation," 2012; H. W. Bland et al., "Stress Tolerance: New Challenges for Millennial College Students," *College Student Journal* 46, no. 2 (2012): 362–75.

41. S. Abraham, "Relationship between Stress and Perceived Self-Efficacy among Nurses in India" (presented at International Conference on Technology and Business Management, 2012), www.ictbm.org; B. L. Seaward, *Managing Stress,* 7th ed. (Burlington, Massachusetts: Jones and Bartlett Learning, 2012).

42. J. S. Lee et al., "Perceived Stress and Self-Esteem Mediate the Effects of Work-Related Stress on Depression," *Stress & Health: Journal of the International Society for the Investigation of Stress* 29, no. 1 (2013): 75–81, doi: 10.1002/smi.2428; C. Eisenbarth, "Does Self-Esteem Moderate the Relations among Perceived Stress, Coping, and Depression?" *College Student Journal* 46, no. 1 (2012): 149–57.

43. G. Chin, "Self-Esteem," *Science* 343, no. 6168 (January 17, 2014): 230; F. Muindi, "Tell the Negative Committee to Shut Up," *Science* 345, no. 6194 (July 18, 2014): 350.

44. M. Friedman and R. H. Rosenman, *Type A Behavior and Your Heart* (New York: Knopf, 1974).

45. S. R. Maddi, "Personal Hardiness as the Basis for Resilience," in *Hardiness*, SpringerBriefs in Psychology 7 (2013), doi: 10.1007/978-94-007-5222-1_2

46. Ibid.

47. L. Poole et al., "Associations of Objectively Measured Physical Activity with Daily Mood Ratings and Psychophysiological Stress Responses in Women," *Psychophysiology* 48, no. 8 (2011): 1165–72.

48. M. Teychenne, S. Costigan, and K. Parker, "The Association between Sedentary Behaviour and Risk of Anxiety: A Systematic Review," *BMC Public Health* 15, no. 1 (2015), doi: 10.1186/s12889-015-1843-x

49. A. Heenan and N. F. Troje, "Both Physical Exercise and Progressive Muscle Relaxation Reduce the Facing-the-Viewer Bias in Biological Motion Perception," *PLOS ONE* 9, no. 7 (2014).

50. G. N. Bratman et al., "Nature Experience Reduces Rumination and Subgenual Prefrontal Cortex Activation," *Proceedings of the National Academy of Sciences* 112, no. 28 (2015): 8567–72.

51. J. Michalak, K. Rohde, and N. F. Troje, "How We Walk Affects What We Remember: Gait Modifications through Biofeedback Change Negative Affective Memory Bias," *Journal of Behavior Therapy and Experimental Psychiatry* 46 (2015): 121, doi: 10.1016/j.jbtep.2014.09.004

52. M. Gerber et al., "Increased Objectively Assessed Vigorous-Intensity Exercise Is Associated with Reduced Stress, Increased Mental Health, and Good Objective and Subjective Sleep in Young Adults," *Physiology and Behavior* 135 (August 2014): 17–24.

53. National Institute of Alcohol Abuse and Alcoholism, "Alcohol and Sleep," *Alcohol Alert* 41 (1998), http://pubs.niaaa.nih.gov

54. I. Ebrahim et al., "Alcohol and Sleep I: Effects on Normal Sleep," *Alcoholism: Clinical and Experimental Research* 37, no. 4 (2013): 539–49, doi: 10.1111/acer.12006

55. G. Colom et al., "Study of the Effect of Positive Humour as a Variable That Reduces Stress. Relationship of Humour with Personality and Performance Variables," *Psychology in Spain* 15, no. 1 (2011): 9–21.

56. H. W. Bland et al., "Stress Tolerance," 2012.

57. I. R. Galatzer-Levy et al., "Coping Flexibility, Potentially Traumatic Life Events, and Resilience: A Prospective Study of College Student Adjustment," *Journal of Social and Clinical Psychology* 31, no. 6 (2012): 542–67.

58. Pryor et al., *The American Freshman*, 2015.

59. M. Mather and N. Lighthall, "Risk and Reward Are Processed Differently in Decisions Made under Stress," *Current Directions in Psychological Science* 21, no. 1 (2012): 36–41.

60. S. S. Deschenes et al., "The Role of Anger in Generalized Anxiety Disorder," *Cognitive Behaviour Therapy* 41, no. 3 (2012): 261–71.

61. L. D. Kubzansky et al., "Shared and Unique Contributions of Anger, Anxiety, and Depression to Coronary Heart Disease: A Prospective Study in the Normative Aging Study," *Annals of Behavioral Medicine* 31, no. 1 (2006): 21–29.

62. B. C. Feeney and N. L. Collins, "A New Look at Social Support: A Theoretical Perspective on Thriving through Relationships," *Personality and Social Psychology Review* (August 29, 2014); J. Ruthig et al., "Perceived Academic Control: Mediating the Effects of Optimism and Social Support on College Students' Psychological Health," *Social Psychology of Education* 12, no. 7 (2009): 233–49.

63. S. Levine, D. M. Lyons, and A. F. Schatzberg, "Psychobiological Consequences of Social Relationships," *Annals of the New York Academy of Sciences* 89, no. 7 (1999): 210–18.

64. 2014 Cisco Connected World Technology Report, "Cisco Business Insights," accessed August 2015, www.slideshare.net; Pew Research Center, "Social Networking Factsheet," 2015, www.pewinternet.org; J. Campisi et al., "Facebook Stress, and Incidence of Upper Respiratory Infection in Undergraduate College Students," *CyberPsychology, Behavior, and Social Networking* 15, no. 12 (2012): 675–81.

65. J. T. Cacioppo and L. C. Hawkley, "Social Isolation and Health, with an Emphasis on Underlying Mechanisms," *Perspectives in Biology and Medicine* 46, no. 3 Suppl (2003): S39–52.

66. G. Miller, "Why Loneliness Is Hazardous to Your Health," *Science* 331, no. 6014 (2011): 138–40.

67. Ibid.

68. NIH/National Center for Complementary and Integrative Health, "Use of Complementary Health Approaches in the US," *National Health Interview Survey*, February 2015, https://nccih.nih.gov/research/statistics/NHIS/2012

69. A. Conrad et al., "Psychophysiological Effects of Breathing Instructions for Stress Management," *Applied Psychophysiology and Biofeedback* 32, no. 2 (2007): 89–98.

70. J. D. Creswell and E. K. Lindsay, "How Does Mindfulness Training Affect Health? A Mindfulness Stress Buffering Account," *Current Directions in Psychological Science* 23 (December 2014): 401–7; J. D. Creswell et al., "Brief Mindfulness Meditation Training Alters Psychological and Neuroendocrine Responses to Social Evaluative Stress," *Psychoneuroendocrinology* 44 (2014): 1, doi: 10.1016/j.psyneuen.2014.02.007

71. M. A. Rosenkranz et al., "A Comparison of Mindfulness-Based Stress Reduction and an Active Control in Modulation of Neurogenic Inflammation," *Brain, Behavior, and Immunity* 27, no. 1 (2013): 174–84; Y. Singh, R. Sharma, and A. Talwar, "Immediate and Long-Term Effects of Meditation on Acute Stress Reactivity, Cognitive Functions, and Intelligence," *Alternative Therapies in Health & Medicine* 18, no. 6 (2012): 46–53.

72. A. W. Li and C. A. Goldsmith, "The Effects of Yoga on Anxiety and Stress," *Alternative Medicine Review* 17, no. 1 (2012): 21–35; A. Bussing et al., "Effects of Yoga Interventions on Pain and Pain-Associated Disability: A Meta-Analysis," *Journal of Pain* 13, no. 1 (2012): 1–9; S. Bryan, G. Pinto Zipp, and R. Parasher, "The Effects of Yoga on Psychosocial Variables and Exercise Adherence: A Randomized, Controlled Pilot Study," *Alternative Therapies in Health and Medicine* 18, no. 5 (2012): 50–59.

73. Mayo Clinic Staff, "Biofeedback: Using Your Mind to Improve Your Health," January 2013, www.mayoclinic.com

74. D. K. Reibel et al., "Mindfulness-Based Stress Reduction and Health-Related Quality of Life in a Heterogeneous Patient Population," *General Hospital Psychiatry* 23, no. 4 (2001): 183–92; R. Sethness et al., "Cardiac Health: Relationships among Hostility, Spirituality, and Health Risk," *Journal of Nursing Care Quality* 20, no. 1 (2005): 81–94.

GETFITGRAPHICS **References**

1. American College Health Association, *American College Health Association–National College Health Assessment II (ACHA-NCHA II) Reference Group Executive Summary Fall 2012*, 2013.

2. Ibid.

3. Ibid.

4. S. B. He et al., "Exercise Intervention May Prevent Depression," *International Journal of Sports Medicine* 33, no. 7 (2012): 525–30, doi: 10.1055/s-0032-1306325

5. Scully et al., "Physical Exercise and Psychological Well Being: A Critical Review," *British Journal of Sports Medicine* 32, no. 2 (1998): 111–20.

Chapter 10

1. National Center for Health Statistics, "FastStats: Leading Causes of Death," updated August 21, 2015, www.cdc.gov

2. D. Mozaffarian et al., "Heart Disease and Stroke Statistics—2015 Update," *Circulation* 131 (2014): e29–e322; D. Mozaffarian et al., "Executive Summary: Heart Disease and Stroke Statistics—2016 Update," *Circulation* 133 (2016): 447–54, doi: 10.1161/CIR. 0000000000000366

3. Ibid.

4. Ibid.

5. Ibid.

6. J. B. Schwimmer et al., "Longitudinal Assessment of High Blood Pressure in Children with Non-Alcoholic Fatty Liver Disease," *PLOS ONE* 9, no. 11 (2014): e112569; C. Friedemann et al., "Cardiovascular Disease Risk in Healthy Children and Its Association with Body Mass Index: Systematic Review and Meta-Analysis," *BMJ* 2012, no. 345 (2012).

7. M. Heron, "Deaths: Leading Causes for 2012," *National Vital Statistics Reports* 64, no. 7 (July 27, 2015); S. L. Murphy et al., "Mortality in the United States, 2014," National Center for Health Statistics, NCHS Data Brief no. 229, December 2015.

8. O. H. Franco et al., "Blood Pressure in Adulthood and Life Expectancy with Cardiovascular Disease in Men and Women: Life Course Analysis," *Hypertension* 46, no. 2 (2005): 280–86; American Heart Association, "American Heart Association Scientific Statement: Combined Behavioral Interventions Best Way to Reduce Heart Disease Risk," July 12, 2010, http://newsroom.heart.org

9. S. Yusuf et al., "Cardiovascular Risk and Events in 17 Low-, Middle-, and High-Income Countries," *New England Journal of Medicine* 371, no. 9 (August 28, 2014): 818–27.

10. Ibid.

11. P. Greenland, E. D. Peterson, and J. M. Gaziano, "Progress against Cardiovascular Disease: Putting the Pieces Together," *Journal of the American Medical Association* 312, no. 19 (2014): 1979–80.

12. H. C. McGill et al., "Origin of Atherosclerosis in Childhood and Adolescence," *American Journal of Clinical Nutrition* 72, no. 5 (2000): 1307S–15S.

13. N. M. van Emmerick et al., "High Cardiovascular Risk in Severely Obese Young Children and Adolescents," *Archives of Diseases in Children* 97, no. 9 (2012): 818–21.

14. C. S. Birken et al., "Association between Vitamin D and Circulating Lipids in Early Childhood," *PLOS ONE* 10, no. 7 (July 15, 2015).

15. H. C. McGill et al., "Association of Coronary Heart Disease Risk Factors with Microscopic Qualities of Coronary Atherosclerosis in Youth," *Circulation* 102, no. 4 (2000): 374–79.

16. American College of Cardiology, "TV Linked to Poor Snacking Habits, Cardiovascular Risk in Middle Schoolers," March 28, 2014; Schwimmer et al., "Longitudinal Assessment of High Blood Pressure in Children," 2014.

17. American Heart Association, "Atherosclerosis," April 21, 2014, http://www.heart.org/HEARTORG/Conditions/Cholesterol/WhyCholesterolMatters/Atherosclerosis_UCM_305564_Article.jsp; "Cardiovascular Disease Risk in Healthy Children," 2012; P. Franks et al., "Childhood Obesity, Other Cardiovascular Risks, and Premature Death," *New England Journal of Medicine* 362, no. 6 (2010): 485–93; Y. M. Hong, "Atherosclerotic Cardiovascular Disease Beginning in Childhood," *Korean Circulation Journal* 40, no. 1 (2010): 1–9; R. E. Kavey et al., "American Heart Association Guidelines for Primary Prevention of Atherosclerotic Cardiovascular Disease Beginning in Childhood," *Circulation* 107, no. 11 (2003): 1562–66.

18. A. G. Mainous III et al., "Life Stress and Atherosclerosis: A Pathway through Unhealthy Lifestyle," *International Journal of Psychiatry in Medicine* 40, no. 2 (2010): 147–61; Mayo Clinic Staff, "Arteriosclerosis/Atherosclerosis: Causes," May 2014, www.mayoclinic.org

19. Centers for Disease Control and Prevention, "Heart Disease Fact Sheet," updated February 19, 2015, www.cdc.gov

20. American Heart Association, "Inflammation and Heart Disease," updated July 2015, www.heart.org

21. Ibid.

22. WebMD, "Homocysteine and Heart Disease," updated February 22, 2014, www.webmd.com

23. A. Ganna et al., "Large-Scale Metabolomic Profiling Identifies Novel Biomarkers for Incident Coronary Heart Disease," *PLOS Genetics* 10, no. 12 (2014): e1004801, doi: 10.1371/journal.pgen.1004801; Emerging Risk Factors Collaboration, "C-Reactive Protein, Fibrinogen, and Cardiovascular Disease Prediction," *New England Journal of Medicine* 367, no. 14 (2012): 1310–20, doi: 10. 1056/NEJMoa1107477

24. A. S. Antonopoulos et al., "Statins as Anti-Inflammatory Agents in Atherogenesis: Molecular Mechanisms and Lessons from the Recent Clinical Trials," *Current Pharmaceutical Design* 18, no. 11 (April 2012): 1519–30.

25. N. J. Stone et al., "2013 ACC/AHA Guideline on the Treatment of Blood Cholesterol to Reduce Atherosclerotic Cardiovascular Risk in Adults: A Report of the American College of Cardiology/American Heart Association Task Force on Practice Guidelines," *Circulation* 129, no. 25, supp. 2 (2014): S1–S45.

26. Centers for Disease Control and Prevention, "High Blood Pressure Fact Sheet," updated February 19, 2015, www.cdc.gov; B. M. Egan, Y. Zhao, and R. N. Axon, "US Trends in Prevalence, Awareness, Treatment, and Control of Hypertension, 1988–2008,"*Journal of the American Medical Association* 303, no. 20 (2010): 2043–50.

27. Centers for Disease Control and Prevention, "High Blood Pressure Fact Sheet," 2015.

28. American Heart Association, "Why Blood Pressure Matters," updated August 4, 2014, www.heart.org

29. Ibid.

30. S. I. Sharp et al., "Hypertension Is a Potential Risk Factor for Vascular Dementia: Systematic Review," *International Journal of Geriatric Psychiatry* 26, no. 7 (2011): 661–69; F. D. Testai and P. B. Gorelick, "Vascular Cognitive Impairment and Alzheimer's Disease: Are These Disorders Linked to Hypertension and Other Cardiovascular Risk Factors?" in *Hypertension and Stroke: Pathophysiology and Management*, eds. V. Aiyagari and P. B. Gorelick (New York: Humana Press, 2011), 195–210.

31. H. Beltran-Sanchez, C. E. Finch, and E. M. Crimmins, "Twentieth Century Surge of Excess Adult Male Mortality," *Proceedings of the National Academy of Sciences* 112, no. 29 (2015), doi: 10.1073/pnas.1421942112

32. American Heart Association, "Understanding Blood Pressure Readings," updated August 2014, www.heart.org

33. S. Kishi et al., "Cumulative Blood Pressure in Early Adulthood and Cardiac Dysfunction in Middle Age: The CARDIA Study," *Journal of the American College of Cardiology* 65, no. 25 (June 2015), doi: 10.1016/j.jacc.2015.04.042

34. Ibid.

35. Mozaffarian et al., "Heart Disease and Stroke Statistics," 2014.

36. Ibid.

37. T. M. Maddox et al., "Non-Obstructive Coronary Artery Disease and Risk of Myocardial Infarction," *Journal of the American Medical Association* 312, no. 17 (2014): 1754–63.

38. Z. M. Zhang et al., "Race and Sex Differences in the Incidence and Prognostic Significance of Silent Myocardial Infarction in the Atherosclerosis Risk in Communities (ARIC) Study," *Circulation* 133 (2016): 2141–48, doi: 10.1161/CIRCULATIONAHA.115.021177

39. Mozaffarian et al., "Heart Disease and Stroke Statistics," 2014.

40. Ibid.; American Heart Association, "About Arrhythmia," updated January 2015, www.heart.org

41. Mozaffarian et al., "Heart Disease and Stroke Statistics," 2014; American Heart Association, "About Heart Failure," updated April 22, 2015, www.heart.org

42. Mozaffarian et al., "Heart Disease and Stroke Statistics," 2014; American Heart Association, "About Congenital Heart Defects," updated January 8, 2015, www.heart.org

43. Mozaffarian et al., "Heart Disease and Stroke Statistics," 2014; American Heart Association, "Heart Disease and Stroke Statistics: At a Glance," 2015, www.heart.org

44. Mayo Clinic Staff, "Stroke: Symptoms and Causes," 2015, www.mayoclinic.org

45. Ibid.; Mozaffarian et al., "Heart Disease and Stroke Statistics," 2014.

46. Mayo Clinic Staff, "Transient Ischemic Attack (TIA)," 2015, www.mayoclinic.org

47. National Heart, Lung, and Blood Institute, "What Are Coronary Heart Disease Risk Factors?" updated June 9, 2015, www.nhlbi.nih.gov

48. Centers for Disease Control and Prevention, Chronic Disease Prevention and Health Promotion, "Tobacco Use," updated April 21, 2015, www.cdc.gov

49. Centers for Disease Control and Prevention, "Smoking and Tobacco Use," updated February 2014; Mozaffarian et al., "Heart Disease and Stroke Statistics," 2014.

50. American Cancer Society, "Secondhand Smoke," revised March 2015, www.cancer.org

51. Mozaffarian et al., "Heart Disease and Stroke Statistics," 2014.

52. Mayo Clinic Staff, "High Blood Pressure Dangers: Hypertension's Effects on Your Body," February 2014, www.mayoclinic.org

53. H. K. Wall, J. A. Hannan, and J. S. Wright, "Hiding in Plain Sight," *Journal of the American Medical Association* 312, no. 17 (2014): 1973–74; S. Kishi et al., "Cumulative Blood Pressure in Early Adulthood," 2015.

54. F. C. D. Andrade et al., "One-Year Follow-Up Changes in Weight Are Associated with Changes in Blood Pressure in Young Mexican Adults," *Public Health* 126, no. 6 (2012): 535, doi: 10.1016.j.puhe.2012.02.005

55. National Center for Health Statistics, *Health, United States, 2010: With Special Feature on Death and Dying* (Hyattsville, MD: US Department of Health and Human Services, 2011), Table 95.

56. N. V. Dhurandhar and D. Thomas, "An Unsolved Question," *Journal of the American Medical Association* 313, no. 9 (2015): 959–60.

57. Mozaffarian et al., "Heart Disease and Stroke Statistics," 2014.

58. Mayo Clinic Staff, "Top 5 Lifestyle Changes to Reduce Cholesterol," accessed August 2015, www.mayoclinic.org

59. Stone et al., "2013 ACC/AHA Guideline," 2014.

60. Healthy People 2020, "2020 Topics and Objectives: Physical Activity," April 2016, www.healthypeople.gov

61. American College of Cardiology, "TV Linked to Poor Snacking Habits," 2014; J. E. Barkley, A. Kepp, and S. Salehi-Esfahani, "College Students'

Mobile Telephone Use Is Positively Associated with Sedentary Behavior," *American Journal of Lifestyle Medicine* 1559827615594338 (July 2015).

62. American Diabetes Association, "Statistics about Diabetes," *National Diabetes Statistics Report, 2014*, released June 10, 2014, www.diabetes.org

63. Mozaffarian et al., "Heart Disease and Stroke Statistics," 2014.

64. Ibid.; Mayo Clinic Staff, "What Is Metabolic Syndrome?" August 22, 2014, www.mayoclinic.org

65. Mozaffarian et al., "Heart Disease and Stroke Statistics," 2014.

66. T. L. Keown, C. B. Smith, and M. S. Harris, "Metabolic Syndrome among College Students," *Journal for Nurse Practitioners* 5, no. 10 (2009): 754–59.

67. J. Schilter and L. Dalleck, "Fitness and Fatness: Indicators of Metabolic Syndrome and Cardiovascular Disease Risk Factors in College Students?" *Journal of Exercise Physiology* 13, no. 4 (2010): 29–39.

68. P. J. Gianaros et al., "An Inflammatory Pathway Links Atherosclerotic Cardiovascular Disease Risk to Neural Activity Evoked by the Cognitive Regulation of Emotion," *Biological Psychiatry* 75, no. 9 (2014): 738.

69. European Society of Cardiology, "Poor Sleep Associated with Increased Risk of Heart Attack, Stroke," June 15, 2015, www.escardio.org; D. Noonan, "The Not-So-Silent Epidemic," *Scientific American* 312, no. 6 (June 2015): 27–28; T. Munzel et al., "Cardiovascular Effects of Environmental Noise Exposure," *European Heart Journal* 35, no. 13 (2014): 829; E. P. Havranek et al., "Social Determinants of Risk and Outcomes for Cardiovascular Disease," *Circulation* 132, no. 9 (2015), doi: CIR.0000000000000228

70. Stone et al., "2013 ACC/AHA Guideline," 2014.

71. A. N. Westover, S. McBride, and R. W. Haley, "Stroke in Young Adults Who Abuse Amphetamines or Cocaine," *Archives of General Psychiatry* 64 (2007): 495–502.

72. Stone et al., "2013 ACC/AHA Guideline," 2014.

73. M. He et al., "ABO Blood Group and Risk of Coronary Heart Disease in Two Prospective Cohort Studies," *Arteriosclerosis, Thrombosis, and Vascular Biology* 32, no. 9 (2012): 2314–20.

74. C. P. Nelson et al., "Genetically Determined Height and Coronary Artery Disease," *New England Journal of Medicine* 372, no. 17 (April 23, 2015): 1608–18; E. Edston, "The Earlobe Crease, Coronary Artery Disease, and Sudden Cardiac Death: An Autopsy Study of 520 Individuals," *American Journal of Forensic Medicine and Pathology* 27, no. 2 (June 2006): 129–33.

75. Mozaffarian et al., "Heart Disease and Stroke Statistics," 2014.

76. US Preventive Services Task Force, "Aspirin Use to Prevent Cardiovascular Disease and Colorectal Cancer: Preventive Medication," April 2016, www.uspreventiveservicestaskforce.org

77. Ibid.

78. Ibid.

79. F. J. Charchar et al., "Inheritance of Coronary Artery Disease in Men: An Analysis of the Role of the Y Chromosome," *Lancet* 379, no. 9819 (2012): 915–22.

80. D. Canoy et al., "Age at Menarche and Risks of Coronary Heart and Other Vascular Diseases in a Large UK Cohort," *Circulation* 131, no. 3 (December 2014), doi: 10.1161/CIRCULATIONAHA.114.010070; E. Gunderson et al., "Lactation Duration and Midlife Atherosclerosis," *Obstetrics and Gynecology* 126, no. 2 (August 2015): 381–90, doi: 10.1097/AOG.0000000000000919

81. M. Sharaki et al., "Which Modifiable, Non-Modifiable, and Socioeconomic Factors Have More Effect on Cardiovascular Risk Factors in Overweight and Obese Women?" *Journal of Research in Medical Sciences* 17, no. 7 (July 2012): 676–80; National Heart, Lung, and Blood Institute, "High Blood Cholesterol: What You Need to Know," NIH Publication No. 05-3290, revised June 2005, www.nhlbi.nih.gov

82. Mozaffarian et al., "Heart Disease and Stroke Statistics," 2014.

83. Ibid.

84. D. G. Murro et al., "Aldosterone Contributes to Elevated Left Ventricular Mass in Black Boys," *Pediatric Nephrology* 28, no. 4 (2013): 2–12, doi: 10.1007/s00467-012-2367-6

85. Centers for Disease Control and Prevention, "Smoking and Tobacco Use: Data and Statistics," updated March 2012, reviewed December 2014, www.cdc.gov

86. American Heart Association, "American Heart Association's Diet and Lifestyle Recommendations," updated August 12, 2015, www.heart.org

87. Ibid.

88. S. Zhao et al., "Intakes of Apples or Apple Polyphenols Decrease Plasma Values for Oxidized Low-Density Lipoprotein/beta2-glycoprotein I," *Journal of Functional Foods* 5, no. 1 (2013): 493–97; American College of Cardiology, "Snacking on Raisins May Offer a Heart-Healthy Way to Lower Blood Pressure," March 25, 2012, www.cardiosource.org; A. Cassidy et al., "Dietary Flavonoids and Risk of Stroke in Women," *Stroke* 43, no. 4 (2012), doi: 10.1161/STROKEAHA.111.637835; American Chemical Society, "Hot Pepper Compound Could Help Hearts," March 27, 2012, www.acs.org; A. Cassidy et al., "High Anthocyanin Intake Is Associated with a Reduced Risk of Myocardial Infarction in Young and Middle-Aged Women," *Circulation* 127, no. 2 (2013): 188–96.

89. Pennsylvania State University, "Monounsaturated Fats Reduce Metabolic Syndrome Risk," March 29, 2013, http://news.psu.edu

90. A. Pan et al., "Red Meat Consumption and Mortality," *Archives of Internal Medicine* 172, no. 7 (2012): 555–63.

91. P. Lagiou et al., "Low Carbohydrate-High Protein Diet and Incidence of Cardiovascular Diseases in Swedish Women: Prospective Cohort Study," *BMJ* 2012, no. 344 (2012): e4026; I. Johansson et al., "Associations among 25-Year Trends in Diet, Cholesterol, and BMI from 140,000 Observations in Men and Women in Northern Sweden," *Nutrition Journal* 11, no. 40 (2012), www.nutritionj.com

92. J. D. Spence et al., "Egg Yolk Consumption and Carotid Plaque," *Atherosclerosis* 224, no. 2 (2012): 469–73.

93. National Institute on Drug Abuse, "How Do Stimulants Affect the Brain and Body?" updated November 2014, www.drugabuse.gov

GETFITGRAPHICS References

1. D. Mozaffarian et al., "Heart Disease and Stroke Statistics—2015 Update," *Circulation* 131, no. 4 (2014): e29–e322, doi: 10.1161/CIR.0000000000000152; D. Mozaffarian et al., "Executive Summary: Heart Disease and Stroke Statistics—2016 Update," *Circulation* 133 (2016): 447–54, doi: 10.1161/CIR. 0000000000000366

2. Centers for Disease Control and Prevention, "Heart Disease and Stroke Prevention— Addressing the Nation's Leading Killers: At A Glance 2011," accessed August 2015, www.cdc.gov

3. Mozaffarian et al., "Heart Disease and Stroke Statistics," 2014.

4. World Health Organization, "Top Ten Causes of Death," updated May 2014, accessed August 2015, http://www.who.int/mediacentre/factsheets/fs310/en/.

Photo Credits

Brief Index